A Textbook of Perioperative Care

For Elsevier

Senior Commissioning Editor: Ninette Premdas
Project Development Manager: Mairi McCubbin
Project Managers: Joannah Duncan and Andrew Palfreyman
Designer: Judith Wright
Illustrations Manager: Bruce Hogarth

A Textbook of Perioperative Care

Kate Woodhead

Independent Operating Theatre Consultant, Leeds, UK

Paul Wicker BSc RGN RMN CCNS PGCert RNT

ODP Programme Leader, Faculty of Health, Edge Hill College of Higher Education, Liverpool, UK

Foreword by

Ian R. Cumming OBE FIBMS CSci FCMI MHSM

Chief Executive, Morecambe Bay Hospitals NHS Trust, Kendall, Cumbria
President, National Association of Theatre Nurses, UK
Visiting Professor in Healthcare Management and Leadership, University of Cape Town, Cape Town, South Africa

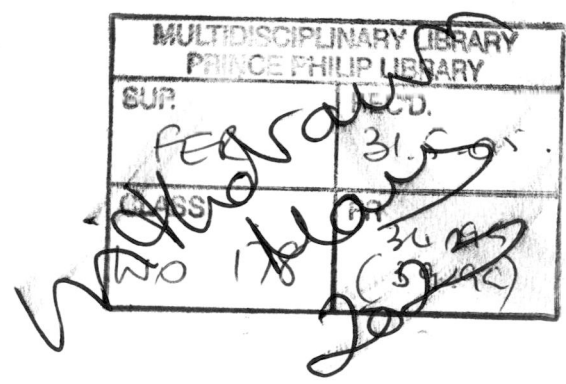
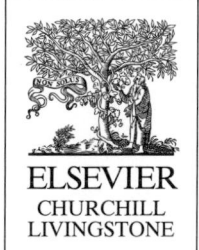

ELSEVIER
CHURCHILL
LIVINGSTONE

EDINBURGH   LONDON   NEW YORK   OXFORD   PHILADELPHIA   ST LOUIS   SYDNEY   TORONTO   2005

ELSEVIER
CHURCHILL
LIVINGSTONE

First published 2005

ISBN 0 443 07285 X

British Library Cataloguing in Publication Data
A catalogue record for this book is available from the British Library

Library of Congress Cataloging in Publication Data
A catalog record for this book is available from the Library of Congress

Notice
Knowledge and best practice in this field are constantly changing. As new research and experience broaden our knowledge, changes in practice, treatment and drug therapy may become necessary or appropriate. Readers are advised to check the most current information provided (i) on procedures featured or (ii) by the manufacturer of each product to be administered, to verify the recommended dose or formula, the method and duration of administration, and contraindications. It is the responsibility of the practitioner, relying on their own experience and knowledge of the patient, to make diagnoses, to determine dosages and the best treatment for each individual patient, and to take all appropriate safety precautions. To the fullest extent of the law, neither the publisher nor the editors and authors assume any liability for any injury and/or damage.

The Publisher

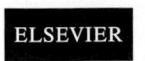 **your source for books, journals and multimedia in the health sciences**
www.elsevierhealth.com

The Publisher's policy is to use **paper manufactured from sustainable forests**

Printed in China

Contents

Contributors

Amanda J. Bassett RGN
Programme Lead – Pre-operative assessment, National Health Service University, London, UK

Maj Liz Bernthal QARANC BSc (Hons) DipNS RM RGN ENB183
Nursing Officer, Queen Alexandra's Royal Army Nursing Corps

Vicki Clark MB ChB FRCA
Consultant Anaesthetist, Department of Anaesthetics, Royal Infirmary, Edinburgh, UK

Jane Donnelly DipHSM RGN RSCN RM NNEB
Senior Sister, Operating Theatre Department, Alder Hey Children's Hospital, Liverpool, UK

Suzanne Fullbrook LLB (Hons) Mphil Barrister (non practising) RN
Senior Lecturer, Law and Ethics, Faculty of Health and Social Care, London South Bank University

Diane Gilmour BN PGCEA DipInfeCon DANS RGN ENB176, 329
Clinical Team Leader (Theatres and Day Surgery), Crawley Hospital, Crawley, UK

Lois Hamlin BN MN(NE) ICCert OTCert RN FRCNA FCN(NSW)
Nurse Manager, Royal Shore Hospital, New South Wales, Australia

Sarah Hart MSc
Clinical Nurse Specialist/Radiation Protection, The Royal Marsden NHS Trust, Sutton, UK

Rita Hehir BA (Hons) MA PGCE RGN RM
Senior Lecturer, ODP Education, Faculty of Health, Edge Hill College of Higher Education, Liverpool, UK

Martin Hind RGN MSc BSc (Hons) PGDE DPSN
Senior Lecturer, Institute of Health and Community Studies, Bournemouth University, Bournemouth, UK

David J. Hurrell BSc MSc FIHEEM AP(S)
Managing Director, Healthcare Science Ltd, Hitchin, UK

Jane Jackson
Consultant Nurse, Assessment Clinic, St Albans City Hospital, St Albans, UK

Melanie van Limborgh MSc PostGradDip ENB176, 182, 998 N33
Lead Nurse Theatres and Trust Decontamination Lead, Main Theatres, Chelsea and Westminster Hospital, London, UK

Caroline MacDonald RGN BSc PGCTLT
Lecturer, School of Nursing and Midwifery, The Robert Gordon University, Aberdeen, UK

Roz McMillan BA RGN
Clinical Lead, Day Surgery Unit, Royal Infirmary of Edinburgh, Edinburgh, UK

Peter Mercer BSc (Hons) RGN
Transplant Service Manager; Transplant Unit, Addenbrookes' Hospital NHS Trust, Cambridge, UK

Judy Mewburn DipHons RGN NSET
MD Operating Theatre Systems; Theatre Nurse, London Bridge Hospital, London, UK

Melanie Oakley BSc (Hons) MSc PGCE RN
Senior Lecturer, Faculty of Health and Social Care Sciences, Kingston University and St Georges Hospital Medical School, London, UK

Mark Radford BSc PGDip RGN ENB183, 998
Clinical Nurse Specialist, Good Hope Hospital NHS Trust, Sutton Coldfield, UK

Jane Reid RGN DPNS BSc (Hons) PGCEA RNT MSc
Dean, Health and Social Care, Somerset Academy, Taunton, UK

Mark Sewart DipHE BMedSci (Hons) ENB176, 998 RGN RMN
Flight Lieutenant, Princess Mary's Royal Air Force Nursing Service, Department of Community Mental Health, Royal Air Force Marham, King's Lynn, Norfolk

Brian Smith BSc (Hons) DipPsych CertEd FAETC RODP
Senior Lecturer in CPD, Faculty of Health, Edge Hill College of Higher Education, Liverpool, UK

Carol Smith BSc (Hons) DipHE RGN
Sister, Main Theatres, Royal Albert Edward Infirmary, Wigan, UK

Gillian Stevenson MBA RGN ONC ENB329
Lead Infection Control Nurse, St John's Hospital, Edinburgh, UK

Paul Whatling BCh MB FRCSEd
Director, Faculty of Medical Informatics, Royal College of Surgeons of Edinburgh, Edinburgh, UK

Paul Wicker BSc RGN RMN CCNS
ODP Programme Leader, Faculty of Health, Edge Hill College of Higher Education, Liverpool, UK

Josie Williams BSc (Hons) DipHE RN FAETC
Former Senior Lecturer, Edge Hill HE College, Liverpool, UK. Lecturer West Midlands ODP Education Centre, Birmingham, UK. Tutor ODP Training Programme, Armed Forces Hospital, Saudi Arabia

Tom Williams MPhil BA DipEd DipHSM DipIOSH FAETC DipIOTT RODP
Former Senior Lecturer, Edge Hill HE College, Liverpool, UK. Senior Lecturer West Midlands ODP Education Centre, Birmingham, UK. Principal ODP Training Programme, Armed Forces Hospital, Saudi Arabia

Jill Yates BSc RGN ENB176 Post grad dip of periop practice (Dist)
Senior Staff Nurse Recovery, Edinburgh Royal Infirmary, Edinburgh, UK

Foreword

Modernization seems to be the buzzword in health care today. At times it feels as if health care is constantly being criticized for having too traditional an approach, for being resistant to change and for not modernizing quickly enough. Yet patient empowerment, clinical governance, extending/expanding roles of staff, controls assurance and risk management, process re-engineering, evidence-based care, and performance improvement are just some of the many challenges (and new terms!) that we have all been faced with in recent years.

Add to the above list those changes that have occurred in the same time frame specific to the operating department, and you will quickly appreciate the enormity of the modernization agenda that has been delivered by all those working in perioperative care. These changes include the type of equipment in use, anaesthetic and surgical techniques, and the roles, training and development of staff. The operating theatres of today must be almost unrecognizable in the way they function to the way they functioned when my mother was a student nurse. What has not changed in this time, however, is the fundamental caring philosophy of all those working in the perioperative arena – whether involved in direct or indirect patient care.

The perioperative practitioner of today needs to have not only practical expertise but also a detailed knowledge and understanding of specific working areas. An appreciation of the particular care needs of a wide variety of patients is also essential. The nature of the perioperative environment also requires individuals to have a broad knowledge of professional accountability, ethics, decontamination, infection control, and leadership and staff management. All of these topics underpin the delivery of high quality evidence-based care that is patient focussed, robust and measurable.

This work provides, in detail, the background knowledge that today's perioperative practitioner will need to succeed in their chosen career. It will undoubtedly help raise the standard of perioperative care that we provide to our patients. I commend it to you wholeheartedly.

2005

Ian R. Cumming

Preface

The times we live in have often been referred to as the 'Information Age'. Indeed, there has never been a time when information has been so freely available, both in paper and in electronic form. This wealth of information also has its pitfalls: it is sometimes difficult to identify the wheat from the chaff; it is a major challenge to be able to find, absorb and apply to practice the highest-quality information available.

The purpose of this book is therefore to offer a comprehensive source of information to support the clinical practice of perioperative practitioners, whether they are nurses or operating department practitioners (ODPs). It offers well-referenced information from credible sources, and acknowledges further sources of reading and the effect on practice of the incredible speed of change facing practitioners today.

The book is written in a clear, authoritative style, and is liberally illustrated with contemporary photographs and diagrams. The patient-centred approach acknowledges the dynamics of modern perioperative practice by focusing on surgical interventions in all the environments in which it is currently practised, including A&E departments, general practice clinics, intensive care units, and at the sites of serious accidents.

Clinical practice in the operating department is becoming increasingly specialist. Any book purporting to reflect accurately the needs of all specialties would be a very large tome indeed. This book does not attempt to do this, but instead concentrates on the principles of practice applicable to any setting and any specialty.

There is a very practical focus. It aims to be the book that nurses and ODPs reach for in order to answer their practical questions but it is not procedure-driven. Instead, it sets out the principles of perioperative practice, from which individual practitioners will be able to develop their own practice techniques.

A Textbook of Perioperative Care has four main sections to assist readers to locate the information they seek and, by organizing the content in a logical, largely chronological way, also reflects the 'journey' patients undertake when they access surgical services. Each chapter sets out key points that help the reader to focus on the main points and topics discussed.

SECTION 1: CORE PRINCIPLES IN PERIOPERATIVE PRACTICE

This section looks at the main underlying principles affecting the care of perioperative patients and reflects many of the priorities that challenge practitioners in today's healthcare community. Topics include accountability and professional practice, leadership and teamwork, risk management, information management, research, ethics and decontamination. The purpose of this section is to identify and discuss the drivers that are making perioperative care such a challenging experience.

SECTION 2: PRINCIPLES OF CLINICAL PRACTICE

This section will take a clinical pathway approach, following the patient from assessment, through anaesthesia and surgery, and finally into recovery.

Each chapter focuses on key issues, such as staff roles in the respective departments, communication and the clinical interventions required to achieve homoeostasis of the body systems. Once again, this section focuses on the principles that underpin the development of good approaches to delivering effective patient care.

SECTION 3: PRINCIPLES OF CARE IN DIFFERENT ENVIRONMENTS

This section reflects the fact that operative procedures are now conducted in a wide range of environments. It builds on the basic principles set out in Sections 1 and 2, focusing on variations from the norm in the different settings. Topics include day surgery, surgery in the community, emergency surgery, and surgery in specialist settings such as endoscopy units and catheterization laboratories.

SECTION 4: PRINCIPLES OF CARE FOR SPECIFIC PATIENT GROUPS

This section focuses on variations from the norm for a variety of specialized patient groups. For example, Chapter 18 gives a comprehensive review of the care of the child in the perioperative environment, including the main principles of care during all the phases of the perioperative journey, the needs of parents and carers, and communication with the child's ward. Chapter 24 reviews the care of perioperative patients with mental illness; an area rarely covered in perioperative texts. Other chapters look at care of the elderly, patients with multisystem illness, and patients who have highly infectious diseases or who are immunocompromised.

This book has been written specifically for perioperative practitioners. It will help to prepare the practitioner for working in an environment that is forever changing: expanding and developing in ways that cannot yet be anticipated.

Read, absorb and apply!

Kate Woodhead and Paul Wicker
Leeds and Liverpool, 2004

SECTION 1

Core principles in perioperative practice

Chapter 1

Accountability and professional practice

Martin Hind

Key points

- Perioperative practitioners require specialist knowledge and skills to provide high-quality perioperative care to their patients
- Practitioners must be able to account for all of their actions and omissions

DEFINITION AND DISCUSSION OF ACCOUNTABILITY IN THE CONTEXT OF PERIOPERATIVE CARE

To be accountable a professional is required to be more than merely responsible for their actions.

Bergman[1] clarified this by explaining how accountability is derived from a set of preconditions referred to as ability, responsibility and authority:

- **Ability** refers to the knowledge, skills and values that underpin the role of the perioperative practitioner in whatever setting they work. Perioperative care occurs in many different settings, with various types of surgical and anaesthetic techniques being employed. These areas require specialist knowledge and skills in order to enable effective practice, and there is no doubt that perioperative practitioners require ability to fulfil this role.
- **Responsibility** refers to the tasks, roles and duties that are assigned to practitioners during their work within the perioperative environment. It links closely with the ability to practise, in that practitioners have many responsibilities within whatever setting they work.

● **Authority** involves having the freedom to make and act on decisions in the exercise of the professional role. The standard of patient care throughout the entire perioperative period relies heavily on the decisions and actions of practitioners. Ability, responsibility and authority are inherent to these activities. There can be no doubt that perioperative practitioners fulfil all of these preconditions to be accountable, rather than just responsible, for their practice. Being accountable places great pressure on the individual practitioner to uphold the best professional standards in whatever setting they practise.

Accountability is rather like gravity: it can be felt but not seen. It is also a complex issue, as there are a number of different ways in which a practitioner may be held accountable. One useful way of revealing this is by considering to whom a practitioner may be held to account for their actions or omissions. It is widely accepted that there are four main modes of accountability: self, legal, contractual and professional.

SELF-ACCOUNTABILITY

This is the personal dimension that cannot really be enforced on the individual from without. It is where individuals judge themselves. It is that sense of right or wrong that people instinctively possess, their own set of morals and values. In the context of perioperative practice, if the practitioner has knowledge, skills and experience then they are perfectly capable of knowing in routine matters what is right and wrong about their practice. Marks-Maran[2] has argued that this mode of accountability is the clarification of personal values and that there can be no prescriptions, laws, codes or job descriptions for moral accountability (see Ch. 2 on Ethics for further discussion on moral and ethical issues). In some instances this is often the toughest mode, as individuals can be too hard on themselves when they reflect on their work.

LEGAL ACCOUNTABILITY

The legal mode of accountability can be divided into criminal and civil law. Perioperative practitioners are accountable to the public through the criminal law and accountable to the patient through the civil law. Criminal charges in relation to care in any arena of health care are rare, but it does sometimes happen. There have, in the past, been cases where healthcare professionals have been convicted of criminal offences that they committed while they were practising. Being engaged in professional practice does not exempt an individual from their responsibilities to society through the criminal law. Peysner[3] has suggested that the area where nurses are most likely to risk prosecution for a criminal offence is where invasive procedures or physical examinations are performed without the consent of the patient. This may lead to prosecution for the crime of battery, or an offence under the Offences against the Person Act of 1861. (The issues associated with consent are also discussed in Ch. 3.)

Negligence

Civil actions occur when a patient sues under the law of negligence; this is sometimes referred to as litigation, and the costs of it are rising every year. One reason for this trend is that patients are becoming increasingly aware of their rights through initiatives such as the Patient's Charter and through the media.

It is well known that the operating department is a risky area and all practitioners need to be constantly aware of the possibilities of litigation. Missing swabs or instruments, diathermy burns, tissue or nerve damage due to incorrect positioning, drug errors, mix-ups with patients, wrong operations and invalid patient consent are just a few of the commonly known risks. In addition to this, increasing pressures on available resources, recruitment and retention problems, communication breakdowns and conflicts among staff are all factors that may influence the occurrence of these risks. All perioperative practitioners have a key role to play in terms of minimizing these risks and ensuring that patients get the best and safest care. Understanding how the law of negligence works may help to achieve this (see Ch. 3 for further discussion on Risk Management issues).

Negligence is defined as a failure in the duty of care owed to another, with resultant harm to that person. Perioperative practitioners need to be aware of three key concepts within the law of negligence:

● Duty of care
● Standard of care
● Causation.

Duty of care The legal test for the duty of care was established in a case entirely unrelated to health care (Donoghue v Stevenson 1932).[4] This case determined that a person must take 'reasonable care to avoid acts or omissions which she or he can reasonably foresee would be likely to injure a person directly affected by those acts'. This means that a duty of care exists between a practitioner and those who could be affected by their actions or omissions. It follows then that a duty of care exists between the practitioner and all patients they are employed to care for. In fact, it is argued that there cannot be a closer legal relationship than that which exists between patients and their carers.[5] While a practitioner is working in their place of employment there is no doubt that they owe a duty of care to patients.

Standard of care Once a duty of care is established the next consideration is the standard of the care given, and this is best explained by considering the Bolam Test. This arises from a case where it was argued that the hospital was vicariously liable for the carelessness of a doctor who gave electroconvulsive therapy to a patient without administering a relaxant drug or restraining the convulsive movements. The patient sustained injuries (Bolam v Friern Barnet HMC 1957).[6] The court sought the opinion of other doctors who worked in this area of practice and they, at the time, supported the actions of the doctor and the case was lost. The key point that arose from the Bolam case was not the clinical situation, but it was the notion that other professionals who normally undertake the role of the defendants measure the standard of care. 'A doctor is not guilty of negligence if he has acted in accordance with a practice accepted as proper by a responsible body of medical men skilled in that particular art' (Bolam v Friern Barnet HMC 1957).[6] Since the early 1980s the Bolam Test has been used in many cases, and it is accepted that this test is now applied to all healthcare professionals. It was also established during the Bolam case that the standard would be that of the 'reasonably skilled and experienced professional'. This indicates that practice may not have to be the best possible, but it must be within the range of acceptable practice and endorsed by practitioners who work in the same field. The actions or omissions of perioperative practitioners are therefore judged legally by their peer group.

The standard of care expected of learners is also an important area to address, as it is inappropriate to apologize to patients about mistakes being made simply because it was a learner who made them. It is important to remember that the term 'learner' means all staff engaged in a learning role. The standard of care by learners was addressed in Wilsher v Essex Area Health Authority in 1986.[7] Wilsher was a premature baby who had a number of clinical problems, including oxygen deficiency. His prospects of survival were poor and he was placed in a special care baby unit. During this time an inexperienced doctor was monitoring the baby's oxygen levels and mistakenly inserted a catheter into a vein rather than an artery. The doctor asked the senior registrar to check their work and the registrar failed to spot the mistake; some hours later, when replacing the catheter, the registrar made the same mistake. In both instances the catheter monitor failed to register correctly the amount of oxygen in the baby's blood and the baby was given too much oxygen, thereby suffering retinal damage. The junior doctor was not found to be negligent, but only because he had asked for his work to be checked. Otherwise he would clearly have been found negligent. However, the senior registrar was found to be negligent (Wilsher v Essex Area Health Authority 1986 All ER 801).[7]

This case determined a key point about the standard of care regarding learners, as it means that inexperience is no defence to an action for negligence. The law requires the trainee or learner to be judged by the same standard as their more experienced colleagues. Although the Wilsher case centred on the actions of doctors the same principle applies to other healthcare professionals, and that would include perioperative practitioners and all learners in the perioperative environment.

Whoever is responsible for the supervision of learners must ensure that the standard of care that patients ultimately receive is maintained at an acceptable level. Conversely, learners should engage in the supervision process themselves by asking for their work to be checked. Supervision should be seen as a two-way process. This would also be true of practitioners who are asked to work in new and unfamiliar areas of practice: there are responsibilities both ways to ensure that the standard of care is not breached. There need to be appropriate arrangements for the supervision of trainees and learners in the perioperative environment which on the one hand allow these learners to obtain experience while on the other hand protecting the standard of care.

It is often very difficult to work out how perioperative practitioners may be accountable when they often work under the direct supervision of surgeons and anaesthetists. Montgomery[8] clarifies this point very well and explains that in a number of cases the courts have acknowledged the fact that healthcare professionals work in teams, in which they have different responsibilities. The idea that each team member is expected to deliver the high standards of care that the team as a whole could offer has been rejected. The courts have rejected the doctrine known as the 'Captain of the Ship', whereby professionals in charge of teams are responsible for the negligence of their members, even though they may not be personally at fault.

If, for example, a swab is left inside a patient during surgery the law recognizes that it was the surgeon's responsibility to have checked that no swab was left inside, rather than to be personally responsible for the scrubbed assistant's error. Whereas the scrubbed assistant may be held liable for the error, the surgeon would be liable for failing to check. The same would apply in the case of the anaesthetic assistant: if the assistant draws up an incorrect anaesthetic dose this does not make the anaesthetist negligent merely because he bore overall responsibility for anaesthesia.[8] The key point here is that professionals are responsible for their own mistakes and not for those of the members of their team.

However, the courts do recognize that a practitioner who relies on the instructions of the surgeon or anaesthetist is not negligent, even if at a later date these instructions prove to be wrong. In other words, a practitioner who carries out an instruction given to them by the doctor, which in hindsight may have been wrong, will not be negligent if it was not obvious at the time that the instruction was wrong. However, practitioners are expected to challenge decisions on either procedural or substantive grounds if it appears, or it is blatantly obvious, that the instructions are wrong. It is no defence for the practitioner to state that they were merely following orders. The law also recognizes that health care can be fraught with emergency scenarios where it may not be possible to follow the standard routine procedure. This is referred to as 'battle conditions', and in these circumstances, should mistakes be made, the situational context would be taken into account.

The standard of care is therefore a key issue in the context of perioperative practice, and there is no doubt that this aspect of negligence is of the greatest relevance to perioperative practitioners.

Causation It is possible for negligence to be established and the patient to eventually lose their case on the issue of causation. This is what happened in Wilshire v Essex Area Health Authority CA (1986), where the baby was given too much oxygen and sustained retinal damage. Although negligence on the part of the registrar was established, it was also found that the baby had an existing condition that could equally have caused the retinal damage. Because it was not clear whether the registrar's negligence or the pre-existing condition had caused the damage, the case was lost.

Vicarious liability

Under the doctrine of vicarious liability, should a patient take action it would be the employers who are pursued by the patient's lawyers, simply because they are more likely to be able to pay any compensation that would be awarded in a successful action. However, if the patient was harmed as a result of the negligence of an individual practitioner, or the practitioner at least played a key role in the mistakes that led up to the incident, then in theory the practitioner could be pursued by the patient's lawyers. To date, there is no record of this having happened. These issues involving vicarious liability raise important points about new and developing roles in the perioperative environment. It is essential that practitioners are fully aware of the boundaries to their practice and that these are clarified and agreed with their employers. Vicarious liability operates on the basis that the practitioner was engaged in the duties that they were employed to undertake. There are many expanded and developing roles within the perioperative environment. These include the surgeon's first assistant, surgeon's assistant, preassessment practitioner, and many varied nurse practitioner roles. It needs to be quite clear to both employers and practitioners the nature and purpose of these roles and the boundaries that are drawn up around them. Role expansion is considered later in this chapter (see p. 8).

CONTRACTUAL ACCOUNTABILITY

The contractual mode of accountability, which involves the law of contract, is a legal relationship between the practitioner and their employer. Under this contract there is a clear legal duty for the employee to carry out the 'reasonable' orders of their employers. Practitioners are responsible for fulfilling all of their contractual obligations as laid down in their job description and within the guidance of the policies, procedures and standards that employers set. These guidelines all serve as parameters to the role, and understanding these parameters is essential if practitioners are going to be in a position to properly account for their actions to their employers. If the practitioner fails to fulfil the reasonable expectations of their employers then the employers can take sanctions against them. Perioperative practitioners are often highly specialized and working in narrow fields of practice. Should an employer ask the practitioner to work in a different area or in a new role, which requires the utilization of new knowledge and skills, it would be reasonable for the employer to provide appropriate training and support for this role. The same conditions would apply if the practitioner were expected to expand their role in some way.

PROFESSIONAL ACCOUNTABILITY

The main reason for adopting this mode of accountability is to protect the patient. The principal function of a professional body is to maintain a register of qualified practitioners and to remove those who are unfit to practise because of a health problem or because of improper conduct. The professional body also normally oversees education and training matters, but perhaps its primary function should be to regulate membership of the profession. This will normally be undertaken in a quasi-judicial process, where a set of rules or code of conduct provides the guiding principles by which practitioners are held accountable and are therefore judged. This is often referred to as professional law.

The two main groups of professional practitioners in the operating department are both registered by professional bodies. Operating department practitioners are now accountable to the Health Professions Council. This is a relatively new registration body which, at the time of writing, is in the early stages of operating.

Nurses are professionally accountable to the Nursing and Midwifery Council (NMC) (formerly the UKCC) in accordance with the principles set out in the Code of Professional Conduct.[9] The NMC states that its mission is to 'establish and improve standards of nursing care in order to serve and protect the public'. The NMC accepts that professional accountability is concerned with weighing up the interests of patients in complex clinical situations. Practices within the perioperative arena reflect these complexities, where practitioners must utilize professional knowledge, judgement and skills to make decisions about patient care. Whatever actions are taken – or not, as the case may be – the practitioner must always be able to justify them. The current code of conduct[9] sets out seven

core principles, all of which have a direct relevance in perioperative care:

1. Respect the patient or client as an individual.
2. Obtain consent before any treatment or care is given.
3. Protect confidential information.
4. Cooperate with others in the team.
5. Maintain professional knowledge and competence.
6. Be trustworthy.
7. Act to identify and minimize risks to patients and clients.

The NMC is charged with protecting the public, and achieves this through professional regulation. The NMC uses the Code of Conduct to set out the standard expected of practitioners. Where an allegation of professional misconduct arises, the NMC judges those before them by the standard of the 'average' practitioner and not against the highest possible standard of professional expertise.[10] The most common examples of professional misconduct that the NMC considers are:

- Physical, sexual or verbal abuse of patients
- Stealing from patients
- Failing to care for patients properly (for employers and managers who are registered with the NMC, this can include failing to maintain an acceptable environment of care)
- Failing to keep proper records
- Failing to administer medicines safely
- Deliberately concealing unsafe practice
- Committing criminal offences.

The NMC also considers cases where practitioners are unfit to practise for health reasons. There are cases where practitioners continue working when they are clearly unfit to practise safely because of a health problem. The NMC provide examples of such problems that might seriously impair a practitioner's fitness to practise; these are:

- Alcohol dependence
- Drug dependence
- Untreated serious mental illness
- Serious personality disorder.

The NMC provides detailed guidance to employers and managers about reporting unfitness to practise.[11]

Being accountable to a professional body is not an easy option. It is arguably the toughest of the external modes of accountability. It imposes standards of practice that often surpass those of the law, or even the practitioner's contractual obligations. This point is best explained by considering the similarities and differences between the different modes of accountability.

Similarities and differences

Although the different modes of accountability can be seen to converge within given practice situations, the key to understanding accountability is to grasp the fact that these modes essentially work in different ways. Although there may be similarities in the way they operate there may also be different outcomes within each mode, because each may be concerned with different aspects of the situation and may also have different standards of proof. This could be illustrated by making a general comparison between the legal and professional modes. Tingle[12] has observed that the law of negligence does not necessarily expect the professional to act as the patient's advocate, whereas a central plank of any form of professional accountability must be the imperative that members act as the patient's advocate in all aspects of their work. It can be seen then that patient advocacy is a critical concept within the professional mode of accountability. A key difference, then, between the legal and professional modes of accountability is that the law of negligence is concerned with setting the minimal standard of care, whereas professional law is concerned with promoting the highest standards of care.[8] A situation might arise when a practitioner is acting within legal boundaries yet at the same time is in breach of their code of professional conduct.

INFORMED CONSENT

Informed consent has both legal and ethical dimensions: the ethical dimensions, in particular the principle of respect for autonomy, are covered in depth in Chapter 2. However, all perioperative practitioners need to be aware of the legal aspects of informed consent.

It is a requirement of the law that competent adults provide their consent before they are touched during the course of any care and treatment they may receive. If consent is not sought then a professional is open to charges of Trespass to Person, in particular Battery. If there was an attempt to seek consent and it was found to be improper, for example where inadequate information was disclosed, then the patient may sue under the law of negligence for a breach of the duty of care to inform the patient. The principles of informed consent are enshrined in the Patients' Charter,[13] which tell patients that they have the right to have any proposed treatment, including any risks involved and any alternatives, clearly explained to them before they decide whether to agree to it.

Beauchamp and Childress[14] identify five elements to consent:

- Disclosure
- Understanding
- Voluntariness
- Competence
- Consent.

These elements serve as a useful framework to consider the importance of the consent process throughout the perioperative period.

DISCLOSURE

Patients undergoing surgery need to be given details about the procedure along with its expected outcomes and associated risks. The level of disclosure is best explained by returning to the concept of standard of care within the law of negligence (see Case Example 'The Sidaway Case').

Case example: The Sidaway case

Amy Sidaway had suffered from persistent neck and shoulder pain and was advised that she would need surgery to her spinal column to relieve the pain. The surgeon warned her of the possibility of disturbing the nerve root but did not warn her of the possibility of damage to the spinal cord itself, even though the surgery would be within 3 mm of it. Amy consented to the operation, which was undertaken with due skill and care. During the operation the spinal cord was damaged and this resulted in Amy becoming severely disabled. Amy sued the surgeon and the hospital governors, alleging that the surgeon had been in breach of his duty of care to inform her of the risks. Under the application of the Bolam Test, Amy lost her case at the trial court, the Court of Appeal and the House of Lords (Sidaway v Bethlem RHG 1985 1 All ER 643).[15]

The Sidaway case demonstrates that it is the Bolam Test that determines the level of disclosure within the consent process. In practice, the agreed level of disclosure may vary, and because of this there may be some disagreement about what is an appropriate level of disclosure. Where differences exist then members of the team should find ways to achieve consensus. Disclosure of information should not be seen as relating only to the surgery and anaesthesia, but would also include all other care that the patient may receive throughout the perioperative period. Perioperative practitioners have a leading role in ensuring that adequate disclosure takes place throughout this entire process.

UNDERSTANDING

Disclosure of information is not enough if the patient fails to understand it. Practitioners need to ensure that their patients understand fully the information given to them about all aspects of their care and treatment throughout the perioperative period. This might include clarifying information given by the doctor, in particular the proposed surgery. There have been concerns raised about the standard and quality of the 'consent for surgery' process, in particular where junior doctors are involved.[16] Perioperative practitioners can play a key part in ensuring that the patient's understanding of their surgery, as well as other aspects of their care, is maintained at a satisfactory level.

VOLUNTARINESS

This relates to the conditions under which consent may be sought. Patients who require surgery are vulnerable to the suggestions of well meaning healthcare professionals who may be clear about what needs to be done. It may be difficult to prevent some degree of 'coercion' in securing consent from a patient, but misrepresentation of the facts or overt manipulation of the patient should be avoided.

COMPETENCE

Consent can only be valid if the patient is competent to give it. Some patients may not be legally or mentally competent to give consent, and this is a complex area which cannot be fully explained in this chapter. However, in the perioperative environment there are a number of specific issues relating to competence that do need consideration.

A patient may be admitted unconscious and in need of life-saving surgery, and it is not possible to seek their consent. In these circumstances the professionals would clearly have a duty to act in the patient's best interest and for the surgery to go ahead, but only if it could be demonstrated that the situation was indeed life threatening.

The same considerations would apply in a situation where, during an elective operation, the surgeon identifies the need for additional surgery, unrelated to that which was agreed to. If the new problem identified was life threatening then it might be justified to perform this additional procedure. However, if it was not a life-threatening problem then, under the law of trespass, it would be wrong for this additional procedure to be performed: the patient would need to be woken up and consulted properly under the usual consent process. Seeking consent from patients in the anaesthetic room may also be problematical, in particular when the patient is under the influence of a 'mind-altering' premedication. It would be very difficult, if not impossible, to demonstrate that all the requirements of a valid consent process had been met in such circumstances. It would therefore be wrong to seek consent from patients under these conditions.

CONSENT

Consent may be either implied or expressed, and both methods can be found during the perioperative period. Implied consent is where the patient indicates through actions that they are willing for a particular act of care to take place, for example holding their arm out for a blood test or blood pressure measurement. Expressed consent can be given either verbally or in writing. Written consent is vastly superior to all other methods of consent giving, as it stands as a permanent record of the consent process: this is of particular use should a case arise at a later date in a court of law.

It is possible that a patient may be anaesthetized and on the operating table when it is discovered that there is no consent form signed, but medical and ward staff are sure that the patient has agreed to the planned surgery. Under normal practices this should not occur, as checking the consent form is a requirement of the preoperative preparation process. However, it is possible that the consent is still valid, as verbal and implied consent are equally valid in law.[17] This might indicate that the procedure could be performed. However, Dimond[17] believes that it would be wiser to ensure that the patient has signed a consent form, and if not, then he or she should be returned to the ward to enable consent to be given. It is stressed, though, that this situation should really be avoided in the first place, with proper and effective consent checking procedures during the preoperative period.

SCOPE OF PROFESSIONAL PRACTICE

In perioperative practice, roles can and do change, and it is important that when such changes occur there is a clear awareness of exactly where the boundaries lie. Surgeons' assistants and first assistants are obvious examples, and these are described elsewhere,[18–20] but whatever roles are expanded the practitioner should be mindful of the key professional principles that underpin such role development.

More generally for nurses, the NMC states that when registered nurses take on responsibilities beyond the traditional boundaries of their practice they must:

- Be satisfied that patient and client needs are uppermost
- Aim to keep up-to-date and develop knowledge, skills and competence
- Recognize limits to personal knowledge and skill and remedy deficiencies
- Ensure that existing nursing care is not compromised by new developments and responsibilities
- Acknowledge personal accountability
- Avoid inappropriate delegation.[21,22]

These principles assert that the practitioner should be more responsive to their patients' needs. It also reinforces the notion of individual accountability by stressing that all practitioners have to be aware of their own competence when expanding the boundaries of their practice. For a more organizational/employment perspective, Younger[23] suggests five aspects that require attention when expanded roles are being developed:

- Parameters of new roles
- Education and training
- Professional implications
- Managerial and personnel issues
- Legal and ethical issues.

In perioperative care these aspects are considered elsewhere,[18,19,24] and readers are advised to access this information for more detail.

RECORD KEEPING IN PERIOPERATIVE CARE

All records made during the perioperative period are potentially legal documents in that they could be used in complaint investigations, professional conduct inquiries, coroner's courts and civil lawsuits. In particular, with ever-increasing litigation, it is even more important that perioperative records reflect the highest standards of care. Ensuring that accurate and comprehensive perioperative records are kept is a key aspect of accountability.

Records are 'any permanent form of information recorded about a patient or client'.[25] Such records may include perioperative care plans, records of care during surgery, drug charts, observation charts, accident/incident forms and transfer records. There are three key principles in respect of record keeping. Records must be:

1. Contemporary
2. Comprehensive
3. Legible and permanent.

CONTEMPORARY

Perioperative records need to be completed as near as possible to the time of the events that they refer to. It may not always be possible to complete records during the process of giving care or responding to incidents, but practitioners must ensure that they complete them in reasonable time afterwards, so that the events are recorded as accurately as possible. The longer the time gap between the event and the recording the greater the likelihood that the events have been misconstrued.

COMPREHENSIVE

Perioperative records should be factual and informative about the events/incidents and should detail the responses and patients' progress. They should serve to clarify the care that was given and not be difficult to understand. For example, 'I took his Resps and Sats and these were okay' is unclear and lacks sufficient detail to clarify to a lay person or solicitor what exactly happened. As a general rule, perioperative records should be written in such a way that the patient themselves could understand them.

LEGIBLE AND PERMANENT

Perioperative records should be legible, abbreviations only being used if they are commonly recognized and well known. Where mistakes have been made these should not be deleted: a line should be put through them to identify the mistake while at the same time ensuring that it can be read at a later date should the need arise. Perioperative records must always be written in permanent form: pencil should never be used and blue pen is not advisable because of its poor photocopying properties.

The NMC has produced standards for record keeping[26] that capture all of the key principles perioperative practitioners should bear in mind in respect of all perioperative records:

- Record keeping is an integral part of nursing and midwifery practice
- Good record keeping is a mark of the skilled and safe practitioner
- Records should not include abbreviations, jargon, meaningless phrases, irrelevant speculation and offensive subjective statements
- Records should be written in terms that the patient or client can easily understand
- By auditing your records, you can assess the standard of the record and identify areas for improvement and staff development
- You must ensure that any entry you make in a record can easily be identified
- Patients and clients have the right of access to records held about them
- Each practitioner's contribution to records should be seen as of equal importance

- You have a duty to protect the confidentiality of the patient and client record
- Patients and clients should own their healthcare records as far as it is appropriate and as long as they are happy to do so
- The principle of the confidentiality of information held about your patients and clients is just as important in computer-held records as in all other records
- The use of records in research should be approved by your local research ethics committee
- You must use your professional judgement to decide what is relevant and what should be recorded
- Records should be written clearly and in such a manner that the text cannot be erased
- Records should be factual, consistent and accurate
- You need to assume that any entries you make in a patient or client record will be scrutinized at some point
- Good record keeping helps to protect the welfare of patients and clients.[26]

Keeping clear and effective records is an essential part of perioperative practice and not an afterthought. Effective record keeping contributes towards maintaining high standards of care while also offering the practitioner a higher level of professional protection.

Accountability places great demands on the practitioner and this chapter has illustrated how such accountability works in perioperative care. The separate modes of accountability can place different levels of demand upon the practitioner, sometimes conflicting, but always aimed at ensuring that the practitioner is able to justify their decisions. This is a fundamental requirement of professional practice and lies at the heart of the best perioperative care.

References

1. Bergman J. Accountability – definition and dimensions. Internat Nurs Rev 1981; 28: 53–59.
2. Marks-Maran D. Accountability. In: Tschudin V, ed. Ethics, nurses and patients. Harrow: Scutari Press; 1993.
3. Peysner J. Litigation. In: McHale J, Tingle J, Peysner J, eds. Law and nursing. Oxford: Butterworth-Heinemann; 1998.
4. Donoghue v Stevenson 1932 AC 562.
5. Fulbrook S. Duty of care. Br J Theatre Nurs 1995; 5: 18–19.
6. Bolam v Friern Barnet HMC 1957 All ER 118.
7. Wisher v Essex Area Health Authority 1986 All ER 801.
8. Montgomery J. Health care law. Oxford: Oxford University Press; 1997.
9. Nursing and Midwifery Council. Code of professional conduct. London: NMC; 2002.
10. Nursing and Midwifery Council. Complaints about professional conduct. London: NMC; 2002.
11. Nursing and Midwifery Council. Reporting unfitness to practise – information for employers and managers. London: NMC; 2002.

12. Tingle J. Perspectives on clinical negligence in the operating theatre. Br J Theatre Nurs 1994; 4: 7–8.

13. Department of Health. The patient's charter and you. Leeds: NHS Executive; 1995.

14. Beauchamp T, Childress J. Principles of biomedical ethics, 3rd edn. Oxford: Oxford University Press; 1989.

15. Sidaway v Bethlem RHG 1985 1 All ER 643.

16. Richardson N, Jones P, Thomas M. Should house officers obtain consent for operation and anaesthesia? Health Trends 1996; 28: 56–59.

17. Dimond B. Legal aspects of nursing, 2nd edn. Hemel Hempstead: Prentice Hall; 1995.

18. National Assocation of Theatre Nurses. The role of the nurse as first assistant in the operating department. Harrogate: NATN; 1993.

19. National Assocation of Theatre Nurses. The nurse as surgeon's assistant. Harrogate: NATN; 1994.

20. Hind M. Surgeons' assistants: a new role for operating theatre nurses. Br J Nurs 1997; 6: 1298–1302.

21. United Kingdom Central Council for Nursing, Midwifery and Health Visiting. The scope of professional practice. London: UKCC; 1992.

22. United Kingdom Central Council for Nursing, Midwifery and Health Visiting. Scope in practice. London: UKCC; 1997.

23. Younger J. Changing roles, changing titles in the perioperative environment. In: Hind M, Wicker P, eds. Principles of perioperative practice. London: Churchill Livingstone; 2000: 140–155.

24. National Association of Theatre Nurses. Developing new roles for non-medical staff within perioperative care. Guidelines for organisations and employers. Harrogate: NATN; 1997.

25. Young A. Record keeping. Br J Nurs 1995; 4: 179.

26. Nursing and Midwifery Council. Guidelines for records and record keeping. London: NMC; 2002.

Chapter 2

Ethical dimensions of perioperative practice

Jane Reid

Key points

- Perioperative practitioners deal with ethical issues on a daily basis
- Ethical reflection is fundamental to the delivery of professional practice
- Ethical dilemmas arise when practitioners face a choice between what they are expected to do and what they think they ought to do
- Ethical theories are an aid to decision making
- The Reid model – a guide to facilitate ethical behaviour for perioperative practitioners

ETHICS DEFINED

Ethics as a concept is inextricably entwined with everyday events, whether in relation to work, the wider world, local communities or family life. Fundamentally, ethics is a feature of all that happens between the peoples of a society as they attempt to do what is right and good by themselves and others.

In the context of perioperative environments, either in the course of providing care for patients or working with colleagues, practitioners are required to make decisions and take action based upon what they regard as good or right and what they believe they ought to do in a given situation.

ETHICS AND MORALS – A DISTINCTION

All too often the terms ethics and morals are used interchangeably, particularly in everyday usage; however, from a formal position it is useful to acknowledge the distinction between the two concepts. Morals (and more specifically the notion of morality) are concerned with the standards of behaviour adopted or promoted by individuals and groups, whereas ethics is a term that is more commonly associated with academic activity, as it is concerned with the study or 'science' of morals. The study of ethics – or moral philosophy as it is sometimes called – involves the theoretical examination of situations and, more importantly, the associated judgements reached by individuals regarding the rightness and wrongness of actions.

However, it is vital that the subject of ethics is not regarded solely as being of importance to theorists and academics, because morality is integral to everyday living and central to the relationships that exist between people and the societies and communities in which they live. Whereas theorists may engage in academic debates that more often than not are remote and faceless, practitioners are challenged to deal with the reality and complexity of ethics as it relates to everyday clinical practice.

An appreciation of difference, informed by ethical reflection, reasoning and understanding, should be regarded as an essential skill for all perioperative practitioners because they are required to work and interact with a variety of people and to function professionally within diverse and complex clinical situations.

VALUING DIVERSITY

Differences between individuals are generated because people are influenced by so many factors, including social and professional norms, culture, custom, religious beliefs and family values. It is this rich tapestry of exposure and experience (the socialization process) as individuals make the journey from childhood through adolescence to take up their adult lives, that influences individual values, attitudes and perspectives.

It is important to recognize that all things are context dependent: few issues can be framed as black or white, right or wrong; there are quite simply no absolutes. What may be judged as right and good in one context by one individual or group may be regarded as wrong and bad by others. Similarly, what is judged as ethical action one day may be regarded as unethical the next.

Another ethical dimension inherent to perioperative practice concerns the advances of medical science. The unrelenting progress of technological development and 'discovery' will continue to challenge the norms, realities and possibilities within the healthcare arena. These factors demand that professionals continue to review and reassess what is possible and, perhaps more importantly, what is judged morally acceptable to the societies in which they live.

To use an illustration from the perioperative world, ethics is akin to recognizing that there are many and varying shades of grey or shadow, depending upon which way the operating light is directed! To play further on the analogy, a priority for the accountable professional is to assess the beam of the operating light, to determine whether it is positioned at the correct angle, facing in the right direction, and sufficiently bright and equal to the task in hand.

The actions of a practitioner standing back, judging the light and angle of an operating lamp and assessing what action is needed, can be equated to the actions of a practitioner engaged in ethical reflection, for the desired endpoint is the same: judging the actions that are required to secure the best results.

It is here, though, that the parallel ends, for ethical reflection is far more complex than assessing the angle of an operating light because it requires more searching questions, and demands that the practitioner accepts ethics as fundamental to the exercise of their caring role. From this position it could be argued that professional perioperative care is indeed 'applied ethics in action'.

ETHICAL REFLECTION: THE BASIS OF PROFESSIONAL CARING

Caring is about doing things for, to and with people. As such, ethical reflection should be regarded as central and fundamental to the delivery of professional practice and the practitioner–patient relationship. The codes of practice that guide the work of professionals associated with the perioperative arena, with their emphasis on acting in the patient's and the public's best interest, imply that ethical reflection is an integral feature of professional decision making and action.

Chapter 1 introduces readers to the concept of responsibility and accountability and outlines the legal dimensions of professional practice and the frameworks within which professionals must work and act. However, morality and the concept of 'being human' demands acknowledgement that there are aspects of life that cannot be prescribed, or externally forced upon individuals. What may be deemed lawful may be judged unethical, and what might seem ethical may be regarded as unlawful. It is this dimension that creates much of the complexity associated with professional caring.

In defining the discrete responsibilities of professional practitioners, as required by their varying codes of practice and the legislative framework, one cannot overlook the need for accountability to one's personal value system, the idea of accountability to the 'self', or the notion of 'unto thyself be true'.

We need only consider the varying perspectives on mercy killings and euthanasia, consent versus informed consent, and attitudes to abortion and the rationing of treatment, to recognize that variance in individual perspective lies at the very heart of professional practice, and, perhaps more fundamentally, is the basis of human caring.

It is this variance in individual perspective (what one's patients or colleagues may consider to be right, wrong, good and bad), as well as an acknowledgement of the 'self' (what one personally thinks or feels to be right, wrong, good and bad), which demands that ethical reflection be at the forefront of professional consciousness and regarded as an integral element of clinical decision making for all professionals.

FRAMEWORKS FOR ETHICAL DECISION MAKING

As we go about our daily lives we face problems and situations that have moral dimensions, for example whether to tell the truth or to lie, be it to a family member, a friend or a recently made acquaintance.

Generally, individuals manage difficult situations by defining the problem, exploring its dimensions, making choices, and taking the associated action however painful or difficult the anticipated implications or outcomes might prove to be.

In general the problems encountered in everyday life are recurring, and as such it is the rich tapestry of social/family rules, directives, parables and virtues that are learned and internalized that provides individuals with a moral guide. Individual moral frameworks are, in the main, used subconsciously, guiding action and decision making subtly and quietly.

Ordinarily these moral guides suffice, largely because people are rarely called to account for, or justify their judgements or the principles that underpin them.

This is less true within the context of professional practice, where individuals by virtue of their position and responsibility are required to account for all decisions reached and all actions taken, moral or otherwise.

Personal and professional values, associated moral justifications and choices are unquestionably brought into sharper focus when practitioners find themselves faced with a moral dilemma.

A dilemma is best described as a choice between two equally unsatisfactory alternatives. It is important to recognize within the context of professional practice that not all dilemmas are moral: for example, some dilemmas arise quite simply because the individual concerned lacks the knowledge or experience as to what would bring about the best outcome.

Similarly, not all moral choices are moral dilemmas, for in some cases practitioners may well know what they ought to do, such as whether to report unsafe practice or unethical conduct: the issue is whether or not they do so.

Practitioners experience conflict when they are expected to act in a manner that is different from what they regard to be right, wrong, good or bad (moral values), or behave differently to how they feel they should (moral principles). For example, a practitioner may feel obliged to report a drunken colleague as unfit for duty. However, they may face a dilemma because the colleague ordinarily enjoys considerable respect and regard within the clinical team, and is experiencing significant domestic pressure because of an acrimonious divorce. The dilemma for the practitioner is to report or not to report the incident and to face the consequences of the associated implications of taking either position.

When practitioners face a moral dilemma, or where they experience what is perhaps better described as 'moral confusion', the situation will result in their asking questions of their internal moral guide. The practitioner will unconsciously refer to this internal guide, expecting it to assist them in their decision making. Questions will centre on what the practitioner believes to be good and right in the situation, and what they feel they ought to do. This process is often referred to as moral deliberation and moral justification.

Moral deliberation involves an appeal to actions that appear morally justified or to arguments that appear to have stronger moral reasons behind them.

Because practitioners are accountable for their actions, they need to be clear about their moral position and the particular ethical argument that they wish to promote or advocate in a given clinical situation. Furthermore, professionals should consider when their internal moral guide is inadequate to the presenting situation, and when a framework or model for ethical reflection may be more useful to their analysis.

ETHICAL THEORIES

A variety of theories, volunteered by philosophers and academics, have been developed over the centuries. The aim of theorists such as Aristotle, David Hume, Jeremy Bentham, Immanuel Kant and John Stuart Mill, to name but a few, was to provide a theoretical position or an ethical stance that might be used to inform decision making. Broadly, each of the theoretical positions is derived from a sequential process in which the theorist outlines the characteristics of individuals, their actions in particular contexts, and the likely consequences of actions taken.

Although wider reading of the subject will highlight a diversity of theoretical perspectives, the two most widely used and applied in health care are deontology and utilitarianism.

DEONTOLOGY

Also referred to as 'duty-based' ethics, this perspective concerns itself with the intrinsic features of an action – 'what one ought to do', or performing that 'which is one's duty'. The theory is concerned with following certain rules or principles irrespective of the consequences, on the basis that consequences can rarely be controlled or predicted.

UTILITARIANISM

Utilitarianism is the better known of the consequentialist theories. In contrast to deontology, this perspective is based on the consequences or expected consequences of an individual's actions, regardless of the intentions or motives in the first instance. Right and good are judged from the position of bringing about the best consequences in a situation, or securing the 'greatest good for the greatest number'.

PRINCIPLES OF ETHICAL BEHAVIOUR

AUTONOMY

Autonomy is derived from Greek autos (self) and nomos (rule), and is concerned with the capacity to which individuals can make choices and decisions regarding their own lives. Linked to notions of 'self-governance' and 'self-determination', autonomy is fundamental to informed consent.

Further to this, the principle of 'respect for autonomy' assumes that people are entitled to hold individual perspectives, views and rights (personal values and beliefs) and use these to make choices and take action. It can be seen, therefore, that whereas the promotion of autonomy is a moral action, autonomous action may equally be judged immoral. For example, a practitioner may exercise his or her autonomy by performing circulating duties for terminations of pregnancy, whereas another practitioner may regard any involvement in the procedures as being immoral.

A crucial consideration for perioperative practitioners with regard to the principle of respect for autonomy concerns the assessment of patients' 'competence' and their capacity and ability to exercise choice.

Linked to ideas of capacity and competence is the notion of paternalism, a concept best described as being related to actions and behaviours that compromise an individual's autonomy. In health care, situations arise where a professional may judge that paternalistic action is in the patient's best interest to safeguard them from harm. To act ethically, practitioners are required to balance autonomy, best interests and paternalism.

It is essential that professionals recognize that patients judged to be non-autonomous are regarded as capable of making some choices. Furthermore, in certain instances, individuals who are clearly autonomous and have the capacity to exercise choice may decline to do so because of ill health, fear or anxiety.

BENEFICENCE

As a principle, beneficence is concerned with doing good and promoting the legitimate interests of individuals. Beneficent action confers an obligation to promote the wellbeing of people, not simply to protect them from harm. By default, beneficence confers further obligation on the part of the practitioner in so far as 'doing good' assumes consideration and assessment of the possible goods likely to be achieved, compared with all possible harms as a result of a given action.

NON-MALEFICENCE

Non-maleficence as a concept relates to the avoidance of harm. Linked to the maxim 'Primum non nocere' (Above all (or first) do no harm), it is inextricably linked to beneficence, for how can one do or promote good unless one has prevented or removed harm?

Practitioners may find it difficult to distinguish between doing good and avoiding harm in some situations, as the circumstances may require the balance of both concepts. Similarly, the two principles may conflict, for example respecting the patient's autonomy and right to refuse a life-saving intervention that the surgeon argues would afford them palliation and additional years of life.

JUSTICE

This principle is concerned with notions of fairness, giving to each his due entitlement and promoting rights to fair treatment and health services.

RULES

Ethical rules are derived from ethical principles and may include:

- Fidelity: to be trustworthy
- Veracity: to tell the truth and not to lie or deceive people
- Advocacy: to speak on behalf of another
- Privacy: to respect access to persons and their possessions
- Confidentiality: to safeguard information arising from the patient-professional relationship.

ETHICAL CODES: GUIDANCE FOR PRACTICE

A great many codes have been developed over time, with the aim of providing benchmarks for standards of behaviour and the specific conduct expected of individuals. Within the context of health care, the standards expected of practitioners must be compatible with the respective society's notion of 'common morality'.

Benjamin and Curtis[1] volunteer that, in the main, codes of professional ethics contain two categories of statement – statements of 'creed' and 'commandment'.

Statements of 'creed' are perhaps better described as 'value belief statements'; they serve to affirm the standards of conduct the profession aspires to, and what is expected in terms of personal commitment, from each of its members. The International Code of Nurses[2] provides an example of statements of 'creed', by describing nurses' fourfold responsibility to 'promote health, prevent illness; to restore health and alleviate suffering'.

By contrast, Benjamin and Curtis suggest that 'commandments' provide a dual purpose. First, they define accepted and acceptable behaviour, thus providing an enforceable minimum standard of conduct that enables a profession to self-regulate and discipline its members. 'Commandments' also serve to guide individual practitioners, indicating in general terms the ethical considerations that should be taken into account when deciding upon personal conduct or when examining the conduct of colleagues. The Codes of Practice of the registration bodies associated with perioperative practice, such as the Health Professions Council, the Nursing and Midwifery Council and the General Medical Council, contain both creed and commandment statements guiding practitioners as to what is expected of them.

In addition to codes specific to each profession, or the ethical code devised and adopted by an employing organization, perioperative practitioners should have an awareness of ethical codes that relate to research:

- The Nuremberg Code (1949)[3]
- The Declaration of Helsinki (1964 and revised in 1975)[4]
- The Human Rights Act (1998).[5]

The Nuremberg Code, which evolved from the trials of war criminals during the Nuremberg Military Tribunals, and the Declaration of Helsinki, were adopted by the World Medical Association in 1975. Both codes provide directives and guidance regarding bio-medical research involving human subjects.

Perioperative staff assisting with, engaged in or aware of research or clinical trials being conducted within their practice setting/sphere of influence, have a moral responsibility, to ensure that the framework of research governance is followed and that the fundamental rights of patients are safeguarded and protected from harm. Research governance demands that practitioners must satisfy themselves that LREC (Local Research Ethics Committee) and MREC (Multicentre Research Ethics Committee) approval for the respective study or trial has been obtained.

Within a framework of research governance practitioners have an ethical responsibility to ensure that:

● Voluntary consent of participants is established
● The focus and anticipated results of the research are beneficial to society
● The participants are accorded the right to withdraw from the study at any point
● Any hazards associated with the research do not outweigh the potential benefits
● Patient confidentiality is maintained and patient dignity respected.

THE PERIOPERATIVE PRACTITIONER–PATIENT RELATIONSHIP

The relationship between the perioperative practitioner and the patient is frequently described as special and unique. This owes much to the privileged position of the practitioner to empower, support, comfort, care for and treat individuals who are rendered vulnerable and distressed by ill health. Practitioners are well placed either individually or collectively to promote the physical, psychological emotional and spiritual care needs of those with whom they come into contact. This position, however, confers certain obligations, and most importantly the need to be observant of the potential for patients to become emotionally dependent at a time when they are most vulnerable, and the obligation to act morally and ethically to safeguard patients' best interests.

Dependency and vulnerability are significant features of the practitioner–patient relationship and relate to the overarching power imbalance that is often a feature of healthcare delivery.

Traditionally, the locus of power has been invested in doctors by virtue of their specialist knowledge, the historical subordination of nursing and allied health professionals, and the particular status medicine has tended to enjoy within society.[6]

The concept of power is succinctly defined by de Jovenal[7] as the 'capacity to make others do what one wants them to do against their own desires and preferences, and against their wills' (p. 50).

Whilst it may be regarded as legitimate for doctors to exert power and influence regarding medical issues, it does not necessarily follow that they should dictate and direct other aspects of care or the actions of practitioners. Consider, for example, the situation of a patient poorly prepared for theatre. If a practitioner discovers that a patient does not understand the consent presented by the doctor for signing, the practitioner has a duty to address the situation and it is within his/her rights to refuse to cooperate with the procedure. Most importantly, the patient needs to be supported and reassured that any qualms they may have voiced are legitimate, and that any questions posed will not result in their being labelled a 'difficult patient'.

Perioperative practice has always been and will continue to be challenging and intense, not least because the situations that practitioners are presented with are often immediate and demand instant decision making. By virtue of their position, practitioners are morally, legally and professionally accountable and thus obliged to always consider the concept of autonomy, the best interests of the patient, and the primacy of the practitioner role as patient advocate.

In seeking to advocate for patients, it is vital that perioperative practitioners are able to distinguish between technical questions, medical authority, the dimensions of their own area of competence, and issues that warrant moral/ethical reflection and debate. In circumstances of an ethical nature that require the determination of right, good, and the patient's best interests, it is important that no one member of the healthcare team is recognized as having particular expertise or permitted to impose their view, by virtue of their position within the team. It is far more appropriate that individuals are recognized as moral agents, and that the views of patient, perioperative practitioner, doctor and allied health professional are accepted as valid and important to ethical deliberation and the decision-making process.

Advocacy assumes that the rights and interests of patients remain paramount. Although considerable debate and comment may be found in the literature regarding the implications and difficulties associated with the concept, practitioners must strive to uphold and promote patients' rights and interests because the perioperative experience itself renders the patient vulnerable.

The particular challenge for perioperative practitioners is that their relationship with the patient is brief and transient, when considered within the totality of the patient's journey. However, this does not negate the responsibility and importance of remaining ethically aware and considerate of respect for the principle of autonomy. Returning to the issue of consent to surgery, for example, irregularities observed in patient documentation cannot be assumed to have been explored or settled in the ward setting or outpatient clinic: any concerns that perioperative staff may have should be followed up and examined with the patient and attending doctor.

USING A MODEL TO GUIDE ETHICAL REFLECTION

THE FOUNDATION TO CLINICAL DECISION MAKING AND THE DELIVERY OF QUALITY PERIOPERATIVE CARE

The perioperative setting is an exciting, demanding and exhilarating place to work owing to factors such as patient dependency, the acuity of the case load, diversity of practice and pressure of work. These factors sit against a backdrop of national agendas, strategic and local developments, advancing technology, and pressures to achieve the very best outcome for patients. Ethical deliberation is one aspect of the decision-making process.

Earlier in this chapter reference was made to 'internal moral guides', which we possess and tap into either consciously or unconsciously as part of the decision-making process en route to specific clinical action.

To organize thinking in relation to complex situations, theoretical models have been developed to encourage a methodical approach to an issue. Models of nursing (such as Roper, Logan and Tierney and Orem), for example, have been a feature of nursing practice and well represented in the literature for some 20 years or so; however, models that facilitate ethical deliberation and analysis of complex ethical situations have in the main been restricted to ethically focused and academic literature, and are arguably less accessible to practitioners on a day-to-day basis.

There is nothing particularly complex about a model: it is merely a theoretical framework proposed by a given individual. It comprises a number of abstract, but often related, sets of concepts that direct the reader to a particular train of thought.

The remainder of this chapter is given over to proposing such a model, as well as presenting a set of examples related to and arising from perioperative practice. They are shared to encourage the reader to engage in case analysis.

THE REID MODEL

Reflections 'on and in' practice have led the author to conclude that clinical decision making which underpins the interventions and actions associated with perioperative care can be eased where practitioners engage in a fourfold approach to ethical questioning and critical analysis of presenting situations:

Step 1: Ethical questions
Step 2: Identifying the domains of the situation
Step 3: Analysis through reflection
Step 4: What to do and how to act.

Step 1: Ethical questions

Step 1 involves the practitioner in posing and examining three ethical questions:

1. What may be judged as good, bad, right or wrong?
2. What should/ought to be done in the presenting situation?
3. What is one's duty?

Step 2: Identifying the domains of the situation

This step of the model involves the practitioner in deeper analysis of the presenting situation by inviting them to consider the three questions in relation to four domains.

In Figure 2.1 and Box 2.1 Reid proposes that four domains are intrinsic features of any perioperative situation. No domain is more important than

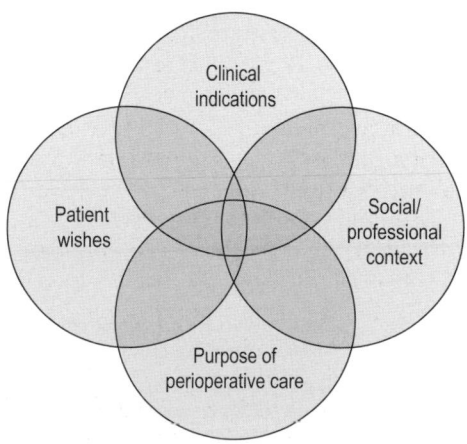

Figure 2.1 Relationship of the four domains intrinsic to perioperative situations.

another: they are merely triggers within the model to prompt evaluation of the specific features of the presenting situation. Evaluation of each domain is dependent upon asking questions of it (Fig. 2.2).

Step 3: Analysis through reflection

To develop the model further, once the variables of the presenting situation have been identified the practitioner is required to structure their reflection by asking particular questions of the presenting situation (Fig. 2.3):

- What matters?
- What are the facts?
- What is the conflict?
- Reflection?

Box 2.1   Description of the four ethical domains

The four *domains* intrinsic to perioperative situations:

Clinical indications   Virtually every situation relates to a patient diagnosis, proposed treatment plan or perioperative intervention.

Patient wishes   Respect for the principle of autonomy should be regarded as fundamental; this requires assessment of the patient's choices, personal values, beliefs and plans. Where these cannot be established (e.g. emergency care of an already unconscious individual), reference to significant others should be regarded as useful, to gain insight into the patient's known wishes, beliefs and value system.

Purpose of perioperative care   The aim of all perioperative intervention is to provide quality patient care that reduces suffering, enhances quality of life, or provides dignity and support to those facing death and their significant others.

Social/professional context   All perioperative situations occur within a social/professional context that extends beyond those immediately involved; this includes the experience of being human, the patient's family/significant others, the legislative framework, the professional bodies and organizational policy.

Clinical indications	Patient wishes
What is the patient's diagnosis/health need?	What does the patient want?
Does the proposed intervention contribute to the patient's wellbeing, or alleviate suffering?	Is the patient competent and do they have the capacity to make a decision?
	Is the patient's decision informed, understood and uncoerced?
	Where the patient cannot make a decision, who will make the decision for them and who/what informs this decision?
Purpose of perioperative care	**Social/professional context**
Can the proposed intervention be described as quality patient care?	What are the factors likely to influence the presenting situation?
Does the proposed intervention reduce suffering or enhance quality of life?	What factors can be influenced by the decision taken?
Does the proposed intervention contribute to a peaceful dignified death and care of significant others?	

Figure 2.2   Evaluation of perioperative domains.

Step 4: What to do and how to act

After analysing a situation in this structured way, practitioners are able to think more clearly about the presenting issues and select a course of action or perioperative intervention and be clear about the rationales and moral arguments that underpin it.

CASE STUDIES

Case 1

Mary Matthews, a 24-year-old woman, presents in the Emergency Department in the late afternoon with severe abdominal pain. A junior doctor attends her and a laparotomy is suggested as the likely intervention. An emergency operation is scheduled within the next 2 hours, and because the surgical wards are busy organizing discharges and creating beds, Mary is transferred directly to the 'holding bay' of the operating department. On arrival she is tearful and distressed, and begs those around her to relieve her pain.

The recently qualified attending practitioner consults the prescription chart, and while he is doing so the duty surgeon telephones advising that she is delayed in clinic and so is unable to see the patient for another hour. The surgeon insists that all analgesia be withheld so that consent can be obtained when she arrives.

Key ethical questions

- What may be judged as good, bad, right or wrong?
- What should/ought to be done in the presenting situation?
- What is the practitioner's duty?

Evaluation of the perioperative domains

See Figure 2.4.

Elements of reflection

See Figure 2.5.

Reflective questions

What matters? This requires an assessment of the issues and the individuals within the situation.

What are the facts? What is known in the situation? This is different from assumptions, presumption and conjecture.

What is the conflict? What aspects of the situation are causing those involved, discomfort and unease?

Reflection? How is this situation similar/dissimilar to past situations that were learned from?

Figure 2.3   Analysis through reflection.

Clinical indications	Patient wishes
Abdominal pain? Unknown cause? Mary is distressed and tearful.	Mary wants to be pain free. Mary is competent but analgesia may compromise her capacity to make an informed decision.
Purpose of perioperative care	**Social/professional context**
To withhold analgesia will cause Mary suffering and is inconsistent with the ethos of quality patient care.	The practitioner is inexperienced and a little unsure of his role and relationship to the surgeon. In emergency situations where the patient's capacity to make an informed decision is affected by drugs, the surgeon may act as the 'agent of necessity' and take action that is in the patient's 'best interest'. The DoH guidelines for consent[8] incorporate documentation for use in instances where the patient's capacity to give consent is compromised.

Figure 2.4   Evaluation of the perioperative domains for Case 1.

```
┌─────────────────────────────────────────────────────┐
│ Reflective questions                                 │
│                                                       │
│ What matters?                                         │
│ Acting as Mary's advocate, acting in Mary's best     │
│ interests, relieving her distress and pain.          │
│                                                       │
│ What are the facts?                                   │
│ On a verbal rating scale (VRS) of 1–10 Mary is       │
│ reporting her pain as 9.                              │
│    The emergency list is not scheduled to start for  │
│ another 2 hours.                                      │
│    The surgeon is unable to attend Mary for another  │
│ hour.                                                 │
│                                                       │
│ What is the conflict?                                 │
│ Wanting to do the right thing for Mary but worried   │
│ about the surgeon's direct order to withhold         │
│ medication until she arrives.                         │
│                                                       │
│ Reflection?                                           │
│ No similar experience to draw upon, but the          │
│ practitioner is conscious of his personal            │
│ accountability, the principles of clinical           │
│ governance and the goals of a patient-centred        │
│ approach to care delivery.                           │
└─────────────────────────────────────────────────────┘
```

Figure 2.5   Analysis through reflection for Case 1.

Discussion

It is recognized that the practitioner may be worried about his inexperience and uncertain of his relationship to the surgeon where this relates to the delivery of quality patient care, but he is aware that the surgeon shares a common misconception that informed consent is invalidated by the administration of certain medications. The practitioner demonstrates knowledge of the consent process advocated by the Department of Health[8] and that consent documentation can accommodate situations where patients are of reduced capacity.

The point in this case should not be whether Mary receives medication or not, but once she does, whether the medication has affected her capacity to give an informed, voluntary, uncoerced consent to the proposed intervention of laparotomy.

The ethical issues involved in this case include assessment of Mary's capacity to make an informed decision and whether she is at risk of inadequate care because of ignorance.

Mary's capacity to give consent, when the surgeon arrives in the holding bay, should be determined by her ability to demonstrate an understanding of the proposed surgery, her ability to listen to and demonstrate understanding of the surgical option and its associated risks, and her ability to express a choice about her care, and not by what

medications she may have been administered in the previous 1–2 hours.

Respect for the principles of beneficence, non-maleficence and autonomy requires the perioperative practitioner to promote Mary's wellbeing and optimize her ability to make a choice, as she is able. Severe pain can impair a patient's ability to listen and understand, so that the validity of consent obtained in such circumstances could be questioned. Withholding analgesia for the purpose of obtaining consent should be regarded as coercive.

Case 2

Susan Mercer, a 43-year-old woman with a history of gynaecological problems, is admitted as a day case for examination under general anaesthetic. Following induction of anaesthesia, the two attending practitioners place Susan in the lithotomy position, discreetly arrange the blankets to preserve her modesty, and position the operative trolley (laid with instrumentation for a dilatation and curettage) in readiness for the surgeon.

The surgeon arrives in the theatre attended by six medical students and suggests that he will examine the patient before scrubbing. The surgeon then invites the students to observe him and calls for someone to remove the blanket that had been covering Susan. As the surgeon conducts the examination he makes comment about Susan's sexual history and attempts to joke with the students about the likely cause of her health problems. The students appear shocked by his coarse language and there is little eye contact among the healthcare team. Within earshot of the perioperative practitioners, the surgeon calls over his shoulder suggesting that the students form an orderly queue and take turns to examine the patient. The surgeon taunts the students from the preparation room, challenging them to consider who will be the most accurate in describing the position and presentation of the patient's uterus.

Key ethical questions

- What may be judged as good, bad, right or wrong?
- What should/ought to be done in the presenting situation?
- What are the practitioner's duties?

Clinical indications	Patient wishes
Gynaecological investigation under general anaesthesia. Susan is positioned in lithotomy, to facilitate surgical access.	Susan is competent and volunteered her written consent to receive anaesthesia and a D&C. It is not known whether Susan is aware that the clinical facility hosts students from the neighbouring medical school. There is no expressed permission on the consent form that Susan has agreed to multiple examination (PV).
Purpose of perioperative care	**Social/professional context**
To permit repeated examination of Susan (as it is not explicitly authorized by her consent) is inconsistent with the ethos of quality patient care and is a violation of her person.	The surgeon is a 'known' and generally respected medical tutor, but the team are clearly embarrassed by his comments about Susan as they are derogatory and disrespectful of her. The practitioners are uncertain about the parameters of the students' visit, particularly in relation to physical examination of patients. They are unaware of any organizational position statement regarding visiting students. The students may feel intimidated by the surgeon and under pressure to follow his instruction (power/coercion).

Figure 2.6   Evaluation of the perioperative domains for Case 2.

Evaluation of the perioperative domains

See Figure 2.6.

Elements of reflection

See Figure 2.7.

Discussion

This situation is sensitive and demanding, as it requires the attending perioperative practitioners to challenge the view that the students should gain experience in physical examination skills by practising on unconscious patients. The practitioners also have to examine their relationship with their medical colleagues and their collective responsibility to safeguard the patient from non-therapeutic intervention.

The situation emphasizes a number of rights and responsibilities for those involved, all of which have to be acknowledged to secure an optimum outcome. Clearly, with reference to the principles of beneficence, non-maleficence and autonomy the attending practitioners must safeguard the rights of the patient to ensure that she is treated respectfully and with dignity.

The scenario highlights the need to safeguard the patient from multiple examination (duty-based ethics) and to challenge the surgeon's argument of 'the greatest good for the greatest number' (consequence-based ethics), and that without practice and experience the students will not develop skills of examination to benefit future patients. Colten et al[9] argue that intimate examination under anaesthesia is of doubtful validity in training students, as it adds little to the mechanical learning acquired when using mannequins and fails to teach the necessary communication skills required for such sensitive examination.

Achieving the right action in this scenario also needs to take account of the surgeon's conduct. It would be very easy for the derogatory comments and critique of the patient's sexual history to influence perceptions of the patient, and for her to be judged as 'less' worthy, or 'less' deserving of a particular standard of care.

The tendency to stereotype, and to adopt tags or 'labels' for patients, creates the potential for professionals to justify their actions through reference to the key features of the label, rather than the intrinsic features of the individual who has been labelled.

Reflective questions

What matters?
- Acting as Susan's advocate by acting in her best interests
- Promoting respect for her as a person and safeguarding her from harm
- Challenging the practice of colleagues whilst maintaining effective team relationships.

What are the facts?
There is no indication on the consent form or in Susan's notes that she has consented to multiple examination for the benefit of student education. There is no therapeutic value to her from repeated examination.

The surgeon has made reference to Susan's sexual history in negative terms and has taunted the students to examine her and to describe accurately the anatomical presentation of her uterus. This situation renders Susan vulnerable and further dependent upon those about her to act in her best interests.

What is the conflict?
The conflict for the practitioners is that they are unaware of any explicit organizational policy regarding the role of students in the operating department, and they cannot find any explicit permission in Susan's notes to justify non-therapeutic multiple examination. Both practitioners regard the surgeon's attitude as judgemental of the patient. Reflecting on their value base, the practitioners are distressed and frame the proposed multiple examination without Susan's consent as 'surgical rape'. Both practitioners recognize that to safeguard Susan's dignity and worth they will be required to publicly challenge the surgeon's instruction to the students.

Reflection?
Neither practitioner has any similar experience to draw upon, but both are conscious of their personal accountability, the tort laws of assault and negligence, the principles of clinical governance and the principle of non-maleficence.

Figure 2.7   Analysis through reflection for Case 2.

Kantian-based ethics require us to view patients as an end in themselves and never merely as a means: to regard and use Susan as a teaching aid should be regarded as unacceptable.

Therefore, the point in this case is not whether the patient should be examined by the students, as clearly the answer should be that she should not, for she has not consented to such, but rather, how the practitioners challenge the explicit instruction of the surgeon that the students should do so.

The surgeon has the right to expect that any criticism of his conduct should initially be made in a private setting, rather than in front of the perioperative team. Ideally, the practitioners should approach him in the preparation room, express their concerns and invite him to reflect on his actions and comments. The goal of this approach is to afford the surgeon the level of respect that the practitioners are seeking for the patient. Where the practitioners are unable to discuss the matter in confidence with the surgeon, they should voice their objection in a non-confrontational way without aggression. Given the obvious discomfort of the perioperative team to the surgeon's initial behaviour, it is likely that the students will acknowledge the voiced concerns and decline the invitation to examine the patient.

An outcome of this situation should be that the perioperative practitioners concerned complete a critical incident form and draw the incident to the attention of their line manager and the Medical Dean. Clinical governance demands that an organizational policy should exist regarding the role and conduct of medical students in the operating department, and that the surgeon should be called to account for his conduct on this occasion.

Case 3

Mr Halliwell is an 84-year-old man who has undergone an emergency hemiarthroplasty. At 2200 hours he is admitted to a recovery unit staffed by two practitioners. Practitioner A is preparing to return her patient to the ward, leaving practitioner B to receive a verbal handover from the anaesthetist and to take a lead in Mr Halliwell's care. Mr Halliwell is hypovolaemic, confused and disorientated, evidenced by his pulling at his oxygen mask and intravenous infusion line. In his distress, Mr Halliwell is shouting out for his wife and flailing his arms. Cot sides and pads have been placed on the bed to safeguard Mr Halliwell from harm. Practitioner B complains out loud that it has been a long shift and that she could do without Mr Halliwell and his 'antics'.

As Practitioner A completes the documentation for her patient, she notes that Mr Halliwell is resisting Practitioner B's attempts to observe and record his vital signs. Rather than assisting her colleague immediately, Practitioner A decides that the recording of her patient's postoperative history is a priority in order to facilitate his return to the ward.

Following discharge of her patient, Practitioner A washes her hands and approaches Practitioner B to assist in the care of Mr Halliwell. As she does so, she observes Practitioner B strike Mr Halliwell on the arm and shout that he is an ungrateful man and that he needs to have his blood pressure recorded.

Key ethical questions

- What may be judged as good, bad, right or wrong?
- What should/ought to be done in the presenting situation?
- What is Practitioner A's duty?

Evaluation of the perioperative domains

See Figure 2.8.

Elements of reflection

See Figure 2.9.

Discussion

Distress, disorientation and confusion are common features when caring for patients postoperatively, not least when caring for the elderly who are compromised by hypovolaemia. This situation does not raise any of the dramatic life and death issues of healthcare ethics, but the way it is dealt with can make a tremendous difference to the lives of those affected.

This situation is without doubt an example of the way in which healthcare ethics are concerned with everyday matters, and with making people's lives and the situations they find themselves in more acceptable to them.

To have to deal with non-compliant patients may of course become frustrating to staff, particularly at the end of a long busy shift when they are tired. However, it is clearly unacceptable to vent frustrations upon the patient. It is difficult to see how the actions of Practitioner B described above could conceivably count as being in the best interests of Mr Halliwell.

Yes, it would be helpful to maintain regular recordings of Mr Halliwell's vital signs; yes, it

Clinical indications	Patient wishes
Mr Halliwell has a fractured neck of femur and has undergone hemiarthroplasty under general anaesthesia. Mr Halliwell is disoriented to time and place. Mr Halliwell is hypovolaemic and dependent on fluid replacement therapy.	Mr Halliwell is distressed and resisting attempts to record his vital signs. It is not known if Mr Halliwell's non-compliance is an attempt to communicate his refusal of treatment or due to his confusion. Mr Halliwell's care plan suggests that he is ordinarily competent.
Purpose of perioperative care	**Social/professional context**
Mr Halliwell requires fluid replacement therapy to compensate his hypovolaemia; his vital signs need recording to determine his recovery from anaesthesia and surgery. Mr Halliwell is disoriented and distressed and is deserving of reassurance, comfort and orientation to the recovery environment.	The unit is staffed by two practitioners of the same grade. Practitioner B reports being tired and appears inconsiderate of the distress exhibited by Mr Halliwell. Mr Halliwell is entitled to receive safe and competent care from Practitioner B, who is professionally accountable for her actions. Practitioner A must act to minimize the risk to Mr Halliwell and should report Practitioner B to a senior person who has the authority to manage her.

Figure 2.8   Evaluation of the perioperative domains for Case 3.

Reflective questions

What matters?

- Acting as Mr Halliwell's advocate by challenging the conduct of a colleague
- Safeguarding Mr Halliwell from further harm and reporting to an authority that the environment of care has failed Mr Halliwell.

What are the facts?

There are two practitioners of the same standing on duty. Practitioner A has observed Practitioner B complain about being tired, complain about the patient's distress, and strike Mr Halliwell as he flailed his arms. Mr Halliwell is visibly distressed and resistive of attempts to record his blood pressure.

Nobody other than Practitioner A observed Practitioner B strike the patient; however, the anaesthetist was in the vicinity when Practitioner B complained of being tired and that she could do without Mr Halliwell's 'antics'.

What is the conflict?

The conflict for Practitioner A is that she feels she should challenge the conduct of Practitioner B, reporting her actions to a senior authority, but there were no witnesses to the incident and she is worried about causing trouble for Practitioner B.

Reflection?

Practitioner A has no past experience to draw upon, but is conscious of her personal accountability, the tort laws of trespass, assault and negligence, the principles of clinical governance and the principle of non-maleficence. Practitioner A is also aware of the duty of care and individual accountability of Practitioner B.

Figure 2.9 Analysis through reflection for Case 3.

would be facilitative of his recovery were he not to tamper with his IVI or his oxygen mask, but not at the expense of striking him, or humiliating him in front of those around him.

Ethics is concerned with the principle of respect for persons, which urges practitioners to look beyond the 'nuisance' of the presenting situation and to consider the humanity of Mr Halliwell and the very humanity that he shares with those caring for him.

Practitioner B has failed Mr Halliwell and herself, for she has spoken to him as if he were a child and struck him as if he had done wrong. This situation demonstrates the relationship between the ethical and legal frameworks, as it highlights an ethical violation of respect for persons and a legal violation of assault.

Practitioner A has observed this act, and so respect for the principles of beneficence, non-maleficence and autonomy demand that she should intervene to the benefit of Mr Halliwell and future patients that Practitioner B is likely to care for.

In the first instance, Practitioner A should reassure herself that Mr Halliwell is receiving appropriate care, and that attempts are being made to orient him to his environment and allay his distress; thereafter she should encourage Practitioner B to reflect on her actions and to learn from them.

The clock cannot be turned back and nothing can change the fact that Practitioner B struck Mr Halliwell, or that she was rude to him, at a time when he was most vulnerable and probably frightened.

The important point in this case is that Practitioner A creates an opportunity to discuss the incident, inviting Practitioner B to analyse her behaviour within the context of standards for professional practice, safeguarding Mr Halliwell's wellbeing and with regard to promoting public trust and confidence in perioperative professionals.

Ideally Practitioner B will recognize her shortcomings and report the incident to her manager, for clinical governance is concerned with developing a 'no blame' culture and learning to effect improvements in patient care.

If Practitioner A is unable to encourage insight, she should voice her criticism and ethical concerns in a non-confrontational way without aggression. If, having been confronted with her shortcomings, Practitioner B fails to acknowledge that her behaviour was unacceptable, or if she shows no remorse for her actions, then Practitioner A should inform Practitioner B that she will report the matter to the relevant manager, and that she will be completing a critical incident form.

There are few practitioners who intentionally hurt or harm patients; in the majority of cases such as this factors such as fatigue and frustration trigger the incident. Reflective learning is a powerful tool and can be used to promote insight and new understanding.

In providing comment upon this case, it is acknowledged that if Practitioner B fails to recognize her shortcomings then informing the line manager and completing a critical incident form may involve serious moral conflict for Practitioner A, not least involving the notion of a breach of loyalty to her colleague.

The fact that there are no witnesses to the incident, and that Mr Halliwell is unlikely to recall being spoken to sharply or struck, places Practitioner A in a difficult position and she will need to appeal to her professional code of practice and her own moral conscience to guide her actions.

This conflict cannot be resolved solely on the basis of one agent exercising authority and power over another, but instead necessitates a cooperative and collaborative approach, which should be at the very heart of perioperative team working.

SUMMARY

Professional caring in the perioperative arena assumes that practitioners see the patient as an equal within the practitioner–patient relationship, not in terms of knowledge and expertise (as clearly the patient is at a disadvantage here), but as a human being, deserving of respect and consideration. Ethical awareness presumes that practitioners respect the principles of diversity and difference, so enabling them to deliver care in a non-judgemental manner that will not diminish the patient as a person. Similarly, teamwork assumes that colleagues whom practitioners work with are afforded equal levels of respect and consideration.

Professional practice therefore demands moral courage, to ensure that the focus of perioperative care remains with the patient. Ethical caring demands commitment and a willingness to undertake actions to the best of one's ability, not merely because one has to, but because one believes that it is ethically right to do so.

References

1. Benjamin M, Curtis J. Ethics in nursing. New York: Oxford University Press; 1981.
2. International Council of Nurses. Code for Nurses. Geneva: ICN; 1973.
3. United States Government. Nuremberg Code. Reprinted from Trials of war criminals before the Nuremberg Military Tribunals under Control Council Law 2 (10): 181–182 Washington, DC: US Government Printing Office; 1949.
4. World Medical Association. Declaration of Helsinki. Tokyo: WHO; 1975.
5. Human Rights Act 1998. Online. Available: http://www.hmso.gov.uk/acts/acts1998/19980042
6. Turner BS. Cited in: Chadwick R, Tadd W. Ethics and nursing practice: a case study approach. London: Macmillan; 1992: 51.
7. de Jovenal B. Cited in: Chadwick R, Tadd W. Ethics and nursing practice: a case study approach. London: Macmillan; 1992: 50.
8. Department of Health. Good practice in consent implementing guide: consent to examination or treatment. London: DOH; 2001.
9. Colten DI, Wakeford R, Kessel RWI, et al. Teaching vaginal examination. Lancet 1988; 2: 375.

Further reading

Beauchamp TL, Childress JF. Principles of biomedical ethics, 4th edn. Oxford: OUP; 2001.

Chapter 3

Risk management

Suzanne Fullbrook

CHAPTER CONTENTS

Key points

- The management of perioperative risk
- The legal framework
- Clinical governance and the management of risk
- Individual accountability and responsibility for risk management

INTRODUCTION: DEFINING RISK MANAGEMENT

In order to define risk management it is first appropriate to define risk: As one commentator has put it: '... risk is the chance of an adverse event ... risk is the combination of the probability or frequency of occurrence of a defined hazard and the magnitude of the consequence of that occurrence.'[1] Management of risk is best, according to Capper, if it is systematic. The advantages include 'clarification of objectives, better understanding of uncertainty, a better response to the unexpected, more effective communication, an improvement in decision making, and the creation and reinforcement of confidence by all staff involved in the process' (p. 31).[1] With these definitions in mind, it is possible to describe the circumstances in which risk management may be undertaken.

Regardless of the environment in which a person works, there will be objects and situations that can potentially cause harm of some description. An example of this is a building site. Contained in such an environment are heavy plant and equipment, chemical substances, noxious and poisonous gases, and many different workers, employed in a variety of trades by different persons or companies. In the absence of a coordinated approach to management of the site, the potential for accidents is vast. Indeed, of all deaths that are workplace related, the construction industry accounts for the vast majority. In the UK in the year 2001 there were 290 workplace deaths recorded: 160 occurred on construction sites.[2]

The environment of an operating theatre can be compared to a construction site in many respects. There is heavy plant, complex and fragile equipment, and many dangerous elements, such as potentially noxious gases, fragile chemical compounds, blood and blood-related products, drugs and other complex liquids. This situation is compounded by many different workers operating in a variety of professional roles, employed by different employers, managers and agencies.

It is therefore necessary to establish laws, rules, procedures, methods and routines whereby an operating theatre, like a building site or any other workplace, can operate such as to ensure the health and safety of all persons who enter and/or are affected by such an environment.

The purpose of this chapter is to identify the laws and other measures needed to establish an effective and appropriate environment to manage risk. By listing all the various routes by which risk management can be undertaken, it is hoped that perioperative practitioners will be able to apply these to their practice, facilitating their producing a safe and healthy environment for themselves, their patients and their colleagues.

LEGAL FRAMEWORK

In the UK the law originates from two sources: statutes, the highest form of law, are made and passed by Parliament; and common law, which works to assist and complement statutory provisions by such devices as precedents and case law.

However, there is a further tier to UK law: that which originates from the European Community, called 'European legislation'. Such laws are incorporated into our legislation and have overarching authority.

In the field of health and safety it is to European legislation that we must first look to understand the laws that bind our behaviour. In 1992, Europe produced several Directives which, when combined with other existing legislation, were designed to cover all aspects of work-related safety. Each Directive was incorporated into UK law by way of a Regulation. Thus, for example, the Framework Directive 89/391 was implemented by the 'Management of Health

and Safety at Work Regulations' 1992.[3] This legislation complements the UK Statutes. The Health and Safety at Work Act 1974 and the European legislation have been interpreted by certain leading cases that have defined and refined how certain provisions are to be implemented.

The fact that we need legislation makes sense if we consider that situations cannot be managed unless those involved have not first understood the rules and the issues involved. We must assess all risks in order to manage the perioperative environment in order to prevent a harm occurring, but we must first understand the nature of our environment or situation, in order to be able to assess the risk factors accurately.

It is important to note at this point that the law relating to risk management is not exclusively directed towards an employer or managing agency. All persons who work in a particular arena are in some way responsible for health and safety. Indeed, the Health and Safety at Work Act 1974 makes this very clear in sections 2 (1) and 7 (2). These sections provide that:

- S 2 (1) … It shall be the duty of every employer to ensure, so far as is reasonably practicable, the health, safety and welfare of all his employees
- S 7 (2) … It is the duty of every employee while at work: (a) to take reasonable care for the health and safety of himself and of other persons who may be affected by his acts or omissions at work.[4]

This exposition has been incorporated into the Code of Professional Conduct produced by the new Nursing and Midwifery Council. Paragraph 8.1 states that: 'You must work with other members of the team to promote healthcare environments that are conducive to safe, therapeutic and ethical practice'.[5] The law leaves it open to the individual company or organization to decide exactly how they will implement the guiding legislation, within certain parameters, although sometimes there are direct rules. For example, the way in which certain substances are stored and handled must comply with the rules that are to be found in the Control of Substances Hazardous to Health Regulations 1992. Noise is controlled by the Noise at Work Regulations 1989.[6]

CLINICAL GOVERNANCE

In order to understand the ways in which health and safety rules have been implemented in the National

Health Service it is useful to first examine the wider principles collectively contained under the umbrella of clinical governance. Clinical governance is the term used to describe the system whereby all areas of health care are objectively assessed to determine where there is a risk to the welfare of patients and staff and others who may be affected in some way, for example visitors to the hospital site. As defined by the RCN, 'Clinical governance is a framework which helps all clinicians – including nurses – to continuously improve quality and safeguard standards of care ... [it] is an umbrella term for all the things that help to maintain and improve high standards of patient care. Clinical governance is not a "thing" – instead it is a framework designed to help doctors to improve clinical standards in the NHS'.[7]

This term denotes a broad response to the issues of health and wellbeing. It is not designed merely to concentrate on physical risks, for example trolleys with malfunctioning wheels or sides, or theatre equipment that is faulty. The remit of clinical governance is that every area and aspect of work is assessed to accurately inform the users of the system where potential problems may occur, in order that those risks can be effectively managed.

There are many mechanisms imported by clinical governance into the health and safety arena so that 'best practice' in a given situation can be undertaken by an informed staff, for example clinical audit, research, evidence-based practice, clinical effectiveness, the evaluation of work environments and the production of guidelines, and the dissemination of knowledge to all who are concerned. So it is with clinical risk management, where 'adverse events [are] detected, openly investigated, and lessons [are] learned'.[8]

RISK ASSESSMENT

Contained within the legislation, one defining statute laid out the rules relating to risk management and risk assessment. Section 3 of the Management of Health and Safety at Work Regulations 1992 lays down the rules for employers as follows:

- S3 (1) Every employer shall make a suitable and sufficient assessment of:
  - (a) the risks to the health and safety of his employees to which they are exposed while they are at work; and
  - (b) the risks to the health and safety of persons not in his employment arising out of or in connection with the conduct by him of his undertaking, for the purpose of identifying the measures he needs to take to comply with the requirements and prohibitions imposed upon him by or under the relevant statutory provisions.[3]

The requirement under S3 is often termed the 'general requirement'. Other regulations contain risk assessment requirements that are more specific. For example, regulation 4(1)(b)(I) of the Manual Handling Operations Regulations 1992[9] imposes three separate obligations on an employer, each of which have to be complied with. First, a suitable and sufficient assessment of all ... manual handling operations has to be undertaken. Second, appropriate steps have to be undertaken to reduce the risk of injury; and third, appropriate steps have to be undertaken to provide general indications, and where reasonably practicable, precise information on risks associated with lifting.

This regulation was the subject of Swain v Denso Marton Ltd (2000)[10] where a man who was an experienced operator lifted a solid metal roller, thinking it was hollow. In the event the roller weighed 20 kg, and the operator's hand was crushed when he could not manage the weight. The court found that there had not been a risk assessment, and considered the ways in which such an assessment could have prevented the injury.

In a healthcare setting the issue of risk assessment has become coupled with, and complementary to, the dimensions of clinical governance. This is important, because the issue of risk assessment is not confined to the employer alone. The progression is as follows: under the principles of clinical governance we are all responsible for the safety and wellbeing of all those affected by our actions.

This approach adopts similar principles to those aired in the case of Sullivan v HWF Ltd (2001).[11] Here, Mr Sullivan (S) fell and suffered a personal injury after kneeling down and tripping on a bolt that had been left on a factory floor. There had been risk assessments made, and specifically, one warned of the risk of leaving bolts lying around. S sued his employer, who counterargued that S was responsible for the implementation of the risk assessment procedures, and therefore responsible for any breaches of the legislation. However, the court found that although S had a responsibility for implementing the procedures he could not be responsible for supervision all day every day. There was a duty on all of the staff to take care of their own safety and that of fellow employees. Interestingly, S was found to be contributorily negligent in that he did not see the bolt on the floor before he knelt down – he had to some extent been responsible for the harm he had suffered.

The risk assessment envisaged by the court must have included all employees checking their own environment and practice before undertaking their tasks. This is not to imply undertaking a formal assessment such as an employer must do, but simply checking one's workplace for potential problems prior to undertaking tasks. Checking the equipment in an operating theatre to ensure it is fully functioning, checking all drugs, checking consent forms, checking staff numbers and skill mixes – these are examples of risk assessments that staff or employees can undertake as routine.

Practitioners must ensure safety at all times. This is achieved by acquiring an understanding of our environment and practice by means of training, research, audit and evaluation. However, an assessment of the risks contained within our environment of work must then be undertaken. As employees, we must report our findings and concerns to managers so that action can be taken to avoid or prevent the potential harm in question. This, however, remains in the theoretical plane if there are no or insufficient procedures in place for the carrying out of a risk assessment and a reporting system designed to convey the findings of the assessment to the appropriate persons or departments.

PROCEDURES

What procedures are necessary for a risk assessment to be effective and to enable the necessary actions to be implemented? The answer would seem to rely once more on the individual employer/organization. In health care, where one turns to the principles of clinical governance one can see that individual organizations, or Trusts/Primary Care Providers (PCPs), are charged with the corporate responsibility of providing the means by which effective risk assessment and management can take place.

It is within the Trust/PCP protocols and guidelines that such issues may be resolved. There are many examples: all Trusts/PCPs will have guidelines as to the safe and effective disposal of clinical waste, the standards of hygiene and infection control required by all staff, the methods for the safe dispensing of drugs and other supplies, and fire management and exit accessibility. However, certain

principles emerge that can inform us of how the legislation and the principles of clinical governance can be applied by us as individuals charged with the duty to assess and manage risk(s).

APPLICATIONS FOR PRACTICE

Employees within the Trust/PCP structure, and others, cannot be expected to know every detail of how the Trust is operating. For example, perioperative practitioners cannot be expected to know the detailed technical workings of all the theatre equipment to such an extent that they could assess it for potential malfunctions. However, practitioners are expected to assess and manage risks in their own individual area, and manage performance within that area in order to reduce the risk of harm. Practitioners must also be sufficiently knowledgeable about current practice and procedure that they are always competent to undertake all the duties that are required. For nurses, this is laid out in the new Code of Professional Conduct[5] in paragraphs 6.1, 6.2 and 6.3, which state that registered nurses must:

- Para 6.1. Keep knowledge and skills up to date
- Para 6.2. Possess the knowledge, skills and abilities required for lawful, safe and effective practice.

Paragraph 6.3 goes on to say that if an aspect of practice is beyond the practitioner's level of competence, then help and supervision must be obtained until the practitioner and the employer consider that he or she has acquired the requisite knowledge and skill (p. 8).

Practitioners must know and understand current legislation regarding all aspects of their work in order to comply with the rules in the Code of Conduct, and that includes issues of health and safety. Practitioners must know the Trust/PCP protocols and guidelines as they affect the running of the operating department, and they must know how to operate all the equipment and medical devices safely. This includes areas such as drugs, their dosages, effects, side effects and storage; other gases, their storage, dosage and route of administration; fire risks/hazards; diathermy; other electrical equipment; and chemical substances. Risks cannot be effectively managed if these areas of practice are not understood, and risk assessments cannot be effectively undertaken.

This is important, as risk assessments must be capable of applying to specific areas of practice.

In R v Cardiff Transport Services (2001)[12] two bus drivers pulled alongside each other in the garage. One driver got out and ran in front of his bus and the other bus, which did not stop in time. The driver sustained fatal head injuries and the Health and Safety Executive prosecuted the company. The Court found that although there had been risk assessments, there had not been one relating to vehicle and staff movements. Such an assessment would have identified three failings within the company and highlighted its unsafe practice.

Practitioners must also know the effects of other members of staff and their contributions to the running of the theatre, for example how the medical, nursing and other theatre personnel interact in respect of their duties, responsibilities and knowledge bases. As all staff are responsible for their own practices, so those practices may affect others.

Harm to staff is a real potential where unsafe practices are allowed to continue, in particular where there are no effective procedures in place for managing risks. In Fashade v North Middlesex Hospital NHS Trust (2000)[13] a theatre sister mixed glutaraldehyde in a plastic bowl. This was left in the room all the time, and the liquid was disposed of into a sink every 7 days. Over time, Ms Fashade complained of eye irritation, nasal irritation, watery eyes, a cough, a tight chest and wheezing.

Six years later during an examination by occupational health, her lung function was found to be decreased. She was off work sick, and when she returned it was to an area where there was no glutaraldehyde, but the damage had been done. By now she was so sensitive to any irritant that she only worked for 3 weeks. An on-site inspection by a health and safety consultant found other irritants. Ms Fashade was retired on grounds of ill health and, now 52 years old, she has a 30–40% disability, with a chance of progressing to an 80% disability needing nursing care. She was awarded £225 000 in damages. A full and effective risk assessment would have revealed the harm being caused to Ms Fashade before such serious problems were allowed to accrue.

In Wells v West Hertfordshire Health Authority (2000)[14] Mrs Wells was a midwife. She had a long history of back complaints and a prolapsed disc. She was sent to work in the delivery suite, and complained to her manager because of the heavy lifting. Her employer did not carry out a risk assessment or send her to occupational health, despite her saying she was injured. She worked on and her condition worsened. The Manual Handling Operations Regulations applied and the Health Authority had failed to carry out an assessment of her individual capabilities, in accordance with Regulation 4(1).

We must also know how what we do affects our patients and other people who might be in the theatre, for example parents of children, family members and observers – maybe medical and nursing students or visiting staff. Most often, people not employed by the Trust would be Agency staff. They are as entitled to protection from harm as staff employed directly, and the Trust would be liable for any harm caused.

Two cases illustrate this.[15] In HSE v Port of Ramsgate and others (1997) a high-level walkway collapsed, killing six people and injuring seven others. The Port Authority was charged under S3 of the Health and Safety at Work Act 1974, which states that employers must conduct operations(s) in such a way as to avoid exposing persons not in their employment to risks to health and safety. They were found liable even though they did not have the technical skill/knowledge to know of the fault in the design.

Likewise, in R v Associated Octel Ltd (1994) an employee of an independent contractor was using acetone when cleaning inside a tank. A light bulb on the contractor's flexible lead broke, causing the acetone vapour to ignite, which in turn caused an explosion. The operative was badly burned as a result of the incident. The House of Lords said that this constituted part of the conduct and undertaking of the employer of the operation, albeit that the worker was not in their employment.

The methods by which material is collected and collated must include training, evaluation, research, assessment and audit. Only by assessing the entire relevant material can practitioners achieve the standards set out in the terms of clinical governance, and thus comply with the laws relating to risk management and assessment under the health and safety regulations.

These are the methods by which practitioners can improve their own performance. There are other formal methods that are employed by Trusts and other health service providers.

OPERATING DEPARTMENT AUDIT TOOLS

As stated, risk management and assessment are elements of clinical governance. As the method chosen to manage care within the health service, it is vital that information is received to monitor outcomes, both of clinical management and of changes invoked by that management.

The methodology by which information is collected and collated is called audit. An audit is performed to establish what an actual situation or set of situations has produced. It is slightly different from research – one is not trying to identify some new trend: rather, one is trying to establish what one has got in order to determine whether or not research into that situation is needed, or at least to inform any proposed research.

How then can an audit best be undertaken? What tools are necessary, and what are the risks? An audit can be undertaken at a particular time – say every 12 months – or it can be an ongoing affair with the data obtained being divided into identified groups. These groups can represent time changes, size, or subject areas. For example, a group may want to establish how long each operating list is taking. This may involve logging each surgical procedure, which over time would reveal the size, nature and duration of each procedure. This information could be used to inform staff levels, skill mixes, medical practitioners, and monies needed to run a competent service. It would not, however, tell you how each diathermy machine had functioned during any given operation. Nor would it tell you how the staff member operating the machine coped during the procedure, nor how many problems – if any – occurred during any particular procedure.

Each audit has to fit the question to be answered, and in this respect audit is like research: the question and the methodology used must be capable of answering the problem addressed. Regardless of this, however, what is crucial to any audit is accurate reporting. Where incorrect reporting occurs the results will be at best meaningless, and often misleading. This could have a serious detrimental effect on patient care.

For some people, the notion of reporting conjures up an image of someone not directly involved with the process under investigation taking measurements and producing their own private report. This is not so. Reporting an event or events first involves record keeping. All health service personnel must keep records of their clients, and each area will have its own requirements as to the particulars involved in their patient care. All practitioners, including nurses, are under a duty to keep good, competent and full records of patient care, which for nurses is stated in the Code of Professional Conduct at paragraph 4.4 (p. 6).[5]

However, in addition to the case summaries and care plans, records are kept of other features of care. For example, records must be kept of all drugs issued to a theatre, and the names, times and other particulars of the person who received the drugs must also be recorded.

Records of day-to-day events that occur in an operating department may assist risk management and assessments by providing an accurate picture of trends as well as documenting the particulars of any individual event. The example of a malfunctioning diathermy machine provides us with a picture of how this may be achieved. Only if records were kept of all of the times when the machine malfunctioned would an audit of the problem be possible. Each record of a malfunction serves to assist in identifying the particular malfunction, and the number of events assist in identifying the scale of the problem.

As is to be expected, it is individual staff members, who are always present when events occur in the operating theatre, who are best placed to make and record the appropriate information. Therefore, systems for such reporting must be in place. An audit will not work if no records are kept, but nor will it work if reports are kept but scattered so that no comprehensive list can be achieved, or are stored away and not given to the appropriate people so that they can begin their assessments.

Lists of things can be kept in an open way and place so that access is easy for all concerned. Such lists will vary according to what is required. For example, there will be lists of machines, their manufacture numbers and their use-by dates if appropriate. It is also important to keep a list of all checks made on the machines: who made them, what they found, and what they did about it. Lists are kept of other tools, for example theatre sets for a particular operation. There will also be needed a list of how the tools are: are they broken, or malfunctioning? Again, the staff who noticed any problem must record the date on which they noticed, their identity, and the action they took to remedy the situation.

Drugs are often used in an operating department in such a way that a dose given to an individual patient will not accurately reflect the amount of that drug drawn up. Some items are drawn up in batches, or at least in large quantities. In order to accurately reflect how much was given to each person, when and by whom, records must be kept to determine not only rates and patterns of usage, but also to identify which drug was used at which time.

This is important because often items, and drugs in particular, are used in vast quantities in a speedy manner. Emergencies are common in operating departments, and so recording the time of delivery of care is essential. It is easy in such circumstances for errors to occur – the wrong drug being given because two drugs were drawn up, left side by side and not properly labelled, for example. Risk management dictates that in order to avoid such a detrimental outcome, proper records should be made and an appropriate risk assessment undertaken before such a practice was allowed to occur.

This would involve communication between all staff who might undertake giving drugs in such situations. It would also involve full and frank disclosure of all adverse incidents, as adverse outcomes to the patient may not be apparent from a set of lists noting the usage rate of a particular drug alone, and therefore the problem may continue unabated, causing serious harm. It is an example that lends itself to the issue of risk management: it is a risk that is well known. It is a risk that has long been identified. However, it is a problem that continues to occur in many places nationwide. It is therefore a good example of how there is still scope for new and innovative systems of risk management to be implemented.

CLINICAL INCIDENT REPORTING

The principles that underlie clinical risk reporting are those contained within the framework of clinical governance. The principle is also outlined in paragraph 8.3 of the NMC's Code of Conduct, which states: 'Where you cannot remedy circumstances in the environment of care that could jeopardise standards of practice, you must report them to a senior nurse with sufficient authority to manage them … This must be supported by a written record' (p. 9).[5]

Where an incident has occurred, a report on the events in question allows for an evaluation and analysis of those events. It is this process that then feeds into the possibility of audit, research and risk assessment. The audit stage comprises an examination of events and a review of how many other events of a similar nature have occurred. It highlights and records the events into an objective format.

The research stage allows for a wider examination of similar events, in the same and other institutions. It also allows for recognition of whether or not many other events of a similar nature have occurred. If one finds that the event in question is a common

occurrence, remedial steps can be taken. Should it transpire that the event is uncommon or even unique, its components can be recorded and the information disseminated to other institutions, so that they in turn can access the information for the management of their institution.

Only when these two stages have been completed can an accurate assessment of the risks involved be undertaken. As stated earlier, there is a duty to undertake a risk assessment, but one undertaken in the absence of all relevant and up-to-date information will necessarily be flawed.

This being so, it is vital that all of the information surrounding the original event is accurately conveyed to the clinical incident report. In all actual events there is a multitude of factors and variables. It is only by having all of the data factually conveyed that one can hope to decipher trends, as well as similarities to and differences from other events.

Practitioners often feel threatened by the idea of producing a clinical incident report, but it is imperative that they are completed. An example might reveal why. For example, during a surgical procedure a person is badly burned during the use of diathermy. The practitioners ring the company that makes the machine, but do nothing else. This event occurs three times during a 2-month period. All of the practitioners take the same course of action, but each time it occurs there is a different set of practitioners on duty. No-one informs the clinical manager. No-one informs their colleagues during a handover report. No-one checks with the company to see if they have visited the department to examine the diathermy machine.

It is easy to see that a breakdown of communication has occurred, but how could a clinical incident report have avoided the difficulties? Well, a report into the first incident, passed on to the manager concerned and the risk management team, would have alerted them to the incident. Action could have been taken at that point. A second report would have alerted them to two facts: first, that the machine in question had not been repaired, and second that there was an ongoing risk to all persons who might have to have diathermy treatment. All practitioners could have been alerted, and the machine taken out of service.

By the time that the harm occurred to the patient, certain assertions could be made:

1. The risk assessment had failed in that the offending machine had not been removed to a place where it could no longer cause harm

2. The system of communications operating within the particular theatre was ineffective and possibly dangerous
3. The Trust/PCP was in breach of its duty under the legislation
4. The health and safety system of reporting to, and working with, manufacturers of theatre plant was defective
5. The person to whom the harm was caused would have good grounds for a complaint and possible legal action for negligence and damages.

Producing a clinical incident report is the first in a chain of actions necessary to achieve safe and effective management of risk. People often think that their report is inconsequential and isolated, and that no change will result from it. This is not so. It is the first response to the event, and a vital one. The personnel in the risk management team cannot be in all places at once. They rely on the 'little reports' to detect trends, so that they can take appropriate action and disseminate the information to those agencies that need it.

Another fallacy is to think that only physical problems need a clinical incident report. This is not so. Bullying in the workplace causing psychological harm is something that can have a devastating consequence on staff morale and competence. This can lead to clinical errors that no-one would suspect as being the result of bullying, but a set of comprehensive clinical incident reports would highlight trends and personnel, and tie the bullying events to any subsequent events causing harm to patients, as well as the original harm to the staff member.

Staffing levels are often highlighted as being a factor in causation where a clinical event occurs. It is much easier to substantiate a claim of understaffing where a record has been kept via the clinical incident reporting system, to tie staff numbers to a particular time when an event occurred. Likewise, staff skill mix, the communication procedures between the various groups of workers in the theatre, and, within the skill mix question, a record of competencies of the staff in any one event can be ascertained and evaluated.

It is therefore vital that the rationale behind clinical incident reporting is understood. It is equally vital that those personnel at the event record all the facts, and then process the documentation to the risk management team. It is vital that a risk assessment of the features leading to the event is undertaken, and that the results are implemented to bring

about change and prevent a recurrence. Lastly, it is vital that information is relayed to as wide an audience as is possible so that other institutions can undertake an informed risk assessment before that particular untoward event occurs in their workplace.

REDUCING SURGICAL RISK

Allied to what has been said above is the issue of reducing a surgical risk. Matters have been considered in a theoretical and wide format, in order that all situations may be envisaged. However, for the purposes of this chapter the investigation of a surgical risk can be more focused. This is because care of the patient undergoing surgery in the operating department is a defined area. All areas of the surgical procedure and the accompanying risk assessments can begin to be implemented from the time that surgery is envisaged, until such times as the anaesthetic is reversed and the patient returned to the ward.

The issue of consent is covered separately below. However, other issues begin from the first time someone comes to the hospital. Staff competency, the physical area where the person will be seen, the type and number of preoperative tests that need to be undertaken, the effectiveness and accuracy of all the communications needed at all stages to ensure that no risks are missed, are all examples.

During the perioperative period itself, such aspects as the physical state of the theatre (clean floors, clean air ducts and vents) must be assessed. The equipment, the accompanying tubes and filters, and the electrical inputs to them must be assessed. All drug therapies and routes of administration, other items of therapy, such as diathermy, swabs, gloves, suture packs and all sterile equipment, must be checked. Fluids, blood and blood products, and all fluid loss must be checked. This list is not designed to be exhaustive: rather it is designed to identify areas where there are risks to the patient and to the staff.

At any stage things can go wrong. There is a duty of care on all practitioners to ensure that they act in a manner that meets the appropriate standard of care. However, if the standard to be met is not appreciated and understood the principle exists in a vacuum. Practitioners acquire an understanding of the correct standard of care through having an informed knowledge of how to operate safely and correctly all of the equipment under their command, and by having an informed knowledge of all procedures and safety requirements. This is all in addition to having an informed knowledge of the needs of the patient, which itself requires a knowledge of the underlying aetiology of their disease or healthcare problems.

Only by observing the above and knowing and understanding the full ramifications of the operating theatre process can practitioners begin to understand how to reduce a surgical risk. Risk assessment and risk management are vital components of safe operating theatre procedure. Without them, practitioners are necessarily sometimes going to be working in a way that incorporates old and/or defective methodology – or worse, no methodology at all. Either way, the risks inherent in a defective system are many and very real.

The health and safety legislation covers all eventualities. The environment of the operating theatre is not a merely practical affair: it includes all aspects of care, because where staff practices are poor or ill informed the consequences can include physical harm being caused. Practitioners who do not understand how to operate a diathermy machine because they did not inform themselves of the correct procedures relating to its use can cause harm to a patient by burning, because the machine, incorrectly used, causes that harm. Therefore, risk assessment of the safe use of a diathermy machine must include an assessment of the competence of the staff who will use that machine.

CONSENT IN RISK MANAGEMENT

Risk management is concerned to avoid harm being caused to a patient, staff member or other person who may be adversely affected by events occurring while they are in a particular place/situation. Although most people would associate risk with health and safety issues, it must not be forgotten that harm is necessarily caused to someone where they have not consented to the procedure being contemplated. Where a person suffers a harm caused in part by their own behaviour, the issue is one of contributory negligence. Therefore, it is important to realize that even where someone has signed a consent form for a surgical procedure they have not consented to being harmed by that procedure.

All surgical procedures involve touching, and often invading a person's bodily integrity. In order to protect against a charge of assault, or even battery, the person who would touch/enter a person's body must first obtain their consent. Section 3 of the NMC's Code of Conduct deals in depth with issues of consent.[5] Chapters 1 and 6 of this book also discuss various aspects of consent.

The consent must be valid and therefore must be informed. In order to achieve the level of informed consent necessary, information must be imparted to the person undergoing the procedure in such a way as to allow them to make an informed choice as to whether or not to undergo the procedure.

The risks of incorrectly obtaining consent to a surgical procedure are many. First, the person who would have the procedure performed on them would have a case for suing the practitioner: the practitioner faces the threat of legal action against them.

Second, it is in the process of obtaining consent that conversations as to the nature of the proposed surgical procedure take place. This is often when the patient can ask questions about the process. This means that the practitioner can reflect and check that all elements of the proposed surgical procedure are correct in all particulars. It is not just an issue of defining the correct limb to be operated on: it is more a case of checking that the patient has indeed correctly understood the nature of the proposed procedure, and the inherent risks involved.

Risk management in this particular case must involve an assessment of the risks to the patient – the risks of their not knowing or understanding the nature of the process, and of their not understanding its risks. Most Trusts/PCPs (where surgery is performed) will produce a form or forms designed to incorporate a checklist of the practical considerations associated with various procedures.

Example of information which these forms record include:

- Identifying the correct limb, area of body or organ that will be the recipient of the surgical procedure
- Obtaining a history of all other illnesses and former surgical procedures, and associated healthcare problems
- Obtaining a list of preoperative tests and the results of those tests.

All of these considerations can be listed to allow the practitioner to ensure that they have been identified and recorded as accurate. In a way, these documents are themselves risk assessment forms: what is being obtained is a checklist of what has to happen or be achieved prior to a surgical procedure, to ensure that the procedure is entered into in a safe manner.

However, a checklist that fails to include a record of the patient's understanding of the procedure, of whether or not they have in fact consented to that procedure, will be rendered ineffective. Therefore, an effective risk assessment must identify the nature of the risk and the methods employed to avoid it. In this case this has to mean a record of how information was imparted to the patient, what information was imparted, by whom, and when. In addition, a record must be kept of how the patient was able to inform the doctor or nurse that they had understood the information and was therefore able to give real consent. This must include the patient's being able to reflect on the information given, such as to be able to choose their response to what was proposed.

CONCLUSION

This chapter has sought to identify some central principles of effective risk assessment and management. The legal sources of the rules relating to risk assessment and management have been identified and explored, as well as the more detailed responses and methodologies employed within the health service. Some examples have been provided to reveal how a risk assessment can be achieved, and the principles of such an assessment and the reasons for it have been contextualized to the realities of the operating theatre situation.

However, the main theme throughout has been to emphasize the reasons why risk management and hence risk assessments are so vital. The role of a risk assessment in effective management has been emphasized, not merely to underline the importance in a legal sense – of complying with the relevant legislation – but to try and impart a firm belief in the validity and power of the assessment of risk.

No practitioner can possibly hope to operate in an arena where no risks ever occur. However, risk management dictates that we all act in such a way as to minimize the risks that will occur, with actions designed to make the operating theatre a safer place for all. These actions are simple, personal and effective if pursued in all areas of personal professional practice. They are: training and reflection, audit and research, assessment and reporting, evaluation and action to alter that which needs altering, and improving areas that represent a potential to cause harm to all who may be affected.

The essential principle of risk assessment is that by undertaking it at the point where there is still a risk of harm, and by acting on its recommendations, one can prevent the harm actually occurring. By acting in such a way at the optimum time, much harm and hurt can be avoided, producing a safe and healthy workplace for all who visit it in whatever capacity.

References

1. Capper P. An overview of risk in construction. In: Uff J, ed. Risk, management and procurement in construction. Centre for Construction Law and Management. London: King's College; 1995: 28.
2. Health and Safety Executive. Health and safety inspectors blitz construction sites across London. HSE Press Release E071: 02. Caerphilly CF83 3CG: HSE Information Services Caerphilly Park; 22nd April 2002.
3. HMSO. Management of health and safety at work regulations 1992 SI 1992/2051 directive – 89/391/EEC. London: HMSO; 1992.
4. Health and Safety at Work Act 1974. London: HMSO.
5. Nursing and Midwifery Council. Code of professional conduct. London: NMC; 2002.
6. Noise at Work Regulations 1989 SI 1989/1790 Directive 86/188/EEC. In: Hendry J, Ford M, eds. Redgrave's health and safety, 3rd edn. London: Butterworths; 1998: 1112.
7. Royal College of Nursing. Guidance for nurses on clinical governance. London: RCN; 1998: 3.
8. Wilson J. Clinical governance. Br J Nurs 1998; 7: 988.
9. Manual Handling Operations Regulations 1992 SI 1992/2793 Directive 90/269/EEC. London: HMSO; 1992.
10. Swain v Denso Marston Ltd 2000 ICR 1079.
11. Sullivan v HWF Ltd 2001 unreported.
12. R v Cardiff City Transport Services Criminal Division 2001 1 Cr App R 41.
13. Fashade v North Middlesex Hospital NHS Trust 2000 unreported.
14. Wells v West Hertfordshire Health Authority QBD 5/4/2000.
15. Akkass R. Tolley's risk assessment handbook. Croydon: Tolley; 1999.

Further reading

Bennett D. Doctors and nurses: asthma and dermatitis caused by latex. J Personal Injury Law 2001; 2/01: 117.

Dimond B. Contractural responsibilities of both the employer and employee. Br J Nurs 2002; 11: 451.

Dimond B. Statuary provisions of the Health and Safety at Work Act 1974. Br J Nurs 2002; 11: 396.

Edwards P. Corporate killing. Healthcare and Law Digest 2001; 165.

Hendry J, Ford M. Redgrave's health and safety, 3rd edn. London: Butterworths; 1998.

Hendry J, Ford M. Redgrave's cumulative supplement. London: Butterworths; 2001.

Latham M. Questions of life and death. Building Magazine; 18 Jan 2002.

McFarlane G. Clinical negligence – risk management and reporting. J Personal Injury Law 2001; 2/01: 164.

Wheeler J. Doctors and nurses: asthma caused by glutaraldehyde exposure. J Personal Injury Law 2001; 2/02: 124.

Regulations

HMSO Provision and Use of Work Equipment Regulations 1992 SI 1992/2932 Directive 89/6551/EEC (amended by Directive 95/63/EC). In: Hendry J, Ford M. Redgrave's health and safety, 3rd edn. London: Butterworths; 1998: 514.

HMSO Personal Protective Equipment at Work Regulations 1992 SI 1989/656/EEC. London: HMSO; 1992.

HMSO Health and Safety (Display Screen Equipment) 1992 SI 1992/2792 Directive 90/270/EEC. In: Hendry J, Ford M. Redgrave's health and safety, 3rd edn. London: Butterworths; 1998: 721.

HMSO COSHHR 1992 and 1994 SI 1992 (now see SI 1996/3138 and 1994/3246) Directive 89/391/EEC. In: Hendry J, Ford M. Redgrave's health and safety, 3rd edn. London: Butterworths; 1998: 846.

Chapter 4

Leadership and teamwork

Lois Hamlin

Key points

- Leadership, management, power, teams and multidisciplinary teams
- Communication, bullying, harassment and horizontal violence

LEADERSHIP

Leadership theories are presented briefly and one, transformational leadership, is used as the suggested framework for managing the team in the operating department (OD). The key to any efficient operating department is an effectively led team that delivers high-quality, timely care to the desired standard and within the resources available; hence the importance of exploring leadership within the operating department. Leaders are not confined to those in formal management positions or authority figures: leaders can and do emerge at all levels in an organization or department, and the effective operating department manager will acknowledge and utilize such valuable assets. However, operating department managers have a highly complex, evolving department to manage and a range of professional and non-professional personnel and activities to orchestrate. Consequently, they need to be effective leaders, now more than ever before. Not only can and should the operating department manager be an effective leader, the operating department itself can be a leading department within the hospital or organization. The operating department is important because of the nature of its work and the resources it consumes. This is particularly so in the independent sector, where it may be the 'engine room' of the hospital, helping deliver profitability.

LEADERSHIP THEORIES

The importance of good leadership cannot be emphasized too strongly. The presence or absence of effective leadership will have a marked effect on the overall functioning of the operating department. Leadership has been written about since the 16th century[1] and talked about since the time of Plato.[2] It is one of the most studied, but least understood, multidimensional concepts in social science. Despite the complexity of the subject, the abundance of theories about it and its confounding nature, leadership is often described simply as the ability to influence others. It is sometimes treated as an abstract concept or process,[3] and occasionally subsumed as an activity of management. There may be ethical or beneficial aspects to it, and leadership may reside within organizations as well as individuals. An example of organizational leadership is the National Association of Theatre Nurses (NATN), which leads perioperative nursing in the UK. It is important to note that leadership differs from management. Examples of leaders in the operating department who are not necessarily managers are theatre practitioners who may act as mentors or preceptors for new staff.

Very early leadership theories dwelt on the leader as hero and the great man (sic) (born to lead).[1] Gradually, following initial research in the early to mid 20th century, trait theory was developed. However, no complete or authoritative list of the physical, psychological and emotional attributes of leaders has emerged. The second significant theory espoused was the behavioural or style theory, which focused on what leaders did in relational and contextual terms. Out of this approach leadership styles such as autocratic, democratic and laissez faire were described. Following on developmentally from the behavioural approach was contingency theory. This approach emphasized that different traits and behaviours were required depending on the situation in which leaders operated. Importantly, followers as well as leaders were emphasized for the first time, and the importance of relationships to effective leaders became evident.

More recently, transformational theory (or integrative approaches) has evolved that focuses on relationships between leaders and followers. This relationship focuses on vision and values, with interactions between leaders and followers that raise each to high levels of motivation and morality.[4] This particular leadership theory has utility for perioperative practitioners, given the nature of their work and their focus on good patient care and outcomes. Additionally, it is an ethically sound approach to leadership.[5] Transformational leadership evolved in the late 20th century and the nursing profession embraced it enthusiastically. This is not surprising, given the urgent need for effective leadership in nursing[6] along with the need for a different kind of leadership.[7]

Transformational leaders display several key attributes, such as being visionary, inspirational and intellectually stimulating. They are also role models.[4] The importance of these attributes cannot be stressed too highly and they will be explored in detail. Before proceeding further, it is important to differentiate between the notions of leadership and management, and to explore the concept of power for operating department managers and their departments.

LEADERSHIP AND MANAGEMENT

Although the terms leadership and management are often used interchangeably in the literature, the two concepts are different.[8,9] It is worth distinguishing between the two, although there is often considerable overlap and controversy surrounding them. Leadership is something more than management[5] and requires more than the attributes of the latter, such as the interpersonal, informational and decisional skills that managers possess, although leaders may also have these attributes. Leadership is something that anyone can engage in, whether or not they occupy a formal management position.[5] Looking at the role of managers, their activities generally fall into four basic categories: dealing with human resource matters; communicating by gaining and disseminating information; networking; and traditional management functions such as organizing, planning, controlling, monitoring and decision making. These are considered standard management capabilities and many texts produce lists of these functions.[3,10,11]

However, despite what is idealized in management texts, Yukl's[12] review of research into the nature of management notes that managers' activities are often fragmented, unplanned and reactive in nature. Further, many managers neither make decisions nor lead.[13] This may even be unavoidable. Although many leaders undertake these management activities, and, arguably, being a good manager is an important facet of leadership,[5] nonetheless leadership requires something more. Key attributes or activities of leaders involve role modelling, being able to inspire and motivate, having and relaying a vision, and respecting and intellectually stimulating followers.[5,12,14–16] The need for both management capabilities and leadership qualities within such a dynamic area as the operating department hardly needs stating.

LEADERSHIP AND POWER

Any review of leadership must examine the concept of power. Without power influence cannot be exerted, and the essence of leadership is influence. The literature characterizes power in various ways.[1,5,12,17] A useful guide describing personal power and positional power will be used for the sake of clarity and brevity. Subcategories within personal power include charismatic (or referent) power, expert power, and power by association. Charismatic power is linked to individuals being able to influence through the behaviour they model (which others want to emulate) and the visions and ideas they project, which inspire others. This perception of power explains how individuals without formal management or leadership positions can exert influence. Expert power is the ability to influence through the possession of knowledge, expertise or judgement; it generates credibility for those who possess it and it is significant. Expertise built up over time in the role of theatre practitioner is frequently, and appropriately, an essential prerequisite for those who wish to influence and/or be operating department managers.

Power by association is somewhat more controversial[5] but is an important source of power. It involves networking and maintaining associations with key influential people and may contain elements of friendship and loyalty, and the ability to do deals.[18]

By contrast, positional power stems from an individual's rank or place within an organization.

One type of positional power is formal authority associated with a specific position. It is sometimes called legitimate power.[5,12] It is more acceptable and easier to use than other forms of power, especially if there is a perceived legitimacy of the person occupying a particular leadership/authority position. Operating department managers usually possess this because of their position. However, how they use that power is crucial. The need for a democratic approach is important. Democratic managers involve others in decision making, believe all team members want to grow and take responsibility, and encourage communication and reward effort. To abuse positional power and authority by not taking the above approach is to become autocratic and, potentially, a bully.[19,20]

Another type of positional power is reward power – the ability to control resources and rewards – and it stems in part from formal authority. However, some rewards, such as praise, recognition and cooperation, can be given by anyone in an organization, irrespective of position. Coercive power is the alternative to reward power. It is the power to withhold rewards or to administer punishments, and is generally viewed as limiting. This has been a brief overview of the concept of power, necessitated by the relationship between leaders having and using power to influence, as operating department managers have a need to be influential in many spheres.

TRANSFORMATIONAL LEADERSHIP

The appeal and suitability of transformational leadership theory for operating department managers relates to the nature of nursing and the work done by the operating department. Transformational leadership theory evolved in the 1970s and 1980s, and key authors and theorists include Burns (1978),[4] Bennis and Nanus (1985),[17] Bass (1985)[21] and Tichy and Devanna (1986).[22] In Australia, Parry (1996) has produced a text on the topic.[5] The profession of nursing appears to have embraced the idea enthusiastically.[1,9,14,15,23–27] This is not surprising, given the urgent need for effective leadership in nursing, highlighted consistently in recent times[1,3,6] along with the need for a different kind of leadership.[8,10,28–30] It should be noted that variations and highly individual interpretations are evident in much of the literature on transformational leadership, which makes it crucial to return to original sources and germinal works.

Transformational leaders display several key attributes, such as role modelling, being visionary, inspirational and intellectually stimulating. First, as role models, they do their job well and are respected. Burns[4] described transformational leadership as a process whereby 'leaders and followers raise one another to higher levels of morality and motivation' (p. 20). Transformational leaders do not use their positions for personal gain but to benefit the workforce or work centre. They display high levels of optimism and enthusiasm, and encourage creativity in their followers. They inspire them. Their followers want to emulate them, a concept that Bass and Avolio[31] call idealized influence. They believe deeply and firmly in themselves and their followers, they have a vision, and they commit to it as well as to their followers. This is very important in a dynamic area such as the operating department. The need to deliver high-level care there demands highly competent practitioners who perform consistently under all conditions, no matter how arduous or difficult. This, in turn, requires a special kind of leadership. Although much of what transformational leaders do constitutes a series of learned behaviours, a mixture of specific actions and objectives, they have something more, something intangible, inspirational, that elevates others. In short, they exhibit a mixture of rhetoric and reality. They communicate positively, and have good self-esteem and self-confidence. They have strong convictions and are often dramatic and expressive, and lead by example.

Second, they are visionary and can clearly articulate their vision and do so often. Their followers become strongly committed because the vision extends their own beliefs and aspirations. Envisioned future states are clearly presented. Importantly, transformational leaders emphasize positive outcomes and goals, and continually reinforce their message. They are genuine in their beliefs and work constantly towards achieving them. For the operating department manager, this means a strong focus on patient-centred quality care delivered to the desired standard.

Third, transformational leaders are inspirational, and by their behaviour and speech enthuse others. They also provide meaning and challenge in followers' work and lives. Fourth, they focus on and believe in their followers (individual theatre practitioners in this case) while not losing sight of the bigger picture or the end game. They know and listen to their followers, they are interested in them and

their needs and, mostly, they are relevant to them and empower them.[17] For example, operating department managers could focus on the professional development of their theatre practitioners and support them in their endeavours.

Finally, they stimulate intellectually, and commit others to their vision. This is because they get their followers to think of problems in new ways. They elicit input and ideas: they do not criticize alternative notions, or force their own solutions on their followers and the problem at hand. They move their followers to self-actualization. Thus, transformational leadership is an interactive, social and interpersonal process. It focuses on enhancing followership, and creating confidence and belief among staff, such that they put achieving the objectives of the leader and the department above self-interest. Transformational leadership is often about changing the culture of organizations, too. This is because transformational leaders recognize the need for change and are change agents.[14] The need for change, for example to address cultural issues such as bullying and harassment, is vital to their ongoing viability. Transformational leaders are also flexible and learn from experience; in fact, they are continual learners. Also, they are disciplined thinkers and careful analysts, but notwithstanding this, as visionaries they trust their own intuition.[2,4,12]

On a cautionary note, transformational leader skills are learned behaviours and some aspects, for example, articulating a vision and inspiring others, could become meaningless if modelled behaviour is different from espoused values.[1,5] Few writers dwell on the shortcomings associated with transformational leadership. However, some write persuasively to suggest that leaders need to switch between the enabling activities associated with transformational leadership and acting forcefully (that is, using the command-and-control approach of positional power) when appropriate.[14,32] This seems contradictory to the notion of empowerment, which is an important facet of the transformational leader, but does offer some insight into the potential shortcomings of this leadership theory. That is, that not all leadership activities can be achieved using only the empowering and inspirational approach associated with transformational leadership. Thus, the significance of this for operating department managers/leaders is that there is a need for flexibility in their approach while adopting a mostly transformational bent.

CONSTITUENTS OF THE TEAM

In the operating department there are various categories of staff, professional and non-professional, and from various disciplines. This includes nursing, medical, technical, ancillary or support workers, various types of health technicians and allied health professionals, such as radiographers. The complexity and highly technical nature of the work of the operating department requires a greater range, diversity and skill mix of staff than previously. The team constituents that are required are determined by:

- The size and layout of the operating department
- Its case load
- The nature and complexity of the surgery performed
- Local (and sometimes other) population demography
- Whether it is a public or private hospital
- The degree of involvement in the teaching and training of various categories of personnel.

Many of the staff in theatre, such as nursing and medical personnel, will have worked in other areas of the hospital prior to moving into the operating department. For others, this may not be the case. What is unusual about the multidisciplinary team in the operating department is that they all come together to form a very cohesive and highly focused group to complete surgical interventions.[33]

NURSING STAFF

The majority of nurses will have completed a broad-based and comprehensive programme of theory and clinical practice related to hospital and community nursing prior to registration. This may include experience in the operating department. Many operating department nurses subsequently gain further, postregistration specialty-specific qualifications. Nurses occupy various roles in the operating department, depending on the size and nature of surgery undertaken within it. Senior nurses are usually managers of the operating department, they often oversee the quality and risk management activities there, and work closely with the division of surgery and anaesthesia, bed management, infection control and sterile services departments to provide optimal patient care. In the operating department they are also responsible for ensuring that organizational policies are enacted, and that departmental policy and procedure, and orientation manuals are current,

evidence based where possible, and incorporate relevant professional nursing standards. This includes standards written by NATN.

MEDICAL STAFF

Various categories of medical staff work in the operating department. Consultant or senior surgeons and anaesthetists are normally contracted to the hospital, with the surgeon usually heading the surgical team. Depending on the size and nature of surgery undertaken in the department, other medical personnel, such as specialist registrars – that is, surgeons in training – may be found. Increasingly, and in line with other developed countries, junior doctors no longer work as part of the surgical team, or their time in the operating department is limited.[34] This has resulted, in part, in increased opportunities for an extended role for the theatre practitioner. This is addressed briefly later in this section.

TECHNICAL STAFF

A variety of technical staff are utilized during surgery. Operating department practitioners undergo a 2-year training programme with theoretical and practical experiences to gain Diploma or National Vocational Qualifications (NVQ) Level 3 in Operating Department Practice (ODP) or Operating Department Assistant (ODA). Other technical staff who may be required include perfusionists, who manage the heart-lung bypass machine during cardiac surgery, and EEG technicians, who may be utilized during complex neurosurgical interventions. Undoubtedly, other categories of personnel and roles will evolve as surgery expands and changes.

GENERAL/SUPPORT STAFF

Other categories of support staff, with a variety of titles, such as nursing auxiliaries or care assistants, also work in the operating department. Many of these complete hospital-based or NVQ programmes. Other staff are also needed in the operating department; they include an overall theatre manager, other clinical managers, clerical staff including data entry clerks, porters, and others such as those who assist with the preparation and supply of sterile goods. Together, all of these personnel form the wider perioperative team. Further details about roles and responsibilities are given elsewhere in this book.

It is important to note that roles and jobs are not static, but evolving. As well as new and developing roles for nurses and others, traditional role boundaries continue to blur. This has occurred for a number of reasons: recruitment and retention issues in nursing; reductions in junior doctors' hours; the changing scope of professional practice;[35] and, importantly, the need for a flexible workforce. These pose both threats and opportunities for perioperative practitioners. For example, the reduction in medical staff in the operating department has allowed the clinical theatre practitioner to develop the extended roles of surgeon's assistant and first assistant. For many scrub practitioners who do not wish to move into educational or managerial roles, this represents an opportunity to continue to grow and develop professionally in a clinical role. Other roles that may develop in the future include the advanced role of independent nurse practitioner, although how this will evolve is unclear. For example, many believe there is a role for perioperative nurses to conduct preoperative assessment independently of the anaesthetist, deliver anaesthesia independently, or complete minor surgical procedures such as endoscopies alone. In many places the latter already occurs.

The ongoing shortage of nurses continues; as in the past, when previous reports, such as the Bevan report, resulted in the introduction of ODPs, so the current crisis will demand alternative solutions. This has resulted in controversies such as healthcare support workers assuming the scrub role. This has been emphasized as inappropriate by most theatre practitioners[36] and NATN does not recommend such practices. However, on legal grounds the role is not the exclusive preserve of nurses or ODPs, and so the issue remains unresolved. Fundamentally, the role of the nurse in the operating department continues to be debated. Whatever their role, it is imperative that all theatre practitioners are competent to perform it. Competence is defined as having the knowledge, skills, values, beliefs and attitudes necessary to perform the activities to the standard expected in employment.

AGENCY AND BANK STAFF

Increasingly, there is a need for operating departments to rely on non-permanent staff to accomplish their activities. Decreasing numbers entering the nursing profession and nurses making lifestyle choices have resulted in fewer theatre practitioners being available or choosing to work permanently in an individual operating department. Consequently, operating departments have to rely on other ways of ensuring they have enough staff, particularly during peak periods. Using agency staff is one solution, but they are expensive and not always available. Some agencies offer only specialist staff, such as theatre practitioners (RGNs, ODPs or ODAs). An alternative approach is for hospitals, or even individual operating departments, to establish their own bank of casual staff. Using bank staff is advantageous as they know the hospital or department, and the costs associated with their use are less than those associated with external agency staff. Whichever method is chosen, the current chronic shortage of theatre practitioners is not going to be resolved overnight. Operating department managers therefore need to take an open-minded approach to staffing issues and be as flexible as possible.

A long-term approach that innovative leader/managers in the operating department can take is to 'grow' their own staff. The aim here is to encourage all, whether undergraduate student or graduate nurse, to come and work in the operating department (or to complete a clinical practicum, if a student).[37] Once there they need to be welcomed into the team, offered appropriate education and support, and given the opportunity to experience work excitement.[38] Predictors of work excitement, such as variety, good working conditions and arrangements, change and opportunities for growth and professional development, can be created by perceptive managers who display the traits associated with transformational leadership. Other innovative ways of raising the profile of the operating department is to plan open days and organize tours for the public. Obviously, these take place when surgery is NOT underway! Other activities to consider include setting up a stand in the hospital lobby, which presents an opportunity to expose the work of the department to the rest of the hospital; do the same in the local shopping centre; or even go on local radio or TV. The value of marketing the operating department should not be underestimated in terms of its impact on subsequent recruitment and staff retention.

THE MULTIDISCIPLINARY TEAM IN THE OPERATING DEPARTMENT

As can be seen from such a diverse and disparate group of professional and non-professional staff, creating effective and cohesive teams to achieve the necessary tasks, namely safe and timely surgical interventions for patients, is challenging. In developed countries there is an increasing shift to use teams, as they represent a better way of utilizing individual skills. Further, there is a move away from directive, hierarchical leadership structures to more participative arrangements with equality among group members, irrespective of role, as a result of changing social values.[39] This is an important consideration. A team can be defined as a group of people with complementary skills who work together to achieve a common purpose, for which they hold themselves collectively accountable.[40] Not all groups of workers are teams. The latter are differentiated by:

- Having a shared goal or reason to work together
- Being interdependent, that is, they need each other's experience, ability and commitment in order to achieve mutual goals
- Being committed to working together
- Being accountable.[41]

As Peter Senge[42] noted, 'show me a team and I'll show you blood sweat and tears'. This is particularly pertinent to the team in the operating department! There are many descriptions of teams and how they are configured, and which describe general patterns of behaviour and stages of development. Earlier theories described team development as forming, storming, norming, performing and mourning (or adjourning).[43] More recent ideas note that teams do not necessarily move in a neat progression through all stages.[39] Development may instead be described as a process of increasing complexity and increasing integration. Each level of development is described by a particular self-identity, moral framework, type of need and cognitive ability.[44] This may be a more useful framework for operating department managers when considering the concept of teams. Nonetheless, teams need to go through various phases as they develop. When creating teams it is important for the manager to begin with the end in mind,[45] to note that teams consistently outperform individuals or random groups, and that an effective team is always worth more than the sum of its parts owing to the synergy it creates.

However, it is acknowledged that not all team members are in a particular team by choice, though this is what all operating department leaders should aim to create. The work of the operating department cannot be accomplished without all members of the team from a number of disciplines working together cooperatively to care for the patient. For this to occur, mutual understanding and an agreed frame of reference are important. Managing teams, particularly those that contain professionals who consider themselves independent and autonomous, requires special leadership skills of the manager. For example, being able to influence rather than resorting to coercion is an important attribute. Involving all members of the team in major strategic and operational decisions, valuing their input, and empowering them to act are also part of the process. It is trite but true that change is the only constant today. As departments – and indeed hospitals and other health services – are reformed and reordered within the wider changes and upheavals in the healthcare sector, so the commitment and support of the team within the operating department is crucial.

For teams to be effective they need to be designed for learning, with leaders/managers framing the challenges that face them in such a way that team members are motivated to learn. Additionally, leaders must create an environment of psychological safety, which will foster communication and innovation.[46] Without this the adoption of new techniques will be slow, as learning is stifled. Given the highly technical and continuously evolving nature of surgery, it is particularly important that teams learn very quickly how to adopt and use new and emerging technologies. This includes areas such as robot-enhanced minimally invasive approaches,[47] or new fields of surgery such as bariatric surgery (surgery for the morbidly obese).[48] Teams also need to be semiautonomous: for example, they need to be allowed to self-roster and work flexible hours, and to meet personal needs as well as departmental needs.[49,50]

What is unique about the operating department is that tightly knit teams accomplish all of their activities, more so than in any other area of health care. Because of this, flexible operating department managers with transformational leadership traits are crucial.

COMMUNICATION

There has never been a greater need for effective communication than now. Globalization and rapidly developing technology and techniques, whether relating to surgery, information technology or telecommunications (and the notion of telehealth), affect the operating department. Good communication assists in ameliorating the negative effects of rapid change. Indeed, good communication is fundamental to effective leadership, and to the management and functioning of the department. It involves exchanges of information between staff and patients, and between individuals and teams, both within and beyond the operating department. Communication can be verbal – the most frequently used method; non-verbal, such as use of body language; or it can be written. Increasingly, information is relayed electronically, such as via personal email. Additionally, the Internet is an increasingly utilized method of communication, for example via electronic bulletin boards and chat rooms. Also, the ability to access information via this route is increasing. Operating department staff increasingly use other electronic means of accessing and sharing information.

EFFECTIVE COMMUNICATION

Effective communication involves the use of appropriate language to convey clear, concise, relevant and timely information. The correct language, spoken or written, the subject matter and the interest or importance of the message are very important. When communication is verbal it requires active listening skills. That is, there must be acknowledgement via gesture, expression and checking of non-verbal clues, to ensure that the message is correctly interpreted and understood. Additionally, probing and questioning skills are needed, and the ability to paraphrase and reflect back messages to further clarify meaning is necessary. Skilled communicators focus on content not delivery, maintain neutrality, and avoid interrupting, or drawing premature or incorrect conclusions. They are also direct and open in their verbal interactions.[51] An important aspect of leading and managing in the operating department is the development of excellent individual communication skills, and ensuring that all staff have the opportunity to develop their communication skills too. This may mean ensuring that, as part of individual practitioners' ongoing professional development, their communication skills are assessed and limitations addressed. There are many excellent training videos, compact discs and other teaching media, which will facilitate staff growth in this area.

BARRIERS TO EFFECTIVE COMMUNICATION

There are a number of barriers to effective communication that must be removed.

Language

Both staff and patients may not speak English as their first language. This has a number of consequences. For patients with a non-English speaking background (NESB) and their family members there is frequently an increased state of anxiety about surgery, beyond that which the perioperative practitioner might normally anticipate. NESB patients are much more sensitive to staff attitudes, body language and non-verbal cues. Those nervous about their ability to cope with difficult situations may be extremely sensitive to signs of tension or irritation in staff. In these circumstances, staff must:

- Be open
- Be patient
- Be receptive
- Speak slowly, softly and calmly, but not in 'pidgin English'
- Show kindness and understanding
- Be aware of and responsive to cultural differences
- Be aware of their own body language
- Whenever possible, use interpreters
- Avoid medical jargon, slang or acronyms.

Many of these actions may also be appropriate for all members of the operating department when dealing with NESB staff. It is important to remember that even English-speaking staff may find the language of the operating department foreign when they first enter the environment. It is important when inducting and orientating new staff that they are given a list and explanation of local jargon and acceptable abbreviations. This will avoid confusion and potential delays occurring during surgery. Medical staff too, especially junior or new ones, must be aware of acceptable abbreviations for surgical procedures, so that the operating lists are understood by all. Importantly, all staff must avoid shouting, swearing and other unacceptable verbal interactions.

Physical

This includes impairments such as hearing loss, and the effect of premedication and other drugs. Elderly patients may be discouraged from bringing their hearing aids to the operating department, which could have a negative effect on their surgical experience. Other physical barriers to communication include excessive noise from a variety of sources. These include audio systems, power tools, such as drills, suction and other equipment, radios, and staff holding unrelated conversations. Any of these can be a distraction for the team or cause distress to the patient. The issue of excessive noise is particularly pertinent when patients are undergoing procedures under local anaesthesia.

Psychological

A number of psychological states, such as anxiety or fear, undermine an individual's (patient or staff member) ability to communicate. Additional stress, whether related to work pressures or to personal matters, will also affect communication negatively.

Serial distortion

This refers to information being incorrectly interpreted.[52] This mostly occurs with verbal communication, particularly when information is relayed to others through intermediaries and, accidentally or otherwise, modified, exaggerated or distorted. The result of misinformation circulating can create stress for patients, their relatives and staff, and give credence to what otherwise should be treated as gossip.

OTHER FORMS OF COMMUNICATION IN THE OPERATING DEPARTMENT

Various written records are kept in the operating department. These include the following.

The patient's medical record

This is a permanent record which notes each episode of care and/or admission for the individual patient. It incorporates the intraoperative care plan or integrated care pathway, and in these are recorded a comprehensive record of the planning, delivery and evaluation of patient care during the perioperative period. These, like the surgeon's operation report, form an integral part of the patient's medical record. It is important that the record of care delivered in the operating department is accurate, concise, legible and contemporaneous. This is particularly important if there is any doubt as to what happened during surgery, or if the patient experiences any adverse event during their time in the operating department, or which could be related to their surgery.

Increasingly, patients are seeking access to their own records and legislation now exists to support this right. This includes the Data Protection Act 1998 and the Access to Health Records Act 1990. These permit living individuals to access various data about their physical and mental health, sexual life, and racial and ethnic origin. Additionally, the concept of an electronic patient record (EPR) is being explored and developed, but issues concerning access and privacy have yet to be resolved.

Theatre practitioners' reports

As indicated earlier, nurses and ODPs keep various records of the care they deliver to individual patients. This includes recording the surgery completed, as well as the surgical count. The count sheet is a vital record and a way of accounting for all items used during surgery, to ensure no foreign body is inadvertently left inside a patient on completion of surgery. The theatre practitioner is responsible for completing all necessary counts and for conveying that information to the surgical team. It is noted in the intraoperative care plan or integrated care pathway; this also records such things as the patient's position during surgery; positioning aids used; the solution used for skin preparation, and the nature and type of electrosurgical unit (ESU) used and position of the ESU indifferent electrode.

The recovery room practitioner's record is commenced when the patient enters the recovery area. It is a record of the care and observations made in the immediate postoperative period, when patients are vulnerable as a result of anaesthesia and surgery. It is also a record of treatments given to relieve pain, nausea and vomiting, and their effectiveness; fluid balance; wound management; and the patient's overall recovery.

The surgical register and other operating department records

It is imperative that all operating departments keep an accurate and permanent record of the nature of all surgeries conducted therein. This is necessary for many reasons, including determining the overall utilization of the operating department. Increasingly, this is an electronic record. Other written information held in the operating department includes:

● **Staff rotas** These are necessary to ensure the right number and type of skill mix is available to staff the operating department adequately. Rotas must be made up sufficiently ahead of time so staff are aware of when they will be on duty, on call and so forth. They must be accessible to all operating department staff and others as deemed necessary by local circumstances.

- **Staff performance development records** All staff in the operating department should undergo regular performance appraisal to ensure they remain competent and are performing the activities as determined by their job description. Performance development activities direct and support staff's professional development needs. This process will help nurses meet NMC standards for PREP or the ODPs Charter, which highlights the requirements necessary to demonstrate ongoing competence.

- **Surgeon's preference cards** These are important records of each individual surgeon's requirements for the various procedures they perform. It is important that these cards are kept up to date. They may be computerized.

- **Team/departmental meetings** Other means of communicating in the operating department include team briefings, staff meetings and the use of newsletters. These are important to ensure a two-way exchange of information. They allow managers to share organizational happenings with all staff so that they are aware of changes and developments within as well as across the department, particularly if the department is large. Individual staff members may also be on various committees internal and external to the operating department, such as infection control, education, research, policy and procedure, and quality improvement. Senior practitioners, managers and others entrusted with committee work must make sure they share information and ideas with the rest of the operating department team, either in meetings or via newsletters. Equally, all team members have a responsibility to bring to the attention of team leaders and managers issues of concern or that affect patient care, from within their individual operating rooms or work areas.

Other channels of communication

All theatre practitioners need to be aware of happenings both within the perioperative setting generally and within the wider healthcare sector. This can occur via membership of organizations such as the National Association of Theatre Nurses (NATN), the Association of Operating Department Practitioners (AODP) and similar professional groups, and via attendance at departmental and hospital in-service sessions, NATN branch meetings and pertinent conferences.

BULLYING, HARASSMENT AND HORIZONTAL VIOLENCE

The vexatious issues of bullying, harassment and horizontal violence in the operating department, despite having long been a problem, have not always been acknowledged or dealt with appropriately. Bullying and harassment are a part of a wider issue, occupational violence. In the healthcare workplace it is not a new concept; although it is known to be a serious problem in the industrialized world[53] it is, in fact, a global phenomenon and on the increase.[19,53,54] It is also a significant issue in nursing.[55] Occupational violence is a multifaceted, poorly enumerated and underreported phenomenon, and subject to various confusing and contradictory definitions.[53] Bullying and harassment are sometimes referred to as internal violence.

Various research findings identify medical staff, managers and supervisors as the main perpetrators of these unacceptable behaviours,[56,58] although co-workers, patients and relatives are also cited in the literature.[54] Further, a culture of silence allows these unacceptable behaviours to continue unchecked, and the incidence is higher than previously assumed or acknowledged.[59,60] Various hypotheses exist as to why bullying and harassment are not acknowledged.[61] These include the fear of retaliation, or that the victim does not realize they are being bullied, or believes nothing can be done about it. Also, complaints are not taken seriously or not properly dealt with.[19] Non-reporting can also reflect the culture of the organization, which can be oppressive. This is particularly the case in organizations which are hierarchically organized, like hospitals. In many jurisdictions, legislation is enacted or health departments and professional associations have issued policy statements advocating zero tolerance of any form of violence against nurses and other healthcare workers.[19,62] The Protection from Harassment Act 1996 prohibits persons from pursuing a course of conduct which they know, or ought to know, amounts to harassment of another. The perpetrator need not be shown to have intended the harm: it is enough that they did it. Managers and employers who are not proactive in preventing bullying, harassment and violence are liable to face legal action from those traumatized by these challenging behaviours.

Defining the terms

It is useful to define terms, although it needs to be acknowledged that there is no final or authoritative definition, and there is some confusion about the terminology, with some overlap occurring.

Bullying   One definition is as follows: repeated and over time, offensive behaviour through vindictive, cruel or malicious attempts to humiliate or undermine an individual or group of employees.[63] The following constitute bullying behaviours:

- Repeated shouting
- Demeaning
- Repeated swearing
- Belittling
- Repeatedly criticizing
- Isolating or marginalizing
- Publicly humiliating
- Monitoring excessively.

It also involves undervaluing, overruling or ignoring. Exposure to these behaviours has a negative effect on an individual's self-esteem, morale, and job satisfaction, and on patient care.[53,54]

Horizontal violence

Horizontal violence is a form of aggressive behaviour among and within oppressed groups. Some authors believe, historically, that nurses have been an oppressed group and have seen themselves as subordinate and second-class compared to other groups of healthcare workers such as doctors. The latter, who have status, prestige and power, are seen to have exploited nurses. As the dominant group, they are also able to enforce their beliefs and values. The powerlessness of the oppressed, and their inability to confront or challenge the dominant group – surgeons, in the case of theatre practitioners – results in the latter taking their frustrations out on each other, with destructive behaviours.[64] This is reflected in passive-aggressive behaviours, such as discouraging the efforts of others and displaying little or no interest in their professional endeavours, scapegoating and sabotage. It is also manifested as bullying and harassment among staff.

Harassment

Most definitions of harassment are broad and include verbal abuse, physical violence, sexual harassment, homicide, any behaviours that create fear, lead to stress or avoidance behaviour in the recipient, and stalking (including electronic stalking) among workers, or between managers and workers.[53] It can also have racial or disability overtones – that is, the physically or mentally disabled or those of minority races (compared to the dominant culture) can be targeted more than others.

One definition is behaviour that is usually unwelcome, unsolicited, usually unreciprocated, and sometimes (but not always) repeated. It makes the workplace or association with work unpleasant, humiliating or intimidating for the people or the group targeted by this behaviour. It can make it difficult for effective work to be done.[65] However, even this definition would make harassment difficult to distinguish from bullying, and in different cultures the word harassment has different meanings. For example, just to further confuse matters in the USA it refers to bullying.

In distinguishing bullying from harassment, the following may be noted: harassment can be a one-off event, whereas bullying tends to be repeated over time, often escalating in intensity. Harassment can have a physical component or a sexual connotation: this includes sexual intimidation, harassment, or actual assault; however, bullying is primarily psychological in nature, at least initially. There is controversy over the gendered nature of bullying, with some saying it occurs equally between men and women; however, in terms of absolute numbers women experience greater rates of bullying and sexual harassment.[66] Finally, harassment, when associated with assault or sexual harassment, can have a criminal element to it, which tends not to be the case with bullying.

In summary, harassment and bullying are similar concepts in that both are an abuse of power in the workplace. There tends to be a gendered aspect to both bullying and harassment, and women are victims more often than men. However, women are also perpetrators of these unacceptable behaviours. Now cyber violence is being reported, with people being harassed and/or bullied via the telephone and email.

In the perioperative setting some authors believe that bullying and harassment are more prevalent.[67–69] They attribute this variously to the geographic isolation of the operating suite, the high stress experienced there, the familiarity and bonding that develops between staff, and the persistent belief that practitioners act only as handmaidens to surgeons and anaesthetists. The issue of harassment of perioperative nurses is not new.[19,70,71] There have been a number of research outcomes over about two decades which identify that perioperative nurses are bullied and harassed. Cox[70] and Tyler and Ellison[69] describe a range of stressors experienced by perioperative practitioners, using terminology such as conflict, abuse, emotional manipulation, personality conflict and lack of support.

When their results are examined more closely, it is evident that bullying and harassment are being described. More recently, the work of Santamaria and O'Sullivan[72] and Michael[56,57] in Australia have highlighted various stressors among perioperative nurses. Santamaria and O'Sullivan[72] identified interpersonal conflict as the leading stressor among the group of perioperative nurses they surveyed, and Michael[56,57] reported many episodes of blatant verbal, physical and sexual abuse and harassment of perioperative nurses. It is, however, important to acknowledge that there are other sources of stress for perioperative practitioners, associated with working in a highly stressful and technologically advanced environment.[73]

The consequences and costs of these behaviours can be profound. Victims can suffer physical and psychological sequelae; additionally, it can affect their jobs and careers. Organizations also experience negative consequences, such as litigation and damage payments. Other effects include:

- Decreased work effectiveness
- Decreased work productivity
- High absenteeism rates
- Low staff morale
- High staff turnover.

This has an adverse effect on the quality and quantity of work produced. Furthermore, the cost in recruiting and training new staff to replace workers who leave can be significant.[74]

Management of bullying and harassment

Any actions taken to stop bullying and harassment are designed to remove the practitioner from the victim role and to reduce or eliminate organizational factors that condone it. Individuals should:

- Document the exact details of the event or events, recording names, dates and precise details in the record[7]
- Discreetly search for other victims and/or witnesses
- Find out about workplace policies and procedures

- Confront the offender and demand that the behaviour stop, and request a purely professional relationship. This approach is considered the most active and assertive response, but many find this difficult to do[19,53,58]
- Make a formal complaint to their immediate supervisor, the human resources department, equal opportunity office and/or union representative.[19,67]

Organizational strategies

As stated earlier, employers can be held accountable if bullying and harassment are not vigorously dealt with and are allowed to permeate the workplace. By implementing a strong policy against all types of bullying and harassment, and maintaining an effective complaints procedure, organizations can avoid being held directly as well as vicariously liable for the unacceptable behaviours of their employees.[75,76] Many authors describe what constitutes an effective bullying and harassment policy as follows:

- Organizations should produce a statement to the effect that a harassing environment is neither authorized nor condoned by the employer. This should enhance employee confidence
- Staff should have a clear understanding of the legal definition and what behaviours constitute bullying and harassment
- Policies should be written that provide the process and contacts for registering a complaint
- Having a policy alone is of no consequence unless it is widely known and publicly displayed
- Education programmes are the best means of prevention, and all staff should attend a training session. In particular, role play is useful, especially for non-managerial staff[77]
- Managers need to be instructed on how to deal with issues and to be aware of corporate and personal liability issues. It is important that they are not judgemental of the victim, and note that individual perception and interpretation determine bullying and harassment.

One of the reasons various forms of bullying and harassment continue is that their very pervasiveness makes them appear normal. However, they are unacceptable behaviours and awareness raising, education and strong leadership are effective at ameliorating their negative effect on all operating department staff. Further, within the NHS a culture of zero tolerance of violence is promoted. In this regard, the role of the operating department manager is crucial in creating and maintaining an acceptable workplace culture aimed at preventing or dealing effectively with bullying, harassment and horizontal violence. This they do by exercising a strong leadership role.

References

1. Girvin J. Nursing and leadership. Basingstoke: Macmillan; 1998.
2. Goffee R, Jones G. Why should anyone be led by you? Harvard Business Review 2000; Sep–Oct: 63–70.
3. Grohar-Murray M, DiCorce H. Leadership and management in nursing. Stamford, Conn: Appleton & Lange; 1997.
4. Burns J. Leadership. New York: Harper & Row; 1978.
5. Parry K. Transformational leadership: developing an enterprising management culture. Sydney: Business and Professional Publishing; 1996.
6. Clinton M, Hendricks J. Issues and trends in nurse management. In: Clinton M, Scheiwe D, eds. Management in the Australian health care industry, 2nd edn. Melbourne: Longman; 1998: 453–475.
7. Porter-O'Grady T. Into the new paradigm: writing the script for the future of health care. J RCN Aus 1996; 3: 5–10.
8. Bennis W. The unconscious conspiracy: why leaders can't lead. New York: Amacon; 1976.
9. Kotter J. What leaders really do. Harvard Business Review 1990; 68: 103–111.
10. Bleich M. Managing and leading. In: Yoder-Wise P, ed. Leading and managing in nursing, 2nd edn. St Louis: Mosby; 1999: 2–20.
11. Vecchio R, Hearn G, Southey G. Organisational behaviour, 2nd edn. Sydney: Harcourt Brace; 1996.
12. Yukl G. Leadership in organisations, 4th edn. New Jersey: Prentice Hall; 1998.
13. Drucker P. The new realities: in government and politics/in economics and business/in society and worldview. New York: Harper & Row; 1989.
14. Dixon D. Achieving results through transformational leadership. J Nurs Admin 1999; 29: 17–21.
15. Dunham-Taylor J. Nurse executive: transformational leadership found in participative organizations. J Nurs Admin 2000; 30: 241–250.
16. Valadez A, Otto D. Role development. In: Yoder-Wise P, ed. Leading and managing in nursing, 2nd edn. St Louis: Mosby; 1999: 21–34.
17. Bennis W, Nanus B. Leaders: the strategies for taking charge. New York: Harper & Row; 1985.
18. Westwood F. Doing deals. Br J Perioper Nurs 2001; 11: 538–541.
19. National Association of Theatre Nurses. Challenging behaviours in the perioperative environment. Dealing with bullying, violence and harassment. Harrogate: NATN; 2002.
20. Woodhead K. Leadership makes a difference. Br J Perioper Nurs 2001; 11: 114–118.
21. Bass B. Leadership and performance beyond expectations. New York: Free Press; 1985.
22. Tichy N, Devanna M. Transformational leadership. New York: Wiley; 1986.
23. Davidhizar A. Leading with charisma. J Advanced Nurs 1995; 18: 675–679.
24. Dunham J, Klafehn K. Transformational leadership and the nurse executive. J Nurs Admin 1990; 20: 28–33.
25. McDaniel C, Wolf G. Transformational leadership in nursing service. J Nurs Admin 1992; 22: 60–65.
26. Trofino J. Transformational leadership: the catalyst for successful change. International Nurs Rev 1993; 40: 179–182, 187.
27. Trofino J. Transformational leadership in health care. Nurs Manager 1995; 26: 42–47.
28. Carlopio J. Holism: a philosophy of organisational leadership for the future. Leadership Quarterly 1994; 5: 297–305.
29. Porter-O'Grady T. Quantum leadership: new roles for a new age. J Nurs Admin 1999; 29: 37–42.
30. Porter-O'Grady T, Krueger Wilson C. The leadership revolution in health care, altering systems, changing behaviours. Gaithersburg, Md: Aspen; 1995.
31. Bass B, Avolio B. Improving organisational effectiveness through transformational leadership. Thousand Oaks, Calif: Sage; 1994.
32. Kaplan R. Leadership that is both forceful and enabling. Leadership in Action 1999; 19: 1–8.
33. Taylor M, Campbell C. The multi-disciplinary team in the operating department. Br J Perioper Nurs 1999; 9: 178–183.
34. National Health Service Management Executive. Junior doctors: the new deal. London: NHSME; 1991.
35. White J, Coleman M. Threats and opportunities facing the theatre nurse. Br J Perioper Nurs 2000; 10: 260–268.
36. Hind M. Healthcare support workers and the scrubbed role. Br J Perioper Nurs 2001; 11: 262–268.
37. Hanlon M. Maximise staff and minimise lists. Unpublished conference paper, NSW Operating Theatre Association, 45th Annual Conference, Sydney: April 2002.
38. Wicker P. Recruitment and retention a personal issue. Br J Perioper Nurs 1999; 9: 84–87.
39. Cacioppe R. Using individual and team reward-recognition to achieve organisational success. In: Wiesner R, Millett B, eds. Management and organisational behaviour. Brisbane: Wiley; 2001: 73–85.
40. Wood J, Wallace J, Zaffane R, et al. Organisational behaviour: an Asia Pacific perspective. Brisbane: Wiley; 1998.

41. Reilly A, Jones J. Team building. In: Pfeiffer J, Jones J, eds. The 1974 handbook for group facilitators. San Diego: University Associates; 1974: 227–237.

42. Senge P. The fifth discipline: the art and practice of the learning organisation. Sydney: Random House; 1992.

43. Tuckman B. Development sequence in small groups. Psycholog Bull 1965; 63: 384–399.

44. Wilbur K. Sex, ecology, spirituality: the spirit of evolution. Boston: Shambala; 1995.

45. Covey S. First things first. New York: Simon & Schuster; 1994.

46. Edmondson A, Bohmer R, Pisano G. Speeding up team learning. Harvard Business Review 2001; October: 125–132.

47. Mathias J. Robots' potential exciting but will technology be affordable? Operating Room Manager 2001; 17: 1–10.

48. Patterson P. Surgery for the morbidly obese requires a special commitment. Operating Room Manager 2002; 18: 1–12.

49. Tanner J, Bailey G. Staff rostering in the operating department. Br J Perioper Nurs 2001; 11: 228–233.

50. Fudge L. Reduced hours and flexitime. Br J Perioper Nurs 2001; 11: 393–401.

51. Westwood F. Leadership and communication: what really works? Br J Perioper Nurs 2001; 11: 190–194.

52. Taylor M, Campbell C. Communication skills in the operating department. Br J Perioper Nurs 1999; 9: 217–221.

53. Mayhew C, Chappell D. Occupational violence: types, reporting patterns and variation between health sectors (discussion paper no.1). Sydney: University of New South Wales, School of Industrial Relations and Organisational Behaviour and Industrial Relations Research Centre; 2001.

54. Howells-Johnson J. Verbal abuse. Br J Perioper Nurs 2000; 10: 508–511.

55. Paterson B, McCornish A, Bradley P. Violence at work. Nurs Standard 1999; 13: 18–23.

56. Michael R. When the specialty becomes a nightmare: workplace traumatic experiences amongst perioperative nurses. ACORN J 2001; 14: 11–15.

57. Michael R. Survive or thrive? The impact of workplace trauma on perioperative nurses: part 2. ACORN J 2001; 14: 14–19.

58. Madison L. RNs' experiences of sex-based and sexual harassment – an empirical study. Aust J Advanced Nurs 1994; 14: 29–37.

59. Mayhew C, Chappell D. Prevention of occupational violence in the health workplace (discussion paper no. 2). Sydney: University of New South Wales, School of Industrial Relations and Organisational Behaviour and Industrial Relations Research Centre; 2001.

60. Mayhew C, Chappell D. 'Internal' violence (or bullying) and the health workforce (discussion paper no. 3).

Sydney: University of New South Wales, School of Industrial Relations and Organisational Behaviour and Industrial Relations Research Centre; 2001.

61. Gilmour D, Hamlin L. Bullying and harassment in the perioperative setting. Br J Perioper Nurs 2003; 13: 17–25.

62. Australian College of Operating Room Nurses (ACORN). Bullying, harassment and discrimination in the perioperative environment. ACORN standards guidelines and policy statements (C4). Adelaide: ACORN; 2003.

63. International Labour Office (ILO), International Council of Nurses (ICN), World Health Organisation (WHO), Public Services International (PSI). Framework guidelines for addressing workplace violence in the health sector. Geneva: ILO, ICN, WHO, PSI; 2002.

64. Hamlin L. Horizontal violence in the operating room. Br J Theatre Nurs 200; 10: 17–25.

65. Australian Public Service Commission. Eliminating workplace harassment guidelines. Canberra: Australian Government Printing Service; 1994.

66. International Council of Nurses (ICN). Workplace violence in the health sector. Geneva: ICN; 2002. Online. Available: http://www.icn.ch

67. Kaye J. Sexual harassment and hostile environments in the perioperative area. AORN J 1996; 63: 443–449.

68. Shibe J. Harassment comes in assorted flavours. Today's Operating Room Nurse 1991; 13: 3.

69. Tyler P, Ellison R. Sources of stress and psychological well-being in high-dependency nursing. J Advanced Nurs 1994; 19: 469–476.

70. Cox H. Verbal abuse in nursing: report of a study. Nurse Manager 1987; 18: 47–50.

71. Buchanan J, Considine G. Stop telling us to cope! NSW nurses explain why they are leaving the profession. A report for the NSW Nurses' Association. Sydney: Australian Centre for Industrial Relations Research and Training (ACIRRT), University of Sydney; 2002.

72. Santamaria N, O'Sullivan S. Stress in perioperative nursing: sources, frequency and correlations to personality factors. J RCN Aus 1998; 5: 10–15.

73. Johnstone L. 1990s surgical technology implicated in the role conflict-inducing stress amongst instrument and circulating nurses. ACORN J 2000; 13: 19–27.

74. Slagle King C. Ending the silent conspiracy: sexual harassment in nursing. Nurs Admin Q 1995; 19: 48–55.

75. Childers-Hermann J. Awareness of sexual harassment: first step toward prevention. Crit Care Nurs 1993; 13: 101–103.

76. Julius DJ, DiGiovanni N. Sexual harassment: legal issues, implications for nurses. AORN J 1990; 52: 95–103.

77. Fiedler A, Hamby E. Sexual harassment in the workplace: nurses' perceptions. J Nurs Admin 2000; 30: 497–503.

Chapter 5

Assuring quality services

Liz Bernthal

Key points

- Quality assurance
- Audit
- Controls assurance
- Evidence-based care
- Clinical effectiveness

INTRODUCTION

Perioperative practitioners face many challenges in their working life and giving the highest standard of care to their patients has always been paramount. The government has demonstrated its increasing commitment to ensuring that quality services are delivered. The publication of many White Papers, such as *Making a Difference,*[1] *Designed to Care: Renewing the NHS in Scotland,*[2] *Putting Patients First in Wales*[3] and *Fit for the Future* (in Northern Ireland)[4] has ensured that delivering high-quality care remains high on governments' agenda in Great Britain and Northern Ireland. Increasing government interest in health care has provided a golden opportunity for perioperative practitioners to continue to improve the quality of care for patients and to make sure it is effective. In the past, patients felt secure that they were receiving quality care from well-trained and experienced practitioners. However, events such as the death of children undergoing cardiac surgery in Bristol have made the public question the care they are receiving.[5] In 2002 clinical negligence claims against the NHS reached £5.89 billion.[6] Now all perioperative practitioners must ensure that they are providing optimum care not only for the benefit of patients but also for their own protection. Practice that is research based is fundamental so that healthcare delivery can be improved; continuing to practise in a ritualistic way because 'things have always been done that way' is no longer justified.

A culture that ensures quality care is being given has seen the greater use of terms such as *quality assurance*, *audit*, *benchmarking* and *clinical effectiveness* being incorporated into everyday practice, and although there are endless publications about these subjects, few discuss what they actually mean. The aim of this chapter is to explain and discuss the terms widely used, as well as the principle of ensuring that perioperative practitioners give quality care that is clinically cost effective. So that quality care can be given and improved, perioperative practitioners should understand what the term quality means so that quality of care given is improved. In addition to this, it is important to understand how to devise and evaluate methods to measure quality, how to investigate and develop practical methods for improving quality, as well as how to motivate others to change their practice, so that the quality of care can be improved. Quality improvement is everyone's responsibility, from perioperative practitioners directly involved in patient care to the Chief Executive, who, with clinical governance, is now accountable for the care given within his or her healthcare organization. Although improving the quality of care is not easy, this chapter hopes to increase perioperative practitioners' understanding of what quality means and so help them to give the quality of care their patients deserve.

This chapter includes the most up-to-date information available at the time of writing. However, it is important to recognize that government initiatives and striving to achieve quality in healthcare is a continually evolving process, and some of the information may become out of date quite quickly, although the principles should remain the same. Perioperative practitioners have a duty to keep themselves updated and abreast of any new government initiatives and developments in healthcare provision, particularly since devolution in 1999, since when individual nations within the UK have developed their own initiatives to improve care.

WHAT IS QUALITY?

There is an increasing expectation in today's society for everyone to receive a quality product from an organization, whether this is good service in a restaurant, for example, or high-quality health care.

DEFINITIONS

There are many definitions from the business world that could be chosen to define quality, such as 'meeting customer requirements' and 'fit for purpose',[5] but these are not entirely suitable for health care. A dictionary definition of quality is 'the degree of excellence of a thing' (Collins).

Specifically, Ovretveit[7] offers a definition appropriate to health care: 'The ability to meet the needs of those requiring the service most, at the lowest cost to the organization and within the guidelines set by higher authorities'. This emphasizes the importance of fulfilling guidelines and the provision of cost-effective care within limited resources in today's climate of cost-conscious health care and market forces.

THE DIMENSIONS OF QUALITY

Maxwell[8] argued that quality in health care has six dimensions:

- Access to services
- Relevance to need (for the whole community)
- Effectiveness (for individual patients)
- Equity (fairness)
- Social acceptability
- Efficiency and economy.

Although these are important, there are several other points that could be included, such as prevention from harm, or improving patient autonomy in making decisions about their care. Donabedian[9] expands the argument that quality cannot be judged by health professionals alone but must include patients' views and preferences. Therefore the involvement of patients in planning and discussing their care is crucial. He stated that quality of care arises from three sources:

- The science of health care
- Individual values and expectations
- Social values and expectations.

MAKING QUALITY RELEVANT

The way in which quality is adapted in an organization will depend on the relationships established with its customers. Failure to provide a quality service will eventually endanger the future aspects of an organization,[10] but increased government spending on health service provision aims to prevent this happening. Since the introduction of an internal market in the 1990s, health service managers have been expected to run their hospitals like any other business, and with government initiatives such as the Patient's Charter[11] and clinical governance,[1] managers are now accountable for the care given. Clinical governance has been defined in the White Paper, *A First Class Service*,[12] as 'a framework through which the NHS is accountable for continuously improving the quality of their services and safeguarding high standards of care by creating an environment in which excellence in clinical care will flourish'. Clinical governance is statutory in the NHS; however, other healthcare providers have incorporated the recommendations given into their day-to-day care management. This indicates that improving quality of care should be at the top of any healthcare provider's agenda, regardless of whether it is statutory or not.

Technological advances, such as the Internet, have eased access to information so that patients are becoming better informed. They are becoming much more involved in discussing the care they expect to receive and have greater expectations and demands than in the past. Therefore, perioperative practitioners need to be able to justify the care they are giving.

DETERMINING THE QUALITY OF CARE GIVEN

In the past the quality of perioperative care was determined by retrospective audits in which any problems could be identified after the event, so it was reactive rather than proactive. However, the current concept of quality requires that effort be directed to ensure that optimum care is given consistently in the first place. Government White Papers such as *The New NHS: Modern Dependable*;[13] *Designed to Care: Renewing the NHS in Scotland*;[2] *Putting Patients First in Wales*;[3] and *Fit for the Future* (in Northern Ireland)[4] as well as *Making a Difference*[1] and The NHS Plan,[14] ensure that quality is crucial and at the heart of the modern NHS. In order to ensure quality care, the drive for evidence-based practice, clinical effectiveness and quality assurance are intrinsically linked. The publication of so many White Papers has emphasized the government's belief that quality is the responsibility of everyone professionally involved in healthcare provision, regardless of their level in the organization. A summary of the most important of the Government White Papers is given in Box 5.1.

EVALUATION OF THE QUALITY OF CARE

Evaluation of the quality of care takes place at various levels within an organization (Fig. 5.1).

'National level' incorporates the government's strategy on health care and its commitment to equality of standards. This includes the National Service Framework, which sets out common standards

Box 5.1   Government White Papers involved with quality assessment since 1983

- 1983 *NHS Management Enquiry.* (The Griffith's report)[55]
- 1990 *Working for Patients*[56]
- 1991 *The Patient's Charter*[12]
- 1993 *Clinical Audit: Meeting and Improving Standards in Health care.*[57]
  A Vision for the Future: The Nursing, Midwifery and Health Visiting Contribution to Health and Healthcare[30]
- 1997 *The New NHS, Modern, Dependable.*[14]
  Designed to care: renewing the NHS in Scotland[2]
- 1998 *National Performance Frameworks.*[58]
  A First Class Service: Quality in the New NHS[13]
  Achieving Effective Practice[40]
  Fit for the Future: A Consultation Paper on the Future of the HPSS (in Northern Ireland)[4]
- 1999 *Making a Difference.*[1]
  Putting Patients First in Wales[3]
  A Health Service of the Talents; Developing NHS Workforce Consultation[59]
- 2000 *The NHS Plan. A Plan for Investment. A Plan for Reform.* London: DOH
- 2001 *The NHS Plan. A Plan for Investment. A Plan for Reform.* (DOH 2000a) *Essence of Care*[15]
  Working Together – Learning Together – a Framework for Lifelong Learning for the NHS[60]

across the UK for the treatment of particular conditions.[15] The role of the National Institute for Clinical Excellence (NICE) in England is to provide patients, health professionals and the public with authoritative, robust and reliable guidance on best practice.[16] Each nation within Great Britain and Northern Ireland has its own regulatory body, such as the Clinical Standards Board for Scotland. The Commission for Healthcare Audit and Inspection (CHAI) is a national body in England that oversees the standards of clinical services and implementation of NICE guidelines and gives guidance on best practice. Every hospital will be visited by CHAI to help ensure that effective systems are in place to improve patient care.[16] Standards set by professional colleges and organizations such as the National Association of Theatre Nurses (NATN) are at this level. The standards set by purchasers, such as Health Authorities, must be achieved by providers (such as hospitals) in order to fulfil their contract with the purchaser. The clinical areas, such as the perioperative environment, have the most crucial effect on the quality of care given, as they have direct involvement with patients. A team approach is essential when quality is monitored so as to reflect the care the patient is receiving. In the past standards have been measured by individual health professionals in isolation from their colleagues, which may not reflect the full picture. A patient undergoing surgery receives care from

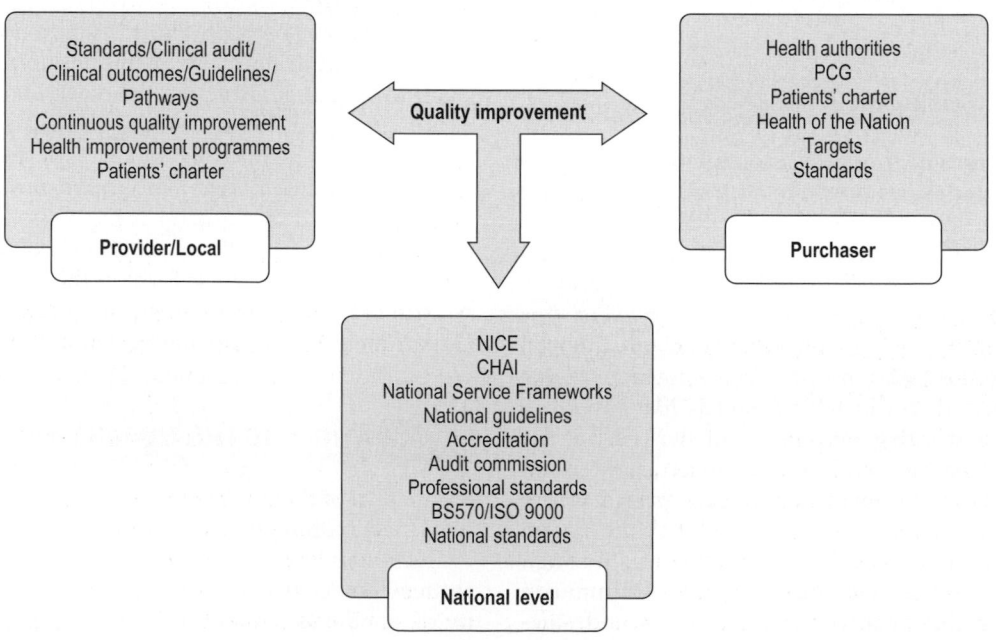

Figure 5.1   The various levels responsible.

Registered Nurses, operating department practitioners (ODPs), healthcare workers (HCWs), surgeons and anaesthetists, all of whom need to give excellent care if a patient is to receive care of the highest standard overall.

Staff must be supported to reach their potential by continuing to develop their knowledge and skills. Of course this concept is not new: Florence Nightingale was already innovative for her time, and recognized the importance of theoretical training to support practical skills.[17]

QUALITY ASSURANCE

Quality care that is value for money is a central focus in current government policies on health care. Quality assurance has become an integral part in the delivery of health care, but what is it?

DEFINITION

The word 'quality' has already been defined, and 'assurance' is defined as 'formal guarantee; positive declaration' (Collins). Therefore, 'quality assurance' is the process of assuring the consumer a standard of excellence by continuously measuring and monitoring it. Quality assurance involves the efforts required to improve a standard if, once it has been measured, it becomes apparent that it could be improved. Therefore, quality assurance aims to guarantee that an acceptable level of quality is being maintained. There are many ways in which this is achieved. For example, setting standards, audit, controls assurance, evidence-based care and clinical effectiveness are all methods that assist in improving standards of care. These will be discussed further in this chapter.

CONTINUOUS QUALITY IMPROVEMENT/TOTAL QUALITY MANAGEMENT

Continuous Quality Improvement (CQI), or Total Quality Management (TQM), as it is also known, is a philosophy that aims to achieve excellence in every aspect of customer service and 'get it right the first time, every time'. The concept of CQI/TQM is quite simple and necessitates that the organization, such as the NHS, has processes in place to ensure that the service and care given to customers (patients) is of a high standard and meets the needs of those customers. Therefore, the management of that organization should show its commitment to providing a quality service by setting up a systematic framework to ensure this is happening. Government White Papers *A First-Class Service*[12] and *The New NHS, Modern, Dependable*[13] support this. In a perioperative setting, like any other healthcare environment, the patients' point of view must be considered so that the high standards of care given meet their needs. This can be achieved by visiting the patients preoperatively so they have an opportunity to discuss their needs, and postoperatively to see if these were met. CQI/TQM also emphasizes that the work environment should stimulate staff to foster pride in the organization and department in which they work; teamwork between all levels of staff and interprofessional collaboration are also important. Perioperative practitioners must be stimulated to increased their knowledge and be willing to learn from previous experience if the quality of care is to be improved.

THE MANAGERIAL PROCESSES

CQI/TQM consists of three managerial processes:

- *Quality leadership* – management commitment to support and develop quality by ensuring funding is available to give a quality service, and resources to train and equip staff to provide such a service.
- *A hospital wide approach* – that quality initiatives are implemented throughout the hospital
- *Continuous measurement and training* – staff are receiving training and development within their own specialty so that they are equipped with the skills and knowledge to provide a quality service.

An organization must support and look after its staff so that they feel valued, as they are more likely to excel in such an environment. Research has shown that patient outcomes and the quality of care are improved in hospitals where professional autonomy and a good working environment are encouraged, and staff have control over their clinical environment and are supported.[18] Aitken et al[18] found that in such hospitals the patient mortality rate was reduced by 7.7%. The authors felt confident that this could not be explained by patient characteristics or any other attributes related to nursing, and was due to an improved quality of care as a direct result of staff giving their best because they felt valued.

QUALITY CIRCLES

A quality circle is a group of between five and eight volunteers working in the same clinical area who meet regularly to identify and solve problems.[19] This differs from clinical supervision, which is reflective in nature and focuses on personal professional development, whereas quality circles develop practice and use the audit process. Quality circles form part of the commitment to CQI/TQM. They originated in Japanese industry and did not come to Britain until 1978, when Rolls Royce found that involving all staff in discussions on quality could reduce costs and improve productivity. The NHS first implemented voluntary quality circles in 1982 following restructuring, in order to encourage greater staff involvement and participation. It can be seen from Figure 5.2 that a quality circle begins by identifying the problem; the process then continues until the problem is solved and management has been informed, and an improvement in standard of care demonstrated.

A quality circle is not hierarchical: members should be encouraged to come from all disciplines and grades of staff within the perioperative environment. Meetings are normally arranged weekly or fortnightly and last for about an hour, regardless of whether or not discussion about the standard selected has finished. Time and money may need to be invested in training so that members of the circle understand their role and a productive quality circle is facilitated.

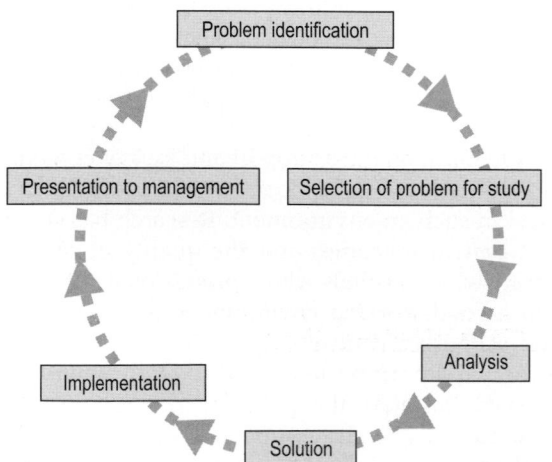

Figure 5.2   Quality circle. (Modified from Robson[19])

STANDARD SETTING

Standard setting is one of the most widely used methods of assessing standards of care. A standard has been defined as a baseline against which to monitor quality and effectiveness.[20] In setting a standard it is important that it does not become a diversion from giving quality care and become an end in itself. It is all too easy to overemphasize the words to be used in setting the standard and for it to be a paperwork exercise rather than concentrating on the actual care being given. All too often, once standards are set they are adapted and written into policy and procedures manuals that are placed on shelves to gather dust and are never consulted. Staff should not become complacent: it must not be assumed that because high standards have been set they are always adhered to. Nor should standards be regarded as static: they should be frequently reviewed and the care given monitored to check that it reflects the standards set as they change.

HOW TO WRITE A STANDARD

A standard must be well written, research based and measurable, as well as written by practitioners directly involved in patient care. An example of a standard could be: 'With immediate effect, this operating department will ensure that all patients (100%) have their body temperature recorded preoperatively on arrival at the operating department so that a baseline temperature is provided prior to surgery. This is so inadvertent hypothermia can be prevented.'

THE 'SMART' PRINCIPLE

Standards should follow the mnemonic 'SMART' principle to be meaningful:[21]

- S – specific
- M – measurable
- A – achievable
- R – realistic
- T – timed.

For example, the standard above fulfils the SMART principle:

- Specific – temperature to be recorded preoperatively
- Measurable – can be measured retrospectively that 100% of patients have had their temperature recorded

- Achievable – should be quite simple to record a patient's temperature on arrival in theatre
- Realistic – it is reasonable to expect that all patients have their temperature recorded
- Timed – 'preoperatively' states the time when this standard is to be undertaken.

Clinical audit is commonly the tool of choice to measure the effectiveness of a standard. This is either completed concurrently, i.e. while the patient is receiving care, or retrospectively when the care is completed, for example when results are correlated to determine whether 100% of patients did have their temperature assessed preoperatively on arrival in the operating department. In this example above it would include the investigation of why 100% of patients were not having their temperature taken pre-operatively if this was the case; and would include the action taken to rectify it, such as purchasing more thermometers. Therefore, standards of care are intrinsically linked with practice, education, management and research.

AUDIT TO MONITOR PERFORMANCE

Audit is the systematic evaluation of care given by comparing it to the ideal standard so that any deficiencies can be rectified and the quality of care improved. It is a cycle of activity involving a systematic review of practice, identification of problems, the development of possible solutions, implementation of change, then review again. NHSME[22] defines clinical audit as follows: 'The systematic, critical analysis of the quality of clinical care. This includes the procedures used for diagnosis and treatment and care of patients and the associated use of resources and the effect of care on the outcome and quality of life for the patient.'

It is essentially a type of peer review, although audit compares current practice numerically rather than just making judgements about the care given. The terms *medical* and *nursing* audit simply reflect which profession is completing the audit; *clinical* audit could be carried out by any health professional who has clinical involvement.

AUDIT CYCLE

Following the 'audit cycle' (Fig. 5.3) eases completion of an audit.

Health professionals use audit every day as they assess and reflect on the care they are giving their patients. In theory, the process of audit itself should improve performance as it encourages discussion about procedures and the care being given, and so focuses practitioners on the standards of care they are giving. King[24] believes that audit helps improve communication, and certainly there is much more teamwork and discussion between different health professionals caring for a patient in planning their care when audit is established. King[24] portrays this even more simply as a cycle of inquiry (Fig. 5.4).

Information on standards to be set can be acquired through literature searches, by discussing with patients what they want, and by discussion with colleagues.

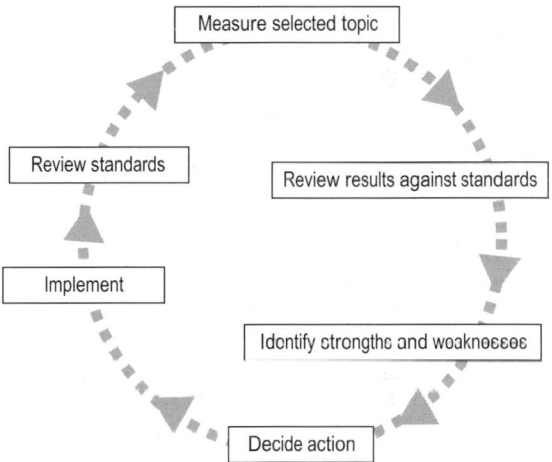

Figure 5.3 The audit circle. (Modified from Malby[23])

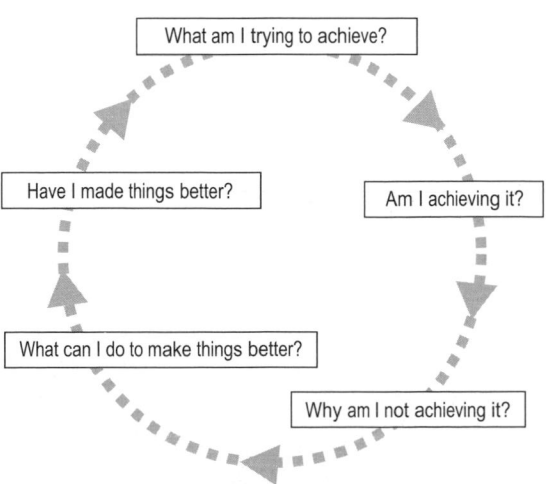

Figure 5.4 A cycle of inquiry. (Modified from King[24])

TRAINING

Although clinical audit has been carried out for many years, with the advent of National Service Frameworks it is likely that staff will be required to undertake audits frequently, and so training is essential. This should be endorsed by senior board members and given to all levels of staff within the organization. Audit works best when it is incorporated into everyday working practices rather than taken on as a paperwork exercise, which so often happens. Whereas standards need to be research based, group discussion is important so that the standards agreed meet and are relevant to the local situation. If completion of a literature search indicates a specific standard is recommended, for example, audit can be used to assess whether this standard is being achieved. Research therefore helps us determine what we should be doing and audit helps us investigate whether we are achieving it. Journals, the Internet and discussion with colleagues are a good source of information.

Motivation and support from all levels of staff is essential. Hudson[25] emphasizes that finding sufficient time is the main problem when completing an audit, and advocates seeking advice in the early planning stage so that the minimum time is wasted (Box 5.2).

An audit should only be completed if staff are prepared to act on the findings and change their practice. Indeed, the ability to change practice is fundamental and shows commitment to improving services and quality of care. Audit can also be used as part of professional development, as it encourages scientific thinking and studying the evidence and research available.

CONTROLS ASSURANCE

Controls assurance requires that Directors of Hospital Boards must ensure that systems are in place to ensure that risks are assessed and properly managed.[21] Local initiatives have developed various strategies to ensure standards of care have been met. Many hospitals have attained external accreditation, such as the King's Fund Accreditation Programme, Charter Mark[26] (a government award scheme for recognizing and encouraging excellence in public service), the ISO 9000 series of quality assurance (the British Standard for quality management systems[26]) or CHI accreditation, so a certain standard of care should be guaranteed.

EVIDENCE–BASED CARE (EBC)

WHAT IS IT?

The last 20 years have witnessed a mounting effort by perioperative practitioners to increase the prevalence of evidence-based practice. Both the nursing profession and the government have recognized the need for this.[27–29] EBC is simply care that is research based. Sackett et al.[30] have defined it as follows: 'Evidence-based care is the conscientious, explicit and judicious use of current best evidence from systematic research through the integration of clinical expertise while making decisions about the care of individual patients'. Evidence-based *practice* is merely practice that provides EBC and combines experience with research, and should be adapted thoughtfully and compassionately to each individual patient and clinical situation. Decisions about care can no longer be based solely on opinion but must be based on research and evidence. The focus of EBC is very much upon the decision-making ability of the individual practitioner, encouraging him or her to replace unfounded opinion and practice with research-based evidence.[31]

WHY CARE IS NOT ALWAYS EVIDENCE BASED

EBC should make perioperative practitioners confident that their care is based on current and appropriate knowledge. However, there is evidence that reality does not match up with the ideal.[32] There are many reasons for this, such as a lack of confidence or skills in critically appraising research; insufficient time because of work commitments; a lack of support from peers, managers and other professionals; as well as a lack of resources. A reluctance to change practice contributes to this – the 'I have always done it this way' syndrome; although there may not

---

Box 5.2   How to make audit effective

- Be clear about what you want to achieve
- Seek advice at the planning stage
- Consider all aspects of the project, such as data collection at the planning stages
- Consider means of making data collection easier and less time consuming, e.g. has it been collected elsewhere before?

be anything wrong with the actual practice, it is important that it is research based and not merely ritualistic.

In order to establish a culture where perioperative practitioners feel comfortable using research to support care, several key components are needed. Individual practitioners require regular clinical exposure and experience, so that they can rationalize the risks and benefits of any particular care they are giving. Any new practice should be supported by research, with the full involvement of the patient. Management should ensure that the staff working in the department are equipped with the skills required to critically appraise the care that they are giving; good communication is essential.

For perioperative practitioners to be involved in evidence-based practice they need to possess a sufficiently sizeable and robust scientific base from which to evaluate the effectiveness of individual care given. It was only in 1972 that Briggs recommended that nursing practice should be research based.[33] Medicine has existed for centuries, but for professional groups established relatively recently in comparison, such as perioperative practitioners, the amount of research that can be accessed may be quite limited, and it may be necessary to study research from other disciplines such as medicine. If research is limited then it is even more important that resources are available to enable practitioners to undertake research of their own so that they are not excluded. Employers should encourage, support and facilitate staff to keep updated and undertake research.

THE EVIDENCE-BASED APPROACH

By taking an evidence-based approach, routine unnecessary practices can be challenged or new roles evaluated. McSherry and Haddock[34] stress that the following processes are required for evidence-based practice to be executed:

- Identify areas in practice from which clear clinical questions can be formulated
- Identify the most relevant evidence from available literature (e.g. through databases)
- Critical appraisal of the evidence for validity and clinical usefulness
- Implement and incorporate relevant finding(s) into practice
- Continue measuring performance against expected outcomes or against peers.

WHY IT IS SO IMPORTANT THAT PRACTICE IS EVIDENCE BASED

Care should be evidence based so that it benefits patients and is clinically effective. If EBC is not practised, care may actually cause harm as well as be non-beneficial.

EXAMPLES OF EVIDENCE-BASED CARE

See Box 5.3

Therefore, by studying the evidence, practice is changed by flushing intravenous sites with saline rather than with heparin, which both benefits patients and is cost effective. (See Box 5.4.)

THE RISKS OF NOT PRACTISING EVIDENCE-BASED CARE

Patient care can be compromised if evidence-based care is not practised. The main reasons why are listed below:

- Personal choice leads to inconsistent care, e.g. the length of time scrubbing: some staff scrub for

---

Box 5.3   Examples of how EBC can be put into practice

Heparin flushes vs saline flushes of intravenous sites to maintain potency and prevent phlebitis for the administration of antibiotics.

Evidence has shown that saline flushes are just as effective as heparin.[35] By using saline instead of heparin, care is improved and risks are reduced, as well as a very great financial saving (up to $218 million annually in the USA, where saline is widely used).[35]

Box 5.4   Treatment for fibroids

In the past hysterectomy was the surgery of choice, with all the risks that major surgery involves, such as haemorrhage, time off work etc., as well as the psychological impact on the woman herself and the inability to have children if still of childbearing age. Research has shown that many of these women were receiving hysterectomy unnecessarily, and could be treated either medically or with hysteroscopy or myomectomy, so that their uterus, and therefore possibly their fertility, could remain intact.

three minutes and others five minutes; some circulating staff wear masks in some specialties, whereas in others not even the scrub team wear them.

• Staff may act as a role model because of their personality, when in fact their practice is not of the highest standard.

• Ritualistic practice, e.g. starving patients from midnight even if the operation is later in the following day; preoperative shaving well in advance of surgery.

• Practice that is out of date.

• The use of a product sponsored by a company regardless of whether the evidence indicates it is the most appropriate.

• Without a strong commitment to giving care based on scientific knowledge perioperative practitioners could lose their credibility with other healthcare professionals whose care is always research based.

Perioperative practitioners are in an ideal situation to be proactive in leading evidence-based care, as they collaborate with several healthcare professionals in the operating department setting.

THE BENEFITS OF EVIDENCE-BASED CARE

Perioperative practitioners know that they should be practising EBC, but it is essential to understand why this is important. Care that is evidence based should:

• Enable an improved quality of care
• Be consistent and standardized, regardless of who provides the care
• Create fewer unacceptable variations in clinical practice
• Avoid ritualistic practice
• Be justified by research
• Be clinically effective
• Be cost effective
• Be less confusing for junior staff who are learning new skills because it is consistent
• Enable policies and procedures to be easily understood and consistent with practice
• Be up to date
• Encourage ongoing monitoring of the quality of care given.

Inconsistency in care can cause confusion, particularly for more junior staff who are learning new skills. For example, some operating departments allow staff to scrub with wedding rings on, whereas others insist that they are removed to reduce the risk of infection.[36] Reading the latest research should answer these questions.

REVIEWING PRACTICE

It is essential that practice is continually reviewed to confirm that it is still of the highest standard and based on current knowledge and thinking. There are often inconsistencies in practice, as has already been highlighted, and this may be the impetus for investigation. For example, a forced-air warming system (e.g. Bair Hugger) has proved to be one of the most effective methods currently used in the prevention of inadvertent hypothermia,[37] yet individual staff often decide themselves which patients would benefit most, which can mean that care is inconsistent. These decisions are often based on personal experience and opinion rather than research, and are therefore not evidence based. Another example is the use of double gloving. Some scrubbed personnel double glove for certain operations but not others, despite considerable evidence that wearing two pairs of gloves provides much greater protection against infection.[38]

Unfortunately, in most departments there are always one or two professionals who demonstrate a reluctance to change their practice, and research can be a powerful tool to encourage them to do so if it can be shown that it is in the patient's or their own interest.

To clarify whether the care being given is evidence based, many questions need to be asked. Beyea[35] recommends the following:

• Who determined the basis for treatment?
• What was the rationale for making that decision?
• What are the clinical implications of this practice?
• Why are we doing this and why are we doing it this way?
• Could it be done better, more efficiently, and more cost-effectively?
• Are these the highest achievable outcomes?

Asking and answering these questions may improve existing practice.

WHERE TO FIND THE EVIDENCE

Finding the evidence often starts in the workplace when the practitioner questions everyday practice.

Finding the time to discover the research for EBC to be practised is difficult, as at present there is no national database to indicate what research has been completed unless a literature search is undertaken. Databases in the library are a good place to start looking for good-quality systematic reviews relating to health and perioperative practice. Librarians are very helpful in retrieving information and some will complete a literature research for you. However, staffing levels in the perioperative environment are often reduced to a minimum, which means there is little possibility of visiting the library in working hours, and as most practitioners lead very busy lives there is also little opportunity to undertake literature reviews and update oneself on the latest research in off-duty time. Therefore, it is essential that any time allocated to finding the latest research is used effectively as possible. Box 5.5 is a guide to where the evidence can be found.

Achieving Effective Practice[39] identifies several activities that can assist in achieving evidence-based practice. These include developing journal clubs or meetings that create opportunities to discuss research findings. The importance of feedback to colleagues

---

Box 5.5   Where to find the evidence

- Libraries
  - Librarian
  - Databases, e.g.:
    - BNI (British Nursing Index)
    - CINAHL (Cumulative Index to Nursing and Allied Health Literature)
    - Cochrane database
    - DARE (Database of Abstracts of Reviews and Effectiveness)
    - ERIC (Educational Resources Information Centre)
    - MEDLINE (Medical Literature Analysis and Retrieval System on line)
    - NAHL (Nursing and Allied Health Literature)
- Clinical audit departments
- Professional bodies, e.g. RCN, NATN, AODP, Royal College of Surgeons
- Information technology centres
- Expert advice
- Voluntary and support organizations
- The NHS Centre for Research and Dissemination (NHS CRD) (York)
- Local universities

---

after attendance at study days and courses is also highlighted. Subscription to research journals is important, for example the *Journal of Advanced Nursing* and *Journal of Advanced Perioperative Care*, as well as the *British Journal of Perioperative Nursing* and *Technic*, which have topics of interest as well as articles that include literature searches completed by others. Such research could create a focus for discussion at the journal meetings.

EVALUATING THE EVIDENCE

EBC cannot occur unless practitioners are skilled in reading, critiquing and analysing research findings. Perioperative practitioners must feel comfortable with the research process, so that they feel confident evaluating and critically appraising the literature available. This is discussed in the chapter on research. To address some of these issues, courses are currently being developed to train staff in the critical appraisal of research. A 4-day workshop run by the Foundation of Nursing Studies (accredited by the RCN) has proved to be very useful. Muhall et al[32] found that 90% of Registered Nurses who had attended the course had the confidence to apply research to practice afterwards, which is particularly impressive, as 85% had had little or no experience of research. For those unable to attend such courses, there is a wealth of literature to assist those less experienced to undertake the review process.[40][42]

IMPLEMENTING EVIDENCE-BASED CARE – PUTTING THE RESEARCH FINDINGS INTO PRACTICE

Putting the research findings into practice can be difficult as it involves changing practice – not only your own but, more demandingly, that of others. Managing change is a topic in itself and there is a wealth of literature available on the subject (for example Wright[43]). The *Effective Health Care Bulletin*[44] is devoted to reviewing the literature. It incorporates getting agreement, getting others involved, giving information, and supporting staff in the process as well as auditing the change in practice to check that it is effective.[45,46] Good communication is essential so that the change process can be planned, and careful consideration of colleagues is paramount, as some staff will welcome a change in practice whereas others may feel threatened by possible alterations in the status quo.

Box 5.6   Monitoring the implementation process

- Initiating implementation
  - Present to management the evidence and proposed changes
  - Agreement to change by staff, management, etc.
  - Preparation of a new policy and procedure document
- Planned change circulated to all staff
- Assessing resource implications
- Develop an action plan
- Implementation
- Evaluation and audit change in practice
- Give feedback to staff

Sackett et al[30] acknowledge that there are four stages to implementing evidence-based practice:

- Identify the problem
- Find the answers through a literature research and critical appraisal
- Implement the changes
- Evaluate the changes.

Box 5.6 is a template for monitoring the implementation process.

EBC provides a framework to question care to make sure it is effective. The most important factor is to ensure that staff are working in an environment that allows them to question their clinical practice and be research minded. Whenever care is given staff need to ask: 'Is this the best way to meet the patient's needs?' If it is not, or you are not sure, then use clinical expertise and research to identify and implement evidence-based care.

BARRIERS TO IMPLEMENTATION OF EVIDENCE-BASED CARE

No matter how much staff are motivated to implement evidence-based practice (EBP) in their department there are many barriers to overcome, from finding time to access the evidence, to convincing others that it should be implemented. Cole et al[46] believe that there are two main barriers to evidence-based practice: that perioperative practitioners have insufficient authority to change care procedures, and that there is a general lack of awareness of relevant research. However, as more and more staff are now

undertaking further study at levels 2, 3 and 4 a greater understanding of how to undertake literature reviews and interpret research should make it easier. Changing and challenging others' practice is probably the most difficult issue; involving them in quality circle meetings may help so that they feel involved in any such decisions. Newman et al[47] have divided barriers into two types, organizational and cultural.

ORGANIZATIONAL

- EBC a low hospital management priority
- Difficulties with teamwork
- Inadequate professional development for staff
- Difficulties in accessing the evidence
- Lack of resources
- Inadequate systems for dissemination
- Lack of innovation.

CULTURE AND PRACTICE

- Motivation to change cannot be assumed
- Ill-defined roles among staff
- Culture in which questioning practice is inhibited.

This emphasizes the importance that staff be well motivated and well supported. Support needs to be provided by all levels of professionals with whom staff are working. It also requires commitment in resources, both financial and, more importantly, of time. This is becoming increasingly difficult in the present perioperative environment of shortages of staff and cost-reducing incentives. However, giving evidence-based care to the perioperative patient is vital. It is a major contribution in providing quality health care, as it provides a framework for questioning our practice, which should be to the benefit of patients.

CLINICAL EFFECTIVENESS

Clinical effectiveness (CE) is another term that is often used, but what is it and how does it differ from evidence-based care? CE is simply ensuring that the care that a patient receives is effective, of high quality and the best value for money, and beneficial. It is fundamental that care given is evidence/research-based for it to be effective. This needs to be supported by education and training, and audits will investigate whether it is effective.

DEFINITIONS

The objective of EBC is to make it more clinically effective, so evidence-based care contributes enormously to clinical effectiveness. Clinical effectiveness has been defined as: 'The extent to which clinical interventions, when developed for a particular patient or population, do what they are intended to do, that is, to maintain and improve health and secure the greatest possible health gain from the available resources'.[48]

The RCN have also defined CE as: 'Applying the best available knowledge, derived from research, clinical expertise and patient preferences, to achieving optimum processes and outcomes of care for patients'.[31]

The terms evidence-based care and clinical effectiveness are often used in conjunction, which can cause confusion. Kitson[31] emphasizes that experts often define the former as a problem-solving tool, whereas more popular authors use it to mean clinical effectiveness. To achieve CE, the government has introduced a framework of clinical governance within NHS organizations in an attempt to guarantee quality services to patients.[1,12,13] This means that how effective care is clinically, as well as how cost effective it is, should be evaluated against national standards. For care to be clinically effective teamwork between all professionals working in the perioperative environment is essential so that clinical information can be shared. Doctors and perioperative practitioners must work collaboratively, sharing each other's knowledge and recognizing the complementary roles that they play in giving individualized quality care. In order to provide CE perioperative practitioners must question their practice in order to improve the outcome for the patient. For example, is it better to shave patients preoperatively or should we be using depilatory creams to prevent the risk of infection? (Most research indicates that shaving causes micro skin abrasions that can predispose to infection.) The mnemonic 'PICO' (patient, intervention, comparison, outcome) can assist in determining CE[49] (see Ch. 9).[49]

PATIENT INVOLVEMENT

In order for care to be clinically effective it is important to involve patients in planning and evaluating their care and to confirm whether they are receiving care that is effective and acceptable to them. In the above example it would be important to ask the patient whether they would prefer to be shaved or to use depilatory cream.

Although it is difficult for patients to evaluate the care they receive during their surgery if they are undergoing a procedure under general anaesthetic, many operations are now performed under local and spinal anaesthesia so patients are awake throughout. Preoperative and postoperative visiting enables patients to discuss any concerns and express their opinions and wishes; patient satisfaction surveys and complaints assess whether patients feel their needs are being met. Patient focus groups are another channel that may facilitate frank discussion. It must be remembered that a lack of complaints or criticism does not mean that patients feel they are receiving excellent care, as some patients are frightened to express their displeasure for fear that staff could become prejudiced against them.

PATIENT OUTCOMES

This is a way of monitoring whether actual practice has been effective.[50] There are many ways in which this can be assessed[51] and patients need to be involved in the process. Clinical audit can be used as a tool to achieve this as well as patient questionnaires. For example, a perioperative practitioner may feel that the analgesia administered to a patient in recovery has been effective, but unless the patient is asked and agrees with this, the analgesia given cannot be assumed to be truly effective.

BENCHMARKING

Benchmarking has been defined as 'professional consensus of best achievable practice'.[52] It allows practitioners to compare the care they are giving with that of others in similar clinical environments. For example, perioperative practitioners should discuss with their patients how they could meet their need for privacy. A comparison group could be set up in which a group of practitioners who work together explore an area of practice that they have identified to compare actual practice against ideal standards recognized by the benchmark. Chapter 7 of *Making a Difference*[1] suggests clinical practice benchmarking as a method to enhance the quality of care. This paper was followed by the document *Essence of Care*,[50] which gives guidelines on how to assess standards of care, and includes

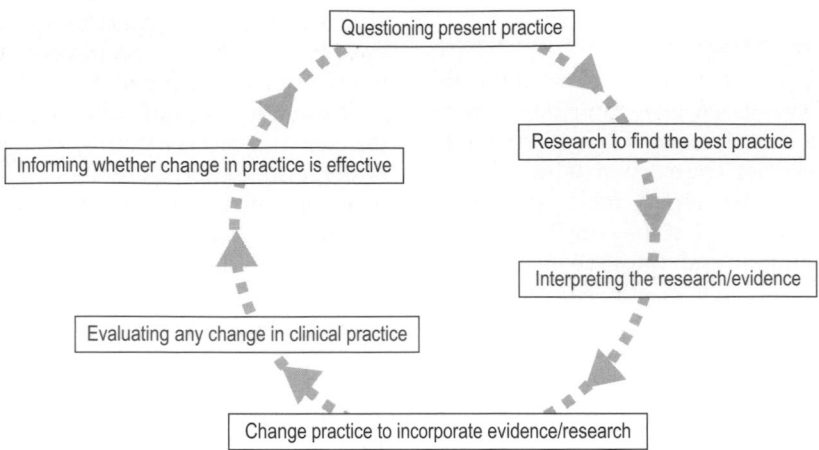

Figure 5.5   The clinical effectiveness. (Modified from Adams[53])

standards for benchmarking eight areas of patient care with instructions for scoring them and using the results to make improvements. It aims to support practitioners in achieving the standards that patients want in fundamental aspects of care, such as pressure ulcers, privacy and dignity. Benchmarking is one of several approaches that can be used to assess standards and help practitioners improve the quality of care they are giving their patients.

CLINICAL EFFECTIVENESS CYCLE

To ensure that care is clinically effective, it is important not only to assess whether the care that is currently being administered can be improved, but also to evaluate whether any change in practice that has resulted is of benefit to patients. Evaluation should be built into any planned change. Evaluation is a process of making a detailed assessment of what has been achieved and how it has been achieved, what is good or bad, and how it can be improved (Fig. 5.5).[53]

Below is a case history as an example of how practice can be improved by questioning it.

Case history: double vs single gloving

Jenny Jones, a junior perioperative practitioner, questioned why double gloving by the surgical team was routine practice in orthopaedic surgery but not in other specialties. The surgical team informed her that double gloving reduced the risk of infection to both staff and patients, as the use of power tools made glove puncture more likely, which increased the chance of transmission of infection. Jenny then questioned the practice of single gloving in other specialties, as she felt that surely staff should reduce the risk of infection to all staff and patients, and recognized that other specialties also used instruments that could make glove puncture likely.

Research to find best practice
Jenny Jones undertook a literature search to investigate the effectiveness of surgical gloves and whether single or double gloving was more appropriate regardless of the specialty. She also investigated current glove leakage and puncture rates.

Interpreting the research/evidence
Jenny concluded from the literature that perforation rates with single gloves were up to 91% and could be reduced to 2.5% if double gloving were used.[38] This could reduce the risk of exposure of the scrub teams to body fluids from 20.8% to 2.5%.[38] She concluded that all the surgical team should double glove for their own and their patients' protection. As care needs to be cost efficient for it to be clinically effective, she investigated the cost of double gloving and found that it would be more cost effective to use the integrated double glove system that incorporated a coloured inner glove, as this was cheaper than using two pairs of traditional gloves.[38]

Disseminating the information
Jenny organized a meeting with all the staff, including surgeons and the theatre manager, to inform them of her findings. The research she had found convinced them that they should be wearing double gloves that

incorporated a coloured inner glove in all specialties rather than just orthopaedics.

Evaluating any change in clinical practice
Three months after the surgical team had double gloved in all specialties an audit was undertaken which concluded that the amount of blood leakage on the hands of the surgical team had dramatically reduced.

Informing whether change in practice is effective
Jenny informed staff of her findings. All staff concluded that it was cost effective and of benefit to both patients and staff for the surgical team to continue to double glove for all specialties, rather than just orthopaedics.

Therefore, by asking a simple question, practice can be improved to become more clinically effective.

To succeed in providing care that is clinically effective, perioperative practitioners, patients and theatre managers need access to the research that has shown what care is effective, and should then support any change in practice that is indicated. This needs to be monitored to confirm that the care is effective and patient care improved. This process requires teamwork between all professionals working in the perioperative environment. It would be useful for any audits such as Jenny's, as well as any research completed, to be disseminated as widely as possible so that other hospitals can benefit from it. This would avoid wasting time by replicating similar studies in different hospitals. Publication in journals such as the *British Journal of Perioperative Nursing* or *Technic* is a good way to disseminate information.

IMPLEMENTATION OF A QUALITY PROGRAMME

Interprofessional collaboration and teamwork are essential if the care of patients is to be improved. For example, it is no good concluding that it is better to double glove when scrubbed if surgeons are not prepared to do this.

CONCLUSION

Quality is a difficult concept to measure and understand, particularly as the number of different terms used can create confusion. Giving quality care that is cost effective is every health professional's responsibility. Perioperative practitioners must continue to really examine, analyse and continually question their practice against new and validated research, so that patients can benefit from the excellent care available. The future of perioperative practice is bright as long as the excellent practitioners already working in the operating department continue to grasp new opportunities, teach others, and learn from each other. Working as a team with other health professionals and patients so that patients feel informed and in control of their care should ensure that the quality of care continues to improve. Patients have a right to expect the highest standards of care possible, and in this age of litigation perioperative practitioners would be foolish not to comply with this. This is in the patients' interest, and it is they that we are here for.

References

1. Department of Health. Making a difference. London: DOH; 1999
2. Department of Health. Designed to care: renewing the NHS in Scotland. London: DOH; 1997.
3. Department of Health. Putting patients first in Wales. London: DOH; 1999.
4. Department of Health. Fit for the future: a consultation paper on the future of the HPSS (Health and Personnel Social Services) (in Ireland). Belfast: DHSS; 1998.
5. Baker R. Principles of quality improvement: Part 1 – defining quality. J Clin Govern 2001; 9: 89–91.
6. National Audit Office NHS (England). Summarised accounts 2002–2003. Online. Available: http://www.nao.org.uk/publications 26 May 2004
7. Ovretveit J. All together now. Health Service J 1994; 104: 24–26.
8. Maxwell JR. Quality assessment in health. BMJ 1984; 288: 1470–1472.
9. Donabedian A. Evaluating the quality of medical care. Millbank Med Q 1996; 4: 166–206.
10. Star A. Quality and quality assurance. In: Hind M, Wicker P, eds. Principles of perioperative practice. London: Churchill Livingstone; 2000.
11. Department of Health. The patient's charter. London: HMSO; 1991.
12. Department of Health. A first class service: quality in the new NHS. London: HMSO; 1998.
13. Department of Health. The new NHS, modern, dependable. London: HMSO; 1997.
14. Department of Health. The NHS plan. A plan for investment. A plan for reform. London: HMSO; 2000.

15. Sale DNT. Quality assurance: A pathway to excellence. Basingstoke: Macmillan; 2000.
16. National Prescribing Centre. Implementing NICE guidance: a practical handbook for professionals. Abingdon: Radcliffe Medical Press; 2001.
17. Nightingale F. Notes on nursing. London: Harrison, 1858.
18. Aitken LH, Smith HL, Lake ET. Lower Medicare mortality among a set of hospital nursing. Image 1994; 22: 72–74.
19. Robson M. Quality circles – a practical guide. Aldershot: Gower, 1984.
20. Sale DNT. Is quality assurance in nursing research based? NT Res 2001; 5: 416–425.
21. Lugon M, Secker-Walker J. Clinical governance: making it happen. London: RSM Press; 1999.
22. National Health Service Management Executive. NHSME letter (93)104. Clinical audit in hospital and community health services. London: HMSO; 1993.
23. Malby B. Clinical audit for nurses and therapists. London: Scutari; 1995.
24. King S. Managing quality assurance in private practice: how to improve standards of patient care. Eur J Chiropractic 2001; 46: 93–94.
25. Hudson B. Making time for clinical audit. Prof Nurse 2001; 16: 26.
26. Cabinet Office. Getting it together: a guide to quality schemes and the delivery of public services. London: MBO; 2001.
27. United Kingdom Central Council for Nursing, Midwifery and Health Visiting. Code of professional conduct. London: UKCC; 1992.
28. United Kingdom Central Council for Nursing, Midwifery and Health Visiting. Guidelines for professional practice. London: UKCC; 1996.
29. Department of Health. A vision for the future: the nursing, midwifery and health visiting contribution to health and healthcare. London: HMSO; 1993.
30. Sackett DL, Rosenburg WMC, Gray JAM, et al. Evidence based medicine. What it is and what it isn't. BMJ 1996; 312: 71–72.
31. Kitson A. Using evidence to demonstrate the value of nursing. Nurs Standard 1997; 11: 34–39.
32. Mulhall A, Le May A, Alexander C. Research based nursing practice. Nurse Educ Today 2000; 20: 435–443.
33. Briggs A. A report of the Committee on Nursing. Cmnd 5115. London: HMSO; 1972.
34. McSherry R, Haddock J. Evidence-based healthcare: its place within clinical governance. Br J Nurs 1999; 8: 113–117.
35. Beyea SC. Why should perioperative RNs care about evidence based practice? AORN J 2000; 72: 109–111.
36. Bernthal EMM. Wedding rings and hospital acquired infection. Nurs Standard 1997; 11: 44–46.
37. Bernthal EMM. Inadvertent hypothermia prevention: the anaesthetic nurse's role. Br J Nurs 1999; 8: 17–25.
38. Bernthal EMM. Two gloves or not two gloves? Br J Perioper Nurs 2000; 10: 102–107.
39. Department of Health. Achieving effective practice. London: DOH; 1998.
40. Papadopoulos M, Rheeder P. How to do a systematic review. South African J Physio 2000; 56: 3–6.
41. Polit DF, Hungler BP. Nursing research principles and methods, 6th edn. Philadelphia: Lippincott; 1999.
42. Sindu F, Dickson R. Literature searching for systemic reviews. Nurs Standard 1997; 11: 145–147.
43. Wright S. Changing nursing practice, 2nd edn. London: Arnold; 1998.
44. National Health Service Management Executive. The effective care bulletin. London: HMSO; 1999.
45. Taylor M. Evidence-based practice in the perioperative environment. In: Hind M, Wicker P, eds. Principles of perioperative practice. London: Churchill Livingstone; 2000.
46. Cole N, Tucker LJ, Foxcroft DR. Benchmarking evidence-based nursing. NT Res 2000; 5: 336–345.
47. Newman M, Papadopoulos I, Sigsworth J. Barriers to evidence based practice. Clin Effective Nurs 1998; 2: 11–20.
48. National Health Service Management Executive. Promoting clinical effectiveness: a framework for action in and through the NHS. London: HMSO; 1996.
49. McCaughan D. Clinical effectiveness as a dynamic process. Prof Nurse 2001; 16: S3–S5.
50. Lipp A. Clinical effectiveness: practical solutions for the new agenda. Br J Theatre Nurs 1998; 8: 32–34.
51. Department of Health. Essence of care. London: DOH; 2001.

Further reading

Adams C. Clinical effectiveness: part five – evaluating clinical change. Comm Pract 2000; 73: 435–438.

Cabinet Office. Getting it together: a guide to quality schemes and the delivery of public services. London: MBO; 2001.

Department of Health and Social Security. NHS management enquiry. London: HMSO; 1983.

Department of Health. Clinical audit: meeting and improving standards in health care. London: HMSO; 1993.

Department of Health. Health service of the talents. Developing NHS. London: DOH; 2000.

Department of Health. National performance frameworks. London: DOH; 1998.

Department of Health. Working for patients. London: HMSO; 1990.

Department of Health. Working together, learning together – a framework for lifelong learning for the NHS. London: DOH; 2001.

Kopp P. Fit for practice. NT 2001; 97: 45–47.

National Health Service Management Executive. Clinical audit: 1994/1995 and beyond. London: HMSO; 1994.

National Health Service Management Executive. Risk management in the NHS. London: HMSO; 1993.

Nelson A. Unearthing evidence of clinical effectiveness. NT 2001; 97: 39.

NHS Executive. Achieving effective practice: a clinical effectiveness and research information pack for nurses, midwives and health visitors. Leeds: NHS Executive; 1998.

Richmond J. Scoring for success. Prof Nurse 2001; 16: 1266–1267.

Squire S. Building a culture of evidence-based care. Prof Nurse 2001; 16: S2.

United Kingdom Central Council for Nursing, Midwifery and Health Visiting. Professional self-regulation and clinical governance. London: UKCC; 2001.

United Kingdom Central Council for Nursing, Midwifery and Health Visiting. Fitness for practice and purpose. London: UKCC; 2001.

Websites

www.medicalaudit.co.uk/
www.ubht.nhs.uk/clinicalaudit/
www.doh.nhsweb.nhsuk/clingov.htm
Evidence-Based Nursing Journal
http://www.evidencebasdnursing.com

Cochrane Centre
http://hiru.mcmaster.ca/cochrane/
NHS Centre for Reviews and Dissemination
http://york.ac.uk/inst/crd

Useful contacts

Association of Operating Department Practitioners (AODP)
112 Malling Street
Lewes
E Sussex
BN7 2RJ
Tel: 01870 7460984
Fax: 01870 7460985
Email: office@AODP.org

National Association of Theatre Nurses
Daisy Ayris House
6 Grove Park Court
Harrogate
HG1 4DP
Tel: 01423 508079
Email: hq@natn.org.uk
website:www.natn.org.uk

Cabinet Office
Quality Schemes Team
Modernising Public Services Group
Trisha Greenhalgh
Room 3.16
Admiralty Arch
The Mall
London SW1A 2WH
Tel: 020 7276 1722
Fax: 020 7276 1704

Centre for Evidence Based Nursing
Department of Health Studies
University of York
Genesis 6
York Science Park
York YO10 5DQ

NHS Centre for Reviews and Dissemination
University of York
Heslington
York YO1 5DD

RCN Nursing and Midwifery Audit Information Service
20 Cavendish Square
London
W1M 0AB

Scottish Intercollegiate Network Administration Support Group (SIGN)
Royal College of Physicians
9 Queen Street
Edinburgh
EH2 1JQ

Getting Research into Purchasing and Practice (GRIPP)
Project Manager
Anglia and Oxford Regional Office
Old Road
Headington
Oxford
OX3 7LF

Departments of Health in UK

England:
Department of Health
Quarry House
Quarry Hill
Leeds
LS2 7UE
Tel: 0113 254 5000
Fax. 0113 254 5800
www.doh.gov.uk

Scotland:
Scottish Executive Health Department
St Andrew's House
Regent Road
Edinburgh
EH1 3DG
Tel: 0131 5568400
Fax: 0131 2442683
www.scotland.gov.uk

Wales:
NHS Directorate
Crown Buildings
Cathays Park
Cardiff
CF10 3NQ
Tel: 029 2082 5111
www.wales.gov.uk/index.htm

Northern Ireland:
Central Services Agency
25 Adelaide Street
Belfast
BT2 8FH
Tel: 028 9032 4431
Fax: 028 9066 8989

Chapter 6

Information management

Paul Whatling

Key points

- Data systems
- Information management
- Utilizing information in perioperative practice

The expression 'information management' is used so freely in modern society that it is easy to assume that everyone knows what is meant by the term 'information'. Most know when information is presented or available, but how does this fit in with everything else that we do?

We are used to dealing with data in many forms when working in health care. The Oxford English Dictionary defines a datum as 'A thing given or granted; something known or assumed as fact, and made the basis of reasoning or calculation'. It is important here to note that the word data is the plural – a misunderstanding commonly seen when people talk and write about data.

So what is information? Smith[1] declared that '... data are random facts, whilst information is the ability to earn (or learn) from such random facts ...' thus suggesting a hierarchical nature. Indeed, it is easy to give examples from health care: the numbers 85 and 50 mean little by themselves, but if you are told that they represent the systolic and diastolic pressures in mmHg of a preoperative patient you immediately infer that you are dealing with a hypotensive patient. Thus the raw data presented have been transformed into information.

As you progress through training you will acquire a knowledge and understanding of how to deal with the low blood pressure, so again we are

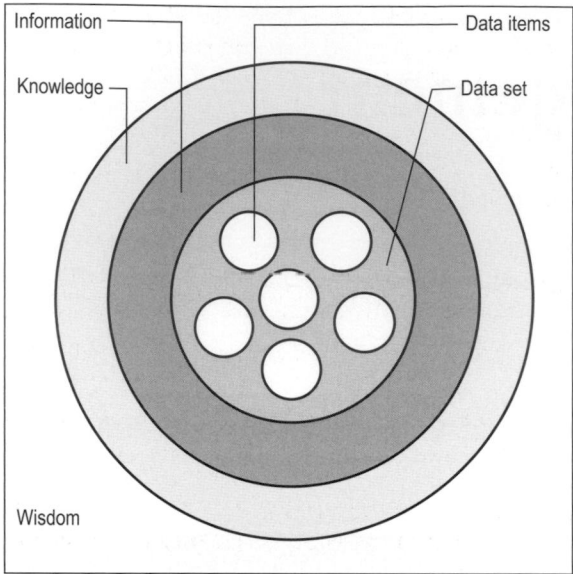

Figure 6.1   Hierarchical relationships.

demonstrating a hierarchy from data through to information and on to knowledge. You will be aware that hypotension may be a result of hypovolaemia, and so infusion of fluids may be appropriate to correct the deficit, but knowing which fluid to give and at what rate often only comes as a result of experience. This refinement of knowledge may be referred to as wisdom.

Some will suggest that the hierarchy from data through to wisdom is a linear one, but probably a better model is that proposed by Godbout,[2] in which he refers to a hierarchical interrelationship between the concepts, with each higher level encompassing the lower ones within it (Fig. 6.1).

The issue of how to manage information is therefore closely related to the management of those data from which information may be derived, and in general the two are inextricably linked. This chapter will explore the issues concerning the storage of data and how this inevitably affects the information that can be derived, but also how a determination of information requirements can help in the design of storage systems. Having developed a strategy for the storage of data, and having defined the information needs, the natural next step is to consider what can be done with the information, how it can be used, how it can be communicated, how it can be evaluated, and how we can pass on information to our patients.

THE ELECTRONIC AGE

It would be unwise not to acknowledge early on in this chapter just how much of an impact the electronic revolution has had on information management in health care. However, it is equally important to stress that the principles that govern the quality management of information apply regardless of whether the medium used is electronic or not. The benefit of electronic systems is that they offer greater access to information, but its management is no different.

It is really only in the last few years that computers have become ubiquitous in operating departments in the UK. Certainly 'dumb terminals' have been around for 15 or more years, allowing access to patient administration data, but it is now common to see highly interactive programs on network desktop PCs allowing scheduling of lists, tracking of patient progress and coding of procedures.

DATA STORAGE

Before we can examine the management of the information, we need to consider some of the issues regarding storing those data from which the information will be derived. Where will they be stored? What will be stored? Who will have access? These are all issues that must be considered prior to developing any information management system.

If you stop and consider what sort of data may be collected in an operating department, you will appreciate that some will be highly sensitive and confidential. Often such data identify details of a personal nature in individual patients, and so there is a need to keep such details confidential and to maintain privacy while allowing access to the data and information where appropriate.

In the UK, the 1998 Data Protection Act addresses these issues,[3] and the full document is available on the Internet. A detailed discussion is beyond the scope of this chapter, but the eight main principles are listed in Box 6.1. Of significance is that this Act specifically extends to include all data that are collected – even paper-based records. The Act covers all data that may be collected on an individual, and focuses on the need to ensure accuracy in collection and the avoidance of processing data without specific consent or need. Processing may be defined as any manipulation of the data in any way, and might include the compilation of a list of patient names, for example into an operating list schedule.

Processing of data within the constraints of the Act is a necessary part of life in managing the information in any operating department. However, the data that may be available to the theatre teams may be very sensitive, and there is therefore a need to maintain confidentiality over and above any data protection. This represents an extension of the seventh principle of the Data Protection Act. In 1997 a team led by Dame Fiona Caldicott published a report on the use of identifiable patient information. The principles to be applied in managing such data are summarized in Box 6.2. The recommendations of the report were implemented in England and Wales and many have been implemented in Scotland too. In summary the recommendations are that there is a single identified 'guardian' in each Trust or health authority who is responsible for ensuring that there is a clear policy for the management of confidential information and that there are mechanisms in place for ensuring that the policy is effective and adhered to.

CROSS-BOUNDARY DATA TRANSFER

Probably one of the biggest revolutions about to take place in health care in the UK since 1948 is the development of a seamless integrated care record service. The feasibility of this is greatly enhanced with developments over the past few years in networking technology and infrastructure, with the advent of high-bandwidth and high-speed data links, which are increasingly wireless.

The ease of transferring data and particularly sensitive or confidential patient data opens up many new issues for the healthcare professional who holds some personal responsibility for the protection of those data. It is true, though, that in general the data held electronically are no less secure than those that were previously held on paper – after all, these could be photocopied and passed on to others, or simply passed around in their original form. However, it is true that data in electronic format are often easier to pass on, with less effort being required and, with the ubiquitous nature of email and personal computers, often less concern as to where such data might be stored by the recipient. The fact is that the issues and responsibilities of the end user are no different in the electronic age than with the previous paper-based systems.

In fact, in many ways it is possible to make data more secure in the electronic age, using secured access systems and also by tracking usage activity, thus enabling an audit trail of access to data and information – something often not possible with paper-based notes. If security and access measures became too draconian it would become impossible for the healthcare system to work effectively, and therefore a balance has to be found between acceptable access and sufficient security. There is often no clear dividing line, and this is recognized in the wording of both the Data Protection Act and the Caldicott guidelines.

Obligations to the other statutory bodies, e.g. the Courts, the Coroner or the police, are unchanged when the data are stored in electronic format.

WHAT DATA SHOULD BE STORED

Although the easy answer would be 'everything', that is often not practical and certainly not always useful. A good clinical example is the measurement of blood pressure in theatre through an arterial cannula: it is possible to record the blood pressure in the patient every few milliseconds and to store these data for analysis later. However, one has to ask if this is really of any use: why would we need such detailed data? Who could possibly want to analyse the change in blood pressure over a period of milliseconds, when perhaps seconds or 10 seconds would be equally valuable? Likewise, in many straightforward cases, blood pressure may be recorded at only 5- or 10-minute intervals. Thus in each surgical case, and at defined points during that case, the anaesthetist decides on the best frequency for collecting data on blood pressure according to the need at that time.

This model can be extended to all data that are collected in health care: it is of no value to collect data that will never be used. There is, though, one very important caveat, which is that it is often not possible to obtain data retrospectively if they were not collected in the first place. Thus it is vital that in determining what data should be collected due consideration be given to the information that will be required at a later date. It is this process of determining the need for information that forms the foundation of good management of that information.

The needs assessment process must take into account the requirements of those who will be using the data and information, and also must consider the impact on those collecting the data. As part of the process it is important to consider carefully how the information will be used, how the data collected will be audited for quality, and how any information will be communicated between practitioners and out to patients.

WHAT WILL BE DONE WITH ALL THE INFORMATION?

In the operating department environment, as in much of health care, the uses to which we put information can be divided into several categories:

- Audit of events and actions
- Decision support, process, reporting and review
- Communication and dissemination
- A foundation for seeking further information.

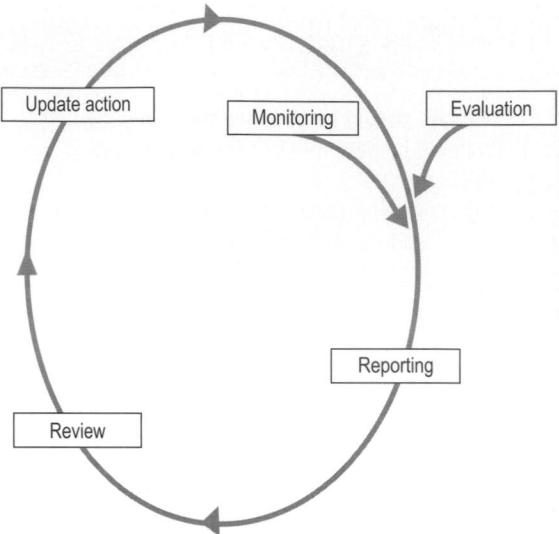

Figure 6.2 The audit cycle.

For each case, a review will be made of the ways in which we can look to effectively manage information, and how the advent of modern computing technology facilitates the process.

AUDIT OF EVENTS AND ACTIONS

In many ways the role of audit can be seen as fundamental to the process of information management. The principles of audit will be familiar to most readers, as will the audit cycle diagram in Figure 6.2. The processes of quality assurance and audit are discussed in detail in Chapter 5.

One of the biggest tasks facing any practitioner who wishes to audit some aspect of work in an operating department is the difficulty in obtaining reliable data. Anyone who has trawled through old dusty theatre ledgers will vouch for the challenges in interpreting handwriting from some years previously, and the lack of consistency in describing fairly standard procedures. Certainly one of the biggest gains from modern computerized systems is that they allow prospective collection of data that can be subsequently reviewed without the manual labour.

The need to review case-mix data has forced a move away from free text descriptions of procedures (as used to appear in the old ledgers) to the standardized approach of coded data using coding schemes such as the International Classification of Diseases (ICD10) and the Office of Population, Censuses and

Box 6.3   Coding schemes

The most commonly encountered schemes may be divided into two categories:

Enumerative

These attempt to list every possible eventuality and attach an alphanumeric coding. There are many possibilities and these lists can become very long and complex.

Examples include ICD-10 (International Classification of Diseases), OPCS (Office of Population, Censuses and Surveys) and Read Codes (before 3.1). These range from the highly specific to the rather general:

- ICD-10
  V32.22 – Occupant of three-wheeled motor vehicle injured in collision with two- or three-wheeled motor vehicle, person on outside of vehicle, non-traffic accident, while working for income
- OPCS-4
  L87.5 – Local excision of varicose vein of leg

The two main difficulties related to these schemes are:

1. The potential for multiple codes that to the practitioner may mean the same things – for example L87.4 is the OPCS code for avulsions of varicose vein – when should this be used and when should L87.5 be used?
2. Difficulty finding a code – either because it does not yet exist or because the route to finding it may not be intuitive, e.g. Tuberculosis of the Lung in ICD-10 is only listed under infectious diseases and not under diseases of the lung.

Compositional

These attempt to resolve some of the issues above by creating a fixed and controlled list of terms which can be linked by the coder with linkage terms such as: ACTS_ON, BY_MEANS_OF, HAS_LOCATION.

These can be constructed to give codes such as: wart-REMOVED_FROM-leg-BY_MEANS_OF-electrocautery. Each of these terms has a code and by building in this way it is possible to develop a complex coding framework with billions of combinations with a relatively small number of terms. There will still be the same potential difficulties of finding codes and also the ability to easily generate nonsense codes, and there are some concerns from clinicians and practitioners over the implementation of these schemes. Perhaps the best known is SNOMED CT (Systemized Nomenclature of Medicine – Clinical Terms), which has been jointly developed by the College of American Pathologists and the NHS (incorporating READ 3.1 and the earlier SNOMED RT).

Surveys classification of surgical operations and procedures (OPCS4) (Box 6.3). Such coding schemes facilitate the comparison of data within and between units and, when linked with outcome data, can prove a valuable resource. The information available from coded data will only be as good as that entered, so it is essential that those entering the data have full training and the necessary understanding of the procedures and processes to be effective.

Many modern systems allow the collection of data continuously and automatically, thereby reducing the likelihood of input errors and missed reports. Furthermore, modern systems can also be designed to monitor the data that is input dynamically, often flagging up to the end users when something is of concern or needs attention. This is a feature of modern anaesthetic equipment that is taken for granted in modern practice, but would you have considered using a similar system to monitor swab usage, patient waiting times or stock monitoring?

So, if computers are so good at monitoring and collecting data, why do we need any human input at all into the information management process? The big problem is usually encountered at the review stage of the audit cycle – all the computers can store all the data, but unless there is human interaction and work to review the data and consider how to implement changes in practice, the computing technology is of no value. One of the best examples of this to be seen in the UK in recent years was the high level of mortality after paediatric cardiac surgery in Bristol in the early 1990s. A recent report by the Bristol Royal Infirmary Enquiry noted: 'Bristol was awash with data. There was enough information from the late 1980s onwards to cause questions about mortality rates to be raised both in Bristol and elsewhere had the mindset to do so existed.' The first five and the last five words are the crux of this very powerful statement – what an important lesson for us all to learn.

DECISION SUPPORT, PROCESS REPORTING AND REVIEW

Questions about decision support will often be answered by practitioners with reference to clinical support systems, for example scoring for appendicitis, or whether to administer thrombolytic drugs to cardiac infarct patients. These systems are important, and computerization of the question, answer and decision process can save valuable time and improve consistency by removing some of the flexibility so often enjoyed by practitioners; whether this is a good thing is debatable. However, a major area of decision support that is often ignored is in process management and process support. The processes of health care are numerous and interlinked in complex ways, and include everything from staff management to stocks and supplies and patient movement control. The role of an Accident and Emergency department duty manager has been likened to that of an air traffic controller at Heathrow, with patients coming in from various directions, circling through various stages of investigation and treatment, before final dispatch in any number of different directions. The same may be said of many an operating theatre suite.

You might ask whether computers can really make very much difference to these processes – after all, modern-style operating departments have been working well for over 100 years (the oldest operating theatre in the UK is in St Thomas' Hospital in London, and was used from 1822 – well before the days of Lister and antisepsis[4]).

The key is in the design of the systems – if the processes of care are properly mapped and understood, it is possible to design systems that will not only facilitate those processes, but also allow for audit and review with a view to implementing changes. Probably the biggest obstacle to date has been the failure to work towards integration of all the systems that are already in place. How many times have you seen a patient's name being entered on a paper-based or computerized system for a typical routine operating list? Would it not be better if there was one central record for patient care that was updated at every event? No longer would the ward staff need to be informed verbally about the sutures used in the skin – this would be entered on the system by the surgeon and that information would be instantly accessible to the ward staff, the GP and the practice nurse, together with a request for a booking appointment to have that suture removed.

Perhaps this is a rather Utopian view, but the technology is certainly available to allow this sort of process management and support. In England, several billion pounds have been set aside to deliver an integrated healthcare system along these lines, and it is only by having the Utopian vision that we can start to move forward.

COMMUNICATION AND DISSEMINATION

Of course it is all very well having all of this information on processes, patient care, mortality, morbidity and numerous other measurable outcomes, but this is of no use unless it is communicated, not only to the staff and healthcare professionals, but also to the patients.

Communication may be through a number of routes, including the traditional paper-based printout of information, but the advantage of electronic systems is the dynamic monitoring of processes and the option for reporting of sudden changes or important developments, or where certain events fall outside a normal range.

This is known as exception reporting, and will be familiar to anyone who has watched a pulse oximeter in theatre for any period of time. The oximeter quietly monitors blood saturation, but every time the recorded level drops below a certain value an alarm sounds, and also, if the machine malfunctions, an alarm sounds. These machines have sufficient reliability that it is perfectly safe not to sit and observe them continuously.

It is not, then, a major step to extend this sort of exception reporting system to some of the other processes in health care – an email notification to an operating department manager that stocks of a particular suture are running low, or that the usage of a given instrument in the last month exceeds the current capacity of the sterile services department. If you then add in the option to code procedures or track staff activity it is clear just how much difference computers can make to the running of an operating department. The major difficulty, though, is in the design of these systems and the prime requirement to ensure that they are fit for purpose and do meet the needs of those actually working in the clinical situation and take into account the working and social practices there. The needs assessment process has often been carried out poorly in the past, but the recognition of its importance is now firmly ingrained: 'Past experience suggests that efforts to introduce clinical information systems into practice settings will result in failures and unanticipated consequences if their technical aspects are emphasized and their social and organizational factors are overlooked'.[5]

As information becomes easier to access, so too can it be disseminated more easily to those outside the immediate clinical environment. This is seen particularly with the recent vogue for league tables of performance in many activities and outcome-related data – particularly from surgical procedures. The ability to generate aggregated statistics at the local, regional and national levels at the 'press of a button' serves as an example of just how accessible information can now be. In parallel with this, there is the formal and informal publication of scientific and research work into the public arena.

We are thus living in an age in which information is available in enormous quantities.

A FOUNDATION FOR SEEKING FURTHER INFORMATION

Anyone who has searched for information – in any format – will be familiar with the experience of following trails and pathways that are of interest, often well away from the original subject. This can be an interesting and enjoyable experience, but also frustrating where achieving the primary goal is delayed. It is inevitable that as more information becomes available from the healthcare process, people will want to study the areas in more depth, explore different avenues and add further to the body of knowledge. The search for information may well be related to a piece of work – perhaps for research purposes – or for audit and development, and is often facilitated now through the use of computerized inventories and cataloguing systems. Whatever the purpose, searching for information should be a structured and planned process in order to achieve the best results.

SEARCHING FOR INFORMATION

There are four main steps in this process:

1. Identify the question that you wish to answer
2. Identify the most likely sources of information for this question
3. Use the relevant search tools to seek the information
4. Apply your search results in your work and review the effectiveness of your strategy.

The first of these is often the most important: 'An approximate answer to the right question is worth a great deal more than a precise answer to the wrong question.' (After John Tukey, late Professor of Statistics at Princeton, USA, credited with inventing the terms 'bit', ubiquitous in modern computing, and 'software').

In days gone by, identifying the most likely sources would involve lists of journals, newspapers and books, often stored in dusty archives. With the increasing use of technology, information is becoming ever more accessible without the need to trawl manually through such archives. Many people are now familiar with the use of the Internet as a means to search for and access information. Search engines are most frequently used and you can read about these online at www.searchenginewatch.com. A more detailed review of search engines is beyond the scope of this chapter.

One of the big problems with using search engines as a means to retrieving healthcare-related data is that the results are often very non-specific, may be totally unrelated to the subject, and there is no measure of quality on many sites. Determining the quality of a website is often a subjective activity in any case – for example the latest update from the Chief Medical Officer posted on the Department of Health website might be taken as very high quality, whereas some of the sites encountered at www.quackwatch.org are likely to inspire less confidence.

Organizations such as the non-governmental 'Health on the Net' or HON Foundation (http://www.hon.ch) state that their mission is to guide laypersons or non-medical users and medical practitioners to useful and reliable online medical and health information. This is achieved through a system of voluntary registration and conformance to a defined set of ethical standards, but is still a long way off becoming the norm.

In addition to using open search engines, it is increasingly common for healthcare professionals to access specialized search databases, often containing detailed catalogues of scientific papers and publications. Such reference lists have been available for a century or more, but in the last 20 years they have become increasingly available in electronic format – originally as compact discs with access limited to libraries, and increasingly now over the Internet and accessible to all, sometimes with a fee, sometimes free of charge.

One of the best known free examples is PubMed, produced by the National Library of Medicine in the USA (http://www.nlm.nih.gov). This contains tutorial material and other related information that provides a helpful introduction to the principles of searching the database and other equivalents. E-learning and training can be a very effective way of disseminating information to disparate groups who may be geographically separated. As with other forms of electronic communication, many of the principles governing this are identical to those in the face-to-face situation. The advantages are principally related to the improved speed of communication and asynchronous access for students, together with an increased level of automated monitoring and exception reporting of the delivery processes.

SUMMARY

This has been a rather whistle-stop tour through some of the key areas of information management. Clearly there is much more one could write about and discuss in a more specialized chapter. It is hoped that this chapter has encouraged you to think and reflect on what we do with data and information in health, and particularly how it impinges on your role in the operating department setting. If this is an area that interests you, there are a number of good courses (many now partly or wholly online) in the UK – for a full list, see the British Medical Informatics Society website at www.bmis.org.

The key message has to be that you should always be thinking about information – what do you need, how can you record it accurately, and what can you do to make it accessible to others with whom you work?

References

1. Smith D. System engineering for healthcare professionals. Half module 216 workbook. Cardiff: Cardiff Institute for Higher Education; 1995.
2. Godbout A. Filtering knowledge: changing information into knowledge assets. J Systemic Knowledge Management 1999. Online. Available: http://www.tlainc.com/articl11.htm
3. Data Protection Act 1998. London: HMSO. Online. Available: http://www.hmso.gov.uk/acts/acts1998/19980029.htm
4. The old operating theatre. 2003. Online. Available: http://www.thegarret.org.uk/
5. Anderson JG. Clearing the way for physicians' use of clinical information systems. Communications of the Association for Computing Machinery 1997; 40: 89.

Chapter **7**

Infection control principles

Diane Gilmour

Key points

- Principles of microbiology
- Transmission of infection
- Prevention and control of infection in the perioperative environment
- Review of current perioperative clinical practices in relation to infection control

INTRODUCTION

The prevention of infection is pivotal to the provision of a safe environment for staff and patients. Microorganisms inhabit the human body, invade tissue and cause disease, yet preventative measures by perioperative practitioners and other healthcare professionals have ensured that such invasion is kept to a minimum in today's operating theatre environment. The changing nature of surgery, technology, and the advancement of anaesthetic and recovery techniques must not detract from the skills and knowledge required by all staff to ensure that the principles of asepsis and infection control are practised in all clinical areas daily.[1,2]

The spread of infection occurs within a sequence of events known as the chain of infection (Fig. 7.1). The aim of preventing and controlling infection is to break the chain by interrupting or removing one or more events.

This chapter will:

- Outline the impact of hospital-acquired infection on both staff and patients
- Briefly describe the theory behind each of the events in the chain

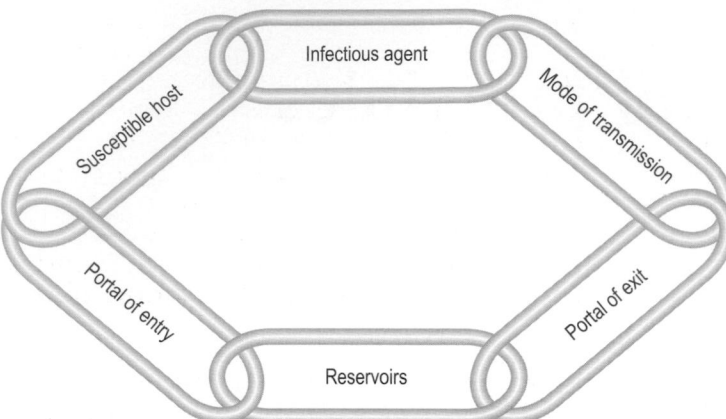

Figure 7.1   The chain of infection.

- Discuss the preventative strategies that can be or are implemented in the operating theatre suite
- Review the literature on infection control methods, including the principles of asepsis, to offer practitioners the opportunity to question and evaluate their current practice.

Infection, in particular hospital-acquired infection, has over the past few years dominated media headlines with 'superbugs' and 'unclean hospitals'. The government has responded to this by announcing and implementing various strategies to minimize the risk to patients, for example Patient Environmental Action Teams, who inspect hospitals on a regular basis, scoring them on the state of their cleaning; the development of national evidence-based guidelines for preventing hospital-acquired infections; a National Audit Office investigation into the management and control of hospital-acquired infection in acute Trusts in England; and the Nosocomial Infection National Surveillance Scheme (NINSS). Such strategies and their subsequent guidance or conclusions have been utilized and applied to the perioperative setting within this chapter.

HOSPITAL-ACQUIRED INFECTION

Over the years health care and its treatment of diseases, medical conditions and surgical interventions has evolved and improved, resulting in an increase in patients' life expectancy. The health service is now successfully treating more acutely ill patients, who are older and have more complex medical problems; such patients are therefore more vulnerable and susceptible to acquiring a nosocomial or hospital-acquired infection (HAI).

This is an infection that is acquired or develops as a result of treatment while the patient is in hospital or another healthcare setting, but which the patient was not suffering from or incubating at the time of admission.[2]

It is estimated that 9% of patients have a hospital-acquired infection at any one time,[3] and that a further 19% develop an infection after discharge.[4] Plowman et al[4] estimate that patients' hospital stay is 2.5 times longer for those who develop a HAI, and that these patients are 7.1 times more likely to die in hospital, depending on characteristics such as age, pre-existing diagnosis and admission specialty.

For the healthcare system the financial burden from HAI cannot be underestimated. In 1986 this was estimated at £111 million,[5] yet Plowman et al[4] estimate that in England this is now £986 million – 9% of the national budget for acute, elderly and obstetric services in England.

The operating theatre department is synonymous with principles of asepsis and aseptic technique, yet nearly 11% of all hospital-acquired infections are found in surgical wounds.[5] In the first national survey in 1980 this figure was 18.9%, and the significant fall in incidence may be due to improved surgical technique, the increased use of antibiotics and the decrease in contamination from microorganisms (for example improved bowel preparation). Ongoing surveillance of surgical site infections reported that the average wound infection for large bowel surgery was 10.6 per 100 operations, compared to 2.5 for total hip replacements and 1.9 for abdominal hysterectomies.[3] Perioperative practitioners may not be aware of the surgical site infection rate until there is a problem, yet 50–70% of surgical wound infections occur post discharge.[3] Madeo et al[6] surveyed day surgery patients and found that 6.1% developed an infection post discharge, the highest rate being in those who had undergone varicose vein surgery. Prolonged procedures, excessive handling and damage to tissues, and poor technique are still important risk factors in the development of surgical wound infection.[2,7]

The incidence of HAI may be seen as a quality indicator of a hospital's performance for both patients and the organization. Prevention is therefore key in ensuring a high-quality service, and this is an important focus for each hospital and its infection control programme. Hospitals will develop audits, targets and objectives for surveillance, review infection control policies, and plan educational activities.[2]

MICROBIOLOGY

Microbiology is the study of living organisms, usually 0.1–1.0 mm in diameter, which cannot be seen by the naked eye or require magnification to view detail.[8]

Microorganisms are found everywhere, often performing essential functions such as in the manufacture of drugs and the production of foodstuffs, as well as harmlessly inhabiting the human body. However, when circumstances and conditions are optimal microorganisms may invade the human body, resulting in an infection (Box 7.1).

Microorganisms are classified in groups, depending upon their similarities in structure, with the first name denoting the group or genus and the second the specific name within that group – the species – such as *Staphylococcus aureus* or *Clostridium difficile*.[2]

The study of microorganisms includes bacteria, viruses, fungi, algae and protozoa, but for this chapter the emphasis will be on bacteria and viruses, as these are the major causes of infectious disease in the operating department environment.

BACTERIA

Bacteria are single-celled organisms with a singular circular deoxyribonucleic acid (DNA) chromosome which multiply by binary fission, that is, the one chromosome becomes two identical copies each within a new cell. However, environmental conditions must be optimum for each bacterium to mature, and these are influenced by nutritional and physical factors (Box 7.2).

Bacteria are classified according to the properties of the cells (Box 7.3, Table 7.1).

VIRUSES

A virus is the ultimate example of a parasite as they are dependent on their host to replicate. A virus is not a cell but a simple strand of nucleic acid (genetic

---

Box 7.1   Definitions

- PATHOGEN – a microorganism that can invade the body and cause disease
- INFECTION – a pathogenic microorganism enters the body, invades the tissues and multiplies, and can cause an infection or disease depending on the host's response to that invasion. The adverse effects of the microorganism entering the body and multiplying are recognized as the signs and symptoms of infection: inflammation, pain, swelling, heat, vomiting, diarrhoea, increased secretions, depending on the affected site
- PATHOGENICITY – the ability of each microorganism to invade and multiply, depending on the environmental conditions and availability of nutrients
- VIRULENCE – a measure of the ability of a microorganism to establish an infection; dependent on a variety of factors and properties that each microorganism possesses – bacteria have slime, or enzymes, or fimbriae or capsules which enable them to adhere to any surfaces, or prevent penetration by the body's defence mechanisms

---

Box 7.2   Nutritional and physical factors for the growth of bacteria

- Energy – usually from the breakdown of carbon compounds
- Nutrients – carbon, nitrogen and inorganic ions
- Water – most die without water, but some are resistant to drying out or form spores
- Temperature – those bacteria associated with the human body multiply at 35–40°C
- pH – most prefer to multiply in neutral solutions pH 5–8
- Concentration of solution – bacterial wall is able to withstand strong and dilute solutions, and within each cell maintains the desired levels of solutes in the cytoplasm
- Oxygen – bacteria vary in their need for oxygen to generate energy. An anaerobe is one that grows in the absence of oxygen and will be killed when exposed to air. A facultative anaerobe is one that grows in the presence or absence of oxygen. An aerobe requires oxygen

material) with a protein coat. They are very small and can only be seen using an electron microscope. Viruses need the genetic material of the host cell to replicate their own, and therefore can only multiply inside living cells. The virus is copied many times within the host cell before being released. The host cell then may be destroyed, but viral infections are short-lived as the host cells quickly multiply and attack the virus. However, some viruses leave their nucleic acid in the host's DNA, where it remains until optimum conditions for cell division occur, thereby causing repeated infections; for example, the varicella zoster virus remains dormant in the nerve ganglion following chickenpox, and when reactivated causes shingles; the herpes simplex virus lies dormant in local nerve cells, reactivating as eye infections or 'cold sores'. Some viruses can cause permanent damage, such as human immunodeficiency virus (HIV), which depletes the immune system.[2,8]

SOURCES AND RESERVOIRS

An infection is the outcome of microorganisms invading and multiplying in tissues and can be transferred from another person or object, or from within that person themselves (Box 7.4).

Microorganisms exist everywhere – in soil, on plants and in and on our body surfaces – yet very few are pathogenic. Some microorganisms inhabit the deep crevices of the skin, sweat glands and hair follicles, as well as internally, and are known as 'normal flora', commensals or resident microorganisms. They prevent pathogenic microorganisms from invading the site and causing disease, are harmless in their own environment, but are potentially pathogenic when transferred to another part of the body (endogenous infection): for example, *Escherichia coli*

Box 7.3   Classification of bacteria

- CELL STRUCTURE – rigid cell wall made of a network of carbohydrates and amino acids which determine the staining properties of the cell, its pathogenicity and the shape
- SHAPE – three distinct shapes: cocci (spherical), bacilli (cylindrical) and helical cells curved like a comma – vibrio – or several curves/spirals – spirilla or spirochaete
- STAINING – Gram-positive bacteria have a thicker cell wall which retains the stain and Gram-negatives discolour the counterstain
- SPORE FORMING – some bacteria, particularly bacilli, when exposed to changes

---

Box 7.4   Infections and definitions

ENDOGENOUS INFECTION – microorganisms that are part of the normal flora cause an infection as a result of impaired defences, or the organism is introduced to an area where it does not usually occur
EXOGENOUS INFECTION – microorganisms acquired from outside the body from another person, object, animal or the environment

---

Table 7.1   Common bacteria and their properties

Bacteria	Properties	Location	Infection
Staphylococcus aureus	Cocci (bunch of grapes) Gram-positive bacillus Facultative anaerobe Non-spore forming	Hair, skin, nasopharynx	Abscesses, wounds, urinary tract, septicaemia
Escherichia coli	Gram-negative bacillus Facultative anaerobe Non-spore forming	Gastrointestinal tract	Urinary tract, wounds
Clostridium difficile	Gram-positive bacillus Anaerobic Spore forming	Gastrointestinal tract	Wounds, hospital-acquired gastrointestinal infections
Neisseria meningitidis	Cocci (in pairs, diplococci) Gram-negative Non-spore forming	Nasopharynx (10% of population carry pathogen)	Meningitis, septicaemia

inhabits the intestines but will cause a urinary tract infection if it enters the bladder (Table 7.1).

Some pathogenic microorganisms enter and invade the body, establishing themselves in a particular site, but do not cause disease. This is known as colonization, and the individual who is colonized is a carrier. Hepatitis B virus can infect the person but not manifest symptoms; 10% of the population carry *Neisseria meningitidis* in their nasal cavity but do not have the signs and symptoms of meningitis.[2]

Additional microorganisms are located on the surface of the skin and are extremely efficient routes for the transmission of infection. Transient microorganisms are easily transferred through direct contact with other people, equipment and body sites to and from hands, and have been implicated in outbreaks of methicillin-resistant *Staphylococcus aureus* (MRSA), respiratory and enteric viral infections. Transient microorganisms are easily removed with good handwashing and cleaning techniques, and practices that will be discussed later in this chapter.[2,8,9]

PORTAL OF ENTRY

The human body has many natural barriers to prevent the invasion of microorganisms – the skin, conjunctiva, lysozymes in tears, the acidity of the stomach, the mucosal lining of the body systems and commensals all defend the body from penetration by a pathogen. Once a microorganism has invaded, it may establish itself at the site of entry or move to another location depending on its own nutritional and growth needs. Once it is established, an infection may occur if the microorganism is able to overcome the body's immune response to that invasion.[2,8] Microorganisms find a variety of

routes to invade the body (Box 7.5), but for the patient undergoing surgery the body's integrity is immediately breached during the management of the airway or the surgical incision.

TRANSMISSION

Fairchild[1] identified that most infections occur postoperatively because the patient's immune system is compromised, their natural defences – mainly the skin and mucous membranes – having been breached, but also through contamination from the environment.

Transmission is the mechanism by which microorganisms are transferred from one place or person to another; however, they are unable to do this themselves and require assistance. The ability of the microorganism to transmit, breach the body's defences and then establish an infection is dependent on its virulence and pathogenicity. For practitioners, establishing the source and the route of transmission is vital to controlling the infection. Transmission can be divided into direct and indirect contact.[1,2,10]

Fluids or body surfaces of an infected individual can be transferred to a susceptible host through direct contact, such as mother to baby in utero. Kissing an infected individual, or contact with respiratory secretions, for example sneezing (tuberculosis, influenza, the 'common cold') may result in the transfer of infection.[2]

Indirect contact occurs when a susceptible host is in contact with contaminated material from another source (object, person). The infected material may be in the air, dust, on the skin or on instruments.

In the hospital environment the commonest route of contact is human, mainly through hands, and this can result in the direct or indirect (touching of contaminated objects then another person) spread of infection. Effective handwashing and scrupulous aseptic technique are efficient ways to break the chain – both are discussed in this chapter.

PORTAL OF EXIT

A microorganism, once having entered, must be able to leave the body in order to continue transmitting the infection to another host. The route of exit is not always the same as that of entry, but secretions and excretions are all important sources of infection. Some microorganisms enter through the mouth and leave through faeces (*Salmonella*), whereas

---

Box 7.5   Some portals of entry

- Inhalation – dust and water droplets carry microorganisms from patients, staff and the environment, and enter the body through the respiratory tract: tuberculosis, influenza
- Inoculation – accidental (needlestick) or deliberate (skin incision, injections) breach of the skin or mucous membranes; also bites: hepatitis B virus, staphylococcal wound infection
- Ingestion – invasion by microorganisms through contaminated water or food into the gastrointestinal tract: *Salmonella*, campylobacter, cholera

another may enter through the nose and respiratory tract and leave the same way (tuberculosis).[2]

SUSCEPTIBLE HOST

All patients undergoing a surgical procedure become susceptible hosts as their immune system is compromised and their defences breached; however, some patients are more vulnerable than others. Mangram et al[7] outlined categories of those patients (Box 7.6) who may be more susceptible to developing a wound infection, and Wilson[2] cited Bowell's patient infection risk assessment tool, both concluding that actions based on such assessments would minimize the risk of potential complications postoperatively.

Box 7.6   Patient risk factors

- Age
- Nutritional status
- Medical history (diabetic, on steroids, obese, vascular disease, liver or renal disease)
- Skin condition
- General hygiene
- Prolonged preoperative stay
- Surgical procedure (type, duration, antibiotic prophylaxis)
- Surgical technique
- Presence of drains, catheters, colostomy or implants
- Intubation

(Adapted from Mangram et al[7])

PREVENTION STRATEGIES

The prevention and control of infection in the operating department is vital to minimize the risk to and preserve the health of patients and staff. All operating department practices related to environmental control focus on achieving an absence of postoperative infection[1,11] and breaking the chain of infection (Fig. 7.2).

THEATRE DESIGN

The design of an operating department is guided by national and professional guidelines (health building notes; design briefing systems), with the size being determined by the function and needs of each individual hospital. Each operating department is divided into zones to control the movement in, and entry to, the theatre environment of staff, patients, visitors, supplies and equipment. The flow of traffic from a clean zone to a dirty one is to prevent cross-contamination between areas,[1,2,10] and the Hospital Infection Society Working Party (HISWP)[12] identified that the cleanest areas were the theatre and lay-up rooms, yet East[13] suggests that research to justify such divisions is limited, and that the education and discipline of staff is more important in reducing and controlling the risk of infection. Movement of staff and patients through the theatre should be reduced to minimize the risk of airborne contamination, theatre doors should be closed to maximize the efficiency and effectiveness of the ventilation system, and walls, floors and doors constructed of robust materials to withstand cleaning and require minimal repair.[1,10,13]

A transfer area or 'holding bay' may be available to receive patients in the department. In the past,

Figure 7.2 Prevention strategies breaking the chain of infection.

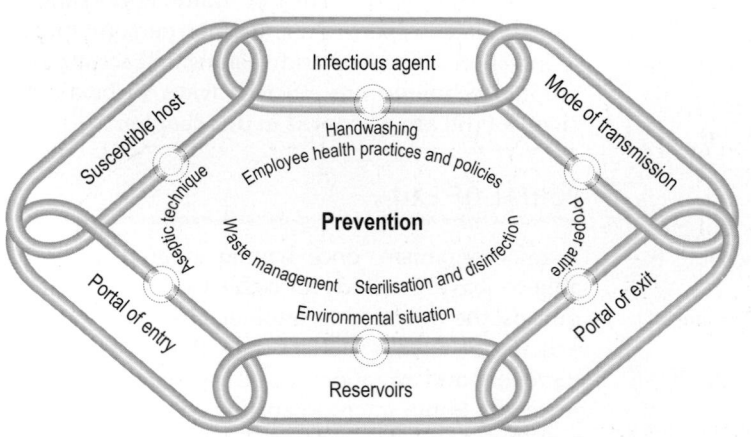

theatre entrances were delineated by red lines and/or adhesive 'tack mats'. Troare et al[14] concluded that bacterial floor counts in a unit were not influenced by the use of an adhesive mat, and Lewis et al[15] showed that transferring a patient from a ward to a theatre trolley did not affect the bacterial count within the theatre itself. The HISWP[12] stated that although moving a patient on their bed in theatre does increase the bacterial floor count, this has limited significance in increasing wound infection rates.

VENTILATION

Airborne contamination in the operating department can be controlled by filtration and ventilation. The ventilation system is designed to control the temperature and humidity of the operating theatre and to dilute microbial contamination and expired anaesthetic gases in the air by effecting at least 20 air changes per hour without recirculation, and by moving air from clean to less clean areas.[1,12,13] Airborne particles may contain dust, skin squames and respiratory droplets, and the level of contamination is dependent on the movements of personnel in the area.[7] Wilson[2] identified that 300 million skin squames are shed per day, and that the main component of dust is skin squames. About 10% of these carry microorganisms, and smaller particles remain airborne for several hours. Large particles may settle on surfaces, furniture or equipment. Smaller respiratory droplets also remain airborne for several hours and may be inhaled.[2] One air

change (every 3 minutes as a minimum) will reduce airborne microbial contamination by 37%.[12]

Ultraclean ventilation systems are used when the risks and consequences to the patient of developing an infection are greater, for example in orthopaedic prosthetic surgery, and provides clean, filtered air vertically on to the sterile field from a filter bank or diffuser directly above the surgical field.[2,7,13]

Mangram et al[7] reviewed research studies on the effectiveness of ultraclean systems and concluded that although infection rates were reduced, the reduction was similar to the patients being given prophylactic antibiotics.

To maintain a positive pressure inside the theatre, forcing old air out of the room through vents close to the floor is vital for an effective and efficient ventilation system, and this can be achieved by ensuring that staff close doors and limit movements within the theatre. The aim of closing the theatre doors is to reduce the movement of personnel and hence reduce microbial airborne contamination, but also to prevent corridor air mixing with cleaner operating room air.[16] Sampling of bacterial counts has allowed researchers to either dispel (red lines, sticky mats) or prove the effectiveness of clinical practice. East[13] found variations with bacterial counts, depending on staff movements and the closing of doors (Fig. 7.3). Ventilation systems must be checked and filters changed regularly.

A temperature of 37°C and high humidity is optimal for the replication of most bacteria, therefore keeping the temperature lower, at 20–24°C, and

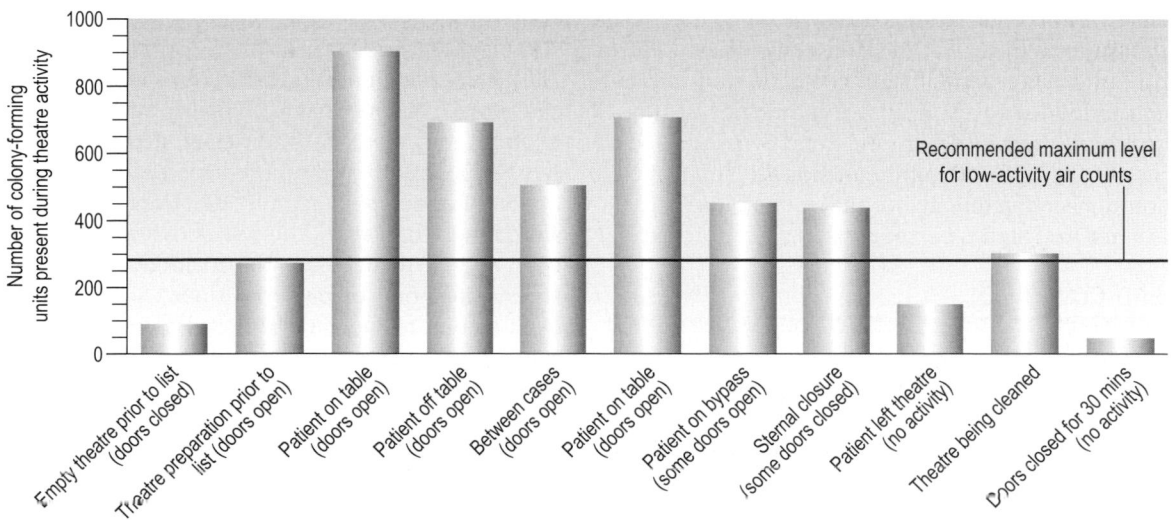

Figure 7.3 Microorganism air counts during different theatre activities. (Reproduced with permission from East[13])

maintaining humidity at 50–55% may inhibit bacterial growth. Patients and staff are able to tolerate low temperatures, and for staff this is comfortable to work in; however, certain patients may require an increase in temperature to prevent hypothermia.[1,10,13]

SURGICAL ATTIRE

Maintaining a clean and safe environment is the aim of all healthcare workers in the operating department, yet they too can be a source of microbial contamination. Microorganisms are shed from exposed skin, hair and mucous membranes, and to minimize the risk to patients, surgical team members wear appropriate clothing.

Scrub suits are preferable to dresses, as they are less likely to cause microbial contamination through open and loose clothing. It is important and research demonstrates this.[7,17] Clothing should be made of a close-woven fabric, such as cotton and polyester, to act as a barrier to prevent the transfer of microorganisms between patients and staff, and laundered at high temperatures without shrinkage or gross deterioration of the fabric. Hospital policies may restrict the personal laundering of scrub suits, but all personnel must wear a clean suit daily, and this must be changed immediately or as soon as possible if it becomes visibly soiled or contaminated (Fig. 7.4).[7,13,17]

Debate continues concerning the wearing of scrub suits outside the operating department, and whether there is a need to wear a cover gown or coat.

The National Association of Theatre Nurses (NATN)[17] recommends that 'all personnel should change into outer clothes when leaving the perioperative environment and don a new set of theatre attire on their return'. The HISWP[12] found insufficient evidence to show that this practice reduced surgical wound infection rates, and concluded that the wearing of theatre attire outside the department should be reflected in hospital policy, to include patients' and staff's perceptions of such practice.

HEAD COVERING

Disposable head covers in different designs and colours are available for all theatre personnel to wear. Made of lint-free materials, they ensure that all head hair is covered and provide a barrier to minimize the risk of microorganism dissemination from staff to patients. However, counter-arguments suggest that an efficient ventilation system would

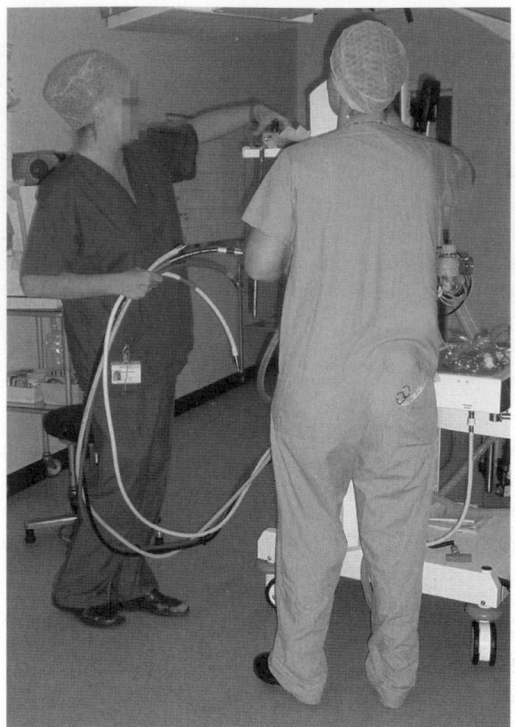

Figure 7.4   Practitioners in scrub suits.

reduce bacterial contamination from hair and skin squames.[18] HISWP[12] recommends that only scrub practitioners and those involved during prosthetic procedures need wear head covers, yet Mangram et al[7] cite wound infection outbreaks isolated from the hair or scalp despite the use of head covers during the procedure.

FOOTWEAR

All theatre personnel should be provided with special protective footwear which is comfortable, easy to clean, and worn only in designated areas. Footwear should also be provided for visitors and students. Theatre shoes should be cleaned daily and stored in a clean area. The use of overshoes has not been shown to decrease the incidence of surgical wound infection or bacterial floor counts, but has been shown to increase bacterial counts on hands during donning and removal. The wearing of overshoes should therefore cease.[7,12,18]

PRINCIPLES OF ASEPSIS

Asepsis is the absence of pathogenic microorganisms on living tissue, and operating team members perform procedures to eliminate and exclude such microorganisms. The correct cleaning of surfaces and equipment and adequate environmental controls all ensure microbial contamination is minimized, but a practitioner's knowledge and skills in adopting and adhering to an aseptic technique and maintenance of a sterile field are also vital in controlling the spread of infection. Rowley,[19] in an earlier study, identified that areas such as theatres, synonymous with asepsis and aseptic technique, appeared to demonstrate poor practices, particularly with regard to handwashing. Mangram et al[7] cite numerous studies that clearly illustrate that a lack of aseptic technique and accidental contamination in the operating theatre has been associated with postoperative infections. All practitioners in every specialty are responsible for ensuring that they have the knowledge and skills to maintain the sterile field, that it is not compromised, that accidental contamination is reported and acted upon, that the environment and working surfaces are cleaned appropriately, and that aseptic principles are understood and adhered to by all staff.

HANDWASHING

Hospital-acquired infection may not be eradicated, but many outbreaks may be prevented through effective handwashing.[20] Transient microorganisms are easily removed through handwashing, and therefore it is one of the most important procedures to prevent the spread of infection.[9] Pinney[21] suggests that although perioperative practitioners are diligent and well practised at scrub techniques they may neglect to apply the same diligence to handwashing. The Codes of Conduct[22,23] state that practitioners must ensure that no act or omission on their part is detrimental to the health, safety and wellbeing of the patient.

Practitioners and other healthcare workers must be aware that hands can become contaminated when handling a patient's bedlinen, when caring for a patient's wound, drain or catheter, and during the disposal of linen and waste, as well as contact with their own body fluids (toilet, blowing nose). Wilson[2] states that transient microorganisms on the hands may be indicative of the environment and the patient: for example, practitioners caring for a patient with MRSA may find the pathogen on their skin for a few hours. The potential for transfer to another patient or member of staff during this time is great, and therefore efficient and effective handwashing is vital.

'Hands must be decontaminated immediately before each and every episode of direct patient contact/care and after any activity or contact that potentially results in hands becoming contaminated'

(Standard 20[20])

The agent of choice and the duration for hand decontamination depend on the purpose – that is, for routine handwashing and between direct contacts with patients, soap and water are effective in removing transient microorganisms and rendering the hands socially clean. In contrast, for a surgical handwash/scrub prior to an invasive procedure, practitioners should use an aqueous antiseptic solution that is effective in removing transient organisms as well as reducing resident organisms to a safe level.[2,9,24] These include chlorhexidine gluconate and povidone-iodine. Both work rapidly, offer persistent activity over a long period, thereby maintaining a low bacterial count under gloves, are safe to use and are accepted by healthcare workers. However, most antiseptic agents can dry the skin and cause dermatitis if used excessively and frequently. If hypersensitivity to either solution is experienced then an alcohol rub/gel may be used following a thorough soap and water wash, which removes physical dirt and transient flora. The correct technique is essential to ensure total coverage of the relevant areas, and the alcohol must be allowed to dry. Alcohol may be more effective than aqueous antiseptics, but on its own has little or no residual effect.[2,9,24]

The mechanical action and friction created when the hands are rubbed together removes soil, dirt and microorganisms, but an efficient and effective technique involves exposing all aspects of the hands, wrists and lower arms (in surgical handwashing) to the soap or agent, particularly the tips and web spaces of the fingers and the outer aspect of the thumb (Fig. 7.5).[25]

Complete coverage of the relevant areas with the agent is essential to ensure adequate antisepsis. For routine handwashing this is 10–15 seconds, but for the surgical handwash it is 2–5 minutes. Recommended practices and guidelines for the timing of the latter vary, but manufacturers state that a total contact time of 2 minutes is as effective as 5 minutes (Hibiscrub and Betadine). Each area of practice must decide on its own policy based on the evidence and best practice[2,9,24] to ensure compliance.

The use of a sterile brush, dry or impregnated, during the surgical handwash is also debatable. The brush aims to remove physical dirt and soil from beneath the fingernails, although manufacturers

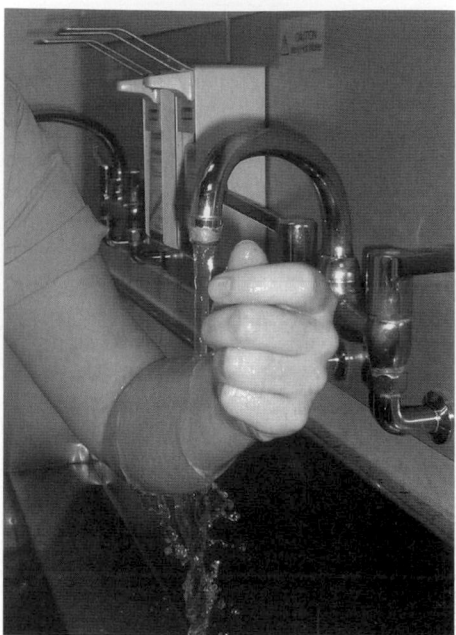

Figure 7.5   Handwashing technique.

now include a nail cleaner with the sterile sponge, which is less abrasive. ICNA recommend that the brush be used on the first application, and only on the nails. Excessive use of the brush may damage the skin, which may increase microbial colonization with resident flora.[9]

Gallagher[26] and Wilson[2] state that skin damage can increase the risk of carriage of pathogenic bacteria, and that therefore to maintain skin integrity hands should be thoroughly rinsed and dried after each wash, and emollient creams or moisturizers applied. Damaged skin, cuts and abrasions must be covered with a waterproof dressing, and practitioners with dermatitis or other skin conditions should be monitored by the occupational health department.

Infection prevention is the goal, irrespective of which antiseptic agent is used or scrub technique practised.

OPERATING DEPARTMENT CLEANING

Cleaning involves the use of detergent and water to remove organic material and its microorganisms. Detergents increase the ability of water to remove soil and dirt by breaking them up. Each hospital should have a policy for the use and dilutions of cleaning solutions, and procedures to ensure correct cleaning methods, as well as maintenance programmes to ensure the regular high-level cleaning of walls, ceilings, floors and other surfaces throughout the operating theatre department.[2]

Within the operating department environment the majority of microorganisms isolated are not harmful and are rarely implicated in outbreaks of wound infection.[1] Practitioners ensure a clean working environment for each patient by cleaning potentially contaminated surfaces in direct contact with the patient, surfaces and equipment involved with the procedure (instrument trolleys), wet mopping the floor, cleaning surfaces after contact with blood and body fluids/tissues, and keeping the doors closed.[2,7,13]

East[13] stated that an operating theatre left unused overnight was virtually sterile before any personnel arrived. Mackrodt[27] concluded that early morning damp dusting did not significantly reduce airborne bacteria, but that routine cleaning reduces and maintains lower levels of *Staphylococcus aureus* throughout the day.

A 'dirty' or known infected case is in practice put at the end of the list and then theatres closed for a period to allow adequate air changes to take place. East[13] and Mangram et al[7] question this, and cite studies that demonstrate no evidence to support such practices. Effective ventilation, positive-pressure air exchanges, adequate cleaning between cases, and efficient and effective decontamination of equipment and instruments diminish the risk of the environment being the source of microorganisms.[13,18] Less than 2% of airborne contaminants from a 'dirty' or infected patient will remain after 12 minutes, therefore resting a theatre for 15 minutes before the next procedure is adequate. In an ultra-clean air ventilated theatre this is reduced to 5 minutes.[12] The HISWP[12] acknowledge that if a 'dirty' or known infected case is scheduled last then this allows adequate cleaning of the environment.

STANDARD PRECAUTIONS

The Control of Substances Hazardous to Health (COSHH) Regulations[28] require employers to assess the risk to staff and patients exposed to and handling any substance hazardous to health, including pathogenic microorganisms.[13,24] Universal precautions introduced in the 1980s to protect healthcare workers from exposure to bloodborne pathogens applied to all body fluids known to transmit or be associated with such pathogens. Such precautions did not include other body substances, which frequently contain other pathogens and may be a major source of infection. The precautions were expanded to

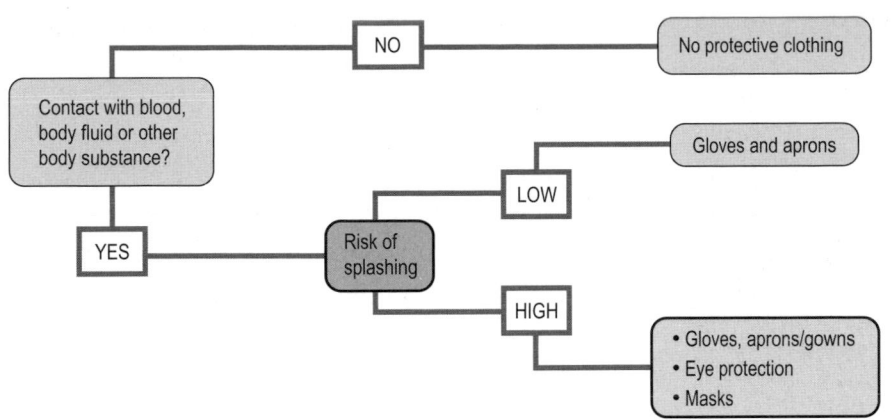

Figure 7.6 Risk assessment and the selection of protective clothing.[2]

include the management and isolation of all body substances, and in 1996 standard precautions replaced universal precautions. These protect patients and healthcare workers from infection risks associated with all body substances.[1,2,13,24]

Standard precautions now recommend that all practitioners and healthcare workers assess the level of risk based on their specific patient activity.[20]

PERSONAL PROTECTIVE EQUIPMENT

Standard precautions recommend the use of personal protective equipment (PPE), including aprons, masks, gloves, gowns and eye protection, depending on the activity and the risk of microbial contamination. Employers have a legal obligation to provide PPE under the Personal Protective Equipment at Work Regulations (1992),[29] and employees should take every precaution to prevent contact with skin and mucous membranes by assessing the risk of exposure to blood and other body substances.[2,24] Protective clothing should be worn when direct contact with body fluids is anticipated, so as to minimize the risk of microbial contamination to both staff and patients[20] (Fig. 7.6).

GLOVES

Gloves protect the hands from contamination while in direct contact with body substances. Gloves must be changed after every procedure (even if several are being performed on the same patient), between patients, and if visibly contaminated. Mahoney[30] found that gloves can reduce the amount of contamination on the hands but do not eliminate it altogether. Since the introduction of universal precautions, healthcare workers have increased their

use of gloves as hand protection, and as a result the number of allergic reactions to latex and cornstarch powder has increased.[31] Latex is preferable owing to its flexibility and resealability. Cornstarch powder was added to gloves to assist in their donning, but practitioners are strongly advised not to use powdered gloves during any healthcare activity.[20] Other materials are available (vinyl, nitrile) and all must comply with European Union (CE) standards, being of an acceptable quality, free from pinholes, and not splitting or tearing easily.[2,20,32] Despite this standard the integrity of the gloves cannot be guaranteed, as many appear to leak and damage may be unseen by the naked eye. Latex has greater resistance to puncture than vinyl, affording greater barrier protection, but alternative materials must be available for those staff and patients who are sensitive to natural latex.[20] The correct removal of gloves at the end of a procedure or following contact with body substances will reduce hand contamination. Gloves should be discarded immediately in a clinical waste receptacle, and the hands washed following removal (see Fig. 7.5).[2] All circulating practitioners dealing with used drapes, specimens, or moving patients from the operating table to trolley or bed after the procedure may be exposed to blood, body fluids and other body tissue contact, and therefore should wear gloves.[18] The increasing use of gloves as protection does not preclude the need for effective handwashing between procedures.[30]

Bernthal,[33] having reviewed the literature, recommends that two pairs of gloves should be worn for every operation. The reason for double gloving is to promote safe practice, protect staff, and reduce the risk of microbial contamination from glove perforation. Bernthal found that gloving perforation rates varied from 38 to 91% when wearing one pair

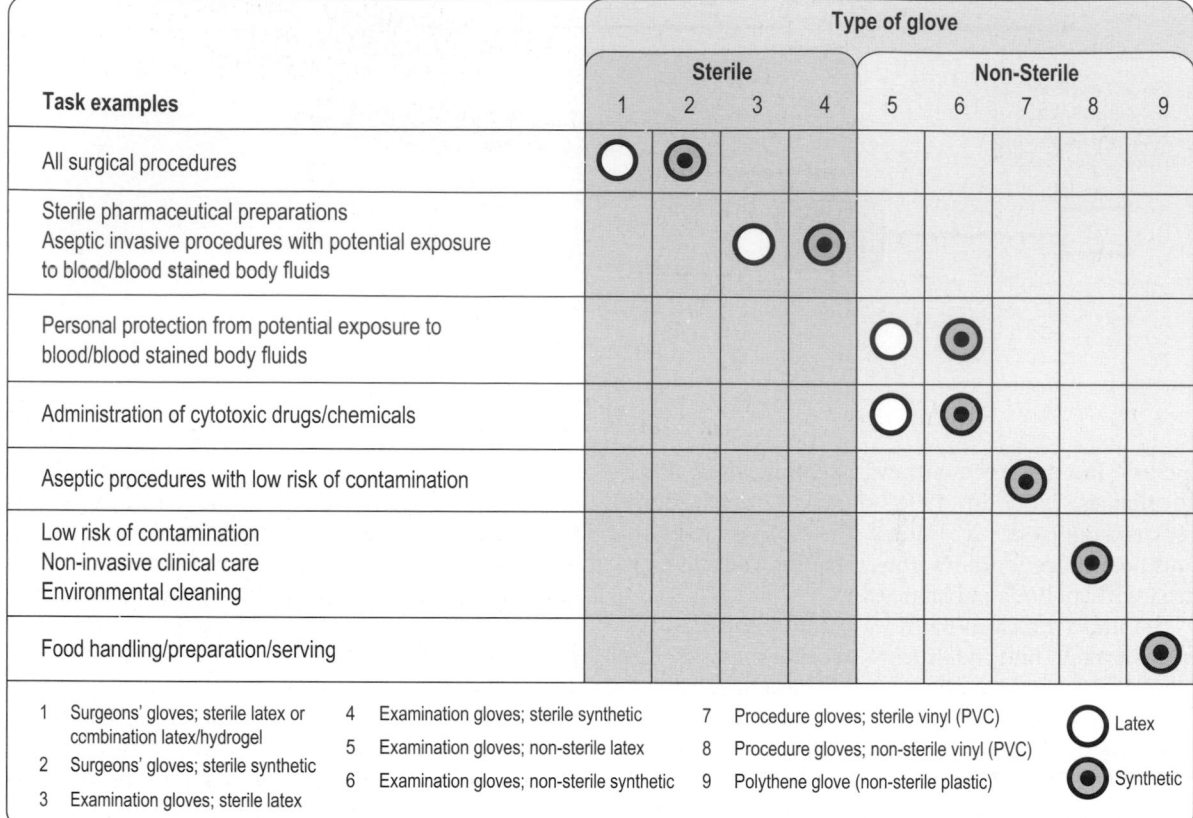

Task examples	Type of glove								
	Sterile				Non-Sterile				
	1	2	3	4	5	6	7	8	9
All surgical procedures	○	◉							
Sterile pharmaceutical preparations Aseptic invasive procedures with potential exposure to blood/blood stained body fluids			○	◉					
Personal protection from potential exposure to blood/blood stained body fluids					○	◉			
Administration of cytotoxic drugs/chemicals					○	◉			
Aseptic procedures with low risk of contamination							◉		
Low risk of contamination Non-invasive clinical care Environmental cleaning								◉	
Food handling/preparation/serving									◉

1 Surgeons' gloves; sterile latex or combination latex/hydrogel
2 Surgeons' gloves; sterile synthetic
3 Examination gloves; sterile latex
4 Examination gloves; sterile synthetic
5 Examination gloves; non-sterile latex
6 Examination gloves; non-sterile synthetic
7 Procedure gloves; sterile vinyl (PVC)
8 Procedure gloves; non-sterile vinyl (PVC)
9 Polythene glove (non-sterile plastic)

○ Latex
◉ Synthetic

Figure 7.7   Making the correct glove choice. (Reproduced with permission of ICNA[32])

of gloves to 2–7% when double gloving, although 60% of perforations remain undetected. The HISWP[12] found that glove perforation did not increase the incidence of infection. Compliance with double gloving is based on a practitioner's personal preference, as many find it uncomfortable and lose dexterity and tactile sensitivity.

APRONS

Plastic aprons are recommended when close contact with the patient may lead to contamination of clothing. In the operating theatre plastic aprons are single-use and discarded and disposed of as clinical waste at the end of the procedure.[20]

MASKS

During a study of 100 caesarian sections Sharma et al[34] found that 23% of scrubbed nurses' masks and 40% of doctors' masks were visibly contaminated with blood splashes. Despite urging staff to

wear protective clothing, they found that in one-third of these procedures staff did not wear goggles or masks. The UK Health Department[35] recommends that masks be worn to prevent exposure to body substances. There are controversy and debate surrounding the efficacy and benefits of wearing a face mask. Edwards[36] reviewed the pertinent literature and concluded that although masks do reduce microbial contamination of the surgical field, their clinical significance to the reduction of surgical wound infections was questionable. Mangram et al[7] also question the benefit to the patient, but identify the benefits of protection to the staff. The HICSWP[12] recommend that scrubbed practitioners undertake a risk assessment and wear masks for their own protection if necessary. The mask should be changed and discarded after each procedure, or if it becomes visibly contaminated with body substances.

'Face masks and eye protection should be worn where there is a risk of blood, body fluids, secretions and excretions splashing into the face and eyes' (Standard 22)[20] (Fig. 7.8).

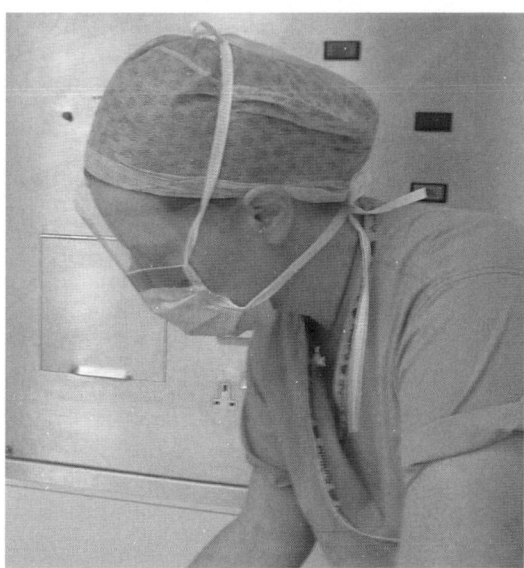

Figure 7.8 Protection for the face and eyes.

EYE PROTECTION

Occupational eye exposure during procedures was significantly higher in those who used no facial protection except a surgical mask.[37] Specific specialties, such as orthopaedics, vascular and cardiovascular, increase the risk to the practitioner of accidental eye exposure,[37] and Sharma et al[34] in their study of caesarian sections, found that 23% of scrubbed nurses' and 40% of doctors' goggles or visors were visibly contaminated with body substances. The UK Health Department[35] recommends that protective eyewear be worn, although anecdotal evidence suggests that practitioners wear eye protection when they are in contact with a high-risk patient or there is a higher risk of body substance exposure. For every procedure the practitioner should assess the risk and take the necessary precautions, but who can foresee the incidence of exposure in any procedure, and should the practitioner or any member of the scrub team wear eye protection no matter what the procedure? (Box 7.7).[37]

THE MANAGEMENT OF WASTE

In England and Wales the average acute hospital of 500 beds produces 10 tonnes of waste a week, including clinical waste.[38] Clinical waste is that which, unless rendered safe, may prove to be hazardous, toxic, or cause an infection to any person coming into contact with it. Clinical waste includes blood bags, human tissue, swabs, dressings, excretions or other body fluids, syringes, needles or sharp instruments if contaminated with the above, and is recovered from hospitals, veterinary practices, surgeries, clinics and pharmacies.[2] The cost of clinical waste disposal is between £180 and £320 per tonne, and costs acute hospitals in England and Wales an estimated £30 million a year.[38] Clinical waste is segregated from household waste to ensure its correct handling, transportation and disposal in accordance with the Environment Protection Act (1990),[39] and to protect staff, patients, the public and the environment from harm. To comply with regulations, hospitals adopted a nationally recognized colour-coding scheme – yellow bags for clinical waste, black for household waste – to ensure that staff segregate waste at source (Box 7.8). All waste transported off site for disposal must be enclosed in approved rigid containers.[2] Staff must be trained in the management and segregation of waste to ensure the wellbeing and safety of staff and patients. Close-suction canisters are single-use disposable units that can be disposed of safely without first disposing of the contents themselves. However, practitioners must ensure that the gel or powder, when used, has solidified the entire contents before disposal, to prevent leakage and spillage.

DISPOSAL OF LINEN

Linen, as clinical waste, must be segregated, transported and disposed of safely in accordance with Department of Health guidelines on Hospital Laundry Arrangements for Used and Infected Linen.[40] Laundry workers sort linen by hand before washing, and it is recommended that linen that may be particularly hazardous (i.e. contaminated with blood, body fluids or excreta) be segregated and placed in water-soluble bags. The bags are then placed directly into the washing machine, thereby minimizing the risk to the laundry worker. The laundry worker may also be at risk of injury if instruments or sharps have been carelessly discarded with the linen. Linen therefore should be labelled at source, so that it can be traced if such an incident occurs.

BLOOD AND BODY FLUID SPILLAGE

Blood and body fluid spillage is a daily occurrence in the operating theatre, and each hospital policy on the management of such occurrences should clearly state the solutions and strengths to be used. Sodium hypochlorite, a chlorine-based solution, is the established one of choice; however, chlorine solutions need to be accurately diluted to be effective (1:1000 for cleaning floors; 1:10 000 for dealing with blood and body fluid splashes). If blood or body fluids are spilt they must be dealt with immediately, but practitioners expose themselves and other healthcare workers to the risk of infection if protective clothing is not worn. A solution of chlorine or the granules must completely cover the spill for a period of time (usually 2 minutes) before being removed with disposable towels and discarded immediately as clinical waste.[2,41] Chlorine compounds themselves also pose a health risk, as splashes may injure the eyes and skin, powders may cause respiratory problems, and in confined spaces toxic fumes may occur.[41] Chlorine should not be used on large urine spillages, as the reaction to the acidic urine releases chlorine vapour.[2,41] Chlorine should not be used on some metals and furnishings, such as operating tables, stools and chairs, as it can corrode the surfaces and tarnish the metal. Chlorine is inactivated by organic compounds such as blood protein, so fresh solutions need to prepared regularly to ensure an effective concentration.

SAFE HANDLING OF SHARPS

Sharps are objects or items that might puncture or pierce the skin when handled, and include needles, bone fragments, blades, sutures, glass, paper and thorns. The safe handling and disposal of sharps forms part of a hospital's clinical waste policy.

- In 1999 Lynda Arnold contracted HIV following a needlestick injury
- Ballard[42] estimates that 25 000–100 000 needlestick injuries occur each year in the UK
- Pratt et al[20] suggest that 16% of all occupational injuries in hospitals are needlestick related
- In a survey[43] 40% of needlestick injuries were sustained by nurses; 20% of all needlestick injuries occurred in the operating theatre.

In the operating theatre the risk of a sharps injury is high, particularly during invasive and surgical procedures, when the passage of scalpels, handling of suture needles and use of sharp instruments such as saws is evident. Sharps injuries can also occur prior to their use, during disposal into an appropriate container, and during disassembly of equipment.[44] Godfrey[43] cited a survey which found that most injuries occurred during the procedure, but 25% took place after use and before disposal.

'Needles and syringes must not be disassembled prior to use or disposal'

(Standard 26[20]).

Solid items such as suture needles and scalpels carry a lower risk of accidental inoculation than hollow sharps such as hypodermic needles.[2] The UK Health Department report in 1998[35] estimated that the risk of transmission of a bloodborne pathogen from an infected worker to an unimmunized healthcare worker following a sharps or percutaneous injury was:

- Hepatitis B virus 1:3
- Hepatitis C virus 1:30
- Human immunodeficiency virus 1:300.

In the USA, legislation in 17 states mandates the use of safer needle devices (automatic needle retraction), and over the past few years manufacturers have developed such devices, for example blade removal devices, safe containers for the storage of sharps, devices to facilitate a no-hands scalpel transfer, and blunt-tipped suture needles.[42,44] Such devices are costly,[44] yet perioperative practitioners can use hands-free techniques for passing sharps[11] by using receivers or trays, which are more readily available within existing resources.

'Sharps must not be passed directly from hand to hand and handling should be kept to a minimum'

(Standard 24[20]).

Double gloving has also reduced the risks of sharps penetrating the skin, thereby minimizing the risk of injury.[33] Almost 40% of sharps injuries in a recent survey occurred while wearing single gloves, 60% when wearing no gloves, but very few when the practitioner was double gloved.[43] Technology cannot prevent sharps injuries, and practitioners' knowledge and skills should ensure a safe working environment by assessing the risks and taking steps to prevent and control those risks.[2,13]

Sharps must be disposed of in a designated container conforming to BS 7320. The units are available in a variety of shapes and sizes, but each must be resistant to penetration or leakage, and made of a material able to be incinerated. Practitioners must ensure that they are sealed when three-quarters full, labelled at source, and disposed of in accordance with hospital clinical waste policy.[2,20]

Perioperative practitioners participate in invasive (exposure-prone) procedures and are at greater risk of acquiring bloodborne viruses through accidental inoculation or splashing to the eyes, mouth or broken skin than many other healthcare workers. However, they are also exposing the patient to an even greater risk by participating in such procedures if they are infected themselves. All practitioners involved in such procedures should be immunized against HBV infection and their response to the vaccine checked. If, after immunization and time, the practitioner does not respond to the vaccine then the occupational health department will assess their risk to patients if they participate in exposure-prone procedures.

Any healthcare worker exposed through a sharps injury must be assessed for their potential risk of infection by the occupational health department or specialist practitioner. All hospitals must have a

---

Box 7.9 Procedure following a sharps injury

- Encourage the wound to bleed
- Wash the area with soap and water
- Cover the area with a waterproof dressing
- Identify the patient the needle or blade was used on
- Inform the person in charge
- Seek advice from occupational health department or out-of-hours Accident and Emergency
- Complete the accident form

---

policy for healthcare workers to follow in the event of such an injury (Box 7.9). It is important for the worker to complete an accident or incident form, including the patient's details, to ensure that if they acquire HBV or HCV or HIV as a result of the injury they will be eligible for industrial injury compensation.

CONCLUSION

HAI cannot be prevented completely and has serious consequences for the patient, but reducing the incidence will benefit both patients and hospital. Surveillance is central to detecting infections and as the foundation for good infection control practices.[3] Perioperative practitioners have an important role in infection control and should work in partnership with other healthcare professionals to influence the improvements to patient care. Infection control is fundamental to a high standard of patient care. Knowledge and skills in microbiology are vital, but better application and adherence to good practice will make a major contribution to achieving that goal.

References

1. Fairchild S. Perioperative nursing: principles and practice, 2nd edn. Boston: Jones and Bartlett; 1999.
2. Wilson J. Infection control in clinical pratice, 2nd edn. Edinburgh: Baillière Tindall; 2001.
3. National Audit Office. The management and control of hospital acquired infection in acute NHS Trusts in England. Norwich: The Stationery Office; 2000.
4. Plowman R, Graves N, Griffin M, et al. Socioeconomic burden of hospital acquired infection. London: Public Laboratory Service; 2000.
5. Emmerson A, Enstone J, Griffin M. The second national prevalence survey of infection in hospitals: overview of the results. J Hosp Infect Control 1995; 32: 175–190.
6. Madeo M, Tomlinson S, Till J, et al. A novel post-discharge surveillance of wound infection after day surgery using NHS Direct. Br J Infect Control 2001; 2: 20–22.
7. Mangram A, Horan T, Pearson M, et al. Guidelines for the prevention of surgical site infection. Infect Control Hosp Epidemio 1999; 20: 247–278.
8. Bannister B, Begg N, Gillespie S. Infectious disease. Oxford: Blackwell Science; 1996.
9. Infection Control Nurses Association (ICNA). Guidelines for hand hygiene. London: ICNA; 1997.
10. Gruendman B, Fernsebner B. Comprehensive perioperative nursing. Volume 1: Principles. Boston: Jones and Bartlett; 1995.
11. Unerman E. Operating room practice. In: Hodge D, ed. Day surgery – a nursing approach. Edinburgh: Churchill Livingstone; 1999.
12. Hospital Infection Society Working Party. Behaviours and rituals in the operating theatre – draft. London: Hospital Infection Society; 2001.

13. East J. Risk management. In: Clarke P, Jones J, eds. Brigden's operating department practice. Edinburgh: Churchill Livingstone; 1998.

14. Troare O, Eschaoasse D, Laveran A. A bacteriological study of a contamination control tacky mat. J Hosp Infect 1997; 36: 158–159.

15. Lewis D, Weymont G, Noakes C, et al. A bacteriological study on the environment of using a one or two trolley system in theatre. J Hosp Infect 1990; 15: 35–53.

16. AORN. Recommended practices for traffic patterns in the perioperative setting. AORN J 1996; 63: 655s–658.

17. National Association of Theatre Nurses. Principles of safe practice in the perioperative environment. Harrogate: NATN; 1998.

18. Parker L. Ritual or reason. NT 1999; 95(Suppl): 60–63.

19. Rowley S. Aseptic non-touch technique. NT 2001; 97: vi–viii.

20. Pratt R, Pellowe C, Loveday HP, et al. The epic project: developing national evidence-based guidelines for preventing healthcare associated infections. J Hosp Infect 2001; 47(Suppl): 81–82.

21. Pinney E. Handwashing. Br J Perioper Nurs 2000; 10: 328–331.

22. Association of Operating Department Practitioners. Code of conduct. London: AODP; 1998.

23. United Kingdom Central Council for Nursing, Midwifery and Health Visiting. Professional code of conduct, 2nd edn. London: UKCC; 1992.

24. Ward V, Wilson J, Taylor L, et al. Preventing hospital acquired infection: clinical guidelines. London: Public Health Laboratory Service; 1997.

25. Taylor L. An evaluation of handwashing techniques: 1. NT 1978; 74(2): 54–55.

26. Gallagher R. This is the way we wash our hands. NT 1999; 95: 62–66.

27. Mackrodt K. Damp dusting in the operating theatre: implications for bacteria counts. Br J Theatre Nurs 1994; 4: 10–13.

28. Health and Safety Commission. Control of Substances Hazardous to Health Regulations 1999. Approved codes of practice. Sudbury: HSE Books; 1999.

29. Health and Safety Executive. Personal Protective Equipment at Work Regulations: guidance on regulations. The Stationery Office; 1992.

30. Mahoney C. The need for a clear policy on glove use. NT 1998; 94: 52–54.

31. Johnson G. Latex allergy: reducing the risks. NT 1998; 94: 69–73.

32. ICNA. Glove usage guidelines. London. ICNA; 1999.

33. Bernthal L. Two gloves or not two gloves that is the question? Br J Perioper Nurs 2000; 10: 102–107.

34. Sharma J, Ekon S, McMillan L, et al. Blood splashes to the masks and goggles during caesarean section. Br J Obstet Gynaecol 1997; 104: 1405–1406.

35. Department of Health. Guidance for clinical health care workers: protection against infection with blood borne viruses. London: DOH; 1998.

36. Edwards P. Contamination of the surgical field – what does the published research say about face masks? Br J Perioper Nurs 2001; 11: 543–546.

37. Pearson T. The wearing of facial protection in high risk environments: the non-compliance of healthcare workers with universal precautions. Br J Perioper Nurs 2000; 10: 163–166.

38. Fielding D. Waste minimisation. Br J Infect Control 2000; 2: 21–23.

39. Environmental Protection Act 1990. London: The Stationery Office.

40. NHS Executive. Health service guidelines: hospital laundry arrangements for used and infected linen. HSG (95)18. London: NHS Executive; 1995.

41. Cooper T. Blood spills: the evidence. NT 1999; 10(Suppl): 65–68.

42. Ballard J. Preventing needlestick injuries: epidemiology, management of exposures and prevention. J Advanced Nurs 1997; 25: 144–154.

Further reading

Plowman R, Graves N, Griffin M, et al. Socioeconomic burden of hospital infection. London: Public Laboratory Service; 2000.

Pratt R. The epic project: developing national evidence-based guidelines for preventing healthcare associated infections. J Hosp Infect 2001; 47(Suppl).

Wilson J. Infection control in clinical practice. 2nd edn. Edinburgh: Baillière Tindall; 2001.

Useful contacts

Infection Control Nurses Association
c/o Fitwise, Drumcross Hall,
Bathgate, West Lothian
EH48 4JT
www.icna.co.uk

National Association of Theatre Nurses
Daisy Ayris House,
6 Grove Park Court,
Harrogate, North Yorkshire
HG1 4DP
www.natn.org.uk

Public Health Laboratory Service, Colindale, London, has specialist infection control nurses in post.

Chapter 8

Decontamination of reusable medical devices

David Hurrell

Key points

- Decontamination
- Sterilization
- Disinfection
- Standards
- Legislation

INTRODUCTION

Decontamination is the term that has been used to embrace all the processes to which a reusable medical device must be subjected before it may be used safely on the next patient. Figure 8.1 shows the lifecycle of a reusable medical device and illustrates all the key stages in the decontamination process.

FUNDAMENTAL DEFINITIONS

Sterilization This may be defined as a validated process that ensures that the probability of a viable microorganism being present is less than one in a million ($p = 10^{-6}$).[2] The validation of the process must necessarily consider the extent and nature of microbial contamination before sterilization (the bioburden). In the absence of actual data it may be assumed that the bioburden consists of not less than 1 million (10^6) bacterial spores that have known, high resistance to the sterilization process. A sterilization process will therefore be designed to eliminate more than 10^{12} microorganisms.[3]

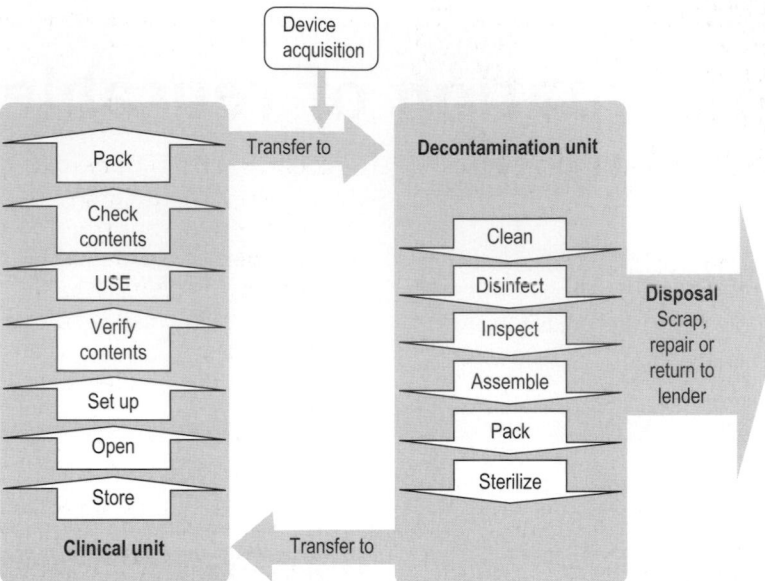

Figure 8.1 Reusable medical device life cycle.

Disinfection Whereas there is widespread agreement on the definition of sterilization there are numerous definitions of disinfection. It is generally accepted that it is 'the removal or destruction of harmful microbes, not usually including bacterial spores'.[4] The lack of sporicidal activity is an oversimplification. There are a number of disinfectant solutions that demonstrate significant sporicidal activity on prolonged exposure and are sometimes referred to as chemical sterilants. With shorter exposure periods these same solutions remain effective against vegetative bacteria, including mycobacteria, fungi and viruses, but will not kill large numbers of bacterial spores, and they may then be referred to as high-level disinfectants.

Cleaning This has been defined as the removal of contamination to the extent necessary for the intended subsequent processing or use.[1]

Validation There is no simple method to verify by inspection or test the efficacy of any of the three elements of the decontamination process concerned with the elimination, or reduction, of microbial and other contamination. In consequence, it is necessary for these processes to be validated, and then each process cycle must be monitored to confirm attainment of the validated parameters (e.g. time, temperature, pressure, concentration of process chemical).

Validation may be defined as a planned and documented demonstration that under operational conditions, controlled within defined limits, the process will consistently and reliably yield product which is in conformance with a predetermined specification.

WHY IS DECONTAMINATION NECESSARY?

Pathogenic microorganisms, and environmental microorganisms that do not invade healthy tissue under normal circumstances, may give rise to infection if introduced directly into the body. In consequence, great care must be taken to ensure that the medical devices and equipment used in the perioperative environment are not a source of microbial contamination.

However, viable microorganisms are not the only source of potential adverse effects.

CREUTZFELDT-JAKOB DISEASE (CJD)

Since the mid-1990s there has been increasing awareness of the possibility for transmission between patients of the novel agents responsible for transmissible spongiform encephalopathies such as variant Creutzfeld-Jakob disease (CJD). These agents are referred to as prions. They are proteinaceous in nature and remain largely unaffected by traditional sterilization and disinfection processes. Because sterilization and disinfection are ineffective against prions the efficacy of decontamination depends almost entirely on the adequacy of the cleaning process.

> **Box 8.1** Categorization of clinical procedures by risk for all types of CJD. (Further risk assessment is being undertaken on the categorization of dental procedures involving tissues that are currently considered low risk.[5])
>
> **High-risk**
>
> - All procedures that involve piercing the dura, or contact with the trigeminal and dorsal root ganglia, or the pineal and pituitary glands
> - Procedures involving the optic nerve and retina
>
> **Medium-risk**
>
> - Other procedures involving the eye, including conjunctiva, cornea, sclera and iris
> - Procedures involving contact with lymphoreticular system (LRS)
> - Anaesthetic procedures that involve contact with LRS during tonsil surgery (for example laryngeal masks)
> - Procedures in which biopsy forceps come into contact with LRS tissue
> - Procedures that involve contact with olfactory epithelium
>
> **Low-risk**
>
> - All other invasive procedures, including other anaesthetic procedures and procedures involving contact with the cerebral fluid

The risk of transmission of CJD between patients is related to both the likelihood of prion protein being present on the surgical instrument and the efficacy of the decontamination procedure. The risk of prion protein being present on an instrument depends on the status of the patient on whom the instrument was used and the nature of the procedure carried out. The risk associated with particular clinical procedures has been categorized into three types: high, medium and low (Box 8.1).

This 'procedure-specific' risk categorization does not preclude the need to assess the 'patient-specific' risk in accordance with the guidance of the Advisory Committee on Dangerous Pathogens and the Spongiform Encephalopathy Advisory Committee on 'Transmissible spongiform encephalopathy agents: safe working and the prevention of infection'.[6]

It must be stressed that this risk categorization refers only to the potential for transmission of CJD (and other transmissible spongiform encephalopathies) and not to the risk of healthcare-associated infection (HAI) in general.

OTHER CONSIDERATIONS

Bacterial and other toxins may cause severe reactions when introduced parenterally. These include the endotoxins, or pyrogens, which are lipopolysaccharides derived from the breakdown of the cell wall of Gram-negative bacteria. Many of these toxins are very heat stable and must be removed by cleaning, as the disinfection and sterilization processes that are in general use cannot be relied upon to inactivate them.

Many of the chemicals, e.g. detergents and disinfectants, used in the decontamination process are themselves toxic or corrosive, and the decontamination process(es) must be designed and operated in a manner which ensures that the residues of the process chemicals, and their reaction products, are removed or reduced to a safe level.

Adventitious particulate contamination has been recognized as a problem for many years. The use of talc to powder surgical gloves was discontinued because the particulate material was found to cause adhesions and granulomas. Any decontamination method should therefore be designed to minimize the risk of adventitious contamination.

The integrity of biopsy specimens is of paramount importance if they are to yield reliable information, which is a prerequisite for accurate diagnosis. When reusable devices are used to take biopsy specimens it is therefore essential that all traces of previous specimens have been removed.

The presence of soiling on reusable medical devices may lead to impaired function or damage to the device. Residues from previous use will make hinged joints stiff and difficult to move, and may obstruct fine-bore lumina or other intricate features of the device.

Even if residual contamination has no known or detectable adverse effect it may still be unacceptable. There can be few patients who would regard the presence of tissues from previous patients, on devices that were to be used on them, as acceptable.

SELECTION OF DECONTAMINATION PROCESS

Instruments used in invasive procedures present a significant risk for healthcare associated infection

Table 8.1   Classification of medical devices by infection risk

Classification	Type of procedure	Level of decontamination required
Critical	Invasive devices that enter tissue that is usually sterile or enters the vascular system, e.g. surgical instruments, biopsy forceps	Requires sterilization
Semicritical	Device contacts intact mucous membrane but does not penetrate sterile tissue, e.g. flexible endoscopes	Requires high-level disinfection (sterilization preferred where practicable)
Non-critical	Device only contacts intact skin, e.g. stethoscope, sphygmomanometer cuff	Can be processed by cleaning (and low-level disinfection where necessary)

(HAI). The extent and nature of the risk is related to:

- The nature of the clinical procedure
- The infection status of the previous patient
- The immune status of the patient on whom the device is to be used.

In most cases no detailed information on the immune status of either the previous or the next patient will be available. It is therefore prudent to adopt procedures that are applicable to all – or to the widest possible range of – potential conditions. The decontamination process to be used should therefore be selected on the basis of the nature of the medical device to be decontaminated and the nature of the clinical procedure.

The decontamination process requirement based on the nature of the clinical procedure is commonly specified as one of three levels. This is based on the classification system first proposed by Spaulding[7] and adopted, with occasional modification, by various workers since (Table 8.1).

As recognized by Spaulding, 'If it were feasible to sterilize all medical and surgical materials in the autoclave or by irradiation, there would be no need to set up these three categories'. However, not all reusable devices can be sterilized by steam, and the number of those that require low-temperature methods is likely to increase with the continued development of complex electronic and fibreoptic devices. In consequence there will be a continuing need for methods that are suitable for thermolabile devices.

PROCUREMENT OF MEDICAL DEVICES

GENERAL

All organizations providing health care should have a documented policy for managing the purchase of medical devices. Once a clinical need has been established, one of the first considerations must be whether the device should be single-use or reusable.[8]

The rationale for the choice of single-use or reusable devices in any particular instance will depend on a number of factors, the overriding one of which should be the performance of the device in use. If both single-use and reusable devices have satisfactory clinical performance the ease with which the reusable device can be decontaminated to the required standard should be considered. If it can be decontaminated satisfactorily then the choice may be based on economic considerations. The total cost for single-use devices needs to be compared with the total cost for reusable devices.

Cost elements for single use devices   (unit price + storage + disposal for the device + disposal of its packaging).

Cost elements for reusable devices – cost per procedure (price for number of units required + repair costs for life of device) ÷ (number of uses) + (cost of decontamination + transport + storage + disposal of packaging).

In many cases the cost of the single-use device will be less than the cost of reprocessing. The use of single-use devices also transfers much of the risk arising from liability for a non-sterile item from the healthcare establishment to the device manufacturer. In an increasingly litigious society this may be a significant consideration.

REUSE OF SINGLE-USE DEVICES

The high cost of many single-use devices and their apparent similarity to devices that are reusable have led many practitioners to consider reprocessing devices labelled by the manufacturer as single-use. The Department of Health cautioned against this practice and stated categorically that single-use devices should not be reprocessed.[9]

Clearly, if the decision is taken to reprocess a single-use device the liability for any adverse effect arising from the use of that reprocessed device will rest with the reprocessor. Without a detailed knowledge of the materials of construction, design performance requirements and environmental tolerances of a particular device it is impossible to ensure that the decontamination process chosen will not adversely affect the device. For example, single-use catheters may be heparinized to prevent problems due to blood clotting. Any cleaning process that would remove residual tissue would also remove the heparin and seriously impair the performance of the device. Many devices that appear superficially as if they could be reprocessed are designated as single-use because they cannot be cleaned effectively. Although they may look clean to visual inspection, electron micrography reveals residual proteinaceous deposits after reprocessing. Similarly, surface damage which may lead to catastrophic failure of delicate devices may be impossible to detect by visual examination.[10]

PURCHASE OF REUSABLE MEDICAL DEVICES

The management process used to control the purchase of reusable devices should include consultation with those involved in all aspects of their use and reprocessing. This is necessary to ensure that the reusable devices purchased will both fulfil their clinical purpose and be compatible with available decontamination equipment and processes.

Medical device manufacturers are required, under the Medical Device Regulations 2002,[11] to provide instructions for reprocessing reusable medical devices. The information to be provided is specified in an International and European Standard.[28]

If reusable medical devices are purchased without due consideration of the decontamination process that will be used there is a serious risk of wasting scarce financial resource on devices which cannot be used or, more seriously, adopting inappropriate decontamination processes which may be ineffective or may damage the device.

Reusable medical devices are manufactured in many different countries and their instructions for use may include reprocessing methods that, despite being common in the country of origin, are not available in the country where they are to be used.

Confirmation needs to be sought from the manufacturer that the proposed process conditions are suitable, for example the sterilization process for devices originating in the USA is often specified as 'gravity displacement steam sterilization at 132°C'; such devices may not be compatible with the porous load sterilization cycle at 134°C used in the UK which, with the allowed tolerances for control and transient superheat, may expose the device to temperatures as high as 142°C.

Factors to be considered when evaluating the compatibility of reusable devices with decontamination processes include, but are not limited to:

- Does the device have one or more lumina, with a large length:bore ratio that would require special methods for cleaning, inspection and sterilization?
- Does the device have one or more lumina or valves that may be occluded or inaccessible during cleaning and sterilization?
- Does the device need to be dismantled prior to cleaning, and if so can it be sterilized when assembled ready for use?
- Are powered devices and electrical devices able to be immersed in water for cleaning? If not, can they be steam sterilized?
- Are the materials, and the combination of materials, used in the device compatible with process chemicals, e.g. detergents, disinfectants (adverse effects may include corrosion, electrolytic attack, absorption of toxic materials, leaching of plasticizer, etc.)?
- What is the temperature used for cleaning, disinfection and sterilization (adverse effects may include melting or softening, plastic memory, differential expansion, etc.)?
- What is the maximum acceptable pressure variation and rate of change?
- Can the device withstand moisture, including immersion in aqueous solutions and/or exposure to steam or high relative humidity (residual moisture may damage electronics or occlude narrow channels in a device)?

LIMITED-LIFE DEVICES

A number of devices on the market are specified by the manufacturer as being suitable for reprocessing only a stated number of times. This operational life will have been determined by studies carried out by, or on behalf of, the manufacturer to determine the maximum number of times that the device can be used and reprocessed without unacceptable risk of failure in use. It is imperative that the reprocessing instructions given by the manufacturer are followed precisely, and that the item is discarded after the specified number of uses even if, superficially, it appears undamaged. This requires an effective tracking and recording system in the decontamination unit carrying out the reprocessing.

IMPLANTS

Many small orthopaedic implants are sold non-sterile and must be sterilized before use. It is common practice for these to be incorporated into the appropriate procedure tray and are sterilized with the surgical instruments. Those that are not used in a particular procedure may then be returned to the decontamination unit with the used instruments and be passed through the decontamination process. This requires careful control to provide the necessary assurance that the decontamination process is compatible with the implants, that the implants do not deteriorate through repeated reprocessing, and that full traceability is maintained. Whenever practicable, these implants should be individually packaged prior to sterilization. If the pack is opened in error, or the implant is used for a trial fit and rejected, the implant should be discarded.

STANDARDS AND LEGISLATION

The Medical Devices Directive MDD/93/42/EEC[12] came into force in June 1998 and was implemented in the UK by the Medical Device Regulations.[11] It provides a system to classify medical devices depending on the level of risk involved with their use, defines essential requirements to be met by medical devices which are placed on the market in the European Union, and specifies conformity assessment procedures for each of the four classification levels. Devices that comply with the Directive, other than procedure packs, must be marked with the CE mark.

The directive does not specify detailed technical requirements but does identify the essential requirements that need to be met. The detailed technical criteria that establish compliance with the essential requirements are specified in harmonized European standards. Thus the essential requirements state that sterile products should be prepared using a validated sterilization process, and this is supported by a series of European standards on the validation of sterilization processes.[13–15,29]

Both sterilizers and washer-disinfectors (WDs) are considered to be medical devices and are classified as Class IIA (where Class I is the lowest risk and Class III is the highest).

The Medical Device Directive[12] applies to the manufacturer of medical devices (such as a surgical instrument or endoscope) that are placed on the market. A hospital sterilization unit may qualify as a manufacturer if a third party, e.g. another Trust, is supplied. Regardless of whether or not the sterilization unit is legally considered to be a manufacturer, the NHS Chief Executive informed all Trusts that sterilization units should meet the technical requirements of the Directive.[30]

The Medical Device Directive[12] also requires that 'if the device is reusable, (the manufacturer must provide) information on the appropriate processes to allow reuse, including cleaning, disinfection, packaging and, where appropriate, the method of sterilization of the device and any restriction on the number of reuses'.

Products that make a medical claim, such as antiseptics, are regulated as medicinal products under the Medicines Act (1967)[16] and Directive 65/65/EEC.[17]

LOCATION FOR DECONTAMINATION

The decontamination process is technically complex, and if it is to be carried out effectively it requires specialist knowledge. Manual washing followed by sterilization of unwrapped items in a simple benchtop sterilizer is unlikely to provide the same standard as that provided by the use of automated washer-disinfectors and porous load sterilizers. The latter cannot be provided economically in a local decontamination unit.

A local decontamination unit is one where reprocessing takes place within, or immediately adjacent to, a clinical unit, and which serves only the clinical units with which it is associated. Until the introduction of centralized sterilization units in the 1960s this was universal practice. The used surgical instruments were decontaminated, by theatre staff, in a room adjacent to the operating theatre. Although this had the advantage of minimizing the number of instruments required it was very labour intensive, provided poor segregation between used and decontaminated instruments, and was not amenable to modern standards of quality assurance.

Current philosophy is that local decontamination units should only be considered where automated and validated equipment, trained staff and appropriate technical and managerial control can be provided. This is difficult to justify on economic grounds unless the devices to be processed are both very expensive and used at high frequency, e.g. fibreoptic endoscopes.

KEY ELEMENTS OF THE DECONTAMINATION PROCESS

The decontamination process can be broken down into a number of discrete elements (see Fig. 8.1). Each element is important, and unless it is carried out effectively, subsequent stages in the process will be compromised. Thus if an instrument is not cleaned properly the subsequent sterilization stage may also fail, because the residual soiling will protect any microorganisms present from the sterilizing process.

CLEANING

The definition of cleaning given earlier ('the removal of contamination from an article to the extent necessary for the intended further processing and use of the item'), although strictly accurate, leaves several problems to be resolved. One needs to determine:

- What contaminants may be present
- The amount of each contaminant that would be inimical to the subsequent intended use
- The method(s) that can be used to monitor attainment of the required standard of cleanliness during both validation and routine monitoring.

Cleaning is, quite obviously, the process undertaken to make something clean. Although we all have a broad understanding of what we mean by 'clean' it is difficult to provide an objective, measurable definition that has wide applicability. In everyday life our concept of 'clean' depends very much on the circumstances: a 'clean' garage would not be to the same standard as a 'clean' kitchen, and we would hope that a 'clean' operating theatre would be to an even higher standard. It is therefore necessary to specify what we intend by the term 'clean' in each particular circumstance. For example, in the

pharmaceutical industry process equipment may be used to make different medicinal products in consecutive batches. The equipment must be cleaned to remove traces of the previous product. In this case the level of cleanliness can be defined in terms of the percentage of the therapeutic dose of the first product that can be detected in the minimum dose of the second product. This not only provides a known level of safety but also leads to an objective analytical method for determining whether cleaning has been effective.

It is important to note that physical removal of soiling from the surface of an item is only the first stage in the cleaning process. If the soiling is simply redistributed on the same item or on surrounding items the impression of cleaning will be illusory. Once removed from the surface the contamination must (a) stay removed and (b) be discarded where it can cause no further problem. (The use of soap in cleaning fabrics provides an example. Although the soap will remove visible soiling it has no component that will stop the redeposition of the dispersed soiling. In consequence, fabrics washed in soap are not 'whiter than white' but take on a grey tone from the evenly distributed redeposited soiling.)

Cleaning considered as an energetic process

Cleaning is a process that requires energy. This may be potentially any combination of three different types of energy, i.e. mechanical, thermal and chemical. Each of these has a role to play, but the extent to which each is needed depends on the type of soil to be removed, the item from which it is to be removed, the material of which the soiled item is made, and the nature of the equipment which can be used and is available.

Mechanical energy
Manual methods
- Wiping is perhaps the simplest form of mechanical energy applied to cleaning. Usually it is combined with chemical energy by using a solvent (e.g. alcohol) or an aqueous solution of detergent. It is used both for environmental cleaning, particularly of work surfaces, walls etc., and for instruments and equipment that cannot be immersed. Unless there is cleaning of the 'wipe' after each application there is often redistribution of soiling, to produce an even layer of contamination. The energy input is dependent on the operator.
- Mopping is similar to wiping but applied to larger areas. It presents the same risk of redistributing

soiling as wiping, hence the strong preference for the 'two-bucket method'. Mopping is generally used for large floor areas. The energy input is dependent on the operator, and mechanical energy is probably secondary to the chemical energy from the water/detergent solution.

Manual/automatic methods   *Brushing* may be manual or automated (e.g. rotary scrubbers for floor cleaning). It is a more vigorous application of mechanical energy than wiping or mopping, and relies to a great extent on the physical characteristics of the brush system. The small cross-sectional area of the end of the 'bristle' allows greater application of pressure from a modest force applied by the operator; the hardness and resilience of the bristle is also important. The nature of the brush may vary from soft pliable hairs used to disperse surface dust to hard bristle, nylon bristle, or even metal wires used to shift hard soiling. Pot scourers made of nylon, or metal, fulfil a similar function as do pipe cleaners used to clean the inner surface of tubular devices. The mechanical abrasion arising from the use of some of these devices (e.g. wire brushes and metal pot scourers) is sufficient to damage the passivation layer on the surface of surgical instruments.

In using any brushing system it must be recognized that there is considerable potential for the generation of aerosols of the soil being removed. This may redistribute the soiling over a wide area and may also be a hazard to human health.

Vacuum cleaning systems are commonly used for environmental cleaning (floors, carpets, soft furnishings, etc.) to remove dust and debris that is not adhering to the surface being cleaned. Wet pick-up vacuum cleaners may also be used in conjunction with mopping or scrubbing. The discharge from the vacuum cleaner must be appropriately filtered if the cleaner is not to be a source of airborne particulate soil.

Compressed air jets are often used for removing surface dust or water from inaccessible parts and components. The removed contaminant is dispersed into the air. In consequence, cleaning by air jetting should always take place in an exhaust ventilation cabinet with appropriate filtration.

Automated methods   *Mechanical agitation* is probably the simplest form of automatic mechanical energy input in self-contained systems and may be provided by rotating the drum of a washing machine, by a rotating agitator, or simply by water flow. The rotating drum method is used commonly in laundry machines (e.g. washer-extractors) but has also been used in washer-disinfectors for surgical instruments. For hollow devices with a lumen, i.e. tubular in form, irrigation of the channel provides the only automated mechanical energy that can be applied directly to the inner surface of the device. The extent of agitation that occurs depends on the turbulence within the flowing liquid. This, in turn, depends on the internal diameter of the channel, the nature of the surface and the velocity of the fluid through the channel. For very long narrow tubes (e.g. flexible endoscopes) the method is generally not as effective as brushing.

In *jet spraying* the items to be cleaned are sprayed with jets of water or detergent solution to dislodge the surface soiling. The water is pressurized using a pump and is recirculated for a predetermined time and then discharged to drain. This method is used by most automated WDs, including both cabinet and tunnel washers, and by dishwashers (both domestic and commercial). The efficacy depends on the spray pattern, jet pressure and liquid volume. It is common practice to use rotating spray arms to ensure uniform coverage of the load. If the WD is loaded incorrectly so that some parts of the load are interposed between the jets and other parts of the load the efficacy will be seriously impaired (this is generally accepted as being the most common cause of process failure in these machines).

Ultrasonic cleaning uses ultrasound to remove soiling from surfaces. Ultrasound is energy in the form of high-frequency vibrations in the material through which it is being transmitted. Sound waves consist of alternate compressions and rarefactions of the transmitting medium, e.g. air or water. When these alternating compressions and rarefactions follow one another in regular succession at a suitable frequency, a note or tone is heard. Sound is audible up to a frequency of about 16 kHz (16 000 vibrations per second, or about five octaves above middle C). Frequencies greater than 16 kHz are referred to as ultrasound. As well as varying in frequency sound waves may also vary in amplitude. For audible sounds an increase in frequency is heard as a higher note, and an increase in amplitude as a louder note.

How does ultrasound clean? The vibrations occurring in the cleaning solution produce pressure changes alternating between high and low pressure. During the low-pressure phase very tiny bubbles of vaporized solution are created which implode violently when the subsequent high-pressure phase occurs. This process is called cavitation. It occurs throughout the cleaning solution and also at surfaces where there is a discontinuity in the surface topography. The dirt is dislodged by the cavitation.

The cleaning solution needs to be formulated to maintain the dislodged dirt in suspension. If this is not done any dirt dislodged may be redeposited on the surface of the items being cleaned.

An ultrasonic cleaner consists of a tank, usually constructed in stainless steel, to the base of which is attached one or more transducers that will cause the panel to which they are attached to vibrate at the required frequency. The frequency signal to the transducer is created by an electronic control board (the signal generator). This may provide a single frequency or a 'sweep' over a range of frequencies. The transducer may be an electromagnetic or piezo-electric device which converts the electrical signal from the generator into mechanical vibration.

The energy input is usually of the order of 10 W per litre of tank capacity. The operating frequency is typically in the range 25–60 kHz. The higher frequencies are usually more penetrating and may be preferred for cleaning devices with smaller crevices and contours.

Operational considerations. The detergent needs to be carefully selected to ensure that it:

- Provides good wetting of the instrument surface to provide effective 'coupling' with the liquid through which the ultrasound energy will be transmitted
- Is low foaming
- Is compatible with the devices to be processed and does not cause corrosion (which is likely to be exacerbated by the ultrasonic action)
- Retains displaced soil in suspension
- Is free rinsing and leaves the minimum residue
- Is biocompatible, with low mammalian toxicity.

The cleaner should not be overloaded, as an excessive mass of instruments will damp the ultrasonic cleaning effect. The same may also occur with elastomeric materials. (The extent to which this may be a problem seems to depend on the elasticity of the material and the frequency being employed.)

Before use the cleaning solution should be de-gassed to remove dissolved air. This is done by operating the cleaner empty for up to 20 minutes. This expels the dissolved air, which would otherwise limit the plosive effect of cavitation by the inclusion of non-condensable gases within the bubbles.

The solution may be heated but the temperature should not exceed approximately 60°C, as high temperatures reduce the penetrative and cleaning effect by allowing the cavitation process to produce much larger bubbles.

The positioning of the instrument basket within the tank should be determined during the validation studies to ensure that it is placed in the optimum position for cleaning efficacy. In many cases the ultrasonic tank has a 'standing wave' formation and the maximum cleaning effect will be at the antinodes, with minimal cleaning occurring at the nodes of the standing waves. The differential effect through the depth of the bath may be determined by the aluminium foil ablation test.[17]

The water in the tank, as with any static water held at temperatures below 60°C, has the potential to become heavily contaminated with microbial growth and should be changed at intervals not exceeding four hours, or when visibly soiled.

Ultrasonic cleaners should only be operated with the lid closed to prevent dispersion of the potentially contaminated cleaning solution as an aerosol. Operators should avoid putting their hands in the tank while it is operating, as the energy is sufficient to cause joint and soft tissue damage. Chronic exposure may cause arthritic conditions.

Chemical energy Contaminants may be removed by dissolving them, i.e. taking them up into solution in suitable solvents. The solvent used may be organic, as in dry cleaning or in swabbing with isopropyl alcohol or, more usually, water or an aqueous detergent solution.

Although water alone is an excellent solvent for a wide range of substances, washing is made more effective by the use of detergents.

Detergents play several roles in the cleaning process. First, by reducing the surface tension of water they allow thorough wetting of the surface, i.e. they act as a surfactant. Second, they will bind to hydrophobic molecules and render them soluble, thereby acting as a detergent. Third, they are formulated with compounds (builders) which are designed to keep the removed soil in suspension. Finally, they may also be formulated to include chemicals that negate the adverse effects of water hardness. These compounds are mostly phosphates, and are largely responsible for the adverse environmental effects that arise from eutrophication of water courses when they are discharged to the sewerage system in significant amounts.

Detergents for use in WDs for medical applications are often formulated to have an additional, or alternative, mode of action and work by breaking down large organic molecules. For example, many detergents for use in surgical instrument WDs contain strong alkali, e.g. sodium hydroxide or potassium hydroxide. These alkalis will cause hydrolysis of proteins and break them down into short-chain peptides and/or amino acids that are more readily soluble in water. Alkali will also react with fats and oils to form 'soaps', which are water soluble. These detergents, although highly effective against the soil on surgical instruments (which is predominantly proteins and fats), are very aggressive. Instruments made of aluminium are readily attacked, and instruments with a black non-reflective finish will be stripped of their coating. Less aggressive formulations (based on sodium carbonate, for example) are available and are sold as 'aluminium safe'.

The same principle of digesting the soil and breaking it down into smaller, more soluble, molecules is the basis of the 'enzymatic' detergents. These are frequently mildly alkaline (the optimum pH for the enzymes in these formulations is often between 7.5 and 8.5) and contain enzymes that will break down proteins, lipids and carbohydrates. Their action is often slower than that of strongly alkaline detergents, and may therefore require a longer contact time.

Note that protease enzymes will not digest the PrP protein, which is the causative agent of vCJD. PrP is in fact isolated from other proteins by digesting them with proteases. PrP is, however, broken down by hot strong sodium hydroxide solutions.[31]

Whatever detergent is chosen must be suitable for the application in other respects. It must be free rinsing so that little residue remains; it must have low mammalian toxicity; it must be compatible with any subsequent processing (see Disinfection); and it must not degrade the cleaning equipment or the items being cleaned.[32–34]

Other chemical agents may also be used in instrument WDs. These include neutralizers used to minimize the effects of strong detergents. These are typically solutions of organic acids (e.g. acetic acid or citric acid) used to neutralize residual alkaline detergent. Surfactants may be used as a rinse aid or rinse aid and lubricant. By allowing the water on the surface of instruments to spread over the surface instead of coalescing into droplets, drying is facilitated.

Thermal energy: elevated temperature Increasing the temperature increases the solvent power of water and hence the amount of dissolved material that it can retain and the speed with which it can be taken up into solution. Elevated temperatures will also soften fats and greases and thus make them easier to remove. In common with other chemical reactions, increasing the temperature will increase the efficacy of detergents (up to an optimal maximum temperature) and increase the efficacy of enzymes (again, up to an optimal maximum). However, excessive temperatures should be avoided in the early stages of a cleaning process where proteinaceous soiling is present. High temperatures, particularly in moist conditions, may coagulate protein and effectively 'bake' soiling on to surfaces. The British Standard for WDs[18] recommends that the initial flushing stage should not exceed 35°C. This is undoubtedly erring considerably on the side of caution, and the maximum temperature of 45°C given in the draft European Standard on WDs[1] seems more realistic.

NATURE OF SOILING

Understanding the nature of the soiling that is likely to be present is the key to ensuring that the cleaning process chosen is effective. For reusable medical devices the soiling will be predominantly body fluids and residual tissue. As previously discussed, this is largely made up of protein and lipids, and from this knowledge it is possible to choose an appropriate detergent and cleaning regimen and an objective quantitative test method for determining the efficacy of the process.

WATER QUALITY

The most obvious attribute of the water used for cleaning which has an impact on cleaning efficacy is its hardness. Hard water will adversely affect the performance of many detergents and will require a specific detergent formulation to deal with the hardness. Also, hard water will cause limescale deposits in the WD. Automated WDs should always be fed with soft water (or water that has been softened). When a base exchange softener is used great care must be taken to ensure that after regeneration with salt the first water drawn off is run to waste. Otherwise the high levels of sodium chloride present may cause rapid and serious corrosion of stainless steel instruments.

For cleaning surgical instruments the manufacturers recommend purified water. This may be prepared by distillation, ion exchange or reverse osmosis (the latter is probably the preferred method). The presence of various dissolved minerals in the water can lead to staining and severe corrosion of stainless steel surgical instruments that may seriously shorten their working life. Contaminants of particular concern, because they cause corrosion, include chloride ions, iron, silicates, etc. The presence of crystalline deposits of mineral salts on the surface of instruments (sometimes called 'water spotting') may encapsulate microbes and protect them from further processing.

For products that are to be used invasively (e.g. surgical instruments) or parenterally (e.g. containers for injections) the water should be low in endotoxins. (Endotoxins are lipopolysaccharides derived from the cell wall of Gram-negative bacteria which, when administered parenterally to mammals, cause a pyrogenic reaction. They are very heat stable and are not destroyed by steam sterilization.)

OPERATIONAL CONSIDERATIONS

MANUAL CLEANING

Environmental

There are some environmental cleaning tasks that, realistically, can only be carried out manually, e.g. cleaning of work surfaces. Others, such as washing floors, could be done manually or by machine. The choice will often depend upon the extent of the task and the particular environment.

Surgical instruments

Recent guidance from the Health Departments in England and Scotland has addressed manual washing of surgical instruments, and a protocol detailing the facilities and processes required has been published.[19]

Any consideration of automated versus manual cleaning must consider a number of aspects: for example, manual cleaning does not require expensive equipment that needs maintenance and periodic testing, but does not provide the consistency available from an automated process; it is highly dependent upon the diligence and skill of the

operator; it cannot be validated; it is not amenable to recording of the critical process variables each time the process is carried out; and, if carried out badly, it may be hazardous to the staff undertaking the task.

What other factors might influence the choice of manual cleaning versus an automated process?

AUTOMATED CLEANING PROCESSES

Automated cleaning processes have the advantage of being, to a great extent, free from variations relating to the skill and diligence of the operator and hence are more reproducible. They are amenable to having the critical process variables recorded, so that there can be objective evidence that an item was cleaned in the prescribed manner, and they can be validated. Automated equipment, such as a WD, is expensive and requires skilled maintenance and testing if its performance is to be kept at the required level. It is therefore only likely to be economic when there is a consistently high demand, e.g. in a centralized processing unit.

Validation of cleaning

In order to validate a process it is necessary to a) specify the process and b) specify the intended outcome so that tests may be carried out to establish whether the process produces the intended result. Once this has been established the critical variables that were used to define the process may be monitored during routine production to ensure that the process is operated as intended.

Critical variables of cleaning processes

The critical variables of an automated cleaning process can be summarized as follows:

- The nature, extent and duration of any mechanical energy in each stage
- Operating temperature in each stage
- The nature and concentration of process chemicals.

For example, for a WD with a jet wash process, the mechanical energy may be assessed by the pump pressure and water flow rate, whereas for an ultrasonic cleaner the relevant variables would be the frequency and amplitude of the ultrasound waves in the cleaning solution.

The intended outcome is, quite clearly, that the soiled items have been cleaned to the standard required. HTM 2030 Validation and Verification[10] gives details of the performance tests to validate the cleaning performance of automated WDs and ultra-sonic cleaners. The validation is based on the use of test soils that are intended to simulate a severe challenge from naturally occurring soiling. These test soils are the same as those given in,[19] and different soils are specified for bedpans, urine bottles, surgical instruments and anaesthetic accessories.

MONITORING CLEANING PROCESSES

Routine monitoring of cleanliness is usually visual. There are commercially available devices intended for use in monitoring the performance of WDs, but currently there are no recognized standards against which the performance of the monitoring system can be judged.

The recommendations in HTM 2030[18] are for monitoring of the critical variables with a suitable recorder (chart recorder or data logger), visual inspection of each load processed, and periodic (e.g. weekly) chemical tests for protein residues.

TESTS FOR CLEANLINESS

The test for cleanliness for surgical instruments, etc. specified in HTM 2030[18] is based on tests to detect protein residues. Three methods are given. The ninhydrin test and the Biuret test are swab tests that are at best semiquantitative but have the advantage that they can be carried out in the Sterile Services Department (SSD) environment. The third method given is the orthophthaldehyde test for proteins, which requires the use of laboratory facilities but is more sensitive than the other two tests.

For environmental surfaces in food preparation areas there are a number of kits on the market for detecting either protein residues (similar to those described above) or the presence of ATP. (ATP is adenosine triphosphate and is a compound present in all living cells. It is detected using an enzyme system called 'luciferinase' (derived from fireflies) which, in the presence of ATP, gives off a flash of light that can be registered by a suitable detector.)

CLEANING AS A PRECURSOR TO DISINFECTION/STERILIZATION

Cleaning will itself remove significant numbers of microbes if these are present. However, the intended use of the product may require a higher level of assurance that the product is free from microbial contamination that could be harmful. Disinfection or sterilization, as appropriate, will then be required.

For disinfection or sterilization to be successful the disinfectant or sterilant must come into direct contact with the microbial contaminant. This will not be possible if the microbes are encapsulated in a layer of congealed organic debris or crystallized in the calcium salts deposited from a hard water supply. The presence of soiling may thus cause failure of the disinfection or sterilization process.

DISINFECTION

Of all the methods available for disinfection and sterilization, heat, especially moist heat, is the most effective and the most widely used. If heat is applied, at temperatures 10°C or more above the maximum growth temperature of the microorganism, all forms of microbial life are destroyed. If this treatment is prolonged for sufficient time, disinfection and then sterilization is effected.

Disinfection by moist heat at temperatures below 100°C, in either the vapour or the liquid phase, is the method of choice in many instances. Again, the use of such methods may be limited by the elevated temperatures involved.

HEAT DISINFECTION

The lethal effects of moist heat are achieved by the irreversible denaturation of enzymes and structural proteins in the microorganism. The temperature at which denaturation occurs varies with the amount of water present, as demonstrated in the data for the coagulation of protein egg albumin:[20]

Egg albumin + 50% water coagulates at 56°C
Egg albumin + 25% water coagulates at 74–80°C
Egg albumin + 0% water coagulates at 160–170°C

So, as the process becomes drier, the temperature required for an equivalent lethal effect increases. In dry heat processes there is only a very limited amount of moisture available (within the microbe), which is insufficient to give a rapidly lethal denaturation effect. The primary lethal process in dry conditions is oxidation of cell constituents. This requires a higher temperature and longer exposure time to achieve an equivalent effect. Thus moist

Table 8.2 HTM 2030 recommended times and temperatures for moist heat disinfection

Minimum temperature (°C)	Minimum time	Equivalent Ao value
73	10 minutes	120
80	1 minute	60
90	12 seconds	120

heat provides an effective and practical method within a reasonable process time. In contrast, dry heat disinfection has virtually no place in our practical options for disinfection.

Moist heat has a broad spectrum of activity for vegetative bacteria, including mycobacteria, enveloped and non-enveloped viruses, fungi and their spores. Among the vegetative bacteria, the streptococci and some staphylococci are more resistant than Gram-negatives. Hepatitis B is one of the more heat-resistant viruses encountered in hospital practice, but is much more sensitive than bacterial spores, which are particularly resistant to heat.

For a moist heat disinfection process, a particular time at a particular temperature can be expected to have a predictable lethal effect against a standardized population of organisms. If particularly resistant organisms are chosen and it is assumed that they are present in numbers in excess of that likely to be encountered in real product, then it is possible to define standard exposure conditions which will always yield a disinfected product in a correctly operated washer-disinfector. Actual exposures can then be related to these standard conditions.

The recommended combinations of time and temperature are shown in Table 8.2.

An alternative method of specifying the required exposure to moist heat has been introduced recently. This is the Ao value.[1] One Ao is equivalent to a 1-second exposure at 80°C. For the same lethal effect the length of exposure required is inversely proportional to the temperature. Thus for every 10°C rise in temperature the exposure time may be reduced by a factor of 10. An Ao value of 600 could therefore be provided by 10 minutes (600 seconds) at 80°C or 1 minute at 90°C.[1,17,18] The draft International and European standard[1] recommends an Ao value of not less than 600 for disinfection of surgical instruments.

CHEMICAL DISINFECTANTS

We have previously considered the Spaulding classification of medical devices as 'critical', 'semicritical' or 'non-critical' according to the degree of risk of infection involved in their use and thus the category of process that should be applied for each class. Let us look again at this classification, but limit our device examples to those that cannot be processed by heat, and our process choices to chemical disinfectants only.

In the USA this approach has been followed in the Center for Disease Control and APIC (Association for Professionals in Infection Control and Epidemiology Inc.) Guidelines, which describe four levels of disinfection:[21]

- *Sterilization*: the destruction of all forms of microbial life, including fungal and bacterial spores (sporicidal disinfectant, prolonged contact).
- *High-level disinfection*: the destruction of all microorganisms with the exception of high numbers of bacterial spores (sporicidal chemical, short contact).
- *Intermediate-level disinfection*: inactivation of *Mycobacterium tuberculosis*, vegetative bacteria, most viruses and fungi, but not necessarily bacterial spores.
- *Low-level disinfection*: destruction of most bacteria, some viruses and some fungi, but cannot be relied to kill resistant microbes such as tubercle bacilli or bacterial spores.

In the UK, disinfectants for use on medical devices are regulated as medical devices (class IIA) under the Medical Device Directive.[12]

RELATIVE RESISTANCE OF MICROORGANISMS TO DISINFECTANTS

The relative resistance of microorganisms to chemical disinfectants is generally regarded as in Figure 8.2, starting with the most sensitive and ending with the most resistant.

This is clearly a generalized scheme: each chemical and its various formulations would need to be assessed for exceptions to the above. Comparative data of a quantitative nature are often difficult to find in the published literature. The data may only apply to ideal test conditions for the chemical, i.e. without added organic soil and with the organism in suspension rather than being tested under

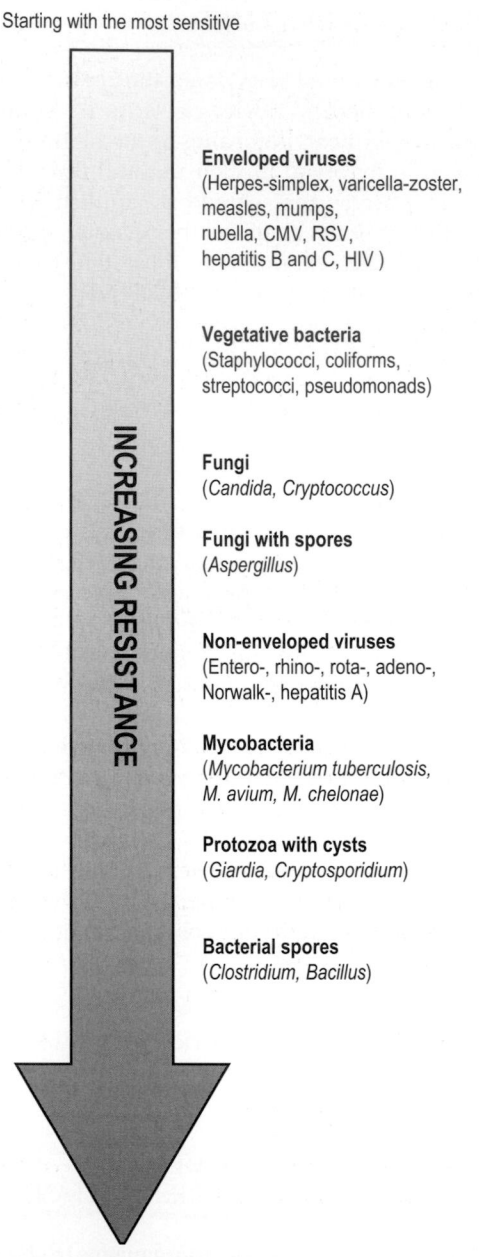

Starting with the most sensitive

INCREASING RESISTANCE

Enveloped viruses
(Herpes-simplex, varicella-zoster, measles, mumps, rubella, CMV, RSV, hepatitis B and C, HIV)

Vegetative bacteria
(Staphylococci, coliforms, streptococci, pseudomonads)

Fungi
(*Candida, Cryptococcus*)

Fungi with spores
(*Aspergillus*)

Non-enveloped viruses
(Entero-, rhino-, rota-, adeno-, Norwalk-, hepatitis A)

Mycobacteria
(*Mycobacterium tuberculosis, M. avium, M. chelonae*)

Protozoa with cysts
(*Giardia, Cryptosporidium*)

Bacterial spores
(*Clostridium, Bacillus*)

Ending with the most resistant

Figure 8.2　Relative resistance of microorganisms.

simulated in-use conditions. The bloodborne virus HIV is, for example, more resistant to chemical disinfectants in its cell-associated state than in the cell-free state.[35] Both may occur in blood from an infected patient.

Historically, much emphasis has been placed in the literature on the sporicidal activity of disinfectants, and only relatively recently has virucidal and mycobactericidal activity been reported quantitatively. For some of the newer products, such as the oxidizing agents superoxidized water (Sterilox) and peracetic acid (e.g. Persafe), there appears to be much less difference in susceptibility between some of the more mucoid Gram-negatives, the mycobacteria and the bacterial spores. We should be alert to the possibility, excluding prions, of disinfectants being developed for which the most resistant challenge is not necessarily the bacterial spore.

BROAD SPECTRUM V NARROW SPECTRUM

For many circumstances in infection control the specific microbial target is not known, and therefore disinfectants which exhibit the widest range of antimicrobial efficacy may be preferred.

In other circumstances, such as antistaphylococcal prophylaxis in a neonatal unit or control of MRSA, more narrow-spectrum products may be chosen to target *Staphylococcus aureus* without causing excessive disturbance to the balance of the normal flora. Other circumstances in which the target is known include blood spillages, where activity against viruses (hepatitis B, hepatitis C, HIV) in the presence of blood is required.

In choosing a disinfectant for a particular task, reliance must usually be placed on the manufacturer's technical data. These data are based on laboratory tests of activity against particular organisms of interest. For many reasons, which are beyond the scope of this chapter, the data from these model systems may bear little relationship to the circumstances in which the disinfectant will actually be used. Great care is required to choose the appropriate disinfectant, and the advice of an experienced and knowledgeable microbiologist should always be sought.

OPERATIONAL CONSIDERATIONS FOR CHEMICAL DISINFECTION

For chemical disinfection to be effective it is imperative that the manufacturer's instructions be followed precisely. The quality of water used for dilution, the concentration used, the storage time after dilution, and the temperature and contact time during the disinfection process must all be controlled within the limits specified. After chemical disinfection it is necessary to remove residual disinfectant. The quality of the final rinse water will determine the quality of the product that will be used on the patient. Detailed specifications for the quality of rinse water required and appropriate methods to control and monitor this quality are described in HTM 2030.[18]

DRYING

If after cleaning and disinfection devices are left wet they will quickly be colonized by environmental microorganisms, which can multiply very rapidly. In a warm room a single microorganism may replicate to give rise to 1000 within 4 hours. Immediately after cleaning and disinfection devices must either be:

- Used immediately (where only disinfection is required, e.g. some fibreoptic endoscopes)
- Transferred immediately to a sterilizer for unwrapped bowls and instruments
- Thoroughly dried prior to storage and/or packaging for transfer to a porous load sterilizer.

The preferred method of drying is by using an automated hot air drier. When the devices have been cleaned and disinfected in an automated WD the operating cycle will usually include a hot air drying as the final stage. Alternatively, a standalone hot air drying cabinet may be provided.

In the absence of a hot air drying facility the devices may be dried by wiping with a suitable volatile solvent, e.g. 70% isopropyl alcohol, or with a non-linting wipe. Leaving devices to drain and air dry should be avoided, as this will allow ample time for contamination to occur.

INSPECTION, ASSEMBLY AND PACKAGING

INSPECTION

Prior to packaging and/or sterilization it is necessary to establish that the devices to be packed are clean, dry, complete, and free from defects that may impair their functionality.

Visual inspection is the only convenient method for verification that devices are clean and dry. This must be carried out under appropriate task lighting, with magnification when necessary. It is apparent that simple visual inspection is not sufficiently rigorous to detect low levels of contamination that

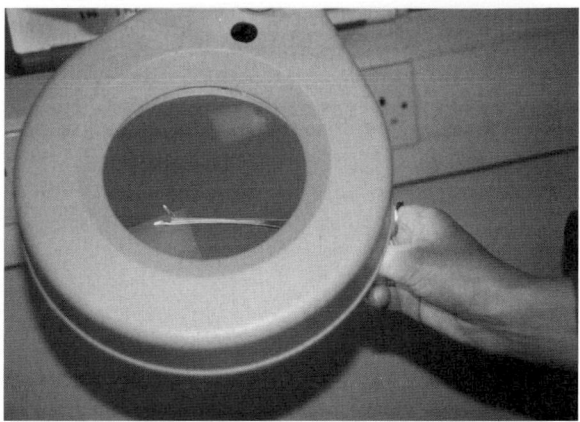

Figure 8.3   Inspection prior to packing.

may still be clinically significant. For this reason, it is imperative that:

- The processing equipment is validated
- The processing equipment is subjected to periodic testing, maintenance and calibration
- The operating cycle is monitored for compliance with the validated parameters.

In addition, cleaned items should be subjected periodically to a more searching quantitative or semi-quantitative test for residual soiling, e.g. the ninhydrin or Biuret tests.

The functionality of the instruments should also be established before they are returned for clinical use. This may be done by simple visual inspection, manipulation or test. These functionality checks should include, but are not limited to:

- Proximation of jaws of forceps, scissors, etc.
- Sharpness of scissors, curettes
- Undamaged edges of osteotomes
- Insulation of diathermy instruments
- Continuity of electrical leads, light cables, etc.
- Operation of power tools.

ASSEMBLY

Instruments that were disassembled for cleaning may need to be reassembled. The manufacturer's instructions should be followed to ensure that the reassembled device can be sterilized effectively. If the device has to be sterilized in the unassembled state then care must be taken to ensure that it is orientated and packed in a manner which will facilitate aseptic assembly at the point of use.

It is common practice to assemble all the instruments required for a particular procedure as a

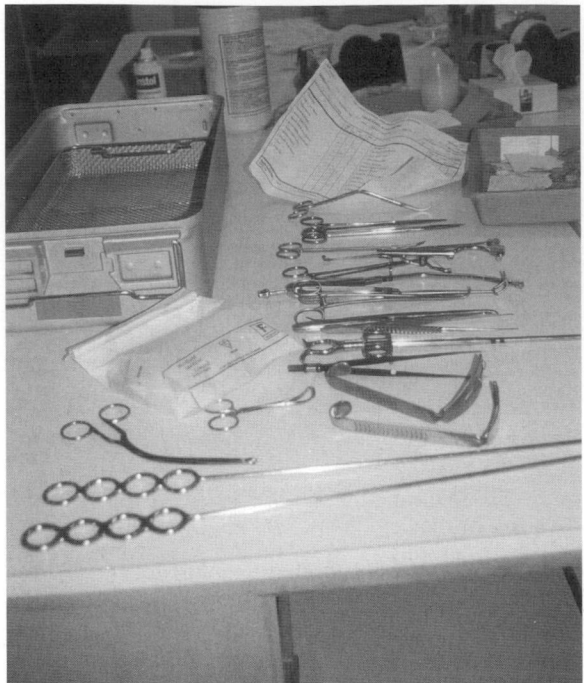

Figure 8.4   Instruments are assembled and checked.

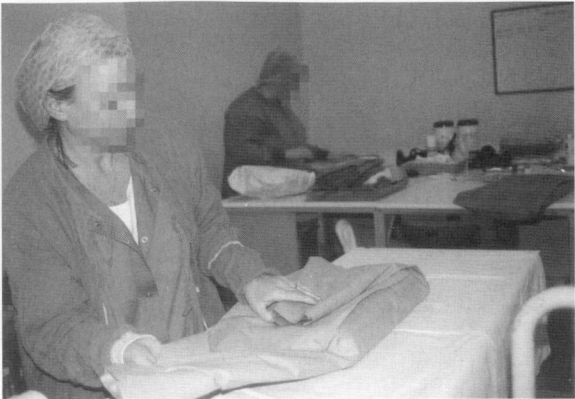

Figure 8.5   Wrapping instrument trays.

single set, with the instruments arranged so that they will be conveniently available in the order required for use. The number and order of instruments to be packed in a single set needs to be determined in the light of the limitations imposed by sterilizer performance, manual handling regulations, and the economics of instrument provision.

PACKAGING

The available options for packaging surgical instruments include the following.

Tray systems, which may be solid or perforated, with a flexible wrap which may be single use (e.g. paper) or reusable (e.g. textiles). At least two layers would normally be used, so that the outer non-sterile layer can be opened to present an inner sterile layer to be handled by the practitioner who has already scrubbed. Wraps consisting of two layers welded together may improve the microbial barrier properties but do not facilitate aseptic presentation.

Although two layers are essential a third layer may also be used to provide a 'dust cover' and additional mechanical protection for the underlying layers. The outer layer may be of reusable textiles, although such material is generally a poor microbial barrier and should not be used for this purpose.

Reusable container systems made of metal or plastic, or a combination of both, are used to contain sets of instruments. The passage of air and steam during the sterilization process may be through a filter or through a system of valves. The microbial barrier properties depend not only on the correct functioning of this filter or valve system but also on the fit of the lid to the base and the condition of the lid seals. Containers of this type offer excellent mechanical protection to the devices during transport and storage, but their integrity depends on stringent maintenance. Many of these containers are difficult to dry in a porous load sterilizer that was set up to process instruments on wrapped trays. If these containers are to be used the sterilization cycle must be programmed and tested with this in mind.

Many complex instruments, e.g. orthopaedic instruments, are supplied by the device manufacturer on graphic trays, i.e. trays with specific retention arrangements for each of the components of the set. These trays are valuable in ensuring that all the components are present and correctly presented, but they are often poorly designed with respect to the sterilization process and are a major cause of wet loads.

Small numbers of devices and individual instruments are usually packed in flexible wrapping materials. These materials should comply with the relevant part of BS EN 868.[22]

Sterilization grade flexible packaging materials can be purchased as paper bags, sheet wrapping material, or reels and pouches with one side of plastic and one of paper. These may be sealed using a heat sealer, or by multiple folds held in place with adhesive tape, or as a self-seal device.

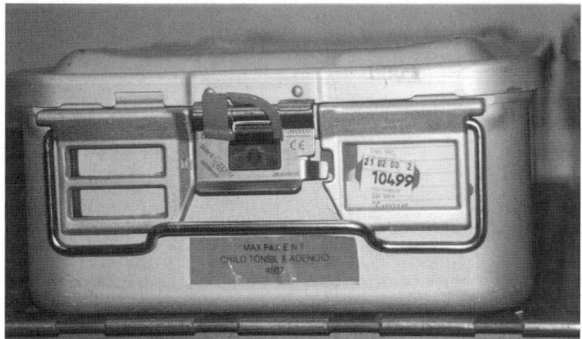

Figure 8.6 Container that is labelled tamper-proof and traceable.

LABELLING

All packed devices should be labelled to show the contents, whether the contents are sterile, the date by which the device should be used and the batch number from which the decontamination processing history can be traced. The preferred method of labelling is to use printed labels; if handwritten labelling is used the information should not be written directly on to the packaging material as this may impair the microbial barrier properties of the material. Alcohol-based spirit markers should not be used, as even after drying, these inks will gas off volatile compounds in the sterilizer and these may interfere with steam penetration.

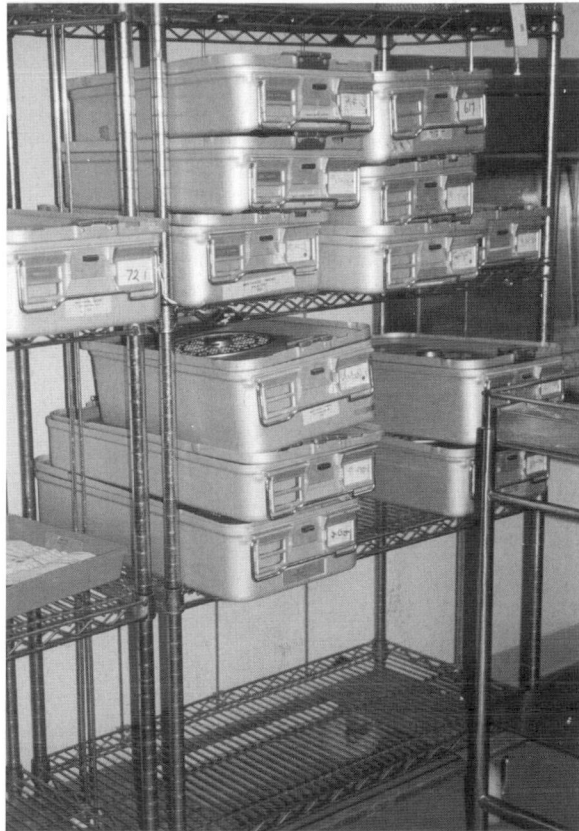

Figure 8.7 Sterilized instrument containers awaiting transfer to theatres.

STERILIZATION

STEAM STERILIZATION

Steam under pressure is the classic sterilizing agent. The various steam sterilization processes are highly effective, comparatively easy and economic to use and control, and are probably the most reliable available. The use of such methods is limited only by the inability of the items to be sterilized to withstand the elevated temperature, contact with moisture, and/or pressure variations that occur during the process.

The relative efficiencies of dry and moist heat

An understanding of the differences in the mode of action between dry and moist heat, and the limitations of each of the processes, is important for the effective application of either.

Under conditions of moist heat, such as saturated steam, sterilization is achieved by the hydrolysis of protein, causing irreversible denaturation. At a given temperature the rate at which denaturation occurs is influenced by the moisture content.

In dry heat processes the primary lethal process is considered to be oxidation,[23] which is a much slower reaction than hydrolysis. However, some hydrolysis will occur due to the water within the microbial cell. The extent to which this occurs depends upon the concentration of free water in the microbial cells, which may be very variable.

Heat resistance of microorganisms

The rate of thermal death of microorganisms may be specified by their D value. The D value is defined as the time taken to reduce the population by 90% under defined conditions, and will depend on the innate heat resistance of the strain, the cultural history, the temperature of the treatment and the recovery conditions. For organisms exposed in liquid suspension the nature of the suspending menstruum will affect the resistance also. For organisms exposed on the surface of dry goods the nature of the substrate may affect the ease with which dry saturated steam is established in the microenvironment of the organism, and thus affect its apparent resistance. Both the culture medium and the temperature of incubation chosen for recovery will affect the number of organisms recovered, and hence the apparent resistance of the organism.

The change of D value with change in temperature is specified by the Z value, which is defined as the temperature change required to effect a ten fold change in D value. For heat-resistant bacterial spores this is generally taken to be 10°C.

A knowledge of the D and Z values enables us to calculate the microbial lethality of any specified steam sterilization process. This can then be used to determine the probability of there being a surviving microorganism and thus evidence that the process has met the criteria for the processed goods to be considered 'sterile'.

Sterile As currently defined in the European Standard,[2] for a device to be labelled sterile it must have been sterilized by a validated process affording a probability of less than 1 in 1 million (10^{-6}) of there being a viable microorganism present.

Sterilization by steam under pressure (Table 8.3)

During steam sterilization of aqueous fluids in containers the steam is used only as an efficient heating medium, the moisture required for moist heat sterilization being provided by the water in the aqueous solution. For steam sterilization of dry goods the materials must be in direct contact with dry saturated steam at the required temperature for the required time. This requires the absence of air.

Saturated steam provides a much more efficient heating medium than either dry heat or boiling water. As saturated steam comes into contact with a cooler surface it condenses and yields the latent heat of vaporization as well as the sensible heat, owing to the difference in temperature between the steam and the surface. At the temperature range of interest – up to 140°C – the latent heat is approximately six times the sensible heat.

The presence of air in steam affects the sterilizing process in several ways. First, for a system at a given pressure the presence of air in the steam will result in a lower temperature. This effect can be calculated by Dalton's law of partial pressures: the temperature of an air-steam mixture corresponds to that expected for steam at a pressure equal to the partial pressure of steam in the mixture. Second, air and steam do not mix readily, and there is a tendency for air to accumulate in the interstices and remote parts of the load, effectively preventing the penetration of the steam. Finally, in a well mixed air–steam mixture the steam component will not be at phase boundary conditions and will not provide such an effective heating medium.

Table 8.3 Methods of sterilization by steam under pressure

Steam sterilizer type	Items that can be processed	Items that cannot be processed
Bowl and instrument (B&I) – mains steam Also known as 'unwrapped instrument and utensil'	Unwrapped solid devices without lumina	Wrapped devices, devices with lumina, hollow-ware (unless correctly orientated in the load)
Benchtop B&I	Unwrapped solid devices without lumina	Wrapped devices, devices with lumina, hollow-ware (unless correctly orientated in the load)
Benchtop vacuum	Singly wrapped devices; devices with short lumina	Double-wrapped devices, textiles and porous goods, devices with long lumina
Porous load	Wrapped goods, devices with lumina, porous materials, e.g. textiles, dressings	Aqueous fluids in sealed containers
Bottled fluids	Aqueous fluids in sealed containers	Non-aqueous fluids, wrapped goods, aqueous fluids in flexible containers
Air-ballasted bottle fluids	Aqueous fluids in sealed containers, flexible or rigid	Non-aqueous fluids, wrapped goods
Laboratory	Culture media, laboratory clothing, wrapped goods, discards	Aqueous fluids in flexible containers

The various types of steam sterilizer are usually classified by the nature of the load they have been designed to process, and are further classified by detailed characteristics of the operating cycle, e.g. the air removal system, the sterilizing temperature.

Air removal options

The air may be removed by upward displacement using the turbulent entrainment of air by steam generated in the chamber (e.g. traditional laboratory autoclaves and electrically heated benchtop sterilizers).

The difference in density of air and steam may be used to remove air from the chamber by allowing the air to be discharged from the base of the chamber in a 'downward displacement' or 'gravity displacement' sterilizer.

Either of these methods is suitable for solid load items with no tendency to trap residual air, e.g. unwrapped solid instruments, or sealed bottles of aqueous fluid. However, when the load consists of wrapped goods, or devices with lumina, air removal using either of these methods is slow and uncertain. Sterilizers to process goods of this type must be equipped with a forced air removal cycle. This is available in two distinctly different types of machine: a porous load sterilizer supplied with steam from an external source (e.g. the hospital supply or a dedicated steam generator), and a benchtop vacuum sterilizer in which the steam is generated within the chamber using electric heating elements. Porous load sterilizers are typically large expensive machines only suited for use in central decontamination units. The benchtop vacuum units may meet some of the requirements for a local decontamination unit but cannot process the full range of items that can be sterilized in a porous load sterilizer.

Most steam sterilizers used for reusable devices are set to operate at a sterilizing temperature of 134°C for 3 minutes, but other time/temperature conditions are available for devices that will not withstand such high temperatures (Table 8.4).

Table 8.4 Recommended time/temperature relationships for moist heat sterilization

Sterilization minimum °C	Temperature maximum	Holding time minimum minutes
121	124	15
126	129	10
134	137	3

In all steam sterilizers the manner in which the devices to be sterilized are loaded into the chamber needs to be controlled if satisfactory results are to be achieved. One of the major causes of wet loads from a porous load sterilizer is poorly loaded and/or poorly packed items. If wrapped items are wet when removed from the sterilizer they should be repacked and resterilized. Wetness or dampness on the packaging may seriously compromise the bacterial barrier properties of the wrapping and reduce the assurance that the contents will remain sterile.

Sterilization by dry heat

The value of heat in the form of fire has been known for centuries as a means of preventing the spread of disease. Dry heat in the form of the Bunsen burner flame, or as an electrothermal heater operating at 800–1000°C, is used in microbiology laboratories to sterilize inoculating wires and loops and to provide rapid decontamination of the necks of culture vessels by 'flaming', although the efficacy of this latter procedure is uncertain.

Industrially and in hospitals dry heat sterilization is used for items that will not tolerate moisture or are impermeable to steam. These include nonaqueous liquids, or semisolids such as glycerin, oils, petroleum jelly and waxes; powdered drug components such as talc and sulphonamides; and glassware and stainless steel equipment.

Dry heat may be less likely to cause corrosion of some materials than steam, e.g. carbon steel sharps (such as some of the microsurgical instruments that, in the past, were used in ophthalmic surgery). This is particularly true if the steam sterilization cycle used exposes the item to significant moisture and heat before the air has been effectively removed.

Materials to be dry heat sterilized must be able to withstand high temperatures, and must also withstand these temperatures in an oxidizing atmosphere.

Dry heat processes typically operate at temperatures between 140°C and 170°C, but temperatures as high as 400°C are sometimes used. The advantage of temperatures above 170°C is that bacterial endotoxins (pyrogens) are destroyed, provided there is sufficient exposure time.

In industrial applications it would be normal practice to carry out cycle development studies to determine the time/temperature relationship that would be optimal for a particular product; this may also take into account the bioburden expected to be

Table 8.5 Recommended time/temperature relationships for dry heat sterilization

Sterilization minimum °C	Temperature maximum	Holding time minimum minutes
160	170	120
170	180	60
180	190	30

found on that product. Alternatively, the conditions specified in the European Pharmacopoeia[24] may be adopted (Table 8.5).

Because of the extended holding times and the long heat-up and cool-down times, dry heat sterilization cycles are very prolonged.

LOW-TEMPERATURE STERILIZATION METHODS

Ethylene oxide

Thermolabile devices produced industrially are sterilized by irradiation or by ethylene oxide. As well as being an effective sterilant ethylene oxide is toxic, carcinogenic, mutagenic, inflammable and explosive. The ethylene oxide process requires careful control if it is to be carried out safely, and demands technical resources that are beyond the scope of most hospital units.[15] If a device needs to be sterilized by ethylene oxide this should be done through a commercial subcontractor.

Low-temperature steam with formaldehyde (LTSF)

Steam in combination with formaldehyde at temperatures below 80°C can also be employed for sterilizing some heat-sensitive items which cannot withstand the higher temperatures involved in steam sterilization. The process was used extensively in the 1970s but fell out of favour. However, new interest in the process is apparent from the publication recently of an European standard for LTSF sterilizers.[36]

Vapour phase hydrogen peroxide (VHP)

VHP can be used as a room-temperature sterilant and has found extensive use in industry for sterilizing isolators used in aseptic manufacturing. Sterilizers employing this technology are being introduced to the healthcare market for processing thermolabile devices. The process allows the sterilization of wrapped goods, and this may in future provide an alternative to liquid chemical sterilants for some devices.[37]

Hydrogen peroxide plasma

At low temperatures and very low pressures, radiofrequency energy may be used to convert hydrogen peroxide gas into a plasma. The hydrogen peroxide is broken down into highly reactive chemical species, such as hydroxyl free radicals, which have a lethal effect on microbial cells. The process can be carried out on wrapped goods and offers the potential to provide a hospital-based alternative to ethylene oxide. There are, however, limitations on the types of device that can be sterilized.[38]

Liquid chemical sterilants

High-level disinfectants, when used with prolonged exposure times, are sometimes referred to as liquid chemical sterilants because they provide a sporicidal effect. Examples include aqueous solutions of compounds such as glutaraldehyde or peracetic acid. They suffer the disadvantage that the devices being processed must be rinsed free of the chemical agent after the sterilizing stage, and thus the microbial quality of the final product is entirely dependent on the microbial purity of the final rinse water. In addition, the devices are processed unwrapped, and therefore the process must take place adjacent to the point of intended use if recontamination is to be avoided. Such methods are a last resort.[39]

STORAGE OF STERILE PRODUCTS

Sterile products must be stored in clean, dry conditions in an area which is not subject to major changes in temperature or humidity and which is free from draughts. Before use the sterile packaging should be examined carefully to ensure that it is intact and undamaged. Any breach in the packaging should be cause for rejection of the product as potentially non-sterile. Sterile goods should be stored so that the label can be read without constant handling, and in date order so that the oldest can be used first (the first-in first-out or FIFO principle).[40]

STERILIZATION INDICATORS

It is common practice to include a colour change indicator on the packaging of sterile products to indicate the status of the product. These indicators, which must conform to EN 867,[25] are used solely to demonstrate that the item has been exposed to the sterilization process. They are designed to change colour well before completion of the sterilization stage, and do not indicate that the item is sterile. Indeed, there are no indicators that will show that a product is sterile. Such an assurance can only be obtained by using a validated sterilization process which is properly controlled and monitored within an overall decontamination process that is subject to the same stringent controls.

MANAGEMENT AND QUALITY CONTROL

Management responsibilities for the different items of decontamination equipment are defined in best practice guidance documents published by the Department of Health.[18,26]

A major source of confusion for theatre staff who do not have detailed knowledge of these documents is the application of the term 'user'. In these documents 'user' refers to the line manager with responsibility for the decontamination equipment (WD, sterilizer, etc.), and not to the person who operates such equipment, nor to the person using the devices processed in the equipment. Thus, if there is a local decontamination unit within a theatre suite, the 'user' who would be held legally responsible for ensuring that the benchtop sterilizer is safe to use, fit for purpose, and properly controlled and operated by trained staff, would be the theatre manager.

The overall management of decontamination is technically demanding and should only be undertaken by personnel with specific training in this field. The management system should be designed and operated in accordance with a formal quality assurance system.[27]

TRACEABILITY

The records kept for the decontamination process should enable retrospective proof that any particular item has passed through each stage of the process satisfactorily. Ideally this traceability should extend to records that enable one to determine on which patient a particular device was used after each processing episode. In setting up such a system care is needed to ensure that there is no possible breach of patient confidentiality.

Ideally, traceability would extend to individual instruments within a set, but there is currently no entirely satisfactory system of marking instruments. Until such systems become available traceability should be based on tracking sets of instruments and individual supplementary instruments.

The records required for tracking and traceability may be kept manually, but such systems are relatively labour intensive and expensive to operate. IT-based systems, where the data are scanned in from barcoded labels and recorded on a database, are cheap to install, convenient to operate, and provide much greater speed and flexibility when tracing the history of a device becomes necessary.[41]

CONCLUSION

In every operating theatre, in every hospital, the tools of the surgeon's trade are sterile instruments. Whether these are provided as single-use instruments or as reusable instruments that are decontaminated between uses; whether decontamination takes place in a central unit or is done locally, it is imperative that the highest practicable standards are maintained. This can only be achieved using trained personnel provided with appropriate validated equipment in a suitable environment under the direction of knowledgeable dedicated management.

References

1. British Standards BS EN ISO 15883: Washer-disinfectors. Part 1: General requirements, definitions and tests. Part 2: Requirements and tests for washer-disinfectors employing thermal disinfection for surgical instruments, anaesthetic equipment, hollowware, utensils, glassware, etc. Part 3: Requirements and tests for washer-disinfectors employing thermal disinfection for human waste containers. Part 4: Requirements and tests for washer-disinfectors employing chemical disinfection for thermolabile endoscopes.

2. British Standards. BS EN 556-1: Sterilization of medical devices – requirements for medical devices designated 'STERILE'.

3. Bigelow WD, Esty JT. The thermal death point in relation to time of typical thermophilic organisms. J Infect Dis 1920; 27: 602.

4. Maurer IM. Hospital hygiene. London: Edward Arnold; 1974.

5. Online. Available: http://www.doh.gov.uk/cjd/dentistryrisk/index.htm

6. Online. Available: http://www.doh.gov.uk/cjd/tseguidance/

7. Spaulding EH. Chemical disinfection of medical and surgical materials. In: Block SS, ed. Disinfection, sterilization and preservation, 4th edn. Philadelphia: Lea & Febiger; 1968.

8. HSC. HSC 1999/179: Controls assurance in infection control: decontamination of medical devices. London: DOH; 1999.

9. HSC. HSC 2000/32: Decontamination of medical devices. London: DOH; 2000.

10. Beck A. Potential reuse? A study of private and professional reprocessing of catheters, guidewires and angioscopes, 3rd edn. Konstanz, Germany: Rontgen and Strahleninstitut; 2001.

11. The Medical Devices Regulations 2002. Statutory Instrument 2002/618.

12. The Medical Devices Directive (93/42/EEC) Official Journal L 169-1993. London: Stationery Office; 2001.

13. British Standards. BS EN 554: Sterilization of medical devices – validation routine control of sterilization by moist heat.

14. British Standards. BS EN 552: Sterilization of medical devices – validation routine control of sterilization by irradiation.

15. British Standards. BS EN 550: Sterilization of medical devices – validation routine control of ethylene oxide sterilization.

16. Medicines Act 1968. (Commencement No. 8) Order 1989. Statutory Instrument 1989 No. 192 (C6). London: HMSO.

17. EEC. Council Directive 65/65/EEC of 26 January 1965 on the approximation of provisions laid down by law, regulation or administrative action relating to medicinal products. OJ L No. 22 of 9.2. 1965: 369

18. NHS Estates. HTM 2030. Washer-disinfectors: Validation and verification – guidance. NHS Estates.

19. British Standards. BS 2745: Washer-disinfectors for medical purposes. Part 1: Specification for general requirements. Part 3: Specification for washer-disinfectors except those used for processing human-waste containers and laundry.

20. NHS Estates. Online. Available: http://www.decontamination.nhsestates.gov.uk

21. Rutala WA. APIC guideline for selection and use of disinfectants. Am J Infect Control 1996; 24: 313–342.

22. British Standards. BS EN 868-1: Packaging materials and systems for medical devices which are to be sterilized (a series of 8 standards of which Part 1 covers 'General requirements and test methods').

23. Ernst RR. Sterilization by moist heat. In: Block SS, ed. Disinfection, sterilization and preservation, 2nd edn. Philadelphia: Lea & Febiger; 1977.

24. European Pharmacopoeia, 4th edn.

25. British Standards. BS EN 867-3: Non-biological systems for use in sterilizers. Part 3: Specification for Class B indicators for use in the Bowie and Dick test.

26. NHS Estates. HTM 2010 sterilization. Guidance. NHS Estates; 1994.

27. British Standards. BS EN ISO 13485: 2001. Quality systems – medical devices – particular requirements for application of EN ISO 9001 (revision of EN 46001: 1996) (identical to ISO 13485: 1996).

28. British Standards. BS EN ISO 17664: Sterilization of medical devices. Information to be provided by the manufacturer for the processing of resterilizable medical devices. 2004.

29. British Standards. BS EN ISO 14937: Sterilization of health care products. General requirements for characterization of a sterilizing agent and the development, validation and routine control of a sterilization process for medical devices. 2001.

30. EL(98)5. NHS Executive letter to Trust Chief Executives 'Medical Devices Directive – CE Marking. England: Department of Health; 23 January 1998.

31. Taylor DM. Inactivation of transmissible degenerative encephalopathy agents. Vet J 2000; 159: 10–17.

32. Proper Maintenance of Instruments, 8th edn. 2004. Germany: Arbeitskreis Instrumenten-Aufbereitung (http://www.a-k-i.org).

33. Instrument reprocessing of instruments in dental practices – how to do it right, 3rd edn. 2003. Germany: Arbeitskreis Instrumenten-Aufbereitung (http://www.a-k-i.org).

34. Working group instrument preparation test series and statements, 1st edn. 2004. Germany: Arbeitskreis Instrumenten-Aufbereitung (http://www.a-k-i.org).

35. van Bueren J, Larkin DP, Simpson RA. Inactivation of human immunodeficiency virus type 1 by alcohols. J Hosp Infect 1994; 28: 137–148.

36. British Standards. BS EN 14180: Sterilizers for medical purposes. Low temperature steam and formaldehyde sterilizers. Requirements and testing. 2003.

37. Klapes N, Vesley D. Vapour phase hydrogen peroxide as a surface decontaminant and sterilant. Appl Environ Microbiol 1989; 56: 503–506.

38. Holler C, Martiny H, Christiansen B, et al. The efficacy of low temperature plasma (LTP) sterilization, a new sterilization technique. Zentralbl Hyg Umweltmed 1993; 194: 380–391.

39. British Standards. BS EN ISO 14160: Sterilization of single-use medical devices incorporating materials of animal origin. Validation and routine control of sterilization by liquid chemical sterilants. 1988.

40. Butt WE, Bradley DV Jr, Mayhew RB, et al. Evaluation of the shelf life of sterile instrument packs. Oral Surg Oral Med Oral Pathol 1991; 72: 650–654.

41. HSC. HSC 2003/032 Decontamination of medical devices. NHS Executive; 2000: 18 October.

Useful Website

British Standards Institute http://www.bsi-global.com

Chapter 9

Research and development

Paul Wicker

Key points

- Perioperative research and evidence-based practice
- Searching for evidence
- Research design – qualitative and quantitative approaches
- The essential steps of the research process

There are many questions that still require answering in regard to perioperative practice. For example, are masks really needed? Do patients benefit from pre-operative visits? Is surgical smoke really harmful? Why do pressure sores develop in theatre? How can pain relief be improved in recovery? What does a patient think about their care during surgery? There are often no high-quality evidence-based answers to such questions and the care that practitioners give is simply based on training, experience and intuition. However, with the move to evidence-based practice there is a need for more robust answers on which to base perioperative care, and this is where research can come into its own.

Research is simply a way of finding answers to a problem. There are many factors that need to be considered in order to do this efficiently, and this is where research can help to ensure that the best-quality answers are obtained.

There are many definitions of what constitutes research, but most have the elements of systematic data collection and the generation of trustworthy or reliable knowledge. One definition by Colin Rees[1] says that research is a systematic activity aimed at extending knowledge through the collection of data in a way that is as objective and accurate as possible.

A danger with trying to describe the value of research in a chapter of this size is that the need to describe the scientific approach to research can appear to support a view of positivism. Positivists believe, among other things, that the purpose of science is simply to stick to what we can observe and measure, and that science – and hence research – is largely a mechanistic or mechanical affair.

Many stereotypes about research arise from this stance – the guy in a white coat working at a laboratory bench mixing up chemicals, the narrow-minded and esoteric researcher, and the ultimate nerd – such as the mad scientists of Hollywood fame. Research can, however, be viewed in a different way where many of those stereotypes of research no longer hold up.

William Trochim describes an alternative to the stereotypical 'mad scientist' view of research in his Research Knowledge Database.[2] This view recognizes that the way scientists think and work and the way we think in our everyday life are not distinctly different. Scientific reasoning and common-sense reasoning are essentially the same process: the only difference is in the degree to which research tries to generate trustworthy answers to questions by following specific procedures to ensure that observations are verifiable, accurate and consistent.

Objectivity is seen as a major requirement of 'good' scientific research. However, every individual is biased, and all observations are affected by personal beliefs, attitudes, knowledge and understanding.

We never achieve perfect objectivity, but we can approach it.[2]

So, in trying to discuss an understanding of the scientific nature of the research method it is important to realize that modern research is rooted in the real world, which is often far less stable and much more complex than any scientific environment. As a result, perioperative research can be embraced by the professions and perioperative researchers viewed simply as people who want to find out good answers to questions in order to improve patient care.

EVIDENCE-BASED PRACTICE

The origin of perioperative research is not normally in the classroom or university but rather in the workplace. Far from being an academic exercise, perioperative research needs to find answers to questions that arise from practice. Very often issues occur from day to day which make a practitioner ask 'why'. The first step in research is therefore that crucial link between something occurring and somebody asking 'why'. If this does not happen then it is unlikely that the problem will ever be addressed or that an evidence-based answer will be found.

The term 'evidence-based practice' (EBP) has been used since the mid-1990s and has been defined as: 'conscientious, explicit and judicious use of current best evidence about the care of an individual patient'.[3]

Evidence-based practice in the perioperative environment involves practitioners reflecting on how they approach their work, identifying areas that

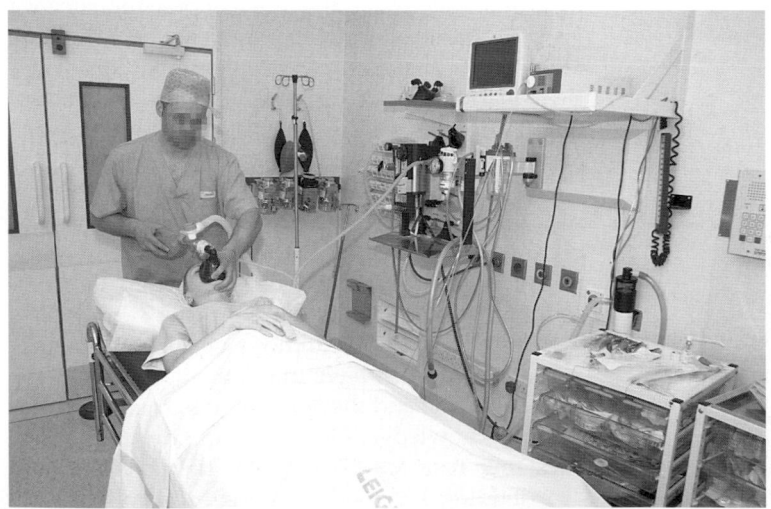

Figure 9.1 The anaesthetic room provides a rich source of inspiration for the development of evidence-based practice.

need improvement, choosing the best way to practise based on the evidence available, and implementing changes for the benefit of patients. Further discussion on evidence-based practice can be found in Chapter 3.

The need for evidence-based practice does not mean that all practitioners should be carrying out research projects. However, it does mean that they should use the best available evidence to assist them to identify best practices for patient care. Evidence in health care can come from a variety of sources, not just research. However, if the practitioner is looking for sources of evidence on which to base practice, then he or she must be able to understand the level of evidence available.

THE HIERARCHY OF EVIDENCE

Fundamental to evidence-based practice is the idea of a 'hierarchy of evidence'.[4–6] This is a model for grading the evidence. Evidence grading is based on the idea that different grades of evidence (study designs) vary in their ability to predict the effectiveness of health practices. Higher grades of evidence are more likely than lower grades to reliably predict outcomes for patients. Thus, a systematic review of randomized controlled trials that show consistent results would be graded as higher-quality evidence than, for example, a small, unicentre research study, a clinical 'opinion' article or an audit of staff

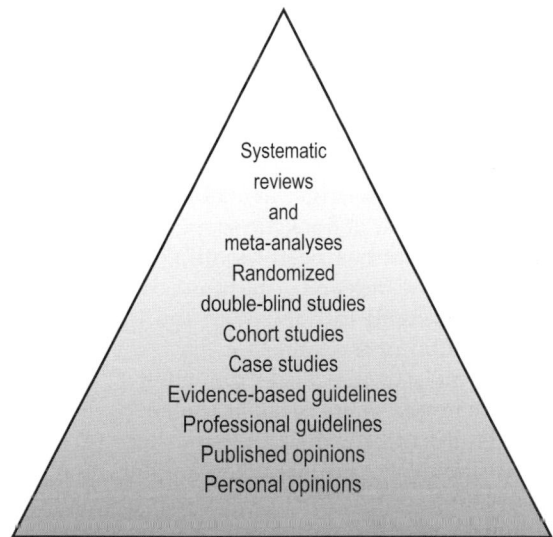

Figure 9.2   Evidence pyramid.

attitudes. Figure 9.2 is an 'evidence pyramid' which shows examples of different types and levels of evidence. The lowest level of evidence is at the foot of the pyramid; this evidence is also present in the greatest quantities. The best evidence, in this example, is at the top of the pyramid – which illustrates that this is also the least available type of evidence in the perioperative field.

High levels of evidence do not exist for all perioperative situations because of the nature of surgical problems and the associated research and ethical limitations. For example, it would be unethical to measure the effect of exposure to dioxane on health by asking one group to be exposed to the chemical while another group is not exposed, as the exposed group would be subject to unnecessary harm. For ethical reasons, the research to answer that question would come from observational studies, which would follow over a period of time patients who have experienced the exposure and compare them with another matched group without the exposure.[7]

The development of perioperative research is therefore a great need for the profession, and it is important that research activities are encouraged.

THE RESEARCH PROCESS

The main aim of a research project is to act as a vehicle for supporting the research activities and ensuring that the original issue is addressed. However, the research activities themselves are crucial to the outcome of the project, and this is the focus of the rest of this chapter.

The research activities must be planned and organized in order to ensure that they are carried out efficiently and that resources are identified. The research must be structured and logical to ensure that factors affecting the answers are all considered. There should also be a way to identify areas of weakness and strength in the research, so that readers can place the answers into context. Finally, the research should be ethical – open and honest, with transparency.[7–9]

Research must therefore be carried out in a robust way that takes into account all these factors, and this is achieved by following the research process. Much has been written about the research process, but most definitions carry the same themes:

- Writing the research proposal – the plan of action

- Identifying and focusing on the issue
- Defining the aims of the study
- Establishing and ensuring its ethical status
- Measuring, collating and analysing the data
- Making conclusions and recommendations
- Reporting and disseminating the findings.

It is this rigorous and systematic approach to the research process that is its strength.

There are several terms that keep appearing throughout research which describe principles that help to ensure that it is robust (strong, solid or thorough) and carried out with rigour (strictly, firmly or carefully). These are reliability, validity and bias.[9]

Reliability refers to the 'stability' of the information. For example, a particular result or measurement should be able to be reproduced under the same circumstances again and again. An analogy would be to consider using an elastic ruler to measure something – not a very reliable way of measuring, even though it may sometimes give the correct measurement. In order to establish reliability the researcher needs to consider factors such as the choice of research tools, and the type of information the study is trying to measure.

Establishing validity involves ensuring that the research activities produce high-quality information. This includes the consideration of issues such as ensuring that the methods used to gather the information are robust, that the evidence is accurate, and that the author is qualified or experienced to make the recommendations or conclusions of the research.

The term 'bias' refers to the activity of identifying elements in the research study that could distort the answer and making sure that they do not. It is impossible to totally eliminate bias, but it must be identified and reduced as much as possible. Bias is very difficult to control in perioperative research because of the huge number of variables that could influence the research. For example, a practitioner who had numeracy problems may introduce a bias into a research project studying an aspect of instrument counts, which would not be present if the practitioner was numeracy literate. If this issue is accounted for in the research design, then the bias can be reduced, or at least the effects of this bias can be understood in relation to the findings of the study. In this example, bias could be reduced by ensuring that only practitioners who displayed a certain level of numerical ability would be eligible to take part in the study. Another example of bias could occur if a research study into the attitudes of clinical staff towards glove use was carried out by a glove manufacturer (with obvious vested interests). Manufacturers go to great lengths to carry out independent research, often by unrelated companies or individuals, in order to reduce this type of bias.

Although elements of reliability, validity and bias may be present in all forms of research, other factors are also important. For example, the findings of a qualitative research study examining the views of individuals may not be objective or unbiased; however, the findings should still be trustworthy, dependable, transferable and consistent.

THE RESEARCH PROPOSAL

One of the first major tasks for the project team to carry out is the development of a research proposal. This is a detailed account of why the research is necessary, what it hopes to achieve, how it is going to be carried out and what resources are required.[1] It is used for various reasons, such as to identify and define all the factors involved in the research project, to obtain permission from employers to carry out the research, and to attract funding. A prime reason for developing a proposal is also to establish the ethical standing of the research in order to satisfy the Ethics Committee that the research is ethical; this is an essential process in every NHS Trust. The proposal normally takes the form of a highly structured essay or report, which closely follows the different steps of the research process.

THE LITERATURE REVIEW

The purpose of the literature review is fourfold: it extends the knowledge of the researcher, it identifies current knowledge available regarding the identified issue, it defines the scope and complexity of the issue that has been identified, and it helps to develop the research questions. The literature review goes hand in hand with the identification and definition of the subject to be researched. For example, an issue may arise from clinical practice, a literature review is undertaken and sheds new light on the issue, which is then refined to account for the new information, the literature review then progresses with a different focus until eventually the issue is defined and redefined until the endpoint is reached, and the focus of the research is identified.

The literature review, therefore, has to be comprehensive in that it draws information from a variety of sources, but also is focused and relevant to the area of interest for the researcher.[10,11]

The literature review attempts to discover everything that is currently known about the issue and define what is still required to be known. It is only after this has been established that the actual questions for research can be stated. Many local libraries offer assistance in literature reviewing, and there is also an excellent series on reading research papers published in the *British Medical Journal* by Trisha Greenhalgh.[12]

The literature review is therefore an important first stage in developing the research proposal and must be carried out thoroughly and comprehensively. A literature review is much more than just collecting and collating a range of articles or books. It incorporates the systematic and critical appraisal of a wide variety of information about the subject.

The skills of critical appraisal are essential for the researcher because of the limitations of all published articles, including research (even major research papers can be flawed). Appraising the information usually takes the form of answering questions in order to try and determine, for example, whether the author is qualified and experienced in the study, whether the information is current and relevant, and whether the process of information gathering and analysis was carried out properly.[13] If the limitations are identified then the value of the information can be identified and the impact on the results, conclusions or recommendations ascertained. There are many ways to critically appraise a source of knowledge, but most of them incorporate a systematic approach to analysing the information in order to ascertain its validity, reliability, currency and relevance to the subject being examined.[14,15]

Currency and relevance have to be assessed by the researcher in terms of their own situation. For example, literature which is over five years old may, in some circumstances, still give insight into an issue, but in other situations may relate to a situation which has now changed. Also, it may be that research on pressure area care in an intensive care unit is relevant to the operating department, or it may not.

Critical appraisal, therefore, is the judgement of the value of the information in relation to the practitioner's own research and area of interest. Researchers use their skill, qualifications and experience to critically appraise the information to assess these issues.

SEARCHING FOR EVIDENCE

The problem with the information age is not finding the information, but rather finding the best information. The Internet has provided a huge library of information which, owing to its sheer size, can be at the same time invaluable and useless. Developing the best ways of searching are therefore incredibly important if hours of time are not to be wasted.[16,17]

The methods used while searching for information are much more complex than on first inspection and should include the following stages:

- Identify the clinical issue
- Format the search question
- Map the search question
- Select appropriate sources of information.

IDENTIFY THE CLINICAL ISSUES

The researcher may require general background knowledge involving the who, what, when, where or why about a particular issue. Background questions are simple questions that produce answers about the basic facts of the issue. Answers to background questions are often in current, regularly updated electronic or print texts, for example, the *British Journal of Perioperative Nursing*, the *Journal of Advanced Perioperative Care* or the *AORN Journal* (published in the USA by the Association of periOperative Registered Nurses), or their associated websites. However, the researcher will also need to search for more detailed information, for example about choice of therapeutic agents, the best diagnostic test for a disease, or the best treatment or care strategy for a particular patient group. This is called foreground knowledge. The foreground questions are more complex than background questions. Answers to these types of focused questions are in primary reports of clinical research or rigorous syntheses of them known as systematic reviews.[17]

FORMAT THE SEARCH QUESTION

Defining the questions that will be used to start the search process is an essential early stage. A useful technique for writing search questions is called PICO – patients, interventions, comparisons, outcomes.[18] This formula provides a structured approach to formatting the question and assists in identifying potential search terms.

To use PICO, divide the questions into four components:

1. Who is affected?
2. What is being done?
3. How are the effects measured and how to compare the effectiveness of different approaches?
4. How effective are the outcomes?

Example of PICO analysis

How effective is diamorphine in the treatment of pain in postoperative patients following major surgery?

Patients   Who is affected? Describe the specific patient population and/or problem context.

For this question, the population is postoperative patients who have undergone major surgery.

Intervention(s)   What is being done? What are the interventions?

In this case, the patient is being offered pain relief using diamorphine. This drug is given in measured amounts (which are easily quantifiable) with a particular result that could be measured physiologically (for example blood levels, blood pressure or heart rate) or subjectively by the patient using a pain scale.

Comparison   How   effective   are   different interventions?

How does diamorphine compare to other analgesics or methods of pain relief?

Outcomes   Define the outcomes that need to be assessed.

The outcomes would normally be what the patient is most interested in, for example whether the drug is effective, if there is something better, and whether there are any undesirable side effects.

Map the question

Mapping the question involves comparing the type of question being asked with the type of information required and where to find it.

The Evidence Pyramid (Fig. 9.2) can be used to map the information required to the types of research studies that will supply it. It can help the practitioner to identify the types of information to use as evidence, from the strongest to the weakest, that are appropriate for the type of question.

To search for the best published studies on a clinical question, move down the Evidence Pyramid to identify the best-quality information that is available.

For the analgesia question above, where the objective is to define outcomes resulting from the use of the therapy in one group of patients compared with its non-use in another, the best evidence will be from randomized controlled trials.[19]

Resources strategy

First, search appraised resources that offer smaller numbers of high-quality materials. For example, the Cochrane Library (http://www.cochrane.org/default.html) offers the Cochrane Database of Systematic Reviews, the Database of Abstracts of Reviews of Effectiveness (DARE), and the Cochrane controlled trials register. Other appraised resources include Clinical Evidence (http://www.clinicalevidence.com), the National Electronic Library for Health (http://www.nelh.nhs.uk) and Bandolier (http://www.jr2.ox.ac.uk/bandolier/index.html). These are 'prefiltered' resources that have critically appraised the information before presenting it on the website. Every word of these small text databases is searchable. It is often best to keep the strategy simple for these databases using single terms, short phrases and synonyms as text words.[18]

Next search for original studies indexed in large databases such as MEDLINE, which contains over 12 million entries). MEDLINE contains the full spectrum of literature reports. The methodological quality of these studies is variable, therefore, to retrieve the highest level of evidence available for a particular question you may need to create a more complex search strategy (using the extended search capabilities of the databases) to replace the simple text word strategy appropriate for a small appraised resource.

Finally, check high-quality websites from accredited sources such as NMAP (http://nmap.ac.uk/), the Health Centre (http://www.healthcentre.org.uk/hc/default.htm), or professional organizations such as the National Association of Theatre Nurses (http://www.natn.org.uk). These sites may contain original research reports but are more likely to provide lower-level evidence that will furnish answers to background questions.

Many of these resources are available through hospital or institution networks, using Ovid or Biomed, for example. The well constructed literature review will show the way to devising the best research question. The research question drives the whole research process and is the next stage to consider.

DEVELOPING THE RESEARCH QUESTION

The main aim of research is to gather data, which can then be analysed in order to answer the research question. If the question cannot be answered through the collection of data, then research cannot be used to find a solution to the clinical problem.

Research studies will define either a question or a hypothesis, or both. There can be one or many questions or hypotheses, and the choice of which to use is determined by the topic being studied and the research method being adopted. The formulation of the research questions or hypotheses is the second key stage in the research process because it defines the general approach to the method of study, which will be either qualitative or quantitative.[5]

There are three basic types of question that research projects can address: descriptive, relational and causal.[20] A descriptive question produces a study which is designed primarily to describe what is going on or what exists. For example, a survey that seeks to identify what percentage of practitioners in a theatre suite carried out preoperative visiting is simply interested in describing something.

A relational question produces a study which is designed to look at the relationships between two or more variables. For example, a research study comparing what proportion of male and female practitioners carried out preoperative visiting is studying the relationship between gender and the use of preoperative visiting.

A causal question produces a study which is designed to determine whether one or more variables (for example time, place of work, education, skill, confidence, etc.) causes or affects one or more outcome variables (for example reduction of preoperative anxiety). For example, a practice coordinator may try and determine whether a teaching programme increased the incidence of preoperative visiting. This would determine whether the programme (cause) changed the incidence of the preoperative visiting (effect). Variables to consider would include, for example, content of the teaching programme, consistency of programme content, variability in workplace, etc.

HYPOTHESES

A hypothesis is a specific statement of prediction which describes exactly what the researcher expects to happen in the study. Not all studies have hypotheses, and they are often used more in quantitative rather than qualitative research. Hypotheses are also more likely to be used when the researchers take a positivist approach to their research.

The logic of hypothesis testing is based on two basic principles:

1. The formulation of two mutually exclusive hypotheses (the hypothesis and the null hypothesis) that, together, exhaust all possible outcomes
2. The testing of these so that one is necessarily accepted and the other rejected.[21]

When the research study is completed, the researcher chooses between the two hypotheses. If the prediction was correct, then the hypothesis is accepted and the null hypothesis is rejected. If the original prediction was not supported in the data, then the hypothesis is rejected and the null hypothesis is accepted.

ETHICAL CONSIDERATIONS

Although research is basically the collection of data in order to answer a question, this simple statement totally ignores the human element.[1] Ethical principles

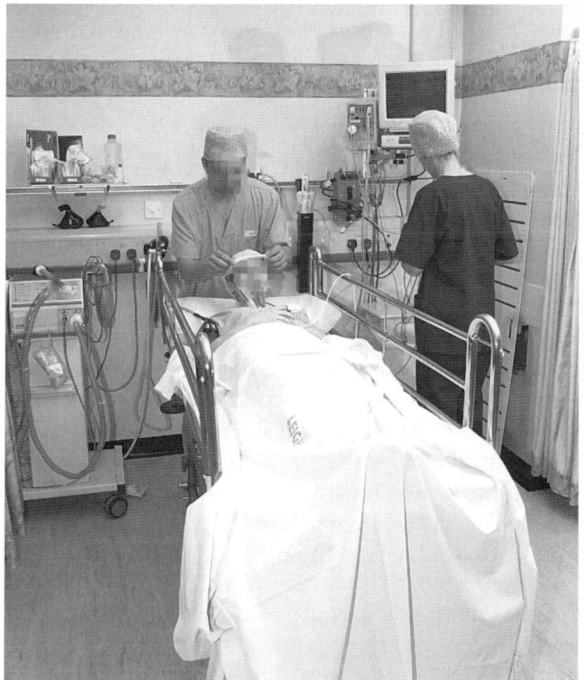

Figure 9.3   Clinical research often uncovers new approaches to the care of the patient.

are covered in detail in most books on the research process, and in the Research Governance Framework[22] published by the Department of Health, which defines the principles of good research practice and is key to ensuring that health and social care research is conducted to high scientific and ethical standards.

HARM VERSUS BENEFIT

Various events in history (such as the treatment of Jews during World War 2) have led the civilized world to believe in the concepts of beneficence – only carrying out research that will do good – and non-maleficence – avoiding harming anybody involved in the research. In order to consider these issues, researchers should look at factors such as cost to individuals in terms of time, pain, money, loss of earnings or dignity; the potential for physical, mental or social harm; and the vulnerability of the patient.[1,21,23]

INFORMED CONSENT

Participants should be fully informed of all aspects of the research they are involved in and be able to give or withhold their consent at any time. This involves looking at issues such as whether the research is part of their normal treatment, what the purpose of the study is, the identity of the researcher, possible harm and benefits, and what use will be made of the results.

CONFIDENTIALITY

Information should be treated with respect. Therefore, issues such as respecting anonymity, limiting access to data, securing documents and destroying original material after use should be considered. The ethics committee are likely to require specific information about the storage, retrieval and security of documents used in the research project.

Other ethical issues to consider include ensuring fairness and respecting dignity, and also fraud in relation to reporting false results.

Every NHS Trust has a local ethics committee, which considers research proposals in terms of their ethical standing. Every research project involving people has to be scrutinized by this committee in order to protect the issues described above, and the Trust also has the authority to investigate the study to ensure that it is following the ethical committee's directions. It is therefore important for the researcher

to develop skills to ensure the ethical standing of the research. If the researcher has any doubt about whether ethical approval is required, he or she should approach their Research and Development department for advice.

THE RESEARCH DESIGN

There is a fundamental distinction between two types of data: quantitative and qualitative. Data are 'quantitative' if numerical and 'qualitative' if not. However, qualitative data can be much more than just words or text, and could include, for example, photographs, videos, sound recordings and so on.[20]

There has been considerable debate over the years about the value and use of the different approaches to research. Quantitative studies produce data that are considered to be 'hard', 'precise', 'realistic' and 'methodical'. Qualitative studies produce data that are considered to be 'perceptive', 'nuanced', 'exhaustive' and 'contextual'. In many ways nursing research has been considered to relate more to the qualitative approach and medical research to the quantitative approach. However, in reality the qualitative/quantitative distinction is often not so concrete, and in many ways qualitative and quantitative data are intimately related to each other.

All quantitative data are based upon qualitative judgments; and all qualitative data can be described and manipulated numerically.[20] For example, a pain scale may produce quantitative results (numbers) from qualitative data (the patient's perception of pain). Therefore, both qualitative and quantitative variables could be included in either a qualitative research study looking at the perception of pain, or a quantitative research study looking at the effectiveness of a particular dosage of an analgesic.

Research data may on occasion be much enhanced if qualitative information is converted into quantitative. Organizing and processing of qualitative information can be enhanced by categorizing the qualitative information into units and numbering. For example, text information (e.g. statements from interviews) could be sorted with other excerpts into piles of similar statements and then measured and manipulated numerically. As an example, qualitative statements about pain could be grouped according to depth of pain, quality of pain, length of painful episode and so on. The resultant figures could then be analysed to give information about the various criteria.

The overall approach to research is therefore dependent on the question asked and the answers required. Although it is true that research studies are rarely truly quantitative or truly qualitative, it is still often useful to define the overall approach. There are many possible approaches to research, three of which are:

- Experimental
- Correlational
- Survey.[24]

EXPERIMENTAL

In experimental research a variable is manipulated to see if it produces or causes a change in a second variable. The former is called the independent variable, the latter is called the dependent variable. For example, a drug (the independent variable) may be given in different dosages to see whether or not a particular side effect (the dependent variable) occurs. The experimental method is often seen as the 'gold standard' for scientific research because it allows researchers to understand and investigate cause-and-effect relationships.

In most instances there may be several factors that could cause changes to the dependent variable. These experiments therefore have to be carried out under highly controlled conditions so that the researcher can be sure that the changes in the dependent variable were caused by the manipulations of the independent variable. For example, a patient may report a lower level of pain not only because the analgesic level in his bloodstream was at the optimal level (the independent variable being manipulated), but also because he is more relaxed, he expects to feel less pain, he would like to leave the hospital, or he wishes to look strong in front of his family.

However, a major limitation is that this method can only be used when it is practical and ethical for the researcher to manipulate the independent variable. For example, it would be neither practical nor ethical to introduce infection into a patient in order to test the efficacy of an antibiotic. Also, experimental studies are often undertaken in highly controlled settings and the results may not reflect what really happens in the real world.

CORRELATION

Correlation is classified as a non-experimental, descriptive method because variables are not directly manipulated as they are in the experimental method. A correlational study is one designed to determine the degree and direction of relationship between two or more variables or measures of behaviour.[24]

Correlation can be used when it is impractical and/or unethical to manipulate the variables. Correlation also can be used as a basis for prediction. For example, if it is known that a certain dosage of drug produces a certain effect, then the effect of a drug can be predicted by knowing its dosage. The value of one variable can be predicted by knowing the value of the other.

However, correlational studies cannot prove nor disprove that the relationship is a cause-and-effect one. For example, a correlational study could not prove or disprove that a certain level of diamorphine in the bloodstream will produce a certain level of pain relief: only the experimental method could do that. It only shows, in a systematic way, that the two variables are related.

SURVEY

There are a multitude of definitions of what constitutes survey research.[25] The survey is another type of non-experimental descriptive study, and does not involve direct observation by a researcher. Rather, inferences about behaviour are made from data collected via interviews or questionnaires. Interviews or questionnaires commonly include an assortment of forced-choice questions (e.g. true/false) or open-ended questions (e.g. short answer essay) to which subjects are asked to respond.[24]

Surveys are particularly useful when researchers are interested in collecting data on aspects of behaviour that are difficult to observe directly (such as attitudes towards preoperative visiting) and when it is desirable to sample a large number of subjects (for example an entire operating department or hospital). Surveys are used extensively in health care, from patient satisfaction surveys, to acceptability of equipment, to usefulness of educational programmes.

The major limitation of the survey method is that it relies on a self-report method of data collection. Intentional deception, poor memory, or misunderstanding of the question can all contribute to inaccuracies in the data. Furthermore, this method is descriptive, not explanatory, and therefore cannot offer any insights into cause-and-effect relationships.

SAMPLING

Sampling is the procedure by which a few subjects are chosen from a population to be studied in such a way that the sample can be used to estimate the same characteristics in the total. The advantages of using samples rather than surveying the whole population are that it is much less costly, quicker, and, if selected properly, gives results with known accuracy that can be calculated mathematically. Even for relatively small samples, accuracy does not suffer even though precision or the amount of detailed information obtained might be affected. These are important considerations, as most research projects have both budget and time constraints.[26]

Determining the population to be targeted is the first step in selecting the sample. For instance, in surveying perioperative patients about their experiences during surgery, the researcher may want to limit the sample to female adults aged between 18 and 40. Because of language constraints, only those patients who can speak and/or read English may be included. Quantitative studies require adherence to specific sampling guidelines, called the Consort Statement, in order to ensure the quality of the study. This statement can be found at http://www.consortstatement.org[27]

Next, the sampling units themselves must be determined; for example, is the research considering one person per operating list, one person per day, entire operating lists, etc? The list from which the respondents are drawn is referred to as the sampling frame or working population.

Third, the method by which the sample is selected must be defined. In probability sampling, the sample is selected in such a way that each unit within the population or universe has a known chance of being selected. It is this concept of 'known chance' that allows for the statistical projection of characteristics based on the sample to the population.

In non-probability sampling, the sample is selected in such a way that the chance of each unit within the population being selected is unknown. Indeed, the selection of the subjects is arbitrary or subjective, as the researcher relies on experience and judgement. As a result, there are no statistical techniques that allow for the measurement of sampling error, and therefore it is not appropriate to project the sample characteristics to the population. Almost all qualitative research methods rely on non-probability sampling techniques.

Sampling is a very important step of the research process because of the influence it can have on the findings, especially if the sample size is too small and is unrepresentative of the population as a whole.

RESEARCH TOOLS

A key step in the research process is the choice of tools used to collect the data.[28]

To choose a tool for the collection of data, the researcher must consider:

1. The data required to answer the question
2. The resources available for the project
3. The advantages and disadvantages of the tool.

Various tools can be used to collect data; many are sophisticated electronic devices which measure physiological parameters or chemical compositions. Others, equally complex, measure behaviours, perceptions and attitudes. Most tools use some form of information technology to enhance their use. Some of the most widely used tools include:

1. Experiments
2. Questionnaires
3. Interviews
4. Observation
5. Records
6. Physiological measurements.[1]

Three tools in particular merit further consideration: experiments, interviews and questionnaires.

EXPERIMENTS

Experiments are used in randomized controlled trials and clinical trials and are often seen as the gold standard of clinical research. Experiments are characterized by randomization, control and manipulation.[28]

Randomization refers to the identification of a random sample which is representative of a particular population. It is therefore a method of ensuring that the distribution of variables has the same chance of being in either group. For example, in a study looking at pressure sores in theatre, the randomization process will ensure that you have the same chance of having overweight, malnourished or diabetic patients in each group.

Control refers to the control over the factors that can cause an effect on the dependent variable.

Studies are divided into two groups, one being the control group and the other the intervention group. The one difference between the two groups is the variable to be studied. The control group will receive standard treatment, and in the intervention group the variable will either be present or absent. For example, in a study looking at the use of patient warming devices, the only difference between the two groups should be the use or non-use of the warming devices. All other factors (for example room temperature, or use of blankets) should be identical.

Manipulation refers to the manipulation of the independent variable – in this case the patient warming device. For example, in this particular study, a device will be used in one group and not in another, and the effects related to one another in an effort to seek a relationship between the use of the device and postoperative patient temperature. This may then be further related to the incidence of postoperative hypothermia.

INTERVIEWS

Interviews are a way of gathering qualitative data, usually from authorities on a subject.[29,30] To conduct a good interview, the researcher must prepare good questions to ask and prepare an interview schedule, which must normally be submitted to the ethics committee. It is also essential to know the reason for the interview and the kind of information that is required to be obtained from the method. This will shape the types of questions that need to be asked. For example, if the purpose of the interview is to obtain answers to background questions about the situation or topic, then questions should be directed towards understanding of the experiences and knowledge of the specific respondent. It would be a waste of time to ask questions that produce answers which could be obtained from a reference source. However, if in-depth information is required which is central to the purpose of the research study then very specific, probing questions must be used and the interview has to be highly structured in order to ensure that high-quality data are produced.

Open questions cause people to give open and full answers. Starting the questions with words such as why, what, when, where, how and if, will lead people to keep talking, and not just answer yes or no. All the questions should be ready before beginning an interview, and should be specific,

brief and clear in order to elicit a similar quality of response. Using the PICO method will help to ensure that questions are well structured.

Because of the human and interpersonal nature of interviews it is important to get the social situation right. For example, the time and place for the interview should be appropriate and the interviewer's attitude should be polite and unhurried.

Taping, or videotaping, the interview is very useful because it can then be reviewed time and again over a period of time. The interviewee's consent is required prior to recording the interview. It is also useful evidence, if required, that the interview actually did take place. Audio recording can be very daunting to respondents, however, and simple measures such as asking the respondent for permission, or allowing them to practise speaking for a while before recording, can help them to relax. Alternatives to electronic recording include taking notes, ticking boxes when words are mentioned, non-participant observation, or writing up the transcript after the interview.

QUESTIONNAIRES

A questionnaire is able to generate large quantities of quantifiable data and is therefore considered to be a quantitative research tool. It is often the main tool used for a research survey. The primary purpose of a questionnaire is to measure the characteristics of a population, and sometimes the relationships between them. A questionnaire is also a good instrument to use to find out what people think – their ideas, opinions, knowledge and attitudes.

Questionnaires work best if they are simple, with short questions. For example, it is best to give people the option of choosing an answer:

1. Do you agree that the padded armrest was more comfortable than the unpadded armrest? (circle one)

Yes   No

2. What do you think about the following statement: 'The preoperative visit was carried out professionally'? (Circle one)

Disagree   Don't care   Agree

3. Which of the following statements most closely matches what you think about the proposal

to introduce preoperative visiting by theatre staff?

1 Very favourable   ☐
2 OK   ☐
3 Neutral   ☐
4 Disagree   ☐
5 Strongly disagree ☐

Although the above examples are very simple, questionnaires can be very sophisticated tools which can glean vast amounts of information. Obvious examples include equipment questionnaires by manufacturers, staff questionnaires relating to pay and conditions, patient satisfaction questionnaires, and in public life, household questionnaires and market research.[25]

DATA ANALYSIS

Once the data have been collected they need to be analysed to provide an understanding of the findings. There are major differences in techniques for analysis, depending on whether the data are qualitative or quantitative. Data analysis is a complex procedure which is beyond the scope of this chapter.

TYPES OF STATISTICS

There are two main classes of statistics. Descriptive statistics describes situations with numbers and inferential statistics makes inferences from the results.[24,31]

DESCRIPTIVE STATISTICS

These take several forms.[1,20,24,31] The main form is looking at what a typical value in a set of data is – in other words the 'average'. The average takes three forms:

- *Mean* – this is the total value of all the units divided by the number of units. In common language this is known as the average. The problem here is that one or two numbers outside the average range (e.g. somebody of 80 in a group where the average is 20) will bias the results.
- *Median* – this is the middle value across a distribution of the data. For example, in a list of 98 numbers of any size it is the 49th number in the list which is median – 50% of the results are above and 50% are below.

- *Mode* – this is the most frequently occurring number. This is the least accurate.

For example, in a group of people 2 are aged 5 years, 1 is aged 20 years, 1 is aged 22 years, 1 is aged 24 years and 1 is aged 26 years. The mode would be 5 years, but this does not represent the average in the group. The median would be 21 years (midpoint is between 20 and 22 years, as there are 6 numbers in the list). The mean would be 17 years.

This situation reveals some of the problems with statistics. For example, a more useful, real-life interpretation of the average age would be between 20 and 26. Similarly, one can see how the extreme numbers (5 years old) skew the average in their favour. In maths this may be a correct interpretation, but in real life this may cloud the conclusions reached by the researcher.

INFERENTIAL STATISTICS

Inferential statistics try to calculate correlation, for example whether two variables form a pattern (e.g. drug dosage and blood pressure), and level of statistical significance, which is the possibility that an outcome could happen by chance. This is known as the P value. In quantitative research, these calculations arise from the numerical results of the control and experimental groups.

There are many other calculations that can be performed on numbers to try and gain an understanding of their significance. For this reason, statistical analysis is often best left to experts.

QUALITATIVE DATA ANALYSIS

There are several different philosophical backgrounds attached to qualitative research which give rise to a wide variety of ways of analysing data. For a full description of qualitative data analysis see *Qualitative Research in Social Work*.[32]

There are several basic differences between data analysis in quantitative and qualitative research. For example, unlike in quantitative research, data analysis in qualitative research may occur before the data collection process has been completed. In unstructured interviews, for instance, analysis should start on what is being said while talking with people; otherwise, the researcher will not be able to decide what questions to ask next in the conversation.

The qualitative researcher must also be aware of the context where the research is taking place. For example, a perioperative practitioner may respond to questions about management quite differently in the middle of an operating room than in a friendly coffee room.

A final point worth reiterating is that the analysis of qualitative data can be just as objective or as subjective as with quantitative data, and in both cases the process of analysis is crucial to the outcome of the study.

DRAWING CONCLUSIONS

The purpose of data analysis is to help in the analysis of the findings while discussing such things as statistical significance and correlations. However, when the analysis is done, the researcher must determine what the main findings of the report really are in order to draw useful conclusions. The conclusion should concentrate on the main findings, as the majority of readers of the research report are likely to be least interested in every stage of the analysis and are more likely to want to know the overall outcomes and how well they answer the research questions. The results will also need to be placed in the context of the literature review and the clinical environment from where the research stemmed.

THE RESEARCH REPORT

The final tasks for the researcher are to write the research report and then to ensure that it is disseminated.

The research report in many ways is like the research proposal – a highly structured essay which covers the detail of the entire project. Typical sections may include background and introductory information, the literature review, the research activities (such as aim, method and results), the discussion, including interpretation of the findings, conclusions and recommendations, and finally any pertinent appendices.

The discussion part of the research report is possibly the most important because it brings together all the research activities in order to answer the question that was first posed. This section should therefore bring the research together and provide an interpretation of the results written in language that is commonly understood, and a summary of the critical conclusions, which are founded in the data analysis. The report will also need to include any strategic recommendations based on the findings of the research which relate either directly to the research question or which may be generalized beyond the scope of the study.[7,28]

Dissemination of the report is important so as to ensure that the results are known by all who could benefit. Dissemination has been greatly enhanced as a result of the Internet, but even so there are a variety of options to choose from, for example reports, presentations, poster presentations, journal publications and book chapters.[24]

CONCLUSION

Research is very simply a way of answering questions to commonly posed questions. Although the research method is becoming more widely known in perioperative circles, there is still much that needs to be done to encourage its use in the generation of high-quality perioperative knowledge, which can then underpin an evidence-based approach to patient care.

References

1. Rees C. Getting started in research. Harrogate: NATN; 2001.
2. Trochim WM. Positivism and post positivism. Research Basis Knowledge Base; 2002.
3. Sackett DL, Rosenberg WM, Gray JA, et al. Evidence-based medicine: what it is and what it isn't. BMJ 1996; 312: 71–72.
4. McKinnell I, Elliot J. The Cochrane Electronic Library: Self-training guide and notes. Milton Keynes: R&D Directorate, NHS Executive Anglia and Oxford; 1997.
5. Joppe M. The research process. Online. Available: http://www.minervation.com/cebm/docs/levels.html#refs 10 Dec 2002.
6. Medical Research Library of Brooklyn. Guide to research methods: the evidence pyramid. Online. Available: http://library.downstate.edu/ebm/2100.htm 3 Dec 2002.
7. Cormack DFS. The research process in nursing. Oxford: Blackwell Science; 1999.
8. Bassett C. Implementing research in the clinical setting. London: Whurr Publishing; 2001.
9. Burns N, Grove S. The practice of nursing research. London: WB Saunders; 1997.
10. Gash S. Effective literature searching for research, 2nd edn. Aldershot: Gower; 2000.
11. Hart C. Doing a literature review. London: Sage; 1998.

12. Greenhalgh T. How to read a paper. Online. Available: http://bmj.com/collections/read.htm 13 Jan 2003.
13. Oxman AD, Cook DJ, Guyatt GH. Users guide to the medical literature. VI. How to use an overview. JAMA 1994; 272: 1367–1371.
14. Parahoo K. Nursing research: principles, process and issues. Basingstoke: Macmillan; 1997.
15. Lobionodo-Wood G, Haber J. Nursing research: methods, critical appraisal and utilization, 4th edn. St Louis: Mosby; 1998.
16. Grandage KK, Slawson DC, Shaughnesy AF. When less is more: a practical approach to searching for evidence-based answers. J Med Lib Assoc 2002; 90: 298–304.
17. Richardson WS, Wilson MC, Nishikawa J, et al. The well-built clinical question: a key to evidence-based decisions. ACP J Club 1995; 123: Nov–Dec123A–12.
18. Condon J. Searching for evidence. Online. Available: http://www.saintjosephdenver.org/courses/FindBestEBM/24 Nov 2002.
19. Markinson A. Randomised controlled trials. Brooklyn: Medical Research Library of Brooklyn; 2002. Online. Available: http://library.downstate.edu/ebm/2200.htm 10 Dec 2002.
20. Trochim WM. Research methods knowledge base. Online. Available: http://trochim.human.cornell.edu/kb/ 10 Dec 2002.
21. Gelling L. Ethical principles in health care research. Nurs Standard 1999; 13: 39–42.
22. DOH. The research governance framework. 2001. Online. Available: http://www.doh.gov.uk/research/rd3/nhsrandd/researchgovernance.htm 12 Jan 2003.
23. Bromhal GS. Research ethics. 2001. Online. Available: http://www.ce.cmu.edu/NetworkU/JEANNE/Public/12-251%20Fall%202000/Research%20Ethics.ppt 25 Nov 2002.
24. Maricopa Community Colleges. Research methods: the laboratory. Phoenix, AZ. 2002. Online. Available: http://www.mcli.dist.maricopa.edu/proj/res_meth/login.html 5 Dec 2002.
25. Moser CA, Kalton G. Survey methods in social investigation, 2nd edn. Aldershot: Dartmouth; 1993.
26. Holloway I, Wheeler S. Qualitative research for nurses. Oxford: Blackwell Science; 1996.
27. Moher D, Schultz K, Altman D. The consort statement. 1996. Online. Available: http://www.consort-statement.org/13 Jan 2003.
28. Network for Research on Experiential Psychotherapies. Online. Available: http://www.experiential-researchers.org/instruments.html 12 Dec 2002.
29. Arskey H, Knight P. Interviewing for social scientists. London: Sage; 1999.
30. Sullivan K. Managing the sensitive research interview: a personal account. Nurse Researcher 1999; 6: 72–85.
31. Clegg F. Simple statistics. Cambridge: Cambridge University Press; 1982.
32. Oka T, Shaw I. Qualitative research in social work. 2000. Online. Available: http://pweb.sophia.ac.jp/~t-oka/papers/2000/qrsw/qrsw.html#s5 13 Jan 2003.

Websites

Website for research methods

Maricopa Community Colleges Research Methods: the Laboratory. Phoenix. http://www.mcli.dist.maricopa.edu/proj/res_meth/login.html

Research tools

Network for Research on Experiential Psychotherapies http://www.experiential-researchers.org/instruments.html

Sampling – the research process

The Research Process
   http://www.ryerson.ca/~mjoppe/ResearchProcess/
Medical Research Library of Brooklyn
   http://library.downstate.edu/ebm/2100.htm

SECTION 2

Principles of clinical practice

SECTION CONTENTS

Chapter **10**

Patient assessment

Amanda Bassett

Key points

- Developing a preoperative assessment service
- Information giving and consent
- Model for improvement

Patients need to know that when they are admitted to hospital their unique needs have been taken into consideration. Indeed, when staff plan for patients it is vital they take into account these many unique wishes and needs. This process may be termed assessment.

Preoperative assessment is the process of assessing patients prior to surgery. Surgical patients need an opportunity to have their medical and social circumstances reviewed before their operation. For instance the patient is having day surgery then travelling times may need to be considered; if the patient is simply having a local anaesthetic then a very detailed preoperative assessment may not be required, but it should be remembered that however small the surgery may appear to a professional, patients still require support and the style of assessment should be tailored to suit them and the organization. Indeed, patients having any surgery need to be assessed preoperatively.[1] This assessment will reveal to both the professional and to the patient events or environments that will need to be considered if optimum results are to be achieved from surgery. It may be that a previously undiagnosed hypertension is identified which can be dealt with prior to operation day. Indeed, without preoperative assessment it is probable that a patient with this condition would be cancelled on the day. This would cause inconvenience to the patient and inadequate utilization of theatres by the organization. Opportunities to talk through their fears and to refer them to other professionals can mean the difference between a patient turning up for surgery or not. Equally the patient may decide that he/she does not want the operation because they do not have enough help in the postoperative period. They may leave it until the operation day to express their concerns, and cancel on the day, meaning theatre time is wasted. Preoperative assessment can ensure that issues such as these are raised before the operation date and are dealt with by professionals who communicate, act on their findings, and make well-informed decisions.

Traditionally many professionals within the hospital have been involved in the assessment process. These include anaesthetists, surgeons, pharmacists, physiotherapists and nurses. Each professional would 'assess' the patient (looking at them from their particular professional viewpoint). The patient may have been required to give similar information to more than one person, or because each person thought it the responsibility of another, information would be missed. This approach does not always work in either the patient's or the organization's favour. However, with continuing initiatives requiring organizations to develop patient pathways, patient-centred services[2] and the need to provide a streamlined service the situation is improving.

Thus in the last 10 years organizations have developed preoperative assessment services. More recently these services have become a focus of how hospitals are able to deliver national targets.[3]

Throughout this chapter we will discuss the key components that lead to successful implementation of these services, and how with well-organized assessment, patients and professionals can predict each unique patient journey and plan for it accordingly (Box 10.1).

AGREEING AIMS AND OBJECTIVES FOR PREOPERATIVE ASSESSMENT

There is no doubt that for many years organizations interpreted the aims of preoperative assessment in different ways and gave such services varying amounts of support. Indeed, it only really started to become important when it was realized that owing to the reduction in junior doctors' working hours[4] there was not going to be time to 'clerk' the patient traditionally. This presented the idea that professionals other than doctors should become involved in the process. Because of the haphazard development of preoperative assessment little has been published about it, although in 1996 Penn et al.[5] wrote that 'Preoperative assessment improves the utilization of day surgery and resources by screening patients for day care'. However, the idea that all patients should be exposed to such a service, and that preoperative assessment should be the key to best practice for surgical patients in particular, has taken longer to address. Owing to a lack of leadership from key stakeholders keen to ensure that their professional identity is maintained and anxious not to make recommendations for other professional groups, little was written on the subject until 2002, when the NHS Modernisation Agency published national guidance.

The Association of Anaesthetists of Great Britain and Ireland also published good practice guidance for their members (2001), and for the first time acknowledged the input of other professionals in the process of preoperative assessment (Box 10.2).

Box 10.1   Key components that lead to successful preoperative assessment services

- Agreeing aims and objectives for preoperative assessment
- Developing staff roles
- Reviewing approaches to patients giving their consent
- Educating patients and information giving
- Involving patient's carers and the family
- Considering physical assessment of the patient, organizing investigations
- Ongoing psychological assessment of the patient
- Acting on information and decision making
- Booking patients for surgery and optimizing available resources
- Measuring for improvement

Box 10.2

'Traditionally the role of the preregistration house officer, preoperative assessment is now widely carried out by nurses or other members of the healthcare team. Non-medically trained staff working to agreed protocols play an essential role in screening patients for anaesthesia and surgery'.[6]

Box 10.3   Key objectives

- Confirm that the patient wishes to have the operation recommended by the surgeon
- Assess the patient's suitability for day surgery
- Assess the patient's fitness for surgery and anaesthesia, including the risk of the combined effects of surgery and anaesthesia
- Ensure the patient fully understands the proposed procedure by further explaining the information provided by the surgeon and providing additional written and oral information
- Provide the opportunity for explanation and discussion – and minimize any fears or anxiety the patient may experience
- Provide information about the preoperative process and any specific preoperative instructions, e.g. who to contact if the patient wants to cancel the operation, any fasting instructions
- Identify any special requirements for the surgical procedure
- Provide an opportunity to discuss with patients any self-help matters to improve the outcome of their surgery (e.g. stopping smoking or losing weight)
- Identify any cultural requirements, and any communication or other special needs
- Assess the home support available to the patient post discharge and identify any special requirements to facilitate prompt discharge

---

Box 10.4   Organizing successful service

When organizing locally a collaborative climate for achieving successful patient assessment, professional relationships and roles need to be examined closely.

- Who is the lead for the service?
- What is it that each staff member is expected to do?
- Can staff make autonomous decisions?
- Do they have access to their multiprofessional peers for support?
- How many different places do patients have to visit?
- Where is the information patients give recorded? And who has access to it?
- Who makes the final decision about when the patient is admitted?
- When is this decision made? And how is it communicated to the patient and to the organization?

Box 10.3 lists the objectives for preoperative assessment service according to the NHS Modernisation Agency.[7] Although these objectives are written with the day surgery service in mind, they can and should be applied to any surgical patient.

DEVELOPING STAFF ROLES

There is no doubt that preoperative assessment services are only successful when they are organized multiprofessionally, and facilitated and led by someone who accepts responsibility for the service and for each patient outcome. It is a matter of debate who this person is, but they are the key decision maker and every service should nominate a lead. Whatever their background, they will be required to work across organizational and professional boundaries. As such they will require sufficient training in

the many decisions required to facilitate a smooth surgical journey for the patient.[8]

If preoperative assessment continues to be organized uniprofessionally the benefits to both patient and organization may not be realized, and such services would only replicate traditional ways of assessing patients' suitability for surgery (Box 10.4).

Clearly, to support this collaborative style preoperative assessment professionals are required to work in a different way, and locally this must be made to work for both professionals and the organization. Criteria should be set to ensure that every professional knows what they are working towards. This will reduce the incidence of organizations making decisions based on one individual's professional opinion.

Changing roles, particularly among the nursing workforce, are common in preoperative assessment. A good place to start when reviewing professional and organizational boundaries is to address opportunities to improve communication. If professionals are working well together they celebrate every opportunity to reflect on their input and to look at what is going well and what not so well. Locally, interfaces need to be set up to support this and should be led by the person who accepts overall responsibility for the service. Opportunities for reviewing the roles of staff can be fully explored in such environments,

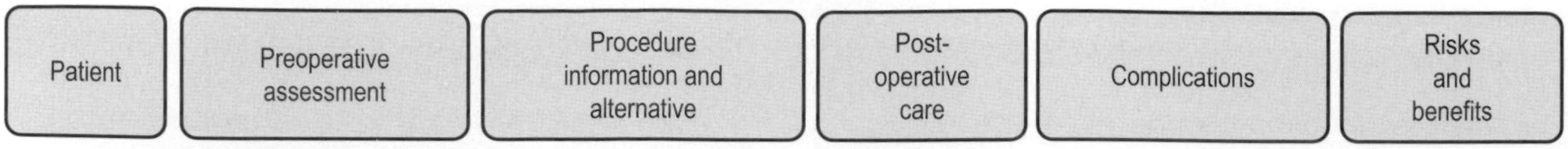

| Patient | Preoperative assessment | Procedure information and alternative | Post-operative care | Complications | Risks and benefits |

Figure 10.1   Patient pathway.

and the blurring of roles offers smoother services for patients, hospitals and their staff.[9]

Importantly, changes in roles require support from both the professions and educational establishments. Education has not kept pace with the rapid development of preoperative assessment services. To date, assessment is covered in different guises in a variety of professionals' training, and as an 'add-on' to some further educational courses. A wide disparity in approach to such services nationally supports the need for developments in training, and a national standard needs to be implemented. To date, most assessors have drawn their knowledge from their initial professional training, local 'on the job' training, visits to professionals in other organizations, and used the limited published work available to develop their roles. More recently *Setting a Standard through Learning*[6] has been developed as a multiprofessional resource to support those in practice. The work is still evolving and will be available from the newly emergent NHS University as an e-learning accredited module.

REVIEWING APPROACHES TO CONSENT

Consent should be obtained by a surgeon who is capable of doing the operation.[10] However, consent is now widely regarded as a process in which many professionals play a part in providing the patient with information on which to make a decision (Fig. 10.1).

Informed consent[10] is when a patient is provided with enough information on which to make a judgement. Current thinking suggests that one professional is not in a position to be able to provide this. Thus preoperative assessment services run by a number of well-educated professionals will provide a conducive environment in which to support the patient during the consenting process. Any discussions with patients should be documented in their notes, and time should be taken to ensure patients and their relatives or carers are furnished with what they need to know. Importantly, any information received by the preoperative assessment professional

---

Box 10.5   Principles of information giving for surgical patients

- Patients understand the aims of preoperative assessment before they attend for the assessment
- Patients acknowledge which information is required for them to present with at preoperative assessment
- Patients understand what is required of them prior to their operation day
- Patients understand the surgical journey and who they can approach at any time for more information
- Patients understand their responsibility in keeping the professional and/or the organization informed of any changes in both their health and their ability to keep appointments

---

should be communicated fully to the surgeon, anaesthetist and other members of the assessment team.

EDUCATING PATIENTS AND INFORMATION GIVING

Providing patients with information as outlined above is very important. As well as facilitating informed consent, information ensures that patients, carers and relatives understand why they need to comply with organizational and professional requests (Box 10.5).

Ensuring information is offered in a timely manner in an environment which ensures that patients use it as a learning experience is most difficult. Hospitals are very busy and often are not a place where patients can learn about their surgery successfully. Although it is acknowledged that patients welcome opportunities to discuss forthcoming admissions, and that it is documented that this may relieve their anxiety,[11] it is worth considering the different ways in which the giving of information can be achieved. Often the patient's own home is a good environment for them to absorb information. Consideration should be given to the fact that information giving is also a continuum, and that patients,

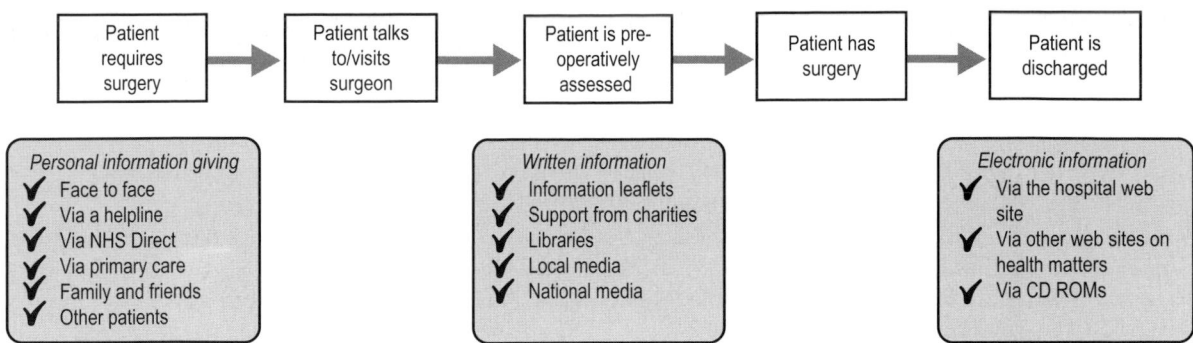

Figure 10.2   Information giving, the patient's journey.

carers and their relatives need to be able to access information at any time (Fig. 10.2).

Assessment services should lead developments in the presentation of multiprofessional material which gives information to patients to ensure the continuity of information and to prevent ambiguity.

It is worth offering patients information at the time they require it and in a style they can understand. It is evident that by doing this the organization can reduce patient-led cancellations on the day of surgery.[6]

INVOLVING PATIENTS AND CARERS IN DEVELOPING PREOPERATIVE ASSESSMENT

Involving patients and carers in developing preoperative assessment services will ensure that services are focused on the needs of local people (Box 10.6). In the past few years there has been much emphasis on achieving this,[12] but in reality it is difficult to put in place. Where preoperative assessment services are led by supported, educated staff using a multiprofessional approach it would appear easier to implement. These staff will appreciate the benefits that such user engagement will bring. For many professionals, organizing preoperative assessment services in isolation involving patients may not seem a priority. However, patient feedback can offer an amazing amount of leverage when talking to other professionals about changes or improvements to services. As always, communication is the key and patients are a great reason to get the surgical journey right. The techniques mentioned in Box 10.6 are all excellent ways for capturing patient comment.

Often a single approach will not be enough to access an adequate number of patients using preoperative assessment services. Just as different patients will require information offered to them in a variety

***

Box 10.6   Opportunities for communication

Patients, carers and users can be involved in the following ways:

- Patient interviews
- Focus groups
- Questionnaires
- Open days
- Comment books
- Pre- and post-admission telephone interviews

***

Box 10.7   Physical assessment of patients prior to surgery

May be split into four main areas.

- Assessment of the cardiovascular system
- Assessment of the respiratory system, including the airway
- Assessment of conditions that a patient may present with and their relevance in preoperative assessment
- Organizing appropriate investigations

***

of ways, so different patients will need other opportunities to share their thoughts regarding services. Roach[13] suggests that a multitechnique approach will offer the most feedback.

CONSIDERING PHYSICAL ASSESSMENT OF THE PATIENT, INCLUDING ORGANIZING INVESTIGATIONS (Box 10.7)

One of the most important aspects of preoperative assessment is establishing whether the cardiovascular system will be able to tolerate the physiological stresses associated with surgery. This depends on the patient's baseline fitness and the degree of any comorbidity'.[6] Throughout Great Britain and across the professions there is fierce debate as to who is best placed to carry out this assessment. In some hospitals, professionals other than doctors can be found to be carrying out physical assessment. However, the professional responsible for physical assessment will need to have a sound knowledge of physiology and anatomy.

'Another important aspect of preoperative assessment is establishing whether it is safe to subject the patient's respiratory system to the rigours of surgery.'[14] As with the assessment of the cardiovascular system, this will include history taking, visual and physical examination, with particular attention to the patient's airway.

The professional undertaking the assessment will need to investigate other conditions that a patient may present with and ascertain how they affect the ability of the patient to survive the stresses of both anaesthesia and surgery. To do this, appropriate investigations may be ordered.[15] The preoperative assessment professional will also be responsible for referring the patient to another specialist (e.g. cardiologist or physician) should this be required, following assessment but before surgery.

Whereas individual patients require assessment prior to surgery, it is apparent that varying levels of physical assessment are appropriate for different patients. Indeed, a generally fit healthy patient (ASA 1 and 2) without any associated medical conditions may not require physical assessment at all apart from general assessment of the airway and anaesthetic grading,[16] and the professional required to do this, as long as they are trained appropriately, may not be a doctor. However, when patients present with multiple conditions and poor respiratory function (ASA 3 and 4) a medically trained member of the assessment team may be required. Distributing patients across the professionals available in a multiprofessional preoperative team in this way will ensure those with the relevant expertise are reviewing the patients that need them most.

COMMUNICATION

The connective threads that weave together successful preoperative assessment are the communication processes with which the preoperative professionals work. Whatever happens, the successful outcome

> ### Box 10.8   Poor communication
>
> Poor communication in preoperative assessment results in:
>
> - Patients not understanding what is required of them at preoperative assessment
> - Patients/organizations unable to plan for surgery and the postoperative period
> - Duplication in recording information
> - Patients not referred for specialist treatment
> - Test results not acted upon
> - Operations being cancelled

of each patient journey depends on professionals acting upon and sharing the information gleaned from preoperative assessment (Box 10.8).

ONGOING PSYCHOLOGICAL ASSESSMENT OF THE PATIENT

Psychological assessment connects with every key component of organizing an assessment service and depends on the ability of professionals to share information. It starts when the consultant first makes the decision to operate, and involves all the professionals involved in the assessment process. Indeed, it may be that a patient is not appropriate for day surgery or, conversely, it could be that a patient would benefit from day surgery and, with support, be better treated in this way. It may be that a social situation requires thought, or that patients need support in helping them become fit for surgery. Whatever form psychological assessment takes it is important that patients' needs are catered for, and this should be particularly addressed through information giving and the consenting process.

ACTING ON INFORMATION AND DECISION MAKING

The success of the assessment of any patient prior to surgery will rest and fall on the decisions made by the assessor, supported by the multiprofessional preoperative assessment team. Criteria should be in place locally to support this decision-making (Box 10.9).

Box 10.9   Criteria for decision making

Identifying local criteria or standard responses to situations should be based on input from professions both in and beyond the preoperative assessment service. It is important to ensure that all patients are treated to a standard, regardless of whom they are seen by.

These criteria should be regularly reviewed to ensure they are robust and achieve the right outcomes for patients and the organization.

Box 10.10   Aims of case studies

In order to achieve their aim case studies should:

- Be short and to the point
- Identify what is not going so well with the current system
- Come up with a solution
- Discuss advantages of the change
- Identify a date or time period to test the ideas
- Reflect and discuss building in other ideas to gain support

Box 10.11   Preoperative assessment opportunities

Preoperative assessment can be delivered in the following ways:

- In patients' homes
- Within primary care
- At one-stop clinics following outpatients in secondary care
- On an appointment basis in a purpose-built area
- Via questionnaires
- Via a telephone service
- Via NHS Direct
- Via digital television

Each patient pathway should be designed and carefully planned, based on the findings during the assessment process. In doing this, the preoperative assessor will act on results of investigations, referrals, and information provided by the patient and other professionals. The consequence of this will be a safe and smooth patient journey, including advance preparation of discharge before surgery has even taken place. In developing preoperative assessment services, professionals should be prepared to question organizational/funding arrangements in order to facilitate the planning of postoperative care.[17] In many areas the patient has to have had the surgery and be in the hospital bed before social care and support can be organized. Case studies should be written up and presented to relevant managers so that organizations can see how current finances constrain the professional's ability to plan care (Box 10.10).

BOOKING PATIENTS FOR SURGERY AND OPTIMIZING AVAILABLE RESOURCES

Unlike any other department or professional within the hospital the assessment service is well placed to organize the operation date for each patient.[18] By ensuring that the patient is on the right list for the correct procedure, and supported by adequate assessment, the preoperative assessment service will provide benefits to organizations and patients, such as a reduction of hospital-led cancellations, patient-led cancellations and patients not attending.[7] Booking initiatives play a major part in developing patient-focused services. After all, patients organize their lives each day and expect to play a part in a timely decision for surgery. In doing this, organizations are able to optimize the use of available resources by matching patient's needs to professional expertise and available equipment, including beds.

There is a place for using information technology in assessment. In some hospitals assessment information is stored directly on a database and shared between the relevant professionals. In others, patients hold their own records and take them to where they are needed. In both cases assessment is a fine example of the opportunities for sharing information among professionals, and this will only improve with the advent of the electronic patient record.[18]

Given the need to ensure that patients are fully involved with their assessment for surgery, different approaches to assessment are needed (Box 10.11).

There will be many local reasons for employing one or all of these approaches, and services will need to be tested and evaluated. There is reason to believe that as long as preoperative assessment staff are well trained then successful preoperative assessment can be delivered via a variety of approaches.

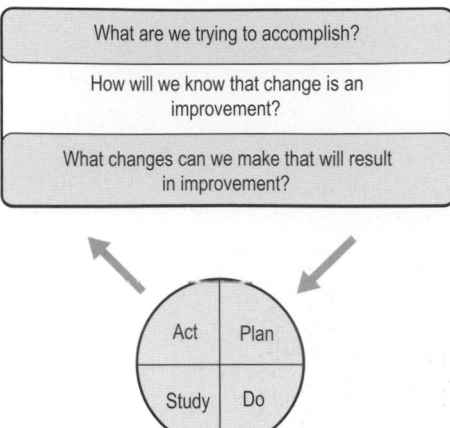

Figure 10.3   Plan, Do, Study, Act (PDSA) cycle.

MEASURING FOR CONTINUAL IMPROVEMENT

Any service that is responsive to patients, professionals and organizational needs will require evidence to ensure that it can provide the proof that things are better. How arrangements are made for the collection of evidence to support service developments will depend on how much time the team, patients and organization allocate to it. In order to improve the profile of the assessment service across the organization, and the impact it has had, resources will need to be allocated to measuring patient outcomes. Traditionally this has not been the role of clinical staff, and indeed training in measuring for improvement has been the responsibility of the audit department. The problem with this is that the facts and figures produced are not connected with the reality of providing a direct service to patients. In order to ensure the information collected is useful and the results are reviewed regularly, its collection needs to be designed by the professionals responsible for assessment. Professionals need to agree on how they will know they have been successful. In preoperative assessment useful tools are ensuring that there has been a reduction of 'did not attends', hospital-led cancellations and patient-led cancellations. There are many models for improvement, but the one that seems to encourage professionals to try out ideas in practice is the Nolan model (Fig. 10.3).[19]

This particular model is simple to understand and provides a culture for experimentation and review. Above all, it is important that services continue to

Box 10.12   Measuring for improvement

Key areas to measure in preoperative assessment are:[7]

- Number of patients who attended preoperative assessment
- Number of patients who did not attend preoperative assessment
- Number of patients who did not attend surgery following preoperative assessment
- Number of overnight stays, with reasons
- Number of operations cancelled on the day of surgery or the day before surgery because:
  - The patient said the appointment was inconvenient
  - The patient no longer wanted the operation
  - The consultant advised the patient that the operation was no longer necessary
  - The patient had a pre-existing medical condition
  - The patient did not follow preoperative instructions
- Number of operations cancelled by the hospital because essential resources (beds, surgeons, anaesthetists, equipment, etc.) were not available
- Staff satisfaction
- Patient satisfaction

develop based on statistical evidence of improvement for patients (Box 10.12).

SCENARIOS
Jane Jackson

The following two scenarios demonstrate what can happen when preoperative assessment is organized either well or not so well.

Case note 1: Mrs A

A 68-year-old woman, recently widowed, is due to undergo bilateral total knee replacement, right first followed by left.

Mrs A has a history of rheumatoid arthritis, the hands, elbows and shoulders being particularly affected. Shopping is difficult, as is carrying or lifting. Hypertension was diagnosed 12 years ago.

A neighbour brought Mrs A to the preoperative assessment clinic. During the interview, it was noted that Mrs A was hypertensive and on recording her blood pressure was found to be 175/108. The blood pressure was remeasured after half an hour and the best of three readings was 170/105. All other observations and examination were within normal limits.

In discussing the procedure and aftercare, it was noted that Mrs A had been experiencing difficulties at home since the death of her husband 3 months earlier. Mrs A lives in a third-floor flat; the lift is not reliable and she finds walking up the stairs with shopping difficult. A neighbour has been helping out.

The nurse in the preoperative assessment clinic discussed various solutions for Mrs A, and ascertained that she had been reluctant to call social services for rehousing, as she thought she might be considered a nuisance, or moved to a residential home. Mrs A agreed that the assessment clinic nurse could telephone social services, discuss the problem of current housing and surgery expectations, and to plan a solution. This was done in the presence of Mrs A, while she was in the clinic. An appointment was made for someone from social services to call on Mrs A the next day.

A telephone call late the next day relayed that social services were indeed able to provide assistance, and placed home care support immediately, with meals on wheels availability as required. As soon as a flat became available on the ground floor Mrs A would have first priority. The department was later informed that Mrs A was moved to her new flat 4 weeks later.

In the meanwhile, Mrs A had been referred to her GP for treatment of her hypertension. She was reviewed in the preoperative assessment clinic 4 weeks after her first appointment and found to be normotensive. Blood samples were taken for full blood count, urea and electrolytes, and a sample for group and save. ECG showed sinus rhythm. X-rays had been updated at the previous visit.

Mrs A could be admitted on the day of her surgery, as planned. Postoperative care was routine and Mrs A was discharged home as expected 5 days post surgery, with Hospital at Home service.

In this scenario the preoperative assessment nurse was able to identify the needs of Mrs A. Having identified those needs, the nurse took action to instigate treatment for the raised blood pressure by writing to the GP, and ensuring that Mrs A would be seen at the clinic 4 weeks later, by which time treatment for the hypertension should have had the desired effect of

lowering the blood pressure to within normal limits. In addition, the nurse identified the social needs of Mrs A which, left unattended, would have resulted in her spending a lengthy period of time in hospital and at risk of becoming more dependent upon the nursing staff, possibly even developing complications associated with long hospitalization, such as infection or deep vein thrombosis.

Case note 2: Mrs B

A 71-year-old woman was due to have an elective revision of right total hip replacement (THR).

Mrs B was referred to the orthopaedic consultant by her GP, with a letter stating that she had undergone a right THR 12 years previously and was now complaining of increasing pain in her right thigh, from hip to knee. Mrs B was seen in outpatients and, following discussion about her previous THR and her current symptoms, was examined and sent for X-ray. The X-ray showed that the shaft of the prosthesis had loosened. Mrs B was informed that she would require a revision right THR, and was placed on the waiting list accordingly.

Six weeks later a theatre space became available at short notice and, as her case was urgent, Mrs B was admitted to the ward without a preoperative assessment. Transport was required to bring Mrs B into hospital; a volunteer driver was found at short notice, and kindly agreed to bring Mrs B in to hospital at 4 pm on the day prior to the expected surgery. An electrocardiograph was undertaken. X-rays of the pelvis were not repeated, as those undertaken in outpatients clearly showed the prosthesis and there was no change in the patient's symptoms.

On admission, Mrs B was found to have an ulcer on her left leg measuring 2 cm in diameter. This had been present for some 7 months and was being dressed by the district nurse. Mrs B was noted to have been diagnosed as hypertensive 15 years earlier, but was well controlled on medication.

During examination by the house officer, Mrs B commented that she had, in recent weeks, developed an increased thirst, and frequency. This had not been mentioned to her GP, as the patient was expecting her hospital appointment. Urinalysis showed large amounts of glucose. A random blood glucose test was undertaken, 4 hours after food, which gave a reading of 18.4 mmol/L.

The HbAlc was 11.4%, but all other biochemistry and haematology readings were within normal limits.

Mrs B had her surgery postponed and was referred to the diabetic team for urgent review and management. A wound swab was taken from the ulcer and sent for microscopy, culture and sensitivity, and Mrs B was referred to the tissue viability nurse.

In this case the lack of preoperative assessment and the short-notice admission resulted in additional work for many departments: admissions, medical records, X-ray department, and the haematology department undertaking routine blood tests on an urgent basis. Theatre time booked for Mrs B would not now be utilized, as there was no further bed in which to bring another elective patient. Equipment for the revision THR, including prosthetics, would no longer be required. Surgeon and anaesthetist would have shortened lists. Mrs B received early referral for her new symptoms of diabetes, and expert attention for her leg ulcer, both of which would continue to be treated in outpatients, following her discharge home, 4 days later.

With preoperative assessment the admission procedure would have been quite different. The nurse in the assessment clinic would have recorded the medical, nursing and social history of Mrs B, and undertaken examination and investigations such as haematology, biochemistry and urinalysis. Swabs would have been taken from the leg ulcer and the GP notified of all results. Referral to the diabetic team and tissue viability nurse would have been made from the preoperative assessment clinic, having first discussed the same with the GP and patient.

Admission for surgery would have been appropriately delayed to enable the diabetes to be controlled and the ulcer to heal. Thus Mrs B would have been admitted at a date appropriate for her surgery, at a time when she would have been in optimum fitness and at less risk of postoperative complications such as infection.

The supporting services for Mrs B's admission – such as admissions, medical records, ward staff, pathology staff and transport, could have been organized to provide their services for an agreed date and time. This would ensure that Mrs B, requiring major surgery, would feel assured that her admission was given appropriate support from the interprofessional team.

References

1. National Council for the Enquiry into Perioperative Deaths. Functioning as a team. London: NCEPOD; 2002.
2. Collaboration and transparency. Getting the patient services clear and connected. London: Salamander Organisation; 2002.
3. NHS Modernisation Agency. Operating theatre guidance. London: DOH; 2002.
4. Department of Health. Junior doctors' hours: the new deal. London: DOH; 1997.
5. Penn S, Davenport H, Carrington S, et al. Principles of day surgery nursing. Oxford: Blackwell Science; 1996.
6. Janke E, Chalk V, Kinley H. Preoperative assessment. Setting the standard through learning. Southampton: University of Southampton; 2002.
7. NHS Modernisation Agency. National good practice on day surgery preoperative assessment. London: DOH; 2001.
8. Association of Anaesthetists of Great Britain and Ireland. Preoperative assessment. The role of the anaesthetist. London: AAGBI; 2001.
9. Munro J, Kinley H. An evaluation of multi-professional roles in preoperative assessment. University of Sheffield/University of Southampton joint publishers; 2000.
10. Department of Health. Good practice in consent implementation guide: consent to examination or treatment. London: DOH; 2001.
11. Smith S. The patient's need for information for a hospital stay. Internat J Nurs Studies 1994; 37.
12. Roach D. Involving patients, carers and users. Buckingham Partnership. (unpublished).
13. Roach D. Techniques for engaging users. Buckingham Partnership. (unpublished).
14. National Institute for Clinical Excellence. Preoperative tests: the use of routine preoperative tests for elective surgery. NICE; June 2003.
15. The American Society of Anaesthesiologists. Patient status score. ASA; 1963.
16. Department of Health. Implementing the new system of financial flows: payment by results guidance. London: DOH; 2003/4.
17. NHS Plan. House of Commons Health Committee; 2001.
18. NHS Executive. The electronic patient record. Leeds: NHS Executive; 1997.
19. Langley GJ, Nolan KM, Nolan TW, et al. The improvement guide. A practical approach to enhancing organisational performance. San Francisco: Jossey Bass Publishers; 1996.
20. NHS Modernisation Agency. National good practice on preoperative assessment for in-patient surgery. London: 2003.

Useful websites

Southampton University www.soton.org.uk
NHSU www.nhsu.org.uk
DOH – NHS Plan www.doh.co.uk
Association of Anaesthetists www.aagbi.org
NICE www.nice.org.uk
NHS Modernisation Agency www.modernnhs.uk

National Association of Theatre Nurses www.natn.org.uk
Royal College of Surgeons www.rcseng.ac.uk
Royal College of Anaesthetists www.rcoa.ac.uk
National Association of Operating Department Practitioners
    www.aodp.org
British Association of Day Surgery www.bads.co.uk

Chapter 11

Care of the patient undergoing anaesthesia

Melanie Oakley and Melanie van Limborgh

Key points

- The role of the anaesthetic practitioner in the context of current developments
- Overview of the preparation of the patient environment, discussing the equipment used and care of the patient once they enter the operating environment
- Pharmacological agents used in anaesthesia
- An overview of emergency anaesthesia

INTRODUCTION

Anaesthesia enables surgery to take place by rendering the patient insensible to pain and sensation, and in the case of general anaesthesia, unconscious. It is a complex science and is a major part of the patient experience when undergoing surgery. Fear for the patient is not always of the impending surgery but of the anaesthetic. Anecdotally frequently asked questions are, 'Will I wake up during the operation?' or 'Suppose I do not wake up at all?' The skill of the anaesthetic practitioner can go some way towards helping the patient combat those fears. They have the knowledge to explain to the patient what is going to happen to them, and they can act as advocate when patients are unable, or too frightened, to speak for themselves. The anaesthetic practitioner will meet the patient as they enter the operating department, be with them through induction of anaesthesia, and stay with them throughout the operative procedure. They will support them as they emerge from anaesthesia and, in some instances if they have the appropriate training, they will go with them to the recovery area. The anaesthetic practitioner takes a holistic approach to caring for their patients.

There are many excellent texts for practitioners working in the anaesthetic field that the reader can go to for more in-depth knowledge of anaesthetics. This chapter only aims to give a broad overview of anaesthetics to give the reader an idea of what is involved, and hopefully encourage them to do some further study (see Further reading).

THE ANAESTHETIC PRACTITIONER

The concept of nurse anaesthetists does not exist in this country despite the flurry of interest a few years ago, when there was a predicted shortfall in consultant anaesthetists.[1] In 1996 the NHS Executive carried out a scoping study[2] which concluded that nurse anaesthetists would not enhance anaesthetic patient care in this country. Added to this, the Royal College of Anaesthetists was fast-tracking senior anaesthetic registrars, and it was predicted that the shortfall would be filled within 2 years. However, at the time of writing the NHS Modernisation Agency in England is in the process of setting up pilot sites for the commencement of non-physician anaesthetist training programmes. These new practitioners will be called 'Anaesthetic critical care practitioners' and will follow a curriculum at Master's level.

As with other areas of the operating department there are two grades of staff working in the anaesthetic area: first, nurses, who have undergone a 3-year general training. Before they commence any form of postregistration study in an aspect of theatre practice they may work as a staff nurse for 6 months to a year, usually rotating round the specialties.

In order to work in anaesthetic specialties, nurses formally must have obtained a National Board course in anaesthetic nursing or equivalent. With the demise of the National Boards this will be in the form of diploma or degree modules in specialist anaesthetic practice. Following the course nurses will consolidate the skills learnt for at least 6 months.

The other grade of staff is the operating department practitioner (ODP), who will have completed a 2-year course in operating department practice. This was originally a City and Guilds qualification, which subsequently became NVQ level 3 and now is at diploma level. This qualification enables ODPs to work in all areas of the operating department.

WHAT IS THE ROLE OF THE ANAESTHETIC PRACTITIONER?

Primarily anaesthetic practitioners are there to ensure that patients are anaesthetized safely, with the least amount of anxiety possible on the patient's part. They are not there to assist the anaesthetist, as appears to be the common misconception.[3,4] The dictionary defines assistant as a 'helper' or 'subordinate worker', (Concise Oxford Dictionary), but this demeans the role of the anaesthetic nurse and the ODP and does not respect them as a professional with specialist knowledge and skills.[5]

The role is multidimensional. Primarily it is to ensure that the patient is well cared for while undergoing invasive procedures. This involves communication skills, an ability to try and put the patient at their ease, and planning individualized care. Advocacy is integral to the role.[5] Added to this the role is becoming increasingly technical, with a need for in-depth knowledge of physiological principles. Finally there is a supervisory role, facilitating the learning of student nurses, trainee ODPs and anaesthetic course nurses. The list is not exhaustive, but clearly this is a highly skilled area of the operating department.

In the UK practitioners can only work in the anaesthetic area if they have an anaesthetic qualification.[4] This means that no prior unsupervised experience can have been gained, although the individual may have worked in recovery.

There is no doubt that with ODPs being trained at diploma level, and with more nurses opting to study at degree level, the role of the anaesthetic practitioner will evolve and there could be many opportunities in anaesthetic practice.

PREPARATION OF THE PATIENT'S ENVIRONMENT

Preparation of the environment in which the patient is going to be received is key to their safe care in the operating department. Therefore, the anaesthetic practitioner should spend a significant period of time on this undertaking. It is essential that when the patient arrives in the department the practitioner has completed this preparation so that their time is devoted to the needs of the patient. In this section, preparation of the anaesthetic room, followed by preparation of the patient, will be discussed. There are many seminal texts examining the equipment used in anaesthesia; thus the purpose of this section is only to give an overview.

Case study 11.1

Learner X was undertaking a course to become an anaesthetic practitioner. His tutor was assessing him during a gynaecology list. The patient arrived in the anaesthetic room and was obviously very nervous. However, X had not finished getting all the equipment ready and so did not acknowledge the patient's presence and continued to set up. The tutor waited a little while to see what X would do, and then stepped in and started to reassure the patient.

Although X was setting up the anaesthetic room safely he did not demonstrate the most important part of the anaesthetic practitioner's role, that of supporting the patient.

When discussing this with X afterwards, the tutor pointed out that he must be aware of how long it took to set up the anaesthetic room. She suggested he should have started earlier, so that all his attention could be focused on the patient when she arrived.

Learner X did not pass his assessment at this point. He worked on his time management skills and passed the assessment on a second attempt.

PREPARATION OF THE ANAESTHETIC ROOM

Before the patient reaches the anaesthetic room the area should have been fully prepared for use. The anaesthetic practitioner should always think of preparing the area systematically to ensure that preparation is complete. One way of preparing an anaesthetic room is the ABC system similar to that used in resuscitation.[6] In this section equipment associated with airway and breathing will be considered, followed by equipment used to monitor the patient's circulation.

THE ANAESTHETIC MACHINE

The anaesthetic machine is essentially a trolley with the means to provide a medical gas supply to the patient. The gas supply is provided by pipeline oxygen, air and nitrous oxide, but in the event of an emergency all anaesthetic machines should have a

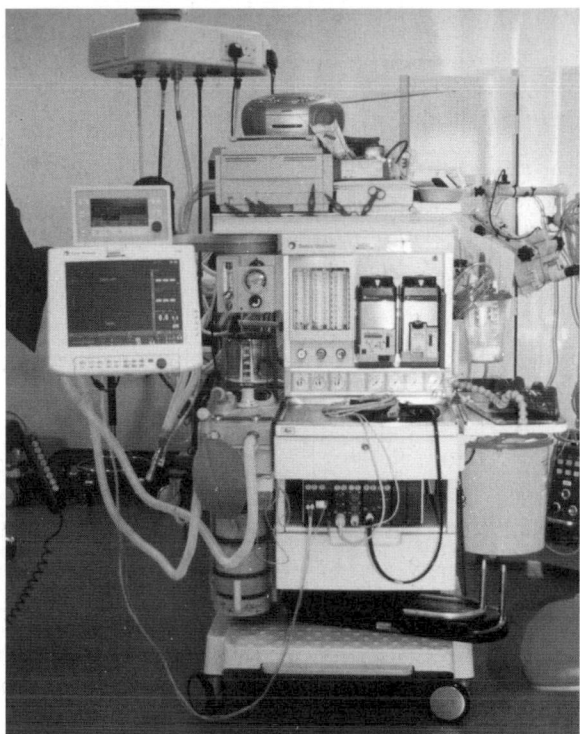

Figure 11.1 Anaesthetic machine in the operating theatre.

cylinder gas supply. Anaesthetic machines have become more technically advanced, with most of the ventilators and monitoring equipment being incorporated into them. However, checking them and making sure they are safe to use is still an integral part of the anaesthetic practitioners' role.

The Association of Anaesthetists provides a standard checklist for anaesthetic machines, and so this chapter will not go into detail.[7] Rather, there will be a discussion on the components of the anaesthetic machine. In most units there will be two machines to check, one in the anaesthetic room and one in theatre (Fig. 11.1). Both will have to be checked prior to induction of anaesthesia. The anaesthetist undertaking the anaesthetic procedure should also check the machines, which in effect means they will have been double checked, thus ensuring patient safety.

ANAESTHETIC BREATHING CIRCUITS

A breathing circuit is used to deliver the anaesthetic agent and medical gases from the machine to the patient via a face mask, endotracheal tube or laryngeal mask airway.[6] The most common anaesthetic breathing circuits in use are the Bain, the circle and the Ayres T-piece.[6] Anaesthetic breathing circuits are normally classified by the Mapleson classification.[8] The circuit should be left ready in the anaesthetic room with the appropriately sized face mask – usually size 4 for a female patient and 5 for a male.

VAPOURIZERS

Anaesthetic vapourizers are used to administer anaesthetic agents such as halothane, enflurane, isoflurane and sevoflurane by means of the anaesthetic circuit, and are used to maintain anaesthesia. They should be checked every time the anaesthetic machine is checked. This includes ensuring that they are working, are correctly attached to the anaesthetic machine, and are full of the volatile agent. Like other medical equipment they require regular servicing.[9]

FLOWMETERS

Flowmeters on the anaesthetic machine should be checked on at least a daily basis. The bobbins in the flowmeter that indicate the level of gases being delivered to the patient should spin freely at the level of the gas being administered, and they should not be cracked or broken.[9]

ANAESTHETIC GAS/VOLATILE AGENT MONITORS

These monitors have now replaced the single CO_2, O_2 and agent monitors, and only need to be calibrated on a regular basis. They work by taking a gas sample from as near to the patient's airway as possible, and the CO_2, O_2 and agent are measured by infrared absorption. Expired carbon dioxide is measured in order to detect whether the patient's airway is compromised by airway adjunct displacement.[6]

VENTILATORS

The ventilator should be reviewed as part of the anaesthetic machine check and may be part of the machine itself, or separate. The ventilator should also have a separate or inbuilt alarm to inform the anaesthetic team if it is not working correctly, or if the patient circuit has become disconnected from it.[10]

PATIENT MONITORING (Fig. 11.2)

The anaesthetic team will routinely monitor the patients' heart rate and rhythm via an electrocardiogram (ECG) monitor. Pulse oximetry will also be

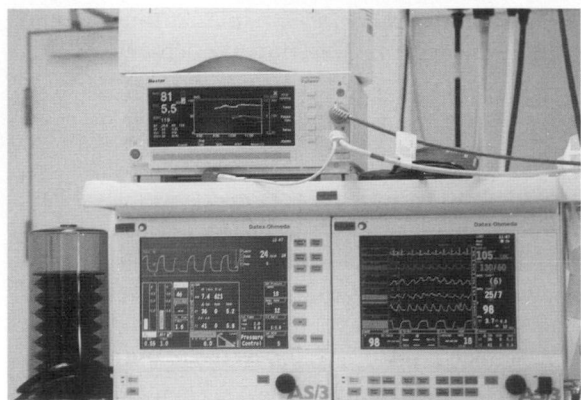

Figure 11.2   Monitoring every physiological parameter during anaesthesia.

employed to measure the level of oxygen saturation in the patient's circulating blood supply. Non-invasive blood pressure monitoring is routine, and equipment for all of these parameters will need to be available. The anaesthetic practitioner must become skilled in interpreting the data seen on the screen, and be able to react in the appropriate manner to those data.[11]

Some patients will require monitoring by more invasive methods, such as arterial blood pressure measurement or central venous pressure monitoring. If this is necessary the anaesthetic practitioner will have to allow sufficient time to prepare all the equipment required, or be able to prepare it quickly and efficiently in the emergency situation.

EQUIPMENT REQUIRED TO SECURE AN AIRWAY

• Laryngoscope – with medium and long blades available. In most instances the medium blade will be used; however, in some situations, when a patient has a longer distance between the oropharynx and the vocal cords in the larynx, the long blade will be used. The laryngoscope should be checked to ensure that the light works, is sufficiently bright for use, and that the blade opens easily.[10]

• Endotracheal tube – three sizes: 7, 8 and 9. A size 8 would be used in a female, a 9 in a male. This facilitates moving down a size if necessary. These tubes should be cut and ready to use. They should be checked prior to use for patency and even cuff inflation.

• Laryngeal mask airway (LMA) – this is a non-invasive form of airway management and is used in many instances instead of the endotracheal tube. Sizes 3, 4 and 5 should be available. They should also be checked for even cuff inflation and patency.[12]

• Catheter mount with filter, for connecting the endotracheal tube/LMA to the breathing circuit/ventilator. Alternatively the endotracheal tube/LMA may connect straight on to the breathing circuit.

• Air syringe – this must be clearly labelled as such to avoid its being used for intravenous injection.

• Tie/tape – after the endotracheal tube/laryngeal mask airway has been inserted this is a means of securing it.

• Gum elastic bougie – this may be used in cases of difficult intubation to place in the trachea under visualization by a laryngoscope; the endotracheal tube may then be 'piggybacked' over the bougie. When the endotracheal tube is in the trachea the bougie will be removed.

• Stylets – may also be used to give shape to an endotracheal tube, such as a reinforced tube, in order to facilitate intubation. After the tube is in place, the stylet is removed.

• Magill's forceps – required with the intubating equipment in case a foreign body requires removal from the patient's airway, or in order to facilitate placing a throat pack in the pharynx or to guide a gastric tube into the stomach.

• Oral/nasal pharyngeal airways – a selection should be available to help the anaesthetist secure an airway in the unconscious patient.

• Local anaesthetic spray – the anaesthetist may wish to use local anaesthetic spray in order not to irritate the vocal cords during intubation.

• Lubricating gel – all laryngeal mask airways and endotracheal tubes should be lubricated prior to insertion.

This list is for an adult undergoing anaesthesia. Obviously for children the equipment would be different (see Further reading).

INTRAVENOUS ACCESS

Intravenous access must be ensured in order to induce anaesthesia and administer fluids during anaesthesia and surgery.

A range of cannulae should be available, although intravenous infusion may not be used for every anaesthetic. It is customary to have a litre of intravenous fluid and an administration set prepared for use. The anaesthetic practitioner should always have

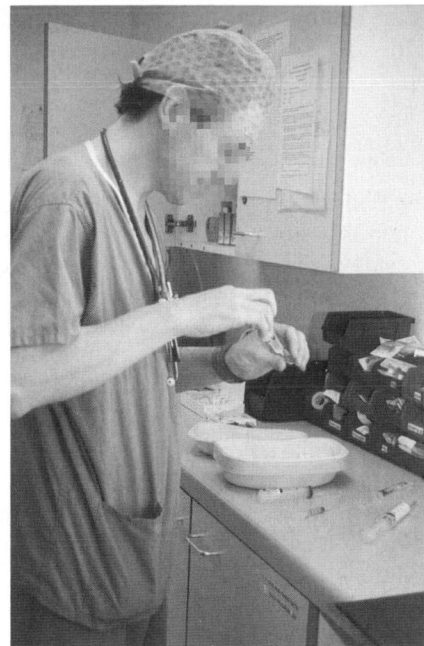

Figure 11.3   The anaesthetist draws up his own drugs.

equipment available to warm intravenous fluid, thereby preventing heat loss. In cases of severe haemorrhage a rapid infuser should be available for the anaesthetic team to use, which greatly speeds the rate and volume of infused fluids administered to the patient. It must be noted that anaesthetists are responsible for drawing up their own drugs (Fig. 11.3).

OTHER EQUIPMENT

Forced air warming or equivalent should be available to help keep the patient's temperature within acceptable parameters. This is especially important for babies and children, and debilitated or shocked patients, but ideally should be used for all patients. If an epidural, spinal or other local/regional anaesthetic technique is to be employed the appropriate equipment must be made available. Before the start of any anaesthetic technique a working defibrillator and resuscitation drugs should be available in case of emergencies.

ELECTRICAL SUPPLY

It is essential that the anaesthetic practitioner understand the action to be taken in the event of a power failure in order to ensure patient safety. A usual check is to ensure that any back-up batteries for monitoring and other equipment are charged.

RECEPTION OF THE PATIENT

When the patient arrives in the area the anaesthetic practitioner should introduce him- or herself. It is best to establish how the patient would like to be addressed, as some people take exception to being addressed by their first name without their permission.

The anaesthetic practitioner should take a handover from the patient's ward nurse and from the patient. This should take place in a manner that preserves the patient's dignity and confidentiality. It would not be appropriate to greet the patient in an open, busy corridor where they might be overheard. Many units now have a specific bay for patients waiting for surgery, where they can wait quietly and be checked into the operating department in a confidential manner. If the anaesthetic practitioner has any queries or concerns, the anaesthetist should be immediately informed before anaesthesia is induced.

When the ward nurse has left, the anaesthetic practitioner will take responsibility for the patient and will not leave them unaccompanied at any time, unless the anaesthetist or another member of the theatre team takes over their care.

Patients usually experience extreme anxiety before anaesthesia and for many different reasons. The anaesthetic practitioner should ensure that they anticipate and address any of the patient's concerns and answer their questions as honestly and sensitively as possible. It may be necessary to include the anaesthetist/surgeon in this conversation, and any concerns the patient has should be documented in the care plan.

If the patient is a child accompanied by a parent or carer it should be remembered that they themselves might be as anxious as the child, and will need support from the anaesthetic practitioner at this time.

The anaesthetic practitioner will need to assess the type of procedure the patient is to undergo and discuss with the anaesthetist the type of anaesthetic technique he or she will be using. It is important the anaesthetist and the anaesthetic practitioner liaise fully regarding the patients they are caring for. The administration of anaesthesia is a partnership that requires preparation and thorough communication to ensure safe and effective care.

When planning the care of the patient undergoing anaesthesia and surgery there are many issues that need to be considered by the anaesthetic practitioner.

- *Age of the patient* – this will affect the anaesthetic procedure, the type of anaesthetic given and the equipment required.[13]
- *Past medical history* – this will be relevant to the type of anaesthetic that will be given. It is important that the anaesthetic practitioner ascertains any drug therapy the patient may be receiving and informs the anaesthetist, as if this is not identified it may be detrimental to the patient.
- *Allergies* – identification of allergies is essential, not only to pharmacological agents but more recently to latex. If allergies are identified prior to anaesthesia, precautions can be taken.
- *Mobility* – problems with mobility are particularly important to identify, as care and attention must be given to the positioning of the patient.
- *Prostheses* should be identified as they may cause problems during surgery, for example if a metal hip prosthesis is not noted a diathermy plate could be placed over it, potentially causing burn injury.[6] Also, a prosthetic glass eye may lead to an error if the anaesthetist wishes to ascertain the level of anaesthesia after induction. All jewellery must be removed or taped.
- *Contact lenses and spectacles* – any contact lenses should be removed, as they may cause damage to the cornea after induction as the natural blink reflex is lost; if contact lenses are present the eye is not able to protect itself. It is equally important that a patient should be able to wear spectacles while in the anaesthetic room, as they must be able to identify who will be caring for them. Also, they should be able to read any documentation, such as the consent form.
- *Hearing aids* – if the patient is wearing a hearing aid the anaesthetic practitioner should allow them to keep it in place. This will ensure that the patient is able to hear what is being said to them during induction and on emergence from anaesthesia; this in turn will decrease the patient's anxiety, as they will be able to communicate with the anaesthetic practitioner and the anaesthetist. The hearing aid can easily be removed when the patient is unconscious if necessary, and replaced on reversal of anaesthesia.
- *Dentition* – dentures do not necessarily need to be removed, as doing so may make it more difficult

for the anaesthetist to maintain an effective airway after induction of anaesthesia. This also leaves the patient with their dignity intact until they are asleep. Poor dentition should be identified, as this could cause a difficult airway problem, and it is essential that the anaesthetist is aware of problems with the teeth so that they can take care when intubating.

• *Nil by mouth status* – the anaesthetic practitioner will need to ascertain when the patient last ate or drank before the anaesthetic is administered. It cannot be taken for granted that the patient is adequately fasted, even if documentation states a particular time of fasting. It is not unheard of for a patient to believe they are adequately fasted but to have been chewing gum, or someone on the ward may have given the patient a drink or something to eat by mistake. Administering an anaesthetic when the stomach is not empty can lead to vomiting or regurgitation (see the section on emergency anaesthesia). Another issue for the anaesthetic practitioner to consider is the length of time the patient has been fasted. Jester and Williams[14] found that many of their patients were fasted for too long. Current consensus on fasting is 6 hours for food, and 2–4 hours for free fluids.[15,16] Best practice suggests that if the anaesthetist prescribes the timing of the last preoperative drink then patients are more likely to be fasted for the optimal period.[14]

• *Documentation* – the anaesthetic practitioner should check that the documentation is complete before anaesthesia is commenced. This should include any relevant blood results, including 'group and save' or 'cross-match', and a sickle-cell test if the patient is in a high-risk group. X-rays should be available, as should a recent 12-lead ECG if indicated. The anaesthetist needs to be informed of any missing information. The anaesthetic practitioner should always check that the patient's consent form for the procedure is signed. Although the consent form itself is not the responsibility of the anaesthetic practitioner, they should check it is available before the induction of anaesthesia, and that the patient understands the procedure they are undergoing – and if not, they should be given the opportunity to ask questions. All details should be cross-referenced with the operating list to ensure the correct patient for the correct procedure. Added to this it is the responsibility of the anaesthetic practitioner to ensure the consent is seen by the scrub practitioner prior to the commencement of surgery.

Case study 11.2

Patient Y arrived in the day surgery unit. He was first on the list for a repair of an inguinal hernia. Staff nurse Z started to admit him and inquired whether he had had breakfast that morning. He said he had not. She confirmed again that he had had nothing to eat or drink that morning, 'Oh yes', he replied. 'I ate a Mars bar on the way in ... but that is not proper food is it?' Clearly, his operation had to be postponed.

This scenario illustrates that although a patient may appear to understand, that comprehension must be checked. Perhaps Y had not been told the importance of not eating or drinking.

ANAESTHETIC PHARMACOLOGY

An in-depth knowledge of anaesthetic pharmacology is of the utmost importance for the practitioner working in the anaesthetic environment. They need to be able to identify which agents are indicated – and more importantly which are contraindicated – in order to advocate for the patient. Advocacy can only happen if the practitioner has this knowledge, which is founded upon up-to-date evidence.

Regarding anaesthetic pharmacology, consideration must be given to how the patient's airway is to be maintained for the duration of anaesthesia. This will guide the anaesthetist in their choice of anaesthetic agents. Obviously this is a simplistic view, and there are many more factors that must be taken into account:

• The type of operation
• The American Society of Anesthesiologists (ASA) classification of the patient based on past medical and anaesthetic history
• Day case or in-patient status
• The age and sex of the patient.

Broadly speaking, if a patient can breathe spontaneously for the duration of their operation their airway will be maintained using a bag and mask (not widely used today) or a laryngeal mask airway. Or the anaesthetist may opt to ventilate the patient for the duration of surgery. Whichever approach applies, the principles of induction, maintenance of anaesthesia and analgesia will be the same. However, when a patient is ventilated a muscle relaxant will be used.

INDUCTION AGENTS

Induction agents induce anaesthesia and can be used to maintain it using intermittent bolus or continuous infusion anaesthesia combined with inhalational agents. Ideally an induction agent should be cost-effective, safe, with a short onset and predictable recovery.[17]

Thiopental

This is a barbiturate induction agent which can be administered intravenously or rectally, but most commonly intravenously. The induction dose is 4–5 mg/kg and induction is smooth, with the patient losing consciousness in one arm-to-brain circulation time. Cardiovascularly it causes vasodilation, leading to a drop in blood pressure. Thiopental is metabolized in the liver. On injection it can cause transient respiratory depression.[17] Thiopental should be avoided in asthmatics as it can cause laryngospasm or bronchospasm.[9]

Recovery following thiopental is smooth, with a low incidence of postoperative nausea and vomiting.[18] It has long been the gold standard of anaesthetic induction agents, as it has a good record of satisfactory performance. However, its use has been superseded with the advent of propofol.

Propofol

Propofol was first released in the 1970s, and Cremofor L was used as the solvent in the propofol solution. However, there were an unacceptable number of allergic reactions and so the product was withdrawn. In the 1980s it was reintroduced in a 1% aqueous emulsion containing soya bean oil and egg phosphatide.[19] Because of the lipid nature of the drug it is painful on injection in the small veins of the hand, and so 1% lidocaine (lignocaine) is added beforehand.[18] Also because of its lipid base, propofol can support bacterial growth if contaminated,[20] and so it should only be drawn up immediately prior to injection.

Propofol can be used as a bolus injection or as a total intravenous anaesthesia technique.[21] It has been demonstrated that the use of propofol as a maintenance agent reduces the incidence of postoperative nausea and vomiting.[17,22]

Pharmacokinetically propofol has a fast redistribution out of the blood. This clearance rate after metabolism in the liver is rapid in comparison with other induction agents, making recovery from anaesthesia swift and leading to earlier discharge from hospital. The widespread use of propofol is one of the major factors in enabling effective day surgery.

Propofol causes hypotension owing to a reduction in systemic vascular resistance. There is potentially significant bradycardia with depression of the baroreceptor reflex. Dose-related respiratory depression may also be observed on induction.[17]

Etomidate

Etomidate is presented in a single bolus of 20 mg in 10 ml. This is because in the past it was used for continuous infusion in intensive care, but it was found that the mortality rate was higher than expected and further investigation demonstrated that etomidate caused suppression of adrenocortical secretion.[9] Etomidate is painful on injection and recovery following administration is poor, with increased restlessness and an increase in postoperative nausea and vomiting.

Etomidate is often used in the ill and elderly, but must still be given with caution as the cardiovascular stability in these patients is often poor. It is metabolized in the liver and plasma, and 2% is excreted unchanged in the urine.[9] Before the advent of propofol, etomidate was used in preference to thiopental because it was more cardiovascularly stable. However, this is now not the case.

Ketamine

Ketamine is not widely used in the United Kingdom, although it has a wider use in North America. One of the benefits of ketamine is that it is an analgesic, and up to 0.5 mg/kg produces profound analgesia without loss of the patient's airway. Because of this it can be used to support patients undergoing painful procedures, such as changing of burns dressings, or physiotherapy for fractured ribs.[17]

When used as an anaesthetic induction agent a dose of 2 mg/kg is given. On induction it increases pulse rate, blood pressure and intracranial pressure. Glycopyrrolate is often given with it because of an increase in salivation. Patients can suffer from hallucinations – termed 'emergence delirium' – in the recovery area, and therefore they should be recovered in a quiet area of the theatre. Benzodiazepine premedications can reduce the incidence of emergence delirium.

MAINTENANCE AGENTS – VOLATILE ANAESTHETIC AGENTS

The precise mechanism by which volatile agents produce anaesthesia is unclear.[17] Many of the characteristics and side effects of these agents are similar. Thus in this section the most commonly used agents in clinical practice will be explored.

Halothane

This is a widely used agent that produces rapid induction of anaesthesia. The drawback with its use is the demonstration of hepatic changes after administration. This is due to 18% of it being metabolized by the liver. Hepatic changes are more likely to be demonstrated after repeated halothane anaesthesia, but only in a few cases.[9] The underlying reason for this remains unclear, although several suggestions have been made, such as a reaction to a metabolite of halothane. The current theory postulates that metabolism of halothane produces trifluoroacetyl (TFA) halide. Through a complex chemical process this results in an inflammatory response in the liver in certain susceptible patients.[23] As a precautionary measure halothane is not administered within 3 months of a previous administration.

Halothane possesses no analgesic effects. On administration it will produce a dose-related hypotension due to vasodilation, depression of the myocardium and conductivity of the heart. Halothane relaxes the pregnant uterus, and so therefore should only be used in very low concentrations in patients who are pregnant. Halothane is a bronchodilator, thus it could be indicated in asthmatic patients.

Enflurane

Enflurane has properties similar to halothane. The main advantage is that only 3% of it is metabolized by the liver, and so it has not been implicated in the hepatic dysfunction related to repeated halothane anaesthesia.

Enflurane is acceptable as a gaseous induction, although more irritant to inhale than halothane. There is a suggestion that enflurane may be nephrotoxic, although this is not confirmed. Thus it is wise not to administer enflurane to patients with renal impairment.[23]

Isoflurane

The advantage of isoflurane over halothane and enflurane is that it does not depress myocardial contractility or conduction. Also, only 0.3% is metabolized by the liver, making it suitable for patients with hepatic dysfunction.

It can also be used as part of a hypotensive anaesthetic technique, because increasing doses of the agent will simultaneously decrease the blood pressure and increase the depth of anaesthesia; this prevents the reflex tachycardia observed in other forms of hypotensive anaesthesia techniques.[9]

Desflurane

Desflurane is one of the newer inhalational agents, which does not appear to have gained wide popularity in clinical practice. It is a rapidly acting agent, but produces too much airway irritation to be employed for inhalational induction. It is associated with increased coughing, breath-holding and laryngospasm.[17] It is similar to isoflurane and associated with rapid recovery, making it suitable for day-case anaesthesia.[9]

Sevoflurane

This is another of the newer volatile anaesthetic agents and appears to be growing in popularity. It is very useful in gaseous induction as it is the least irritant to the airway of all the inhalational agents.[17,23]

As with enflurane, there is some evidence to suggest sevoflurane is nephrotoxic, but this has not been demonstrated in the clinical situation.[17] However, it is best avoided in patients with renal impairment. Two and a half per cent of sevoflurane is metabolized by the liver.

It has been noted that the newer inhalational agents (desflurane and sevoflurane) need to be used at low flow rates when the circle anaesthetic system is used. However, it may be that toxic metabolites limit the use of sevoflurane in a closed circuit in combination with soda lime.[9]

To summarize, all inhalational agents have, to a lesser or greater degree, side effects for the patient. It can be seen that the selection of volatile agents is multifactorial, and they should be chosen according to patient benefit and the balance of risks.

ANALGESICS

This section will look at analgesics used for the duration of anaesthesia. There are many other analgesics, which are used as part of a balanced anaesthesia technique, but they are not within the scope of this chapter.

FENTANYL

Fentanyl is a synthetic opioid derived from pethidine. It is used mainly during anaesthesia because it is short acting and is a severe respiratory depressant, neither of which characteristics are desirable in the recovery phase. With smaller doses of fentanyl, respiratory depression will last up to 30 minutes; with larger doses it may be prolonged for up to 2–3 hours. Fentanyl has relatively few side effects. Its use via the epidural route has gained widespread popularity. It appears that when given extradurally its action is potentiated and can last up to 4 hours.[24]

ALFENTANIL

The main use of alfentanil is in day surgery, as it is very short acting and is used as part of a total intravenous anaesthesia technique. It is a respiratory depressant, but its effects are less profound than those of fentanyl.

REMIFENTANIL

This is a relatively new opioid analgesic designed for use as part of an intravenous anaesthesia technique. It is short acting and wears off within minutes of its being withdrawn. The side effects are similar to those of fentanyl.

MUSCLE RELAXANTS

Muscle relaxants fall into two categories, depolarizing and non-depolarizing. These terms relate to their mode of action at the neuromuscular junction. In order to understand muscle relaxants it is important to examine the normal nerve impulse.

Motor neurones are long cells which originate in the spinal cord or the midbrain. The nerve impulse or action potential is transmitted down the nerve axon, jumping from one node of Ranvier to the next until eventually it reaches the neuromuscular junction. This is where the nerve axon and the muscle cell come into close contact with one another, but do not touch. In order for the action potential to be carried across to the motor endplate a neurotransmitter called acetylcholine is used. Acetylcholine is produced in the synapse from acetyl and choline moieties. Acetylcholine is released when the action

---

Box 11.1   The normal nerve impulse

- Nervous impulses originate in the anterior horns of the spinal cord
- The nerve impulse moves along the nerve axon by electrical conduction
- The axon then branches into nerve terminals, each of which comes into contact with one muscle cell. The nerve structure closest to the muscle is the synapse, which is opposite the endplate
- The physiological gap is bridged chemically by acetylcholine, which migrates across the synaptic cleft and binds selectively at the endplate
- There is a change in membrane permeability
- Sodium [Na+] moves into the cells
- Potassium [K+] moves out of the cells
- There is a change in potential known as endplate potential
- Depolarization spreads through the muscle and calcium ions, which are intracellular reservoirs of calcium, are released from the endoplasmic reticulum
- The muscle contracts
- Repolarization takes place, which restores the endplate to its resting potential
- Acetylcholine is destroyed by cholinesterase

---

potential reaches the nerve terminal. It then migrates across the synaptic cleft and binds selectively to the motor endplate. This causes a change, which produces opening of the ion channels. Sodium [Na+] moves into the cell and potassium [K+] moves out. The inflow of Na+ causes depolarization of the endplate, which in turn produces a muscle action potential and causes calcium ions to be released from the endoplasmic reticulum, which leads to muscle contraction (Box 11.1).[25] Acetylcholine is rapidly removed from the neuromuscular junction by cholinesterase and the membrane returns to its resting potential.[23]

Depolarizing muscle relaxants

The only depolarizing muscle relaxant used in the United Kingdom is suxamethonium. The actions of suxamethonium can be explained by its chemical structure being similar to that of acetylcholine. Thus suxamethonium is said to 'mimic' acetylcholine, and when given, the cell membrane becomes permeable

Box 11.2   Advantages of suxamethonium

- Works within 30 seconds
- Gives optimal intubating conditions
- Does not need to be reversed, as it is broken down by plasma cholinesterase within 3–5 minutes

Box 11.3   Complications of suxamethonium

- Fasciculation
- Myalgia (muscle pains)
- Hyperkalaemia
- Bradycardia
- Raised intraocular and intragastric pressure
- Prolonged neuromuscular blockade – acquired and inherited plasma cholinesterase deficiency
- Malignant hyperthermia
- Anaphylaxis

to sodium and potassium and so depolarization takes place. Suxamethonium is removed from the neuromuscular junction by plasma cholinesterase.[26]

The advantages of suxamethonium are that it works within 30 seconds and gives optimal intubating conditions. Therefore it is the drug of choice for a rapid sequence induction, where the gap between induction of anaesthesia and intubation needs to be as short as possible. The other advantage of suxamethonium is that it does not need to be reversed, for as previously mentioned it is hydrolyzed by the enzyme plasma cholinesterase (Box 11.2). Conversely, this can also be a disadvantage, as some patients have an inherited plasma cholinesterase deficiency and are unable to remove suxamethonium from the neuromuscular junction.

There are many complications when using suxamethonium (Box 11.3). According to Harper,[26] because of the many complications there is a need for a non-depolarizing muscle relaxant which is short acting without the side effects. He calls this the search for the 'Holy Grail'.

Non–depolarizing muscle relaxants

Atracurium This is a synthetic non-depolarizing muscle relaxant. It is unique in that it is metabolized by the Hofmann elimination reaction – meaning the breakdown takes place at a pH of 7.4 and a temperature of 37°C. Atracurium is also broken down by esterases in both the plasma and the liver. The onset of action is between 2 and 5 minutes, with duration of action of between 25 and 40 minutes. Patients will begin to breathe spontaneously after this, although most anaesthetists will use a reversal agent. Bradycardia may occur during surgery. Histamine release may be a problem with larger doses, but not with normal clinical doses.[27]

Mivacurium At a molecular level mivacurium is similar to atracurium, having a benzylisoquinolinium structure. It is the only non-depolarizing muscle relaxant to undergo metabolism by plasma cholinesterase, meaning that it is cleared rapidly from the plasma, thus facilitating a short duration of action. What directly follows on from this is that a patient who has reduced plasma cholinesterase levels is susceptible to the duration of action of mivacurium being prolonged, as may occur with suxamethonium. The maximum block will be reached after about 4–5 minutes, with a duration of action between 10 and 20 minutes. It is usually unnecessary to use an anticholinesterase for reversal. There are no significant changes in the cardiovascular response, although there can be a drop in blood pressure due to histamine release.[27]

Vecuronium This is a synthetic steroid-based muscle relaxant derived from pancuronium. It is supplied in a freeze-dried powder which is dissolved in water. Once made up it can be kept for 24 hours. It is eliminated through the kidneys. It has an elimination half-life of 60 minutes, which is relatively long. The clinical significance of this is that accumulation may occur following larger doses, especially in patients with renal failure. Onset of action is approximately 2 minutes and a normal intubating dose lasts 20–30 minutes. The patient will begin to breathe spontaneously, but an anticholinesterase can be used. It has a clean cardiovascular profile, with very little histamine release in normal clinical doses.[27]

Pancuronium This was the first steroid-based non-depolarizing muscle relaxant, but without the hormonal activity. It is metabolized in the liver. Where there is renal or hepatic impairment the duration of action may be prolonged. A maximum block is achieved after between 2 and 4 minutes and duration of action is about 25–60 minutes. It is reversed with an anticholinesterase. It has very few side effects, but tachycardia, hypertension and increased cardiac output may be observed. Pancuronium does not release histamine.[27]

Rocuronium A steroid-based non-depolarizing muscle relaxant which has been relatively recently introduced into clinical practice. It is eliminated principally in the liver, unchanged. Thus in patients with hepatic dysfunction the duration of action is increased. Intubation is possible within 60 seconds and its duration of action is about 30–40 minutes. Reversal is with an anticholinesterase. As yet few side effects have been reported.[27]

REVERSAL OF NON–DEPOLARIZING MUSCLE RELAXANTS

Non-depolarizing muscle relaxants are reversed by an anticholinesterase such as neostigmine. There are four mechanisms whereby an anticholinesterase will influence neuromuscular transmission:

- Inactivation of cholinesterase
- Modification of the depolarization of the motor nerve terminals
- Increased release of acetylcholine
- Direct effect at the postsynaptic cholinoceptors.

Of these four by far the most important is inactivation of the cholinesterase.[28] If we return to the normal physiology of the nerve impulse (action potential), acetylcholine is destroyed by cholinesterase. Neostigmine, in simple terms, inhibits cholinesterase, allowing more production of acetylcholine, or it replaces the non-depolarizing muscle relaxant in the receptor sites at the neuromuscular junction, hence the blockade is overcome.

Neostigmine has side effects such as bradycardia, increased peristalsis and increased salivation, and so glycopyrrolate is given with neostigmine. This gives less initial tachycardia than atropine and better protection against subsequent bradycardia.

EMERGENCY ANAESTHESIA

For the patient undergoing emergency anaesthesia a variety of problems may ensue. First, the patient is unprepared for surgery both physically and psychologically. Second, in the majority of cases patients are hypovolaemic and need urgent fluid replacement. The most important potential problem for patients relates to the need to protect the airway during induction of anaesthesia in the absence of an appropriate period of fasting. Patients who are not fasted prior to anaesthesia and have undergone a traumatic event will suffer from delayed gastric emptying. They are thus at risk of aspirating their stomach contents and developing aspiration pneumonitis.[29] A New York obstetrician first described aspiration, and in obstetric patients it is referred to as Mendleson's syndrome. When applied to the non-obstetric population it is called acid aspiration syndrome. The incidence of aspiration is 1–6/10 000, with a mortality rate of 5%. However, what is more worrying is that silent regurgitation is thought to occur in 25% of patients undergoing anaesthesia.[30] This section considers emergency induction, looking specifically at rapid-sequence induction.

WHO IS AT RISK?

- Obstetric patients
- Trauma patients
- Patients with a history of reflux or hiatus hernia
- Patients with gastrointestinal obstruction
- Obese patients
- Any patient where there is a history of delayed gastric emptying.

The aim of any emergency induction is to prevent the aspiration of stomach contents, and ways of doing this include:

- Emptying the stomach prior to induction
- Inducing anaesthesia in the head-up tilt position
- Inhalational induction in the left lateral head-up tilt position
- Consideration of a local anaesthetic technique if possible
- Neutralize the stomach contents with the use of ranitidine and sodium citrate.

However, the most common technique for emergency anaesthesia is a combination of neutralization of stomach contents and rapid-sequence induction.

RAPID-SEQUENCE INDUCTION

This entails the use of cricoid pressure or Sellick's manoeuvre. This involves compressing the cricoid cartilage, which in turn is pressed against the 5th or 6th cervical vertebrae. Sellick described the application of cricoid pressure using three fingers, with the thumb and the middle finger either side of the cricoid and the forefinger applying the pressure.[31] The reason for the use of the cricoid is that it is the only complete ring of cartilage, all the others being C shaped.

There has been debate about the force with which the pressure is applied.[32] It is now generally accepted that 30 N of pressure is sufficient to prevent regurgitation.[33] It has been demonstrated that a force greater than this will cause airway obstruction.[34] The sequence of events is as follows:

- Ensure all equipment is ready and available and the suction is on and under the pillow
- Ensure intravenous access
- Position the patient in the 'sniffing the morning air' posture
- Preoxygenate for 3 minutes
- Locate the position of the cricoid, explaining to the patient what is happening as they will be extremely anxious
- As the induction agent is being given and the patient loses consciousness, apply cricoid pressure
- Cricoid pressure should not be removed until the endotracheal tube has been checked for its position
- If the patient vomits the anaesthetist will make the decision to remove the cricoid pressure. The patient is then at risk of aspirating. If cricoid

pressure is maintained they are at risk of a ruptured oesophagus (Boerhaave syndrome).[35]

Rapid-sequence induction is a skilled procedure at a time when the patient is at greatest risk. The anaesthetic practitioner must demonstrate skill, an ability to be calm under pressure, and be empathetic to the needs of the patient.

CONCLUSION

This chapter has demonstrated that the practice of anaesthetics is complex and technical. The role of the anaesthetic practitioner is highly skilled, the most important role being care of the patient at a vulnerable time. All patients need someone with them who is able to be empathetic and meet their needs. However, anaesthetic practitioners do not work in isolation: they are part of a team of people who want to give the best care to the patient during the perioperative period. These include the anaesthetist, the surgeon and the surgical practitioner. There is scope to build upon the existing role of the anaesthetic practitioner and enhance the care given to patients undergoing anaesthesia and surgery still further.

References

1. Bailey R. What's in a name? Nurs Standard 1995; 10: 23–24.
2. NHS Management Executive. Professional roles in anaesthetics: a scoping study. London: HMSO; 1996.
3. MacRae W. The team approach to anaesthesia. Br J Theatre Nurs 1996; 6: 9–10.
4. Association of Anaesthetists of Great Britain and Ireland. Assistance for the anaesthetist. London: Association of Anaesthetists of Great Britain and Ireland; 1989.
5. Oakley M. The anaesthetic nurses' perception of their role. Anaesth Recovery Nurse 1999; 5: 6–8.
6. Morton NS. Assisting the anaesthetist. Oxford: OUP; 1997.
7. Association of Anaesthetists of Great Britain and Ireland. Checklist for anaesthetic apparatus. London: Association of Anaesthetists of Great Britain and Ireland; 2004.
8. Griffiths R. Breathing circuits and their uses. Br J Perioper Nurs 2000; 10: 55–59.
9. Simpson PJ, Popat MT. Understanding anaesthesia, 4th edn. Oxford: WB Saunders; 1999.
10. Davey A, Moyle JTB. Ward's anaesthetic equipment, 4th edn. London: WB Saunders; 1999.
11. Spiers C, Stinchcombe E. An introduction to cardiac monitoring and rhythm interpretation. Br J Anaesth Recovery 2002; 3: 8–14.
12. Millar JM, Rudkin GE, Hitchcock M. Practical anaesthesia and analgesia for day surgery. Oxford: Bios Scientific; 1997.
13. Parker A. Care of the older perioperative patient. Br J Anaesth Recovery 2002; 3: 16–20.
14. Jester R, Williams S. Pre-operative fasting: putting research into practice. Nurs Standard 1999; 13: 33–35.
15. Hung P. Pre-operative fasting. NT 1992; 88: 57–60.
16. Chapman A. Current theory and practice: a study of pre-operative fasting. Nurs Standard 1996; 10: 33–36.
17. Van Decar MT. Anaesthetic drugs. Sem Perioper Nurs 1998; 7: 29–38.
18. Fryer JM. Intravenous induction agents. Anaesth Inten Care Med 2001; 2: 277–281.
19. Weksler N, Rozentsveig V, Tarnoploski A, et al. Commercial propofol solutions: is the more expensive also the most effective? J Clin Aneasth 2001; 13: 321–324.
20. Seeberger MD, Staender S, Oertli D, et al. Efficacy of specific aseptic precautions for preventing propofol-related infections: analysis by a quality-assurance programme using the explicit outcome method. J Hosp Infect 1998; 39: 67–70.
21. Sanders LD, Isaac PA, Yeomans WA, et al. Propofol induced anaesthesia. Anaesth 1988; 44: 200–204.
22. Gunawardene RD, White DC. Propofol and emesis. Anaesth 1988; (Suppl): 65–67.

23. Harper N. Inhalational anaesthetics. Anaesth Inten Care Med 2001; 2: 241–245.
24. Pleuvry BJ. Opioid mechanisms and opioid drugs. Anaesth Inten Care Med 2001; 2: 450–455.
25. Donati F. Physiology: nerve, junction and muscle. In: Harper NJN, Pollard BJ, eds. Muscle relaxants in anaesthesia. London: Edward Arnold; 1995: 1–12.
26. Harper NJN. Suxamethonium. In: Harper NJN, Pollard BJ, eds. Muscle relaxants in anaesthesia. London: Edward Arnold; 1995: 55–76.
27. Pollard BJ. Non depolarising muscle relaxants. In: Harper NJN, Pollard BJ, eds. Muscle relaxants in anaesthesia. London: Edward Arnold; 1995: 77–96.
28. Harper NJN. Reversal of neuromuscular blockade. In: Harper NJN, Pollard BJ, eds. Muscle relaxants in anaesthesia. London: Edward Arnold; 1995: 135–155.
29. Dawson PR, Crockford S. Anaesthesia and aspiration pneumonitis. Br J Theatre Nurs 1996; 6: 37–39.
30. Davies P, Warwick J. Regurgitation, vomiting and aspiration. Anaesth Inten Care Med 2001; 2: 358–361.
31. Sellick BA. Cricoid pressure to control regurgitation of stomach contents during induction of anaesthesia. Lancet 1961; 2: 404–406.
32. Palmer JH, Ball DR. The effect of cricoid pressure on the cricoid cartilage and vocal cords: an endoscopic study in anaesthetised patients. Anaesth 2000; 55: 260–287.
33. Vanner R. Techniques of cricoid pressure. Anaesth Inten Care Med 2001; 2: 362–363.
34. Hartsilver EL, Vanner RG. Airway obstruction with cricoid pressure. Anaesth 2000; 55: 208–211.
35. Andrews PLR. Physiology of nausea and vomiting. Br J Anaesth 1992; 69(Suppl): 2s–19s.

Further reading

Craft TM, Upton PM. Key topics in anaesthesia. Oxford: Bios Scientific; 2001.
Gregory GA, ed. Paediatric anaesthesia, 4th edn. London: Churchill Livingstone; 2001.
Radford M, Countie B, Oakley M. Advancing perioperative practice. Cheltenham: Nelson Thornes; 2004.
Rushman GB, Davies NJH, Cashman JN. Lee's synopsis of anaesthesia, 12th edn. Oxford: Butterworth-Heinemann; 1999.
Steward DJ, Lerman J. Manual of paediatric anaesthesia, 5th edn. Edinburgh: Churchill Livingstone; 2001.
Smith I, ed. Day case anaesthesia. London: BMJ Books; 2000.

Useful contacts

Association of Anaesthetists of Great Britain and Ireland
http://www.AAGBI.co.uk
Association of Operating Department Practitioners
http://www.AODP.org

British Anaesthetic and Recovery Nurses Association
http://www.barna.co.uk
National Association of Theatre Nurses
http://www.natn.org.uk

Chapter 12

Care of the patient undergoing surgery

Carol Smith

Key points

- The roles of the perioperative team
- Care of the patient during the intraoperative period
- Identifying perioperative risks
- Planning individualized holistic care

THE ROLES OF THE PERIOPERATIVE TEAM

The perioperative practitioner has a multifaceted role. The main aim is to provide holistic, evidence-based and clinically effective care and support to the patient during the perioperative experience. The practitioner must do this in a challenging environment, alongside other members of the multidisciplinary team, while acting as the patient's advocate and maintaining accountability for his or her own actions.

The team leader maintains overall coordination of the perioperative team during the operating session and it is his or her responsibility to delegate duties to the rest of the team according to their knowledge, skills and learning needs. Williams[1] suggested that the best examples of teamwork in the NHS are to be found in the perioperative environment. The roles undertaken by perioperative practitioners include scrub practitioner, circulating practitioner, support worker and anaesthetic practitioner. The perioperative team also includes other professionals, such as surgeons, anaesthetists, technicians and radiographers, and it is this diversity that makes the multidisciplinary team so dynamic.

The scrub practitioner has a variety of roles aimed at supporting the perioperative team. He or she dons appropriate protective clothing, such as mask, hat and eye protection, and then scrubs and gowns according to local procedure. The practitioner then prepares the sterile trolley using an aseptic technique. A vital part of preparation to be a scrub practitioner is to develop a knowledge and understanding of the planned operative procedure.[2] A major responsibility of the scrub practitioner is to maintain a sterile environment while assisting the surgeon throughout the procedure, ensuring the swab, needle and instrument counts are correct.

Good surgical technique is an essential skill that needs to be developed in order to ensure the best care and protection of the patient from injury. During any procedure there are certain safety factors to consider, with the use of items that may cause injury to the patient or surgical team. For example, diathermy forceps must be kept in the holster and only removed when required; after the surgeon has used them they must be replaced in the holster. At no time must they be left on the patient, as this may result in burns. The scalpel and its blade must be placed in a receiver which is then offered to the surgeon when required; the surgeon takes this instrument out of the receiver themselves and replaces it after use, to avoid injury to the patient and the scrub practitioner if passed from hand to hand. Needles are mounted on a needle holder and passed to the surgeon when required, handle first, and should not be left on the patient.

The circulating practitioner (or circulator) assists with the operating room preparation before the operating list commences. The operating room must be clean, have all the equipment for the procedures, all the instrumentation required, and any consumables, such as swabs and sutures, must be available.

The circulator also assists with the preparation of the trolley and with the continuous supply of consumables used throughout the procedure. The circulator, together with the support worker, also takes part in activities such as transferring and positioning the patient, connecting up any equipment used, managing the processing of surgical specimens, and completing perioperative documentation.

The anaesthetic practitioner is responsible for supporting the anaesthetist during the administration of the anaesthetic, and also for delivering direct care aimed at maintaining the patient's comfort and safety during anaesthesia. The anaesthetic practitioner also usually works alongside the circulator to support the patient throughout the surgical procedure.

The operating department is well known as an area of high risk, and practitioners must be aware of the possibility of harm to the patient and consequent litigation. The loss of swabs and instruments, diathermy burns, tissue and nerve damage, and incorrectly completed consent forms are just a few of the ever present risks.[3]

Although there are many other areas of potential risk, the following have been highlighted as being of particular concern to perioperative practitioners:

- Establishing the correct patient details
- Transferring the patient
- Surgical positioning
- Management of pressure areas
- Preventing deep vein thrombosis
- Preventing hypothermia
- Preventing diathermy burns
- Maintaining infection control
- Maintaining dignity
- Managing body piercings
- Ensuring swab, needle and instrument counts
- Communication
- Completing documentation
- Care planning.

ESTABLISHING THE CORRECT PATIENT DETAILS

Ensuring that the correct patient arrives for the correct operation, correctly prepared, is one of the key roles of the perioperative team. An operating list must be obtained with the consultant surgeon's name, the operating room number, date and start time and, as a minimum, the following information for each operation:

- Patient's name
- Unit number
- Date of birth
- Ward
- Surgical procedure.

Changes to the order of the operating list must be avoided, but in exceptional circumstances, for example if the patient needs an ECG or X-ray prior to the operation, then it may be necessary to change the order so as to utilize the surgical time efficiently. In such cases it is important to communicate the details to all areas in the operating department and to all staff affected by the changes.

The patient should be given sufficient information by the medical staff to be able to give informed consent, either on the ward or in a preoperative clinic. The patient then needs to be sent for in adequate time to allow appropriate checks to be made on leaving the ward, entering the operating department, and in the anaesthetic room. Before the procedure commences the patient should be correctly identified by the scrub practitioner, who may be seeing the patient for the first time at this point. The circulator should show the scrub practitioner the name and unit number on the outside of the case notes and check this information with the consent form. The consent form must clearly state the following information:

- Patient's name
- Unit number
- Date of birth
- Surgical procedure, including side if appropriate
- Patient's (or guardian's if appropriate) signature and date
- Signature of the doctor who has explained the procedure.

(For further discussion on the requirements for valid consent see Ch. 1.) The information on the consent form should be compared with the operating list to ensure that all the perioperative team agrees that they have the correct patient for the corresponding procedure. If there are any discrepancies this must be brought to the surgeon's attention before the start of the procedure. Another common precaution against accidental surgery is to mark the site of surgery with an indelible marking pen.

Assessing the implications of any allergies is an important part of the checking-in procedure. The patient will have already completed a preoperative questionnaire before coming to the operating room, which includes a question about allergies. During the usual checking-in procedures patients are also asked to verify this information, which is documented on the care plan. This information must be pointed out to the scrub practitioner before the start of the procedure, as consideration must be given to areas such as skin preparation and dressings.

Patients can become sensitive to latex, a substance found in many products in the operating department, such as gloves, masks, cannulae and syringes. Reactions can range from minor skin irritations to respiratory symptoms, and even in extreme cases respiratory arrest. Latex allergic reactions, including anaphylaxis, are occurring with greater frequency.[4] However, unless the patient is aware of the allergy then there is no way of knowing of their sensitivity in advance. Therefore the patient's skin must be checked at the end of the procedure for any reactions. Allergic reaction to latex is also an increasing problem among perioperative practitioners, and there have been reports of up to 43% of practitioners developing this allergy.[5]

TRANSFERRING THE PATIENT

The patient is brought in to the operating room either on a trolley or on a bed, which is lined up with the operating table, making sure that the brakes are on and the height of the table is the same as that of the trolley or bed. All staff must be familiar with safe techniques for transferring the patient. There are three common methods of lateral transfer system:

- Easyslide
- Patslide Patient Transfer
- Samarit Roll Board.

The same principles are used with all equipment. Patients are transferred in three easy steps:

1. The device is placed underneath the patient as he or she is gently rolled to one side
2. The patient is then rolled into a supine position during the transfer across to the operating table
3. The patient is then rolled the other way to remove the device.

The Easyslide is a quilted, padded tube which slides across itself and has a washable nylon cover. Disposable plastic covers are supplied, allowing it to be changed for every patient and thereby preventing cross-infection. This system is recommended for transfer from trolley to table only.

The Patslide Patient Transfer (Figs 12.1A,B) is ideal for transfer on to the patient's bed, it is lightweight and resilient, radiolucent, and can be easily cleaned with detergent.

The Samarit Roll Board offers the same advantages as the Patslide, and it can be folded away and hung up. This mechanism can be used from table to trolley or from table to bed (Figs 12.2A,B). It is the only system that can be used when the patient is required to be transferred on to a clean sheet following surgery.

All staff using these methods must follow the moving and handling procedures according to local

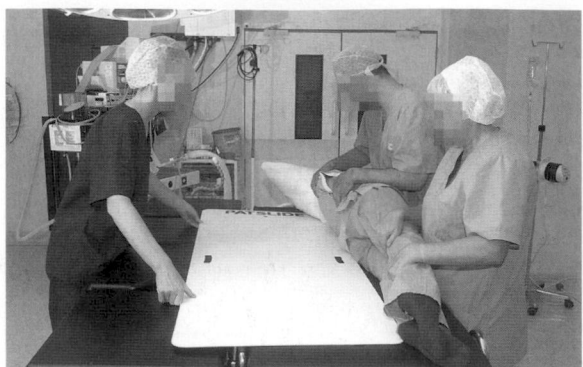

Figure 12.1A   Patslide patient transfer.

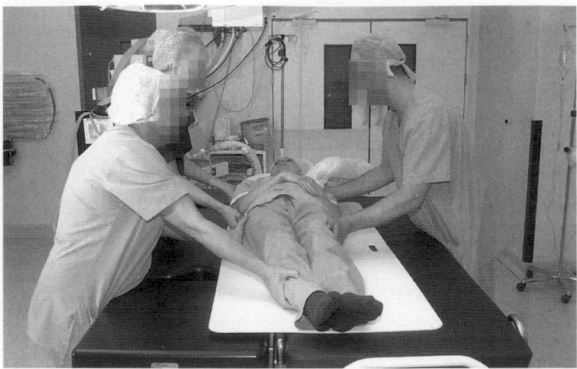

Figure 12.1B   The patient is moved.

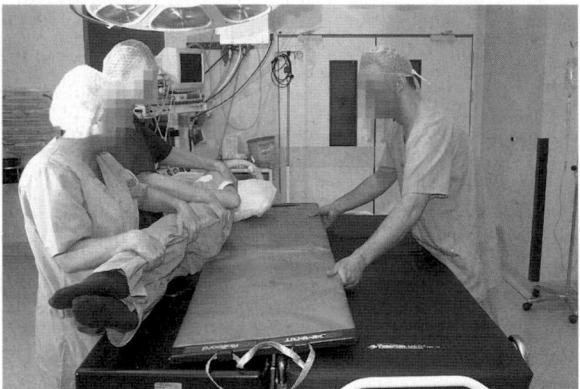

Figure 12.2A   The patient is rolled.

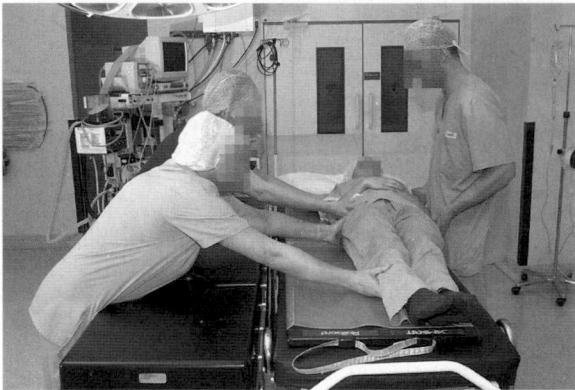

Figure 12.2B   The patient is moved across.

policy, and be trained in the safe transfer of patients using these devices.

As with all patient transfers, the anaesthetist should coordinate the team in order to ensure that the patient's airway is maintained. Care must be taken with medical devices attached to the patient, for example infusion lines or urinary catheters, in case they become dislodged during the transfer.

Practitioners should be aware of the potential injuries that can occur while moving and handling patients. All jewellery should be removed, including rings and wristwatches. Fingernails must be short to avoid accidental scratching, and consideration given to whether staff identity cards are worn.

SURGICAL POSITIONING

It is essential that all practitioners are aware of the potential hazards of moving and positioning the anaesthetized patient.

The patient must be positioned correctly according to the procedure being performed. Adequate

numbers of staff are required and all must be fully trained in the positioning of patients for surgery. Various pressure-relieving devices are used depending on the position adopted. Gel mats are positioned on the operating table before the patient is transferred. Arm supports with padding are often used to prevent arms from falling, unless the anaesthetist prefers the arms stretched out on a board to facilitate intravenous access. The patient must be placed on a clean dry sheet which is smooth and wrinkle free. Common positions used for surgery include:

- Supine
- Trendelenburg
- Reverse Trendelenburg
- Lithotomy
- Lateral
- Prone.

The most commonly used position is supine, where the patient is flat on his or her back. This position is also used for transferring the patient from, for example, the operating table to a bed. Heel supports are often used to prevent pressure on the patient's heels and calves.

The Trendelenburg position is supine with a head-down tilt and is generally used for lower abdominal surgery. This is particularly useful in gynaecology, where the contents of the abdominal cavity fall under gravity towards the diaphragm, making the organs more accessible to the surgeon.

Reverse Trendelenburg is a head-up tilt used for head and neck, and ear, nose and throat procedures.

The lithotomy position is where the patient is supine with the legs raised and feet placed in stirrups. The lower end of the table is removed. This position is often used in gynaecology procedures and for lower bowel procedures, such as sigmoidoscopy and haemorrhoidectomy. Before lifting the legs the practitioner must obtain permission from the anaesthetist, and both legs must be lifted simultaneously by a practitioner on each side of the patient, holding one hand under the patient's heel and the other hand behind the knee to avoid any injury to the hips and jarring of the knee joints. The hips and knees are flexed and the feet placed in the stirrups on the outside of the poles.

The lateral position is used to position the patient on his or her side. Pillows are placed between the patient's legs along with small gel mats, and restraint straps are used to keep the legs in place. A pelvis support is attached to the table, generally in the area of the patient's stomach; a lateral support is also used in the patient's back, and a gutter arm support used for the arms. This position is often used for nephrectomy, thoracic and lumbar spine procedures.

When prone, the patient lies on his or her front on pillows positioned under the chest, sacrum and legs, and supported with straps. The head is positioned to one side to allow access to the airway, and the arms are supported with boards. This position is often used for spinal surgery.

MANAGEMENT OF PRESSURE AREAS

Patients undergoing surgical procedures are at increased risk of developing pressure sores. The length of time spent on the operating table, the surgical position adopted, the patient's temperature, and moving and handling techniques[6] influence the chance of developing a pressure sore. A pressure sore may be defined as an area of necrosis caused by excessive and prolonged pressure.[7] Waterlow[8] states that pressure sores are caused by the death of

tissue when the blood supply to the capillary bed is occluded. Occlusion stops the tissue from being supplied with nutrients, and also prevents waste products from being removed. Damage to the skin can also occur by friction when poor moving and handling techniques are used. Areas at high risk are the sacrum, spine, elbows and heels.

Various pressure sore prevention gel pads are available, such as mats, ankle supports, heel supports, head rings and boots.

While moving the patient an assessment of their skin can be made and any observations of bruising or redness can be documented preoperatively, and the same postoperatively on the care plan.

The patient's temperature contributes to the development of pressure sores, as Scott[9] stated that hypothermia can lead to peripheral shutdown and cell hypoxia; therefore, intraoperative interventions should not only focus on the reduction of interface pressures but also on the maintenance of normothermia.

It is always possible that the scrub team may lean on the patient during surgery: this must be prevented in order to prevent injury to the patient.

DEEP VEIN THROMBOSIS

The perioperative patient is susceptible to deep vein thrombosis (DVT) for a variety of reasons, including prolonged periods of inactivity and the effects of anaesthesia and surgery on the body's normal physiology. Venous thromboembolism may be the most common preventable cause of death in hospitalized patients.[10] The relief of pressure on the calves by heel supports, gel mats and pillows may help to reduce the possibility of DVT, but there are two main techniques used for the prophylaxis of DVT:

- Antiembolism stockings
- Intermittent pneumatic compression.

Antiembolism stockings have been providing baseline prophylaxis for many years. They are available as knee length or thigh length. However, thigh-length stockings can form constrictive bands if not worn correctly, and are more likely to cause complications such as skin necrosis and arterial thrombosis.[11]

The DVT prophylaxis system (Fig. 12.3) is an intermittent pneumatic compression apparatus consisting of inflatable leggings which are wrapped

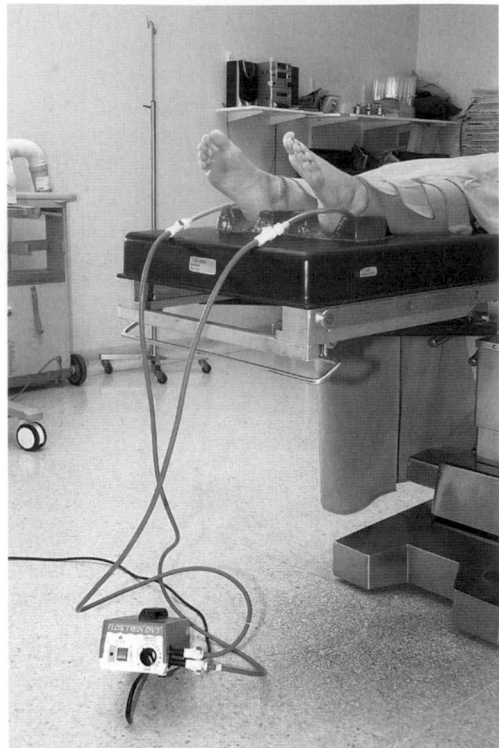

Figure 12.3   The Flowtron DVT prophylaxis.

around the patient's calves preoperatively and fastened with Velcro. Once the patient is on the operating table and has been positioned accordingly, he or she is then connected up to the pump, which can be placed under the table by tubing with snap-lock connectors, which help to prevent accidental disconnection. Should disconnection occur, an audio alarm sounds. The external pneumatic compression system inflates the stockings with air for 10–15 seconds, followed by deflation of 45–50 seconds. The pump operates on a 60-second automatically timed cycle. This compresses the veins and aids return of the blood to the heart, thus reducing stasis of blood in the venous system. The recommended level of pressure required for DVT prophylaxis is 40 mmHg.[12]

HYPOTHERMIA

Perioperative patients are always at risk of losing body heat during surgery. Age, duration and type of surgery are some of the factors that influence the fall in core body temperature. Administration of an anaesthetic causes temperature-regulating mechanisms in the hypothalamus to be depressed: this inadvertent compromising of homoeostatic mechanisms frequently leads to the development of hypothermia.[13]

The perioperative practitioner should keep the patient covered up as long as possible, only folding back the sheet to apply the diathermy plate and the DVT prophylaxis system, until the surgeon is ready to prepare the skin. Only the surgical site should be exposed, unless there is a good reason for exposure, such as anaesthetic access.

The temperature in the operating room can usually be controlled locally. The ideal temperature for patient and staff comfort is between 20 and 22°C. However, convective heat loss occurs as a result of air currents. If precautions are not taken to prevent heat loss, the patient's temperature could initially drop from about 0.5 to 1.0°C owing to the vasodilating effect of the anaesthetic agent and the body redistributing its heat. As the surgery commences a further drop in temperature takes place. Patients whose temperature drops below 34°C are often subjected to discomfort and have a longer postoperative recovery. Temperatures below 34°C may be life threatening, therefore action must be taken. There are two main methods which are generally used for warming the patient:

- Conductive heating systems
- Forced warm air systems.

A conductive heating system uses a heating pad which is placed on the operating table underneath a gel mat, which it warms. The heating pad is set to 39°C in order to prevent intraoperative hypothermia. The pad is flexible and can be easily rolled up for storage; it is radiolucent and can easily be cleaned with detergent. It is connected to the control unit, which can be placed under the table and switched on prior to surgery. This can be left switched on for a full operating list and will keep the gel mat at a constant temperature throughout the day. Care must be taken not to fold the pad, as this can damage the heating elements.

Forced warm air systems are now established as the most effective method of preventing and treating heat loss in surgical patients.[14] These can be obtained in a variety of different sizes depending on the surgery. Warming blankets can be used either over the patient's legs or over the top of the body. They are made of a soft flexible fabric which allows custom draping according to the procedure being undertaken; the adhesive edges secure the blanket to the patient, allowing maximum skin

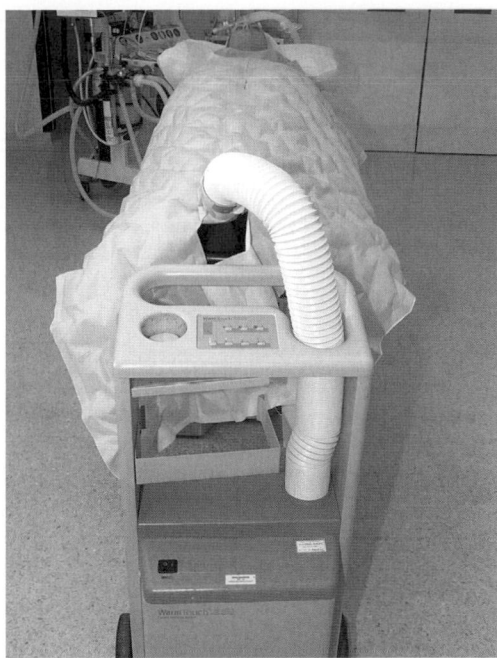

Figure 12.4   The forced ward air system.

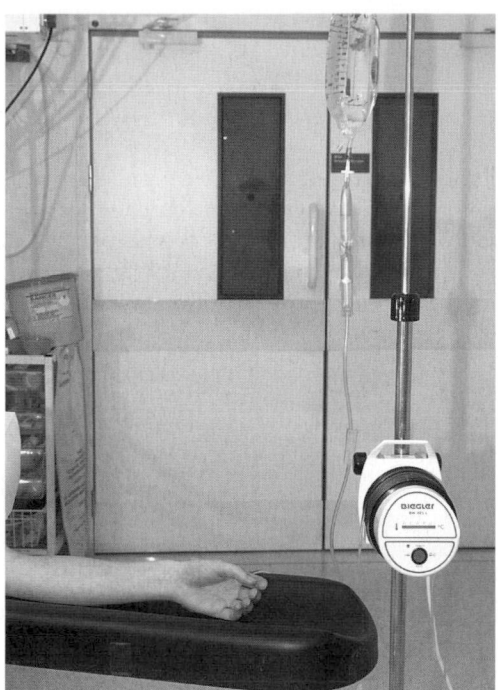

Figure 12.5   Blood warmer.

surface coverage without interfering with or allowing air to blow into the field of surgery. The warming unit is placed on the floor and the nozzle is connected to the inlet hole on the blanket, which is then inflated with warm air at a temperature of 38°C. As the blanket inflates the warm air escapes from the underside, thus warming the patient with immediate effect. This system can also be used in the recovery area (Fig. 12.4).

Alternatively, a heat-retentive insulating drape can be used over the patient's body. Head covers are also available. These are also radiolucent and antistatic.

Any intravenous fluids can go through a blood warmer (Fig. 12.5), and the anaesthetist monitors the patient's temperature using a temperature probe. Abdominal washouts and bladder irrigation should be stored in a warming cabinet well before the start of the list so that they reach the required temperature before being used.

ELECTROSURGERY (DIATHERMY)

Electrosurgery (diathermy) is one of the most commonly used tools in the operating department for maintaining or producing a bloodless field.[15] It is used to coagulate bleeding vessels, thereby providing haemostasis, and to cut through tissue. Current

flows from the electrosurgical generator to the active electrode, through the patient's body tissues to the return electrode, and then back to the generator (diathermy machine). There are two pedals attached to the machine, a blue one for coagulation and a yellow one for cutting; the surgeon activates the diathermy by standing on the appropriate pedal. If finger-switch diathermy is being used, there are blue and yellow buttons on the instrument. Bipolar diathermy is used mainly on peripheral areas of the body when fine coagulation is required. The active and return electrodes are combined within the one instrument, the current passing down one side of the instrument and returning up the other.

Before the start of the procedure the perioperative practitioner must make sure that the patient is not touching any earthed metal objects, such as the operating table or IV stands. Under certain circumstances, for example if the patient plate becomes detached, current can pass through that area when the diathermy is activated, resulting in a burn to the skin where it is touching the earthed metal object.

Reusable patient plates should be avoided as they pose a risk due to faulty cleaning and maintenance, and modern disposable plates are designed to be practically foolproof. A new, unused, disposable plate should be applied to the patient each time.

Usually the best place to attach the plate is the leg, although any clean, dry, hairless, muscular area is appropriate. It must not be placed over any scar tissue or bony prominences, or in touch with any external orthopaedic implants (e.g. external fixators), or touching any earthed metal object, such as the operating table. Shaving can cause damage to the skin and should be avoided if at all possible – in most cases the practitioner should be able to find another suitable area. The purpose of the patient plate is to provide a safe return path for the electrosurgical current. Disposable gel electrodes have a soft, hydrogel conductive adhesive and a non-conductive adhesive border surrounding the conducting surface to prevent any skin preparation or bodily fluids coming into contact with the conductive area. Most electrosurgical pads are now single-use items.

Care must be taken to prevent pooling of the skin preparation solution around the site of the return electrode: if this happens then a new plate must be applied. The plate must be checked to ensure it is still in contact with the skin if the patient needs to be moved during the procedure. Most modern generators have an alarm system which will activate if the plate becomes detached. If the alarm sounds, all connections and parts of the electrosurgical system should be checked to ensure that they are properly connected or attached.

Setting up the electrosurgical system is not a complex affair, but there are several tasks that must be carried out to ensure patient safety. A holster, which is fastened to the drapes, should be used to store the active electrode. The forceps should be attached to the cable, which is then passed to the circulating practitioner, who connects it up to the machine before it is switched on. The scrub practitioner will check that the generator is on the correct settings for the surgery being performed.

It is preferable to use an aqueous solution to prepare the patient's skin, but if the surgeon prefers to use an alcohol-based solution then it is necessary to make sure that the skin is dried prior to the start of the procedure. The patient's body heat can cause alcohol-based solutions to form a highly inflammable vapour, which can collect underneath waterproof drapes.

Throughout the surgery it is the scrub practitioner's duty to replace the forceps in the holster after the surgeon has used them. They must never be left on the patient, as the surgeon could accidentally stand on the foot pedal at the wrong time, causing a burn. At the end of the procedure the diathermy plate should be removed and the patient's skin checked for signs of accidental burns.

Surgical smoke is created when tissues are heated by the electrosurgery. Both staff and patients are exposed to this hazard. Surgical smoke contains three primary components:

- Particulate matter consisting of carbonized tissue, blood, infectious viruses and bacteria
- Steam
- Toxins.[16]

This risk can never be completely eliminated; however, various methods can be used to reduce the risk, for example:

- The use of high-filtration face masks
- Use of a surgical smoke vacuum unit
- Avoidance of high-power waveforms
- Efficient ventilation systems for the operating room.

INFECTION CONTROL

Although a great deal of time and effort is spent in cleaning the inanimate objects of an operating room, one of the greatest infection risks to patients is from their own bacteria.[17] Therefore, the preoperative preparation of the skin plays a very large part in reducing the risk of infection. The aim of skin preparation is to reduce the risk of postoperative wound infections: it removes microorganisms from the skin and inhibits their recolonization, encouraging primary healing of the surgical wound.

Before skin preparation can commence, the surgical site should be assessed in relation to its potential for infection. Hair may need to be removed from around the incision area; ideally this should be done before the patient's arrival in the operating room. If it is necessary to perform hair removal in the operating room then this must be done according to local protocols. Inappropriate hair shaving techniques can cause skin abrasions, and this can provide an opportunity for microorganisms to grow. The shaved hair must be removed from the site, otherwise it may contaminate the wound. Any abrasions or rashes must be recorded on the patient's care plan.

The selection of skin preparation is normally the surgeon's preference; however, if the patient has an allergy to the agent it must not be used, as this may cause a skin reaction, and an alternative must be found. If the skin appears to be sensitive to the preparation used then this must also be recorded in the care plan.

Preparation of the surgical site is performed by the surgeon or the scrub practitioner, who is competent in skin preparation techniques, using a swab on a sponge holder. The size of the incision is taken into consideration when preparing the surgical site, allowing for the incision to be extended if necessary and for the insertion of drains. The skin preparation is achieved by starting at the incision site and extending to the periphery, when the sponge holder and swab are discarded. The preparation site has to be large enough for the possibility of movement of the drapes during the procedure.

The surgical team scrub and gown up in order to reduce the spread of microorganisms from the team to the patient, and also to protect themselves from contamination with blood or body fluids. Most hospitals now use a preset tray system, where the instrumentation comes ready packed from a sterile services department. Any supplementary items that are added to the tray during the procedure are taken by the scrub practitioner using an aseptic technique to avoid contaminating either themselves or the trolley (Fig. 12.6). This will be discussed in further detail later in the chapter under 'Swab, Needle and Instrument Count'. It is the scrub practitioner's responsibility to maintain a sterile environment throughout the procedure and any breach in sterility must be dealt with immediately. At the end of the

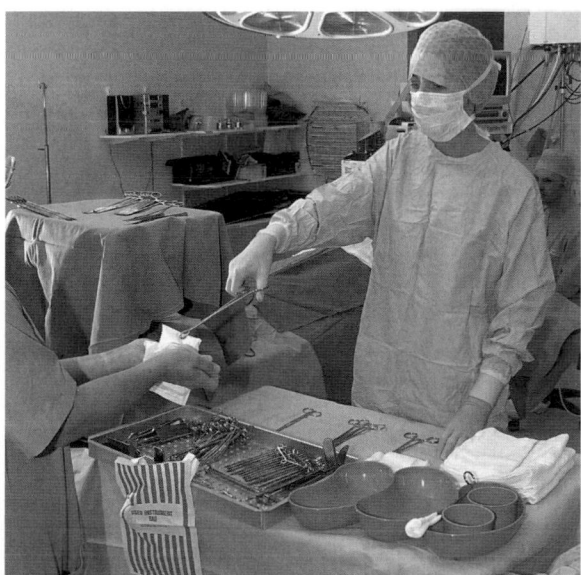

Figure 12.6 Supplementaries are taken by the scrub practitioner using the aseptic technique.

procedure a sterile dressing is applied to the wound before the drapes are removed from the patient.

DIGNITY

Patients' dignity must always be considered. This can be maintained by leaving the patient covered with the sheet until the surgeon is ready to start preparing the skin, and then only the area to be prepared is exposed. Care must be taken not to leave patients uncovered without reason.

BODY PIERCINGS

Body piercing and the wearing of body jewellery is becoming increasingly popular. Patients should be encouraged to remove their jewellery before surgery, particularly if it is close to the surgical site. However, some patients do refuse, and in this case they may present two main problems when undergoing surgery: infection, and injury to themselves.

Items of jewellery could be a source of infection as they can easily become contaminated with bacteria, especially if they are not kept clean. Injury can occur if the jewellery becomes entangled in drapes or accidentally pulled out. The site of the piercing should be checked preoperatively and recorded on the perioperative care plan, and checked postoperatively for any injuries. Other dangers include loss of the item caused by it falling out or becoming misplaced, and there is also a small risk of diathermy burns if the item lies near the site of surgery and accidentally comes into contact with the active electrode.

CHECKING OF ACCOUNTABLE ITEMS

Although the surgical team often requires what is referred to as a 'swab check', in actual fact there is a range of accountable items that need checking. All items listed below used by the surgical team during any operative procedure must be included in the count; these can include:

- Instruments
- Swabs, all of which must be X-ray detectable
- Needles
- Slings
- Patties
- Pledgets

- Blades
- Hypodermic needles
- Diathermy blades
- Nylon tape
- Bulldog clips.

Items are checked before the start of the procedure when the trolley is being set up, at the commencement of the closure of the first layer of the cavity, and at the commencement of the skin closure. This task is always performed by two people, the scrub practitioner and the circulator, at least one of whom must be qualified and experienced. The aim of this procedure is to account for all items and is an essential responsibility of the scrub practitioner in order to prevent the retention of foreign bodies.[18]

At the start of the procedure the scrub practitioner ensures the pack's sterility by checking the packaging of the sterile instrument tray for any tears or other damage, and that it is within its expiry date. The practitioner then opens the sterile instrument tray, and the trolley is set up using the aseptic technique. All the instruments on that tray are checked against a sheet containing the list of instruments and their quantity. Any discrepancies are recorded on the check sheet before the start of the surgical procedure.

When the scrub practitioner is satisfied that everything is correct and in working order the circulator passes any extras that are required, according to the surgeon's preferences and using an aseptic technique. All extra instruments are checked for sterility before opening, and are recorded on the instrument check sheet. The scrub practitioner's and circulator's names are also recorded on the sheet. The scrub practitioner counts the Raytec swabs (commonly 7×5 cm or 10×10 cm) in batches of five, with the circulator also checking that the X-ray detectable line (Raytec line) is present. If a pack of swabs does not contain the correct number then they are removed from the operating room and a new pack is counted in. Swabs must not be cut or altered in any way, as this can lead to discrepancies in the count. All items listed above are recorded on a whiteboard, and any more accountable items that are added during the procedure are also added to the board, as indicated (Fig. 12.7).

All small swabs and pledgets should be used on a sponge holder or forceps, but if during the procedure an item is used loose in the cavity as requested by the surgeon, then this must be recorded on the board as a reminder to the scrub practitioner. When

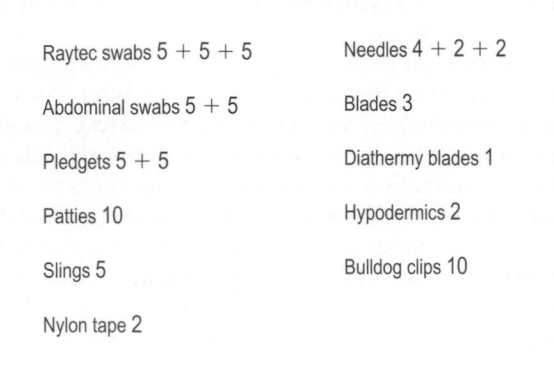

Raytec swabs $5 + 5 + 5$	Needles $4 + 2 + 2$
Abdominal swabs $5 + 5$	Blades 3
Pledgets $5 + 5$	Diathermy blades 1
Patties 10	Hypodermics 2
Slings 5	Bulldog clips 10
Nylon tape 2	

Figure 12.7   Example of a White Board.

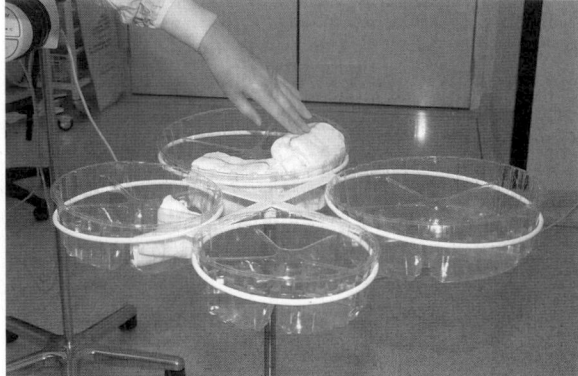

Figure 12.8   The CMS Swabsafe container.

the item is removed from the cavity and accounted for it can be erased from the board.

The method of discarding used swabs is according to local policy, an example of which is the CMS Swabsafe container system (Fig. 12.8). There are two different sizes of container to accommodate Raytec swabs and abdominal swabs, each container being divided into five sections. These containers are placed in a carousel, which can be positioned where the scrub practitioner can discard the used swabs themselves, thus reducing the handling of dirty swabs by the circulator. When discarding a used Raytec swab the scrub practitioner must check that two swabs are not stuck together; they are then folded and placed in the Swabsafe container. The same applies to the abdominal swabs, which are folded in four, rolled up, the tape wrapped around and the swab then placed in the container. When they are filled with five swabs the circulator places a lid on the container and removes it from the carousel, replacing it with a new one. All discarded items must remain in the operating room until the completion of the operation. This system also allows the swabs to be weighed in order to estimate blood loss.

At the start of the closure of the first layer the scrub practitioner and the circulator check all items on the tray, together with items discarded, including all swabs in the Swabsafe containers. Adequate time must be allowed by the surgeon to perform this task. On completion of the count the scrub practitioner informs the surgeon that the count is correct. If there are any discrepancies at this stage then the scrub practitioner must inform the surgeon immediately of the missing item and a recount be performed; the closure of the wound must be delayed until the item is found. Only when the missing item is recovered can the surgeon recommence the closure.

On completion of the count the circulator records this in the operating room register and the patient's records, with their signature. Practitioners involved in the count should be aware of exactly what they are checking and the medicolegal implications of signing for this procedure.[19] Another count is performed at the start of the skin closure, and this is also signed for by the circulator. Should there be any interruption during the count, it must be recommenced. If a thorough search of the missing item fails to locate it then an X-ray must be taken before the patient leaves the operating room.

At the end of the procedure everything is accounted for again to ensure that it is all discarded according to local policy, and that everything is removed from the theatre before the start of the next case. The instrument check sheet is signed again and sent back to the sterile services department with the instrument tray. Any disposable sharp instruments, blades and needles are disposed of in the sharps bin according to local policy. Should any instruments break during the procedure this must be recorded on the instrument check sheet and all the parts accounted for and returned with the tray, with instructions for repair or replacement.

COMMUNICATION

Good communication skills are an essential part of the perioperative practitioner's role, as good communication is essential in such an acute and rapidly changing environment. There are two methods of communication used in the operating department, verbal and non-verbal.

Verbal communication consists of spoken instructions, either face to face or via a telephone message. If a practitioner receives a message which concerns the patient it is important that it be passed on immediately. 'Operating room etiquette' (the unwritten code of operating room conduct) states that the surgeon must never be approached directly while operating, and all communication must go through the scrub practitioner. The circulator approaches the scrub practitioner, who then passes it on at an appropriate time to the surgeon. Any less important messages can wait until the surgeon has finished the procedure.

Non-verbal communication consists of written instructions in the patient's care plan, documenting the care given. This will be discussed in more detail under 'Care planning'. Other written communication includes policies, protocols and departmental documentation in the form of computer records and the theatre ledger. This will also be discussed further in the following section.

DOCUMENTATION

As with all aspects of care, accurate and legible records are an important part of the practitioner's role. Record keeping is important for two reasons:

- The safety and wellbeing of the patient
- The legal and accountability aspect pertaining to the staff into whose care the patient is entrusted.[20]

Documentation in the operating department includes the following:

- Operating lists
- Surgeons' preference sheets
- Policies/protocols
- Theatre ledger (operating register)
- Computer-held records
- Care plans/pathways.

The operating list is displayed in the operating room at the beginning of the day. This provides the perioperative practitioner with information regarding instruments, equipment, the operating surgeon, and the ages of patients, helping him or her prepare for some of the needs of individual patients.

Surgeons' preference sheets provide the practitioner with information regarding the surgical requirements, such as blades, swabs, sutures, and specific instruments and equipment. This increases efficiency by helping practitioners prepare the requirements prior to the start of the list, thereby avoiding delays that could prolong patients' procedures.

Written policies are an essential requirement, as they identify standards of practice to ensure that all practitioners are working to the same level. They are a useful aid for teaching and learning for both new and experienced staff.[21] It is the responsibility of all perioperative practitioners to familiarize themselves with new policies and protocols – ignorance of the correct policy is no defence against negligence.

The operating room ledger (or operating register) is a record of the patient's details, the procedure undertaken and the personnel involved. It is often used in court and may be used in evidence to support allegations of assault or negligence against the practitioner or hospital (see Chs 1 and 3 for more discussion on the need for documentation). Information includes:

- Start and finish time
- Date
- Name
- Age
- Ward
- Operation
- Type of anaesthetic
- Category of operation
- Consumables used
- Instrument trays
- Signatures of circulator and scrub practitioner
- Consultant
- Surgeons
- Anaesthetist
- Implants/drains/catheters.

Electronic records are also becoming more popular as technology advances. These contain the same information as above, but have the added benefit of providing easier access to information, and can provide reports such as average lengths of operating lists, percentage of overruns, average times of specific operations, etc. These records are invaluable in providing operating department managers with information to increase efficiency and effectiveness.

The patient care plan is an important feature in the planning and implementing of patient care and stays with the patient as he or she progresses through the suite.

Documentation of the patient's care during surgery provides a full account and evidence of the care they received. It can also be used for audit purposes, and can act as a reference should any complaints or legal matters arise in the future.

CARE PLANNING

There are two main purposes for perioperative care plans:

1. To provide information that will help practitioners identify any special needs or concerns of the patient
2. To record perioperative care that has been given in order to ensure accountability and continuity of care throughout this phase of the patient's treatment.

Figure 12.9 illustrates common parameters of care which are recorded, and shows how the information obtained at a preoperative visit can be used to plan the patient's care during their surgical procedure.

Perioperative patients require evidence-based, individualized holistic care. The care plan provides the practitioner with information that will identify any potential patient problems and will help them prescribe, plan and deliver care for the entire perioperative period, in order to ensure that care delivered is a continuous process.

Information for the care plan can be gathered at a preoperative visit, or in some cases (such as when emergency surgery is required) during the immediate preoperative period. As changes in practice and the needs of the patient occur, the perioperative practitioner can respond by updating the care plan accordingly. It identifies any special requirements of the patient as regards transfer and positioning, any concerns that they may have about their forthcoming surgery, and any problems that might occur as a result. It is an effective method of communicating instructions between departments within the operating suite.

There are four main sections required in the care plan:

- Reception
- Anaesthetic room
- Operating room
- Recovery.

On arrival in the operating department the patient is identified as the correct patient by checking the details on their identity band, and that all relevant

THEATRE CARE PLAN

Patient's Name [   ]   Unit Number [   ]

Date of Birth [   ]   Ward [   ]

RECEPTION

IDENTIFICATION
Case Notes/Addressographs ☐   Identity band ☐   Unit number corresponds   Yes ☐   No ☐

CONSENT
Self ☐   Relative ☐   Other (please state)...

ORIENTATION
Alert ☐   Sedated ☐   Lethargic ☐   Confused ☐   Non-responsive ☐

SPECIFIC NEEDS/PROBLEMS e.g. allergies, medical conditions
....

FASTING TIME.......................................

PRE OPERATIVE TESTS
ECG ☐   X-ray ☐   Bloods ☐   Other (please state)................................

BLOOD
None ☐   Group and Save ☐   Cross matched ☐   Number of units...............
Location.........................

WATERLOW SCORE NOTED
☐

PERSONAL BELONGINGS

	Removed	Returned to ward	Retained by patient
Hearing aid			
Glasses/Contact lenses			
Inhalers			
Dentures			
Jewellery			
Other (please state)			

Reception practitioner.. Date.................................

Figure 12.9 Theatre Care Plan.

ANAESTHETIC ROOM

MONITORING

ECG ☐ Item number.....................

Pulse oximeter ☐ Item number.....................

ANAESTHETIC TECHNIQUE

General ☐ Sedation ☐

Local infiltration ☐ Spinal ☐

Epidural ☐ Caudal ☐

Regional block.............................

AIRWAY MAINTAINED

E.T. tube ☐ Size..........................

Laryngeal mask ☐ Size..........................

Anatomical mask ☐

Oro/pharyngeal Airway ☐

Oxygen via face mask ☐

CANNULATION

Venflon: In situ on arrival ☐ Inserted ☐

CPV ☐ Arterial cannulae ☐

EYE PROTECTION

Tape ☐ Eye pad ☐ Shield ☐ Other ☐

OTHER INFORMATION

Naso-Gastric tube Size.................

....

Please state...

....

Anaesthetic practitioner...

Figure 12.9 (*Cont'd*).

OPERATING ROOM

MONITORING

ECG/BP ☐   Item number...............................
Gas analysis ☐   Item number...............................
Other ☐   Item number...............................
Tourniquet ☐   Time on.................
                    Time off.................

METHOD OF TRANSFER

Easyslide ☐
Patslide ☐
Samarit Roll Board ☐
Other ☐

POSITION ON OPERATING TABLE

Supine ☐   Prone ☐
Left lateral ☐   Right lateral ☐
Lithotomy ☐   Lloyd Davis ☐
Modified Lithotomy ☐   Trendelenburg ☐
Other......................

TABLE ACCESSORIES

Warming mattress ☐   Elbow retainers Left ☐ Right ☐
Pelvis support/Lateral support ☐   Armboards Left ☐ Right ☐
Fracture/Hip table ☐   Headring ☐
Shoulder pad ☐   Other.......................

PRESSURE RELIEVING DEVICES/ACCESSORIES

Gel mat ☐   Gel boots ☐
Gel pad ☐   Pillows ☐
Ankle support ☐   Flowtron leggings ☐
Other.....................

SKIN PREPARATION

Betadine aqueous ☐   Betadine spirit ☐
Chlorhexidine aqueous ☐   Chlorhexidine spirit ☐
Weak Iodine ☐   Tisept ☐
Other.....................

Figure 12.9 (Cont'd).

INCISION

Midline: Upper ☐   Gridiron ☐
              Lower ☐   Kocher ☐
Pfannenstiel ☐   Transverse ☐
Nephrectomy ☐   Hip: Left ☐   Right ☐
Endaural ☐   Postaural ☐
Neck ☐   Other............................

DRAINS

Suction ☐   Size............... Site............. Quantity..............
Tube ☐   Size............... Site............. Quantity..............
Corrugated ☐
Other.............................
Wound infiltration ☐   ☐ %   ☐ ml

SKIN CLOSURE

Absorbable ☐   Non-absorbable ☐   Clips ☐   N/A ☐

DRESSINGS

Airstrip/Mepore ☐   Melolin ☐   Blue dressing swabs ☐
Gamgee ☐   Mefix ☐   Velband ☐
Crepe ☐   Kling ☐   POP ☐
Cotton wool ☐   Other.............................

SUPPLEMENTARY

Packs ☐   Size............... Site.............
Splints ☐   Size............... Site.............
Urinary catheter ☐   Size...............
Other..

OPERATION PERFORMED

Actual...
....
Swabs/needles and instrument count correct ☐
Tourniquet/diathermy site checked and clear ☐   Yes ☐   No ☐
Pressure areas checked and clear   Yes ☐   No ☐
Comments...
....

PATIENT TRANSFERRED   Bed ☐   Trolley ☐

Scrub practitioner............................. Circulating practitioner................................

Figure 12.9   (*Cont'd*).

RECOVERY ROOM

LEVEL OF CONSCIOUSNESS
Recovery score................ On admission

Time................

AIRWAY STATUS
IPPV ☐   Extubated at...........hrs.

Intubated/ventilated via Waters circuit ☐   Extubated at...........hrs.

Intubated/self-ventilating via Waters circuit ☐   Extubated at...........hrs.

Ventilated/anatomical face mask via Waters circuit ☐

Laryngeal mask ☐   Removed at...........hrs.

Oro/pharyngeal airway ☐

Oxygen therapy.........litres/min via mask ☐

Other................

Oro/pharyngeal suction ☐

Comments...

MONITORING
Pulse oximeter ☐   Item number................

ECG ☐   Item number................

Blood pressure ☐

INTRAVENOUS INFUSIONS
Blood transfusion ☐

Fluid balance chart completed ☐

WOUND OBSERVATIONS
Wound/Wound dressing checked ☐

Drain site checked ☐

Drainage recorded ☐   Quantity....................

Observation of affected limb(s)

Colour ☐   Movement ☐   Sensation ☐

POP in situ and checked ☐

Comments...

ANALGESIA GIVEN IN RECOVERY
Analgesia given as prescribed ☐

ANTIEMETIC GIVEN IN RECOVERY
Antiemetic given as prescribed ☐

Figure 12.9 (Cont'd).

OTHER DRUGS GIVEN IN RECOVERY

Drug.........   Dose............   Route...........   Time.........   Given by..........

Drug.........   Dose............   Route...........   Time.........   Given by..........

Drug.........   Dose............   Route...........   Time.........   Given by..........

URINARY CATHETER

Urine measured and amount documented on admission   ☐

Urine output measured hourly ($<$40 ml hr inform medical staff)   ☐

Bladder irrigation carried out   ☐

Comments..

PRESSURE RELIEF/ACCESSORIES

Waterlow score noted   ☐

Patient nursed on ward bed   ☐

Pressure relief mattress in situ   ☐

Skin integrity assessed hourly   ☐

Flowtrons in situ   ☐

Warm touch/blanket   ☐

CONDITION ON DISCHARGE

Recovery score...................

Vital signs are within patient's own normal limits   ☐

Pain score on discharge..................

Intravenous fluid prescription sheet completed   ☐

Wound/wound drains checked   ☐

Drug regimes completed   ☐

Case notes/X-rays available   ☐

ADDITIONAL INSTRUCTIONS TO WARD

Oxygen therapy on return to ward   @.........%   Duration.................

Other..

....

Recovery practitioner...

Figure 12.9   (*Cont'd*).

documentation is accompanying them, such as the case notes and any X-rays. The information on the consent form must correspond with the operation listed, be fully completed with the patient's details and the operation to be performed, and be signed and dated by the patient and the doctor who has explained the procedure.

For the consent to be informed, patients should be given the amount of information needed to make an informed choice about a given treatment[22] (see Ch. 1 for a detailed account of the principles of consent). In the case of a patient being unable to give consent, the doctor who is performing the procedure must sign the appropriate consent form for this purpose. This is only in exceptional and specific circumstances: it does not give the surgeon the right to do whatever they wish to the patient. If the patient is under 16 the consent form should be signed by a parent or guardian. However, any person under 16 who is considered mature and intelligent enough to understand the nature of the treatment is also regarded in law as capable of giving consent: this is termed 'Gillick competence'.[23]

The orientation of the patient is observed, any specific needs, such as inhalers, should accompany the patient, and any essential personal belongings necessary to communicate, such as a hearing aid or glasses, should be present.

Specific medical problems are identified and recorded, and any allergies noted and passed on to the scrub practitioners so that they can select appropriate skin preparations and dressings. The fasting time is also recorded, and if the patient has had any preoperative tests, such as ECG, X-ray and bloods, whether the patient has been cross-matched, how many units are available, and the location of the stored blood.

All the above information is collected, documented in the first section and signed by the practitioner receiving the patient in the department.

Once the patient enters the anaesthetic room and is anaesthetized the anaesthetic practitioner is responsible for completing this section as regards monitoring and anaesthetic technique.

Following entry into the operating room the patient is transferred and positioned for surgery. The circulating practitioner records the method, position and any accessories used. At the end of the procedure the actual operation performed is documented by the scrub practitioner, the swab, needle and instrument counts are verified as being correct, and that the diathermy site and pressure areas are checked and are undamaged. This section of the care plan is signed by both the scrub and circulating practitioners.

The care plan then follows the patient through to the recovery area, where monitoring and administration of drugs are recorded; this section is signed by the recovery practitioner on the patient's discharge from the operating suite.

CONCLUSION

The modern perioperative practitioner faces a variety of challenges as they care for their patients. Modern surgery is faster and more complex than ever before, and the role of the practitioner must constantly change and develop in order to respond to pressures such as increasingly complex technology, increased throughput of patients, and changes to skills mix and staffing levels.

The care and support of the patient while they undergo the operative procedure can only be achieved by practitioners practising safely and efficiently as part of the perioperative team. This chapter has illustrated some of the many challenges facing practitioners as they provide care to the perioperative patient during their surgical procedure.

References

1. Williams M. Teamwork in healthcare: time for review. Br J Theatre Nurs 1998; 8: 19–24.
2. Taylor M, Campbell C. The multi-disciplinary team in the operating department. Br J Theatre Nurs 1999; 9: 178–183.
3. Hind M. Clarifying accountability in operating theatre practice. Nurs Standard 1997; 12: 44–45.
4. Jackson D. Latex allergy and anaphylaxis – what to do? J Intraven Nurs 1995; 18: 33–52.
5. Booth B. Hidden dilemma. NT 1994; 90: 46–48.
6. Starritt T, Ewing E. Implementing good practice in the prevention and management of pressure sores. Br J Theatre Nurs 1999; 9: 60–63.
7. Bridel J. Pressure sore risk in operating theatres. Nurs Standard 1993; 7: 4–10.
8. Waterlow J. Operating table. The root cause of many pressure sores? Br J Theatre Nurs 1996; 6: 19–21.
9. Scott EM. Hospital acquired pressure sores as an indicator of quality: a research programme centred in the operating theatre. Br J Theatre Nurs 1988; 8: 19–24.

10. Hull RD, Raskob GE, Hirsh J. Prophylaxis of venous thromboembolism: an overview. Chest 1986; 89(Suppl): 375.
11. Sadler P. Prevention of deep vein thrombosis and pulmonary embolism. Anaesth Inten Care Med 2000; 1: 20–21.
12. Davis B. Towards 2000: a new age in DVT prophylaxis. Br J Theatre Nurs 1999; 9: 116.
13. Morley-Foster P. Unintentional hypothermia in the operating room. Can Anaesth Soc J 1986; 33(4): 516–527.
14. Cuifo D, Dice S, Coles C. Rewarming hypothermic postanaesthesia patients: a comparison between a water coil warming blanket and a forced-air warming blanket. J Post Anaesth Nurs 1995; 10: 155–158.
15. Wicker P. Electrosurgery in perioperative practice. Br J Theatre Nurs 2000; 10: 221–226.
16. Hoglan M. Potential hazards from electrosurgery plume. Can Operat Room Nurs J 1995; 13: 10–16.
17. Taylor M, Campbell C. Patient care in the operating department (2). Br J Theatre Nurs 1999; 9: 319–323.
18. Taylor M, Campbell C. The multi-disciplinary team in the operating department. Br J Theatre Nurs 1999; 9: 178–183.
19. Taylor M, Campbell C. Surgical practice. In: Clarke P, Jones J, eds. Brigden's operating department practice. Edinburgh: Churchill Livingstone; 1998.
20. Jarman B. Care plans for the operating department. Br J Theatre Nurs 1992; 25: 477–484.
21. National Association for Theatre Nurses. Operating department records. Harrogate: NATN; 1999.
22. Taylor B. Parental autonomy and consent to treatment. J Advan Nurs 1999; 29: 570–576.

Useful contacts

J Nesbit Evans & Co Ltd
Woden Road West
Wednesbury
West Midlands
WS10 7BL
021 556 1511

Tyco Healthcare UK Ltd
154 Fareham Road
Gosport
Hampshire
PO13 0AS
01329 224000

Daniels Healthcare
72-80 Akeman Street
Tring
Hertfordshire
HP23 6AF
01442 826881
http://www.daniels.co.uk/patslide.htm

Vital Signs
Sussex Business Village
Lake Lane
Barnham
PO22 0AL
01243 5553000
http://www.vital-signs.com

Huntleigh Healthcare Ltd
310-312 Dallow Road
Luton
Bedfordshire
LU1 1TD
01582 413104
http://www.huntleigh-healthcare.com

Central Medical Supplies Ltd
CMS House
Basford Lane
Leebrook
Leek
Staffordshire
ST13 7DT
01538 399541
http://www.centralmedical.co.uk

Chapter 13

Care of the postanaesthetic patient

Jill Yates

Key points

- Skills and care in the recovery room
- Care of the patient from preoperative assessment to postoperative discharge
- Common postoperative complications

The recovery room is a specialized area within the operating department where patients recover after surgery. Over the years, recovery care has developed from a brief period of observation to a prolonged and active period of monitoring in a specifically designed clinical area.[1] It is a unique place caring for patients at varying levels of consciousness which requires staff to have appropriate specialized clinical skills and knowledge. The necessity for dedicated skilled recovery practitioners has increased as surgical procedures have become more complex and numerous.[1] The latest guidelines from the Association of Anaesthetists of Great Britain and Ireland recognize the speciality of this area and recommend that at least one member of staff has an Advanced Life Support certificate, with all staff being encouraged to attain an appropriate airway management qualification.[1]

STAFF EDUCATION

The provision of a satisfactory quality of care during recovery from anaesthesia and surgery relies heavily on investment in the education and training of recovery room practitioners. The Association of Anaesthetists of Great Britain and Ireland[2] recommended that all practitioners who work in the recovery area should have received appropriate training and possess a nationally recognized qualification above that of either Registered General Nurse or NVQ level 3 in Operating Department Practice. They also recommend that if advanced life support training is not possible then the minimum standard should be an English National Board (ENB) qualification (ENB A94 Post Anaesthetic Recovery) or equivalent for all grades of staff. At the time of writing, this document has not been updated to account for the demise of the ENB and the development of postregistration recovery courses by higher education institutions.

These documents do, however, highlight the requirement for post basic education which is in line with the ethos of lifelong learning. Practitioners who routinely work in the recovery area must develop a wide range of clinical skills including, for example, the ability to practise:

- Airway management
- Intravenous drug administration
- Venepuncture/cannulation
- Invasive monitoring
- Defibrillation
- Epidural top-up.

These clinical skills require the provision of a comprehensive training programme with regular updates and support in the clinical area. There must be a training programme and clinical supervision that will allow staff to develop or maintain clinical skills as required. All practitioners must have an understanding of anatomy, physiology and pharmacology in order to recognize potential complications associated with recovery practice and to provide a high standard of patient care.

PREOPERATIVE VISITING

Patients are often visited by a perioperative practitioner before surgery in order to make personal contact, which will help to facilitate the emotional support of the patient, and to gather information that is often omitted by the surgeon or anaesthetist. Information collated regarding the patient's physical and mental wellbeing is as important as their past medical history and aids with the patient's care during their perioperative experience. It could be argued that recovery practitioners are the most suitable team members for this role, as they have a high level of contact with conscious patients. Utilizing a preoperative visit allows the practitioner to collect information to plan individual care while also providing information for the patient to reduce anxiety prior to surgery.[3] Such visits are not always possible in emergency surgery or if patients are critically ill. These visits can be carried out on the ward or at the preassessment clinic prior to surgery. During the visit, information relating to pre- and postoperative pain control can be given to patients, with the addition of written material to read. Preoperative visiting is time consuming and requires resources, but it is an essential service for patients and potentially minimizes delays during the theatre list if specific equipment can be located before the patient enters the department.

The information collected then has to be disseminated to the perioperative team, which could be done in a briefing prior to the start of the operating list.

THE POSTOPERATIVE RECOVERY AREA

The recovery room is a peaceful patient-centred environment where patients can recover from anaesthesia. The area should have natural light to aid assessment of patients' skin colour, be well ventilated to remove exhaled anaesthetic agents, and be separate from the theatre area to reduce the amount of noise and activity. The area is usually divided into bays, each of which has the basic equipment required to manage a patient immediately postoperatively.

RECOVERY PRACTICE

The main aims of recovery practice are to care for the patient while providing intensive support in the immediate postoperative phase. Initially this involves airway support with monitoring of vital signs and detailed patient assessment. As the patient regains consciousness and is able to maintain his or her own airway, the emphasis of care shifts to continued patient assessment and the relief of symptoms such as nausea and pain, and to the provision of emotional support.

EQUIPMENT

It is essential that the following equipment is checked daily, clean, and ready for use. The minimum equipment required for a recovery bay is outlined below. This selection of equipment would allow a recovery practitioner to receive a patient, start routine monitoring, assess the patient's needs, provide individual care and manage the patient's airway. Extra equipment will probably be required if the patient has an existing disease (such as diabetes, for example) prior to surgery.

- Oxygen supply, twin flowmeters, tubing
- Fixed and variable-performance oxygen masks, nasal catheters
- Mapleson C breathing circuit with angled connector
- Capnograph
- Anaesthetic face mask with filter, a full range of oropharyngeal airways
- Suction unit with tubing, Yankauer ends and a full range of suction catheters
- ECG monitor, electrodes
- Pulse oximeter
- Automatic blood pressure measuring equipment
- Selection of swabs, adhesive tape, syringes, needles, cannulae
- Syringe to deflate cuffs of airway adjuncts
- Disposable gloves, vomit bowl, tissues
- Sharps disposal bin, waste bin
- IV pole
- Pressure bag
- Full range of crystalloid and colloid infusions
- Infusion pumps
- Thermometer
- Clock with sweep hand
- Telephone and emergency call system.

The following equipment should be available in the immediate recovery area to deal with deteriorating/changing condition in the postoperative phase:

- Arrest trolley with emergency drug box, defibrillator and reintubation equipment
- A range of nasopharyngeal airways
- Manual sphygmomanometer with stethoscope and range of blood pressure cuffs
- Invasive monitoring – arterial, CVP monitors and transducers
- Anaesthetic machine and ventilator with disconnector alarm
- Blood warmer
- Bronchoscope
- Cricothyroid puncture set
- Equipment for blood gas sampling
- Peripheral nerve stimulator
- Chest drain set and clamps
- Glucometer

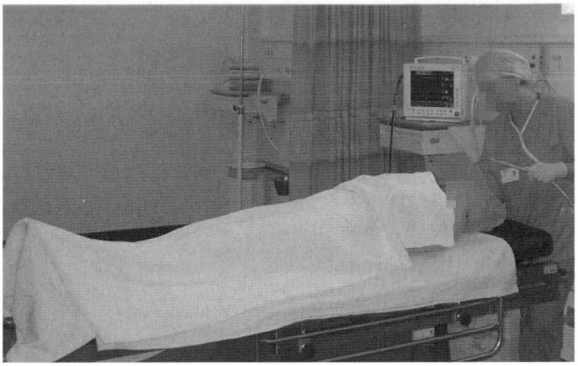

Figure 13.1 A typical modern recovery bay, showing some essential equipment.

- Blood fridge
- Portable suction and oxygen
- Forced air warming device with blanket
- Electric fan.

The following drugs must remain easily available for use in emergency situations:

Cardiac arrest
- Adrenaline (Epinephrine) 1:10 000 (1 mg/10 ml)
- Atropine sulphate 1 mg/10 ml
- Atropine sulphate 3 mg/30 ml
- Calcium chloride 10% (10 ml)
- Amiodarone 300 mg/10 ml.

Reintubation
- Suxamethonium – has to remain in drug fridge.

Anaphylaxis
- All staff must be able to locate the anaesthetic protocol for treating patients with malignant hyperpyrexia. The protocol will involve factors such as the use of dantrolene, cold fluids and ice.

RECOVERY MONITORING

A high standard of monitoring should be maintained until the patient is fully recovered from anaesthesia. Clinical observations are often supplemented by the use of the following monitoring devices, depending on the patient's condition.[4]

PULSE OXIMETRY

A pulse oximeter non-invasively measures the arterial haemoglobin oxygen saturation in the blood and the pulse rate. Normal arterial oxygen saturation values are above 95%. This monitor is a valuable addition to the clinical skills of skin colour observation and assessment of respirations, as it will detect a significant number of episodes of oxygen desaturation which are often visually undetected by an observer.[10] The readings are not in real time and will be a reflection of the patient's past condition which, although providing an early warning of developing hypoxaemia, requires immediate intervention before hypoxia develops.

The monitor uses a sensor to emit red and infrared light, which passes into the tissue and the detector measures the amount of light absorbed. The detector can determine the percentage of oxyhaemoglobin in the arterial haemoglobin by measuring and analysing the difference in the absorption of light between oxyhaemoglobin and deoxyhaemoglobin. The sensor is placed on the periphery where there is a good arterial pulse; common sites are the fingers, toes and ear lobes. The assumption taken from this reading is that if the patient's periphery is well oxygenated then their vital organs are too. There are a few complications with this monitoring system, including pressure injury after prolonged use, which is avoided by regular inspection and rotation of the probe site; this condition is mostly seen in intensive care units. Factors that can affect the accuracy of recordings include poor peripheral circulation; hypothermia; agitation or excessive movement; extraneous light; carbon monoxide poisoning; methaemoglobinaemia; and opaque nail polish.[5]

NON-INVASIVE/INVASIVE BLOOD PRESSURE MONITORING

Blood pressure is measured either invasively or non-invasively depending on the condition of the patient and the surgical procedure being performed. The most common method is automatic blood pressure monitoring. The blood pressure cuff is usually placed over the brachial artery because of its accessibility during surgery. The popliteal or posterior tibial arteries could also be used. These machines are set to cycle and will sound an alarm if the systolic and diastolic pressures register outside the preset range. Non-invasive blood pressure measurements are not as accurate as invasive monitoring, and will become increasingly inaccurate if the patient is unable to stay still, is obese or oedematous, or they have a decreasing circulatory blood volume.[5]

In the event of mechanical failure or to check automatic readings, an aneroid sphygmomanometer with inflatable cuff and stethoscope is required for standard auscultatory blood pressure monitoring.

Invasive monitoring of blood pressure is commonly obtained via cannulation of the radial artery. The pressure within the artery is transmitted via a column of fluid to a transducer. The transducer converts the pressure into an electrical signal that can be converted into millimetres of mercury (mmHg) and displayed on the monitor with an arterial waveform. Arterial blood pressure monitoring is continuous and indicated for haemodynamically unstable patients. Reliable monitoring depends upon correct calibration and reliable equipment. Unreliable readings can be a result of kinking/clotting of the arterial catheter, catheter positioning, and air in the system.[5]

ELECTROCARDIOGRAPH

Electrocardiograph (ECG) monitors measure the electrical activity of the cardiac muscle. This activity is conducted via electrodes fixed to the patient's skin and then amplified electronically and displayed as a trace on a monitor.[5] The practitioner observing the monitor will be required to interpret basic cardiac rhythms and relate any ECG changes to the effect that this may have on the patient's condition.

CENTRAL VENOUS PRESSURE

Central venous pressure (CVP) provides an estimation of the patient's circulating volume and is equated to the right ventricular end-diastolic pressure. It is transduced (converted from mechanical movement to electrical signals) in the same way as arterial pressure, and produces a waveform on the monitor. Routes for central venous cannulation are the right cephalic vein, the internal/external jugular vein or the subclavian vein. By monitoring the adequacy of the central venous return, blood volume and right ventricular function, an assessment can be made of the adequacy of the fluid replacement regimen. The average reading is 0–8 mmHg.[6]

If a more accurate measurement of cardiac output is required a pulmonary artery catheter can be inserted. This is the most invasive method of measuring right arterial, pulmonary arterial and pulmonary artery wedge pressures. Although pulmonary artery catheters are not often used routinely in patients who are cared for in the recovery room, they are often used during extensive operative procedures and in the intensive care unit.[6]

CAPNOGRAPHY

A capnograph measures the end-tidal carbon dioxide (CO_2) level. This is done by attaching a sample line to a port on the filter above the endotracheal tube. The CO_2 is passed into a photodetector, which measures the amount of infrared radiation absorbed by the CO_2 and calculates the CO_2 value after the gas has passed through a sample chamber, multigas filter and detector. An end-tidal CO_2 waveform is produced which will change as a result of rebreathing or airway disease.[5] This is a useful assessment of adequate ventilation and allows the monitoring of any modification to normocapnia as required.

TRANSFER OF THE PATIENT FROM THE OPERATING ROOM TO THE RECOVERY ROOM

During transfer to the recovery area the patient must be accompanied by the anaesthetist and at least one operating room practitioner. The anaesthetist and practitioner will hand over care to the recovery practitioner and supply the following information:

- Identity of the patient
- Details of the operative procedure, including the presence of drains, sutures, dressings, etc.
- Anaesthetic technique and perioperative drugs administered
- Summary of the patient's condition, including relevant pre-existing disease
- Significant perioperative events (for example extensive haemorrhage)
- Postoperative orders from the surgeon and the anaesthetist.

PATIENT ASSESSMENT

Continual patient assessment is the key to high-quality recovery practice, with the main aim being to identify the best way to restore the patient's natural homoeostatic balance as soon as possible. The assessment involves examining each body system individually and collating the information to achieve a complete picture, allowing appropriate interventions to be carried out with a full understanding of the patient's condition. The level of complexity of the assessment is dependent on surgical specialty, the

monitoring required and the condition of the patient; however, the principles of assessment are the same.

In their practice guidelines for postanaesthetic care the American Society of Anesthesiologists[7] recommend that periodic assessment and monitoring of respiratory rate, airway patency, oxygen saturation, pulse rate, blood pressure, temperature, drainage, bleeding, urine output, mental status, pain, and nausea and vomiting should all be routinely considered. Where specific monitoring is recommended, for example arterial blood pressure monitoring, the duration of the intervention will be dependent on the patient's clinical status.

The initial assessment of airway, breathing and circulation (ABC) begins as soon as the patient enters the department. This assessment should be performed by the anaesthetist and recovery practitioners to provide a baseline for assessment in recovery, and is usually performed while positioning the patient on his or her bed and attaching monitors. After this rapid initial assessment the practitioner and anaesthetist will discuss the specifics of the anaesthetic and any postoperative orders. All patients should be breathing spontaneously before the anaesthetist leaves the recovery room.[8]

The recovery practitioner's initial priority is maintenance of the patient's airway. If the patient is unconscious, with their airway being supported by an airway adjunct, then they require intensive monitoring, one-to-one, with a second practitioner being available as required.[1]

Initially, following general anaesthesia most patients are placed in a lateral position, as this will facilitate drainage of any secretions/stomach contents and prevent the tongue being drawn by gravity against the posterior wall of the pharynx, until laryngeal reflexes return. Patient positioning depends on past medical history, the operative procedure performed and the type of anaesthetic given; not all patients require to be in a lateral position.

The practitioner will then perform a detailed assessment of the patient, starting with the respiratory system by looking at ventilatory patterns, oxygen saturation and airway adjuncts in situ. Blood pressure, heart rate and rhythm will reflect the status of the cardiovascular system, with renal function being assessed by intravenous input and output from urinary catheter or any drains. Neurological function is assessed by the responsiveness of the patient to external stimuli. A core temperature, visual check of skin condition, pain, nausea and sedation scoring will complete baseline recordings.

All patient observations are normally recorded initially every 5 minutes until stable, and then at least every 15 minutes. Documentation of these observations allows for the identification of changing trends in the patient's condition.

RESPIRATORY ASSESSMENT

Respiratory function is closely monitored to ensure adequate ventilation for tissue oxygenation and cellular respiration. The depth, rate, noise and effort of respiration are all important factors in respiratory assessment. Changes in oxygen consumption and carbon dioxide production stimulate the central nervous system to alter the rate and depth of breathing, allowing arterial carbon dioxide, oxygen levels and pH to remain stable. Stretch receptors and sensory nerves in the lungs, pain, emotional responses, fever and sepsis also alter the pattern of breathing.[9]

The depth of breathing equates to the amount of gas being moved in and out of the respiratory passages with each breath: this is normally about 500 ml during normal quiet breathing. If the patient is attached to a C circuit their ability to deflate the reservoir bag, combined with capnography, is an indication of good respiratory function. Shallow respiration, when the patient is unconscious, can be a sign of continuing depression from anaesthesia and/or analgesia. In the conscious patient, shallow breathing can be the result of poor positioning, incisional pain, obesity or pre-existing lung disease.[10]

Respiration should be quiet and effortless; if it is noisy this indicates a problem. There are recognized noises that indicate a problem/obstruction in different parts of the respiratory tract. Gurgling indicates an accumulation of mucus/secretions, which should be removed promptly by suction. Crowing may indicate laryngospasm, which could result in partial or complete closure of the trachea by paralysis of the vocal cords; complete laryngospasm is silent. Wheezing can indicate bronchospasm, which occurs most often in patients with pre-existing pulmonary disease.[10]

The rate of respiration of a normal adult is 12–20 breaths per minute, and a minimum of 8–10 breaths per minute is preferred prior to extubation of an endotracheal tube. Ten breaths per minute are also normally considered to be the minimum before receiving intravenous opiates.

The above combine to be an assessment of respiratory function, which in the postoperative period is altered most frequently by airway obstruction.

Case study 13.1: Laryngospasm

A 42-year-old man was transferred into recovery following laparoscopic cholecystectomy. There was nothing of note in his past medical history. Routine monitoring was connected – ECG, BP and SaO_2. The patient was intubated and breathing spontaneously on admission to the recovery area. Oral suction was performed and the anaesthetist extubated the patient and administered oxygen via a face mask.

As he tried to breathe the patient made a crowing noise. This was due to the intrinsic laryngeal muscle reflex closing the larynx, thus obstructing the flow of air to the lungs. The patient was regaining consciousness and becoming distressed, so he was reassured.

Actions taken
The anaesthetist used an anaesthetic face mask and C circuit with high-flow oxygen to apply positive pressure to relax the larynx and allow oxygen to pass into the trachea and lungs. This eased the spasm, so the anaesthetist prescribed for the oxygen being administered to be humidified. After 10 minutes the patient still felt that his breathing was difficult so the anaesthetist prescribed 1 mg of adrenaline (epinephrine) to be nebulized with 1 ml of saline 0.9% in order to vasoconstrict and hence shrink the swollen airway mucosa. This removed the spasm completely and the patient began to breathe quietly and easily.

Other potential outcomes
If laryngospasm is complete and is not relieved with positive-pressure ventilation within 1 minute the patient will require to be intubated. This is achieved by administering a short-acting muscle relaxant to relax the smooth muscle of the larynx and an induction agent so an endotracheal tube can be passed as required.

Anaesthetic drugs used in emergency intubation
Suxamethonium – a short-acting depolarizing muscle relaxant particularly used for rapid-sequence intubation. Onset: 10–30 seconds. Duration: 1–5 minutes.

Propofol (induction agent) – smooth induction, rapid recovery and no hangover effect; is noted to have possible antiemetic effects.

Thiopentone – ultrashort-acting barbiturate induction agent; generally provides smooth induction.

These drugs are used in combination with other anaesthetic drugs depending on the condition of the patient.

When adequate respiratory function is established then the anaesthetist can extubate the patient. The patient's respiratory function must be monitored closely, with the anaesthetist being available to deal with any complications.

COMMON RESPIRATORY PROBLEMS

Airway obstruction

A common postoperative airway obstruction occurs in the upper airway at the pharyngeal level as a result of the patients' tongue falling back into the pharynx. This is more likely to occur when patients are supine and relaxed, and is due to the muscular composition of the tongue, some of which originates from the mandible. Therefore, in a paralysed or unconscious patient the mandible falls posteriorly and subsequently takes the tongue with it. Patient positioning alone may prove insufficient, and the practitioner should employ the head-tilt/chin-lift manoeuvre, which lifts the tongue and epiglottis away from the pharyngeal wall. A sustained jaw thrust may be required if this does not clear the airway. If this fails to relieve the obstruction then creating an artificial airway by inserting either an oropharyngeal (via the mouth) or a nasopharyngeal airway (via the nose) may be required.[10]

Airway obstruction from the larynx downward is chiefly due to laryngospasm, bronchospasm or particulate matter such as stomach contents from vomiting or regurgitation. Other possible causes of obstruction include soft tissue oedema resulting from allergic reaction or mechanical trauma.

Oxygen

Oxygen (O_2) is administered routinely after surgery to maintain adequate levels in the arterial blood. The amount, duration and device used to administer the oxygen depend upon the procedure and the patient. Routine postoperative oxygen is administered via a variable-performance Hudson mask delivering approximately 40% oxygen. This mask works by drawing air in via the patient's respiratory effort; however, the actual concentration of oxygen received by the patient depends upon the ventilatory pattern. Nasal cannulae are an alternative

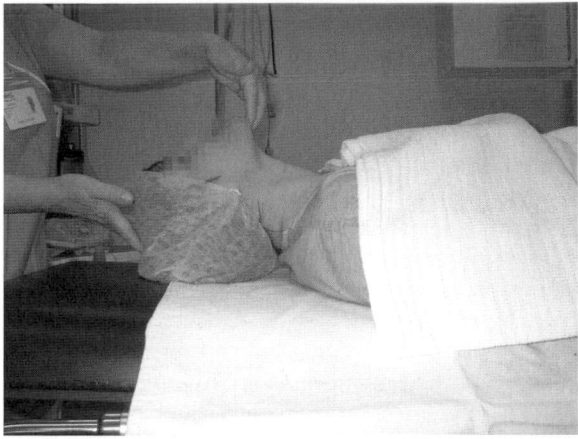

Figure 13.2   Demonstration of the head tilt/chin lift manoeuvre, which lifts the tongue and epiglottis away from the pharyngeal wall.

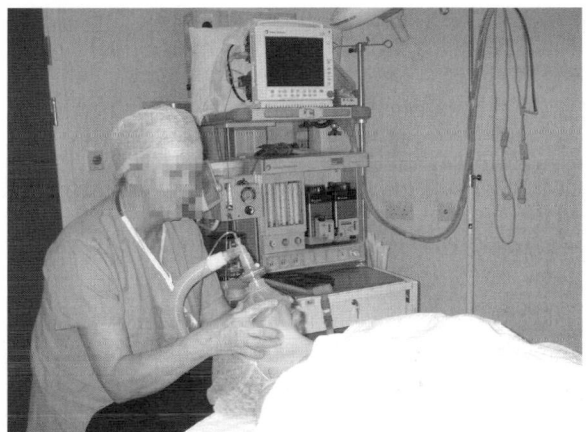

Figure 13.3   Maintaining a patient's airway while delivering oxygen via a face mask. Note the jaw thrust which helps to maintain an open airway.

to a variable-performance mask, being less claustrophobic and generally well tolerated by patients. Low oxygen flow rates are required to prevent damage to nasal mucosa.

If the patient has lung disease a more precise mask can be used with a fixed performance, for example a Venturi mask. These masks deliver a constant concentration of oxygen because air is drawn into the mask by oxygen flow at a constant ratio and independent of the ventilatory pattern.[10]

Hypoxia

The function of the respiratory system is to deliver oxygen to and to eliminate carbon dioxide from the tissues, using blood as the exchange and transport medium. Any respiratory complication will, if uncorrected, lead to hypoxaemia (inadequate arterial oxygenation) and/or hypercarbia (retention of carbon dioxide). Hypoxia is a state where there is inadequate provision of oxygen reaching the tissues, even in the presence of oxygenated blood.

Respiratory inadequacy in the immediate postoperative period may be caused by respiratory depression from narcotics and potent anaesthetic agents, residual paralysis from muscle relaxants, pain, hypothermia or airway obstruction. The result may be hypoxia, hypercarbia and respiratory acidosis. Signs and symptoms of hypoxia include a reduced oxygen saturation level (hypoxaemia), and restlessness and confusion that indicate impaired cerebral oxygenation. The increased use of pulse oximeters allows hypoxia to be recognized early before cyanosis develops.

Postoperative hypoxia can be prevented by administering adequate analgesia, oxygen, and maintaining normothermia. Another simple measure to enhance the provision of oxygen is good positioning of the patient and encouragement to take adequate breaths.[10]

CARDIOVASCULAR ASSESSMENT

Blood pressure

The three principal factors influencing blood pressure (BP) are cardiac output, peripheral resistance and blood volume. These factors combine together to maintain circulation and tissue perfusion. Postoperative changes to all these factors will occur because of the stress of surgery, anaesthetic drugs, core body temperature changes and perioperative fluid losses. Blood pressure is regularly monitored to identify any trends towards hypotension or hypertension in the postoperative period.

Postoperative hypotension is common and can be caused by anaesthetic factors, such as spinal/epidural anaesthesia, patient positioning, intraoperative or postoperative blood loss, pre-existing medical conditions and poor lung ventilation. Hypotension is defined as a blood pressure of less than 20% of the preoperative recording. The clinical signs associated with hypotension are a rapid thready pulse, disorientation, restlessness, oliguria and peripheral vasoconstriction.[6]

A hypertensive blood pressure recording can also be caused by the effects of anaesthesia, respiratory insufficiency causing carbon dioxide (CO_2) retention,

pain/anxiety, and delirium on emergence from anaesthesia. Hypertension is defined as a blood pressure 20% higher than the patient's preoperative level. The clinical signs associated with hypertension – headache and altered mental status – will determine the severity, as often hypertension can be asymptomatic.[6] Hypertension must be considered in the context of the patient's condition and medical history, as the increasing strain on the myocardium may not be tolerated by those with cardiac disease.

Short-term control of BP is performed by the baroreceptor reflex, which is sensitive to changes in BP, and by the chemoreceptor reflex, which is sensitive to changing levels of O_2, CO_2 and hydrogen ions, so it is important to maintain oxygenation.[9] If the patient has lost a significant amount of circulating volume perioperatively then the sympathetic response will promote the release of vasoconstrictive hormones in an attempt to increase arterial blood pressure.[9] This is a longer-term effect, but if the patient is not supported with fluid replacement at this stage then it can lead rapidly to hypovolaemic shock.

Before any methods are employed to raise/lower blood pressure it is important to establish the cause of the problem. Decisions to treat an altered BP should be based on trends rather than a single reading, and high/low readings should always be rechecked. All the other information about the patient should be considered, for example respiratory effort, conscious level, heart rate, SaO_2 reading, wound checks, urine output, information from the operating theatre and pre-existing disease. This will usually determine the cause of the hypotension/hypertension, allowing an intervention to be carried out and the anaesthetist to be informed as appropriate.

Heart rate

It is important to assess the patient's radial pulse for rate, regularity and strength, as this gives basic confirmation of adequate cardiac output while initiating touch between practitioner and patient.

Two common dysrhythmias found during the recovery period are sinus bradycardia (slow heart rate) and tachycardia (fast heart rate). Bradycardias are commonly caused by hypoxaemia, hypothermia and vagal stimulation. Atropine is administered to increase the heart rate and usually no further treatment is required.[6] Tachycardia usually decreases if the cause is treated; some of the causes include pain, anxiety, drugs, hypoxaemia, hypovolaemia and increased temperature.

Cardiac arrest

The common precipitating factors in cardiac arrest in the perioperative area are hypoxia, excessive anaesthetic agents, hypovolaemia, hypotension and pre-existing medical conditions. Prompt intervention is required, with cardiopulmonary resuscitation commencing rapidly to ensure the best patient outcome. Cardiac arrest teams are common in every acute area and should be called for every emergency, including those occurring in recovery. Figure 13.4 is an algorithm often used for the resuscitation of patients.

RENAL ASSESSMENT

Fluid balance

The anaesthetist will prescribe an intravenous therapy fluid regimen to fulfil the individual patient's requirements, replacing fluid lost during preoperative fasting and during surgery. The normal adult requires 2000–2500 ml of fluid per day to ensure an adequate renal function.[9]

Patients are observed during their postanaesthetic recovery for signs of hypovolaemia or circulatory overload. The signs and symptoms of hypovolaemia include pallor, a weak thready pulse, increased heart rate, falling blood pressure, peripheral vasoconstriction, oliguria and thirst. The cause of the hypovolaemia must be ascertained, monitored, and signs of improvement assessed. Postoperative haemorrhage is the most common cause of hypovolaemia in the recovery room.

The opposite of hypovolaemia is circulatory overload, where patients become vasodilated, breathless, tachycardic, show increasing blood pressure and have a full bounding pulse. This can lead to adult respiratory distress syndrome, which is caused in this situation by pulmonary oedema causing the gas exchange in the lungs to be impaired, resulting in hypoxia.

In both cases patients require to be reviewed by an anaesthetist and have their fluid regimen altered appropriately.

Case study 13.2: Haemorrhage

A patient enters the recovery area after an abdominal operation where the blood loss was 1200 ml. The patient is extubated, responsive to voice, peripherally vasoconstricted, cool and pale (temperature 34.2°C). There are two peripheral lines, one with a blood transfusion in progress and the other giving crystalloid fluid. The anaesthetist has requested a haemoglobin check after the blood transfusion. The patient is breathing spontaneously, slightly hypotensive (90/56) but stable, heart rate 90–100 bpm. The recovery practitioner places a forced air warming blanket on the patient and also warms intravenous fluids to increase the patient's temperature. The patient has a wound drain and a urinary catheter in place.

The blood loss from the drain is persistent (100 ml in 5 minutes) and the patient becomes restless, increasingly hypotensive (60/90), and the heart rate increases to 120 bpm.

Actions taken
The drain is observed constantly, with the blood loss recorded and anaesthetist and surgeon informed. The rate of intravenous fluids is increased, under anaesthetic orders, to assist loss of circulating volume, blood and synthetic volume expanders are used (Gelofusine), and oxygen level increased to prevent hypoxia. The patient continues to haemorrhage and is returned to theatre.

The anaesthetist supports blood pressure with a vasoconstrictor sympathomimetic and increases fluid input. Once the patient is in theatre an arterial line, CVP line and temperature probe are inserted; a urinary catheter is already in situ.

Maintenance fluid replacement of 2 ml/kg/h. The patient would require blood gas, clotting and coagulation screen: the result of these tests would indicate whether they required a continuing blood transfusion ± clotting factors. The haemorrhage arrests in theatre with further blood loss of 3500 ml, and the patient returns to recovery for assessment.

Possible outcomes
Cardiac/respiratory arrest may occur if the patient continues to bleed. If patient is overtransfused adult respiratory distress syndrome may develop, leading to hypoxia which may require artificial ventilation to raise the alveolar partial pressure of oxygen, thus increasing the gradient for diffusion to occur. Postoperatively intensive care is indicated if the patient remains unstable from a cardiovascular, respiratory or metabolic point of view. High–dependency care may be required if invasive monitoring is necessary.

This patient was stabilized in the recovery unit and because of difficulties with blood clotting was transferred to an area of high dependency, returning to the ward after 2 days.

ADULT ADVANCED LIFE SUPPORT

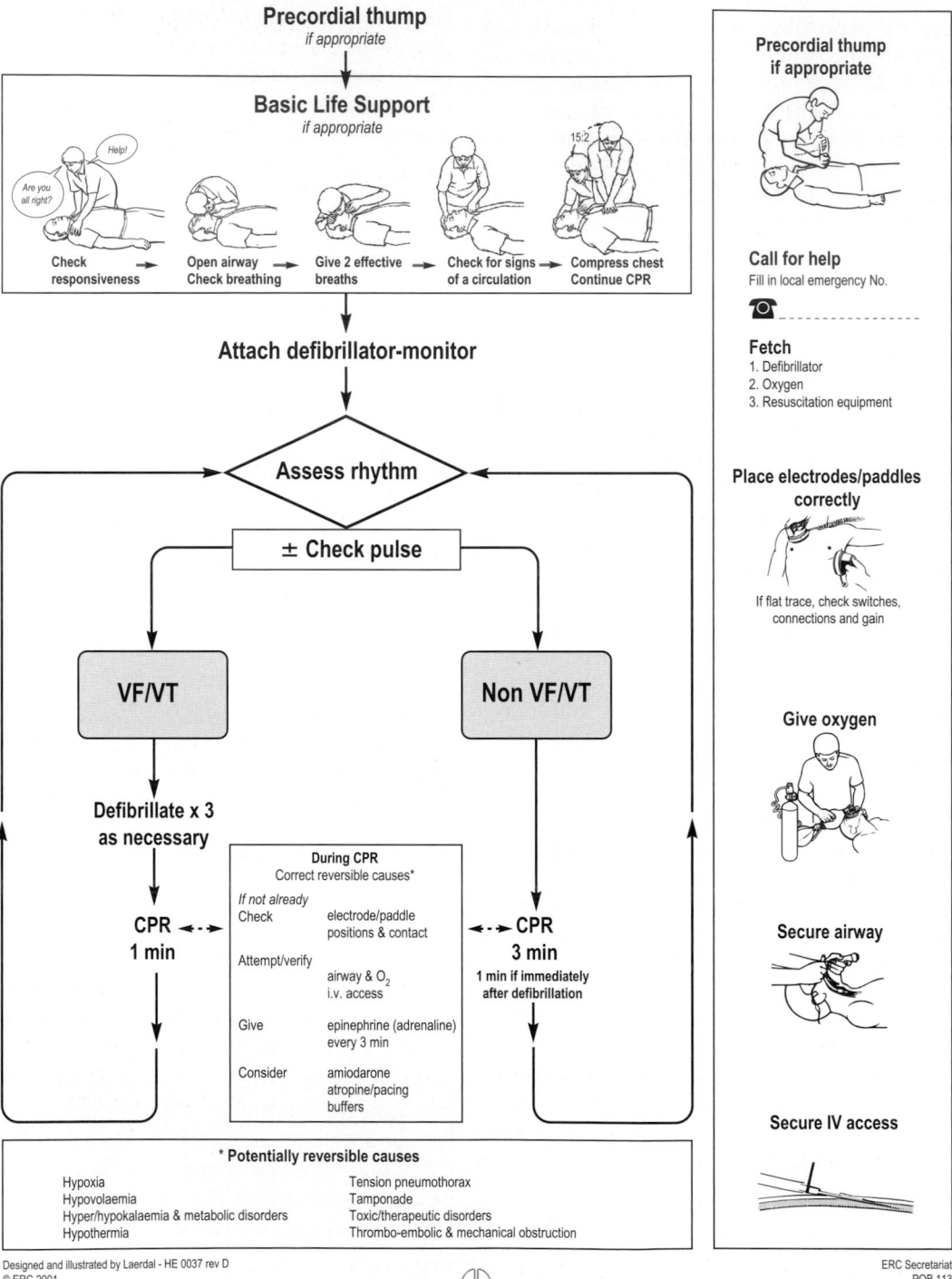

Precordial thump
if appropriate

Basic Life Support
if appropriate

Check responsiveness → Open airway Check breathing → Give 2 effective breaths → Check for signs of a circulation → Compress chest Continue CPR

Attach defibrillator-monitor

Assess rhythm

± **Check pulse**

VF/VT

Non VF/VT

Defibrillate x 3 as necessary

CPR 1 min

During CPR
Correct reversible causes*

If not already
Check — electrode/paddle positions & contact

Attempt/verify — airway & O₂ i.v. access

Give — epinephrine (adrenaline) every 3 min

Consider — amiodarone atropine/pacing buffers

CPR 3 min
1 min if immediately after defibrillation

* Potentially reversible causes

Hypoxia
Hypovolaemia
Hyper/hypokalaemia & metabolic disorders
Hypothermia

Tension pneumothorax
Tamponade
Toxic/therapeutic disorders
Thrombo-embolic & mechanical obstruction

Designed and illustrated by Laerdal - HE 0037 rev D
© ERC 2001

European Resuscitation Council

ERC Secretariat
POB 113
2610 Wilrijk (Antwerp)
Belgium
tel.: +32 (0)3 8213616
fax.: +32 (0)3 8284882
website: www.erc.edu

Precordial thump if appropriate

Call for help
Fill in local emergency No.
☎ _____

Fetch
1. Defibrillator
2. Oxygen
3. Resuscitation equipment

Place electrodes/paddles correctly

If flat trace, check switches, connections and gain

Give oxygen

Secure airway

Secure IV access

Figure 13.4   Recognized protocol for resuscitating patients. (Reproduced with permission of European Resuscitation Council)

Negative outcome

With no intervention the reflex sympathetic drive switches off, causing the blood pressure and cardiac output to drop. The supply of oxygen to the tissues starts to fail, ischaemic intestine and pancreas release cytokines and leukotrines into the circulation, depressing the heart and damaging the capillaries. The results are a progressive circulatory collapse with profound tissue hypoxia, leading to ischaemia and then death.

Urinary catheter

Urethral catheters are inserted after surgery to observe fluid output. The minimum amount of urine produced per hour to ensure adequate kidney perfusion/function is 30 ml;[9] less than this should be reported to the surgeon.

Patients who are not catheterized should be observed postoperatively for urinary retention, as anaesthesia/surgery can reduce bladder tone. Patients who are suspected of having urinary retention will complain of pain and restlessness, and may also have a bradycardia and be hypotensive. The recovery practitioner will assess for a distended bladder (a bladder scanner can be used), and if the patient cannot void urine they may require to be catheterized on instruction from the surgeon.

NEUROLOGICAL ASSESSMENT

Most patients do not require a formal neurological assessment either prior to or after surgery, but are assessed for understanding of their situation, sedation, and obeying commands after regaining consciousness. Changes to neurological status postoperatively are greatly dependent on the age and preoperative condition of the patient and the duration and outcome of anaesthesia and surgery. When neurological assessment is required postoperatively the Glasgow Coma Scale is the most commonly used clinical assessment of consciousness. It was devised as a formal scheme to overcome the ambiguities that arose when assessing unconscious patients.[11]

SKIN AND WOUND MANAGEMENT

The wound site should be checked regularly for bleeding. If there is minimal bleeding or seepage through the dressing, a pressure dressing can be applied on top of the original one. The original dressing is left intact to minimize potential infection.

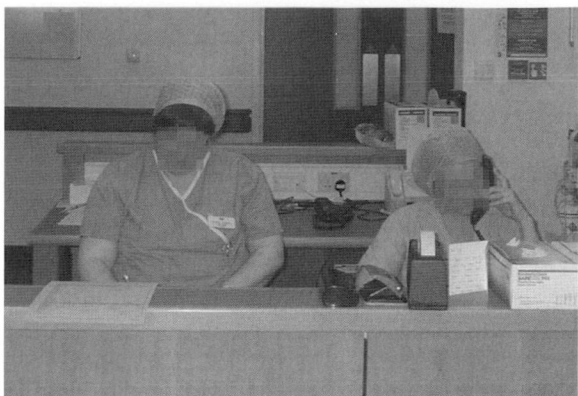

Figure 13.5   Recovery practitioners require a range of skills from essential record keeping to life saving skills such as airway management.

Any wound drains/stomas should be labelled and the nature and amount of contents charted regularly. The surgeon must be informed of any concerns, e.g. swelling of the wound site, which could indicate haematoma or sudden losses through drains.

PRESSURE AREA CARE

An assessment of pressure areas should be made using a recognized assessment tool, combined with the practitioner's clinical judgement. Waterlow[12] continues to be a universal assessment tool in pressure area care. Patients' scores increase (become worse) with the duration of surgery and then stabilize in the recovery room. Patients must be placed on an appropriate pressure-relieving mattress both during surgery and postoperatively to minimize the risk of developing pressure sores.

TEMPERATURE

Patients entering the recovery area after major surgery should have their temperature checked routinely. The optimum temperature for metabolic processes to occur is 36–37°C. Values lower than this will reduce the rate of chemical reaction, as physiological systems function most effectively if body temperature is held constant or close to the optimum.

HYPOTHERMIA

If the patient's temperature is below 36°C they are termed hypothermic. Hypothermia has been shown to increase the risk of surgical complications such as coagulopathy, morbid cardiac events and a decreased resistance to wound infections.[13] These risks are greater in frail, elderly patients undergoing extensive operations.

General anaesthesia totally abolishes the behavioural responses that are important in normal thermoregulation, for example shivering and vasoconstriction. This is due to the combined effect of the drugs administered during anaesthesia, resulting in anaesthetized patients becoming poikilothermic, with body temperatures being determined by the environment. Redistribution hypothermia (where body temperature balances with that of the immediate environment) is the major cause of hypothermia during the first hour of neuraxial or general anaesthesia.[14]

To achieve normothermia patients can be warmed gradually using a forced air warming device, which is currently the most effective non-invasive option.[14] Hypothermic patients may also receive supplemental oxygen postoperatively to assist with increases in oxygen demands caused by shivering as they try to increase their temperature.

PAIN AND NAUSEA ASSESSMENT

Pain is an individual, subjective experience with the only reliable assessment being the patient's own perception of it. However, objective assessment of pain, in order to define the level of analgesia required, is a routine part of postoperative care and is evaluated in combination with temperature, pulse, blood pressure, sedation and nausea scores.

Common pain scoring tools include the visual analogue scale, the verbal descriptor scale and the verbal numerical rating scale.[18] Verbal descriptor scales require patients to score their pain as 'none, mild, moderate or severe'. Patients are asked to score their pain out of 10 when using a verbal numerical scale, or to place a mark on a line of increasing pain intensity when using visual analogue scales. The use of these tools is limited in the immediate postoperative phase but they are invaluable when the patient is conscious and orientated to their surroundings, allowing pain scoring to become more accurate.

Similar scales are used for the assessment of nausea and sedation. All three scores are considered when administering analgesics to patients.

POSTOPERATIVE NAUSEA AND VOMITING (PONV)

Postoperative nausea and vomiting are still common causes for increasing the patient's stay in the recovery room. The risk factors include a previous history of PONV, travel sickness or migraine; gender, with women being more susceptible; type of operative procedure (abdominal operations are considered more emetogenic); anaesthetic agent used; and amount of opiates given.[15]

Anaesthetics cause nausea and vomiting because anaesthetic agents and narcotics affect the vestibular apparatus, thus affecting balance. Morphine, lack of oxygen, dehydration and electrolyte imbalance also stimulate the vomiting centre in the medulla. Most anaesthetists give prophylactic antiemetics during surgery, because as well as nausea and vomiting being unpleasant for the patient they reduce the risk of aspiration in the immediate postoperative period.

Patients suffering from PONV also require good basic care and careful handling. Basic care, such as offering mouthwashes, opening windows, privacy and washing the patient's face, is not research based but will show the patient empathy and caring.[15]

Prevention

- Identify those at highest risk
- Use prophylactic antiemetics
- Keep anaesthetic time to a minimum
- Avoid hypoxia and dehydration
- Keep postoperative movement to a minimum
- Be cautious with postoperative oral fluids
- Avoid unpleasant smells, sights and sounds
- Use other analgesics to reduce the amount of opiates administered postoperatively.

Acupressure is also advocated for the control of postoperative nausea, with the pressure point being in the midline on the anterior aspect of the forearm 2–3 inches from the proximal skin crease of the wrist. Acupressure is non-invasive but is only helpful in relieving nausea: it is not indicated if the patient is actively vomiting.

PAIN MANAGEMENT

Effective pain management is essential on humanitarian grounds as well as improving morbidity associated with the patient's illness or surgery. The Royal College of Surgeons of England and the College of Anaesthetists, in a combined report,[16] concluded that pain was still a common and significant problem in hospitals.

Pain, the stress response to injury and the inflammatory process induced by a surgical wound are inextricably linked and amplify each other. Poor postoperative pain control contributes to patient morbidity and mortality, with effective pain relief reducing morbidity by enabling early mobilization and discharge from hospital.[17] Severe pain reduces movement, which increases the risk of deep venous thrombosis, pulmonary embolism, damage to areas susceptible to pressure, constipation and muscle wasting. Respiratory complications can arise if pain prevents deep breathing and coughing. Pain increases the activity of the sympathetic nervous system and produces tachycardia and hypertension, which increase the myocardial oxygen demand and the risk of myocardial ischaemia. Acute pain also prevents beneficial sleep and rest, causing patients to become fatigued, demoralized, and reducing their confidence in the staff providing the postoperative care.[10]

Good pain management relies on basic principles of individualized regimens with multimodal analgesia, as this limits the dose of any one therapy and hence the side effects; regular analgesia; regular assessment of pain; and regular prescription review.[18]

PARACETAMOL AND NON-STEROIDAL ANTI-INFLAMMATORY DRUGS

Non-steroidal anti-inflammatory drugs (NSAIDs) and paracetamol should be used as components of a multimodal approach to postoperative analgesia. Paracetamol has antipyretic activity and NSAIDs have anti-inflammatory activity, which makes for an effective analgesic combination. Both drugs, however, have contraindications that make them unsuitable for certain groups of patients.[18]

OPIOID ANALGESICS (Box 13.1)

Opioid analgesics are used to relieve moderate to severe postoperative pain. The key principles with this group of drugs is titration of dose against desired effect, pain relief, and minimizing unwanted effects.[17] The side effects include respiratory depression, increased sedation leading to airway obstruction and hypoxaemia during sleep, nausea, vomiting, constipation, pruritus, hallucinations and urinary retention.

There is no compelling evidence that one opioid is better than another, but there is evidence that pethidine has distinct disadvantages when given in

---

> **Box 13.1   Commonly used opiates**
>
> Morphine sulphate can be administered intravenously, intramuscularly, subcutaneously or sublingually. Morphine is a stable drug if titrated to effect, having minimal effect on blood pressure, heart rate and rhythm when hypoxia is avoided.
>
> Diamorphine is metabolized to morphine in vivo, but it approximately doubles the strength of morphine, e.g. 5 mg of diamorphine is equal to 10 mg of morphine.
>
> Fentanyl is a synthetic opioid which is 50–100 times more potent than morphine, and has a rapid onset with peak effect in 5–10 minutes, with analgesia lasting 20–40 minutes if administered intravenously. It is metabolized in the liver to inactive metabolites.
>
> Alfentanil is another analogue of fentanyl that is about one-tenth as potent and has one-third the duration of action of fentanyl.
>
> Tramadol is a centrally acting analgesic agent which produces analgesia by an opioid effect, and by also enhancing the serotoninergic and adrenergic pathways. It is less potent than morphine and appears to have fewer opioid side effects.

---

multiple doses owing to the accumulation of its metabolite norpethidine. This metabolite acts as a central nervous system irritant, ultimately causing convulsions, especially in patients with renal dysfunction.[19]

Morphine and similar opioids have the active metabolite morphine-6-glucuronimide. In renal dysfunction this metabolite can accumulate and result in greater effect from a given dose, because it is more active than morphine. This is not a problem with titration but can be a complication with an unconscious patient.

PATIENT-CONTROLLED ANALGESIA

This is an established method of providing postoperative analgesia where the patient titrates the drug dose intravenously within set parameters, thereby avoiding numerous intramuscular injections. Patient-controlled analgesia (PCA) also overcomes delays with opiate administration due to controlled drug regulations and staffing shortages. The anaesthetist will prescribe the drug and concentration, the bolus dose, the time between boluses, and administer a loading dose prior to use. This may include, as an example, morphine sulphate 100 mg diluted in 50 ml of normal saline (2 mg/ml) with a 2 mg bolus and a 5-minute lockout period. Antiemetics can also be added to the infusion, but there are many different opinions as to whether this practice is beneficial to the patient. Infusion devices used will vary between hospitals. The risks with this regimen are those of opioid administration combined with potential errors in preparing the infusion and programming the infusion device. The infusion device must always be positioned at or below the level of the patient's heart, with an antisiphon valve used to prevent rapid discharge of infusion contents due to gravitational effects. If intravenous fluids are being administered through the same cannula there must be a non-return valve on the intravenous limb to allow the opioid boluses to be administered. Most patients will be prescribed supplemental oxygen while using a PCA to minimize the risks of hypoxia.[18]

If the patient's respiration becomes severely depressed then opioid administration should be stopped and the administration of naloxone, a pure antagonist, considered. Naloxone reverses the depressant and analgesic effects of narcotics. Naloxone should be titrated until the patient's respiratory pattern improves and sedation levels decrease, then the analgesic regimen should be reviewed and the patient observed closely for further signs of respiratory depression.[18]

EPIDURAL ANALGESIA

Epidural analgesia is an effective technique for the control of postoperative pain, with proven evidence that it improves the patient's outcome after major surgery by reducing the incidence of deep vein thrombosis, pulmonary and cardiac morbidity.[20] Local anaesthetics are administered to produce sensory, motor and sympathetic blockade, and opiates are administered for analgesic effect. Opioids and local anaesthetics have a synergistic effect, so that lower doses of each are required for equivalent analgesia with fewer adverse effects.[21] The risks associated with an epidural (dural puncture, infection, haematoma, nerve damage), those of the local anaesthetic (hypotension, motor block, toxicity) and those of the opioid (nausea, sedation, urinary retention, respiratory depression, pruritus) combine to require these patients to be observed postoperatively in

specialized areas in the ward or high-dependency area. There is also an added risk of the wrong dose being administered, so increased surveillance is required to prevent unwanted side effects.[22] Epidural infusions can also be patient controlled as required.

There are numerous regional blocks that can be performed depending on the site of the surgical incision. Other sites for continuous regional anaesthesia include the paravertebral space, the intrapleural space, the brachial plexus, or the site of a major nerve. The potential complications of these methods are the same as for epidural infusions.

DISCHARGE TO WARD

Either an anaesthetist or a recovery practitioner assesses the patient for discharge, following clear discharge criteria. There are many scoring systems in use, but a common one is the Aldrete system.[23] This is a score of activity, respiratory function, cardiovascular activity, consciousness and oxygenation. The importance of the score is related to the environment that the patient is being discharged into. For example, a high score is required for discharge to the ward area, whereas a lower score is acceptable for discharge to a high-dependency unit.

The American Society of Anaesthetists[8] recommends that each patient care facility should develop individual discharge criteria, and recommends several general principles that should be incorporated:

- Patients should be monitored until discharged
- Patients should be alert and orientated, with any altered mental status returned to their baseline
- Vital signs should be stable and within acceptable limits.

When the patient is discharged from the recovery room there must be a detailed handover of care from the recovery practitioner to the ward nurse, as follows:

- Patient is identified
- Procedure performed and surgeon's instructions relayed
- Intraoperative details described – blood loss, wound closure, dressing, drains in situ, urinary catheter
- Anaesthetist identified and anaesthetic described – including intraoperative analgesia, antiemetics, antibiotics, anticoagulants, intravenous fluids, invasive monitoring

(for intensive care or high-dependency unit) and anaesthetist's instructions

- Details of the patient's condition during their time in recovery, including blood pressure, pulse, respirations, pain score, nausea score, sedation score, temperature
- Both practitioners check wound dressing, drains, urinary catheter, intravenous infusions in progress and infusions running
- Both practitioners will check that analgesia, intravenous fluids, anticoagulants and any other medications have been prescribed.

The patient can only be transferred to the ward when the recovery practitioner and ward nurse are satisfied that their condition is stable and suitable for the level of supervision offered in the ward area. Oxygen may be required during transport. If the patient is being transferred to intensive care or a high-dependency unit the anaesthetist may accompany them.

ALTERNATIVE THERAPIES

There is a current trend to provide alternative therapies to patients in the hospital setting which will complement their medical management. Relaxation therapy, reflexology, aromatherapy, massage and music are all complementary therapies that could be useful to deal with the stress of surgery. Substantial anecdotal evidence is available to support the benefits of these therapies to postoperative patients, but there is a lack of research-based evidence.

Music therapy has been researched to the greatest degree, and numerous studies show that music can distract and relax patients postoperatively, functioning as a satisfier, but none of the studies offered a credible relationship between music therapy and a reduction in pain or analgesic requirements.[24–27] The studies reviewed did, however, provide research evidence to suggest that music therapy can be used to relax patients during the perioperative period and function as a satisfier. This evidence is of sufficient strength and potential patient benefit to be applied to alter clinical practice. Music therapy seems ideal for use in the recovery room to relax patients and improve the environment by acting as a distraction from any excess environmental noises.[28]

This chapter only briefly outlines the basics of recovery practice, but hopefully will act as a good foundation for new practitioners. Recovery practice is rewarding as it allows practitioners to work autonomously and use their acquired knowledge and skills to provide the best care during a time when the patient's condition is often rapidly changing. This stimulating and challenging area of perioperative practice provides a perfect environment to facilitate the development and introduction of evidence-based approaches to patient care.

References

1. Association of Anaesthetists of Great Britain and Ireland. Immediate postanaesthetic care. London: Association of Anaesthetists of Great Britain and Ireland; 2002.
2. Association of Anaesthetists of Great Britain and Ireland. The anaesthetic team. London: Association of Anaesthetists of Great Britain and Ireland; 1998.
3. Reid J. Preoperative information giving: an essential element in perioperative practice. Br J Theatre Nurs 1998; 8: 23–29.
4. Association of Anaesthetists of Great Britain and Ireland. Recommendations for standards of monitoring during anaesthesia and recovery. London: Association of Anaesthetists of Great Britain and Ireland; 2000.
5. Ward C. Ward's anaesthetic equipment, 4th edn. London: WB Saunders; 1998.
6. Davoric G, Franklin C. Handbook of haemodynamic monitoring. Philadelphia: WB Saunders; 1999.
7. American Society of Anesthesiologists. Practice guidelines for postanesthetic care. Illinois: American Society of Anesthesiologists; 2001.
8. Aitkenhead AR, Smith G. Textbook of anaesthesia. Edinburgh: Churchill Livingstone; 1996.
9. Clancy J, McVicar A. Physiology and anatomy: a homeostatic approach. London: Edward Arnold; 1995.
10. Drain CB. The postanaesthesia unit. A critical care approach to postanaesthesia nursing, 3rd edn. Philadelphia: WB Saunders; 1994.
11. Sternbach GL. The Glasgow coma scale. J Emerg Med 2000; 19: 67–77.
12. Waterlow J. Calculating the risk. NT 1988; 83: 38–60.
13. Frank SM, Fleisher LA, Breslow MJ, et al. Perioperative maintenance or normothermia reduces the incidence of morbid cardiac events: a randomised clinical trial. JAMA 1997; 277: 1127–1134.
14. Sessler MD. Complications and treatment of mild hypothermia. Anaesthesiol 2001; 95: 531–543.
15. Arnold A. Postoperative nausea and vomiting in the perioperative setting. Br J Perioper Nurs 2002; 12: 24–30.
16. Royal College of Surgeons of England and the College of Anaesthetists. Commission of the provision of surgical services. London: Royal College of Surgeons of England and the College of Anaesthetists; 1990.

17. McQuay HJ, Moore RA. An evidence-based resource for pain relief. Oxford: OUP; 2000.
18. Lothian University Hospitals NHS Trust. Guidelines for the management of acute pain, 7th edn. Edinburgh: Lothian University Hospitals NHS Trust; 2002.
19. Szeto HH, Intrurrisi CE, Huode R, et al. Accumulation of norepidrine, an active metabolite of meperidine, in patients with renal failure or cancer. Ann Inter Med 1977; 86: 738–741.
20. Ballyntyne JC, Carr DB, deFerranti S, et al. The comparative effects of postoperative analgesic therapies on pulmonary outcome: cumulative meta-analyses of randomised controlled trials. Anaesth Anal 1998; 86: 598–612.
21. McQuay HJ. Epidural analgesics. In: Wall P, Melzack R, eds. Textbook of pain. London: Churchill Livingstone; 1994: 1025–1034.
22. Bates DW, Cullen DJ, Laird N, et al. Incidence of adverse drug events and potential adverse drug events. JAMA 1995; 274: 29–34.
23. Chung F. Discharge criteria – a new trend. Can J Anaesth 1995; 42: 1056–1058.
24. Taylor L, Kuttler K, Parks T, et al. The effect of music in the postanaesthesia care unit on pain levels in women who have had abdominal hysterectomies. J Perianesth Nurs 1998; 13: 88–94.
25. Zimmermann L, Nieveen L, Barnason S. The effects of music interventions on post-operative pain and sleep in coronary artery bypass patients. Nurs Pract 1996; 10: 153–170.
26. Heiser R, Chiles K, Fudge M, et al. The use of music during the immediate postoperative recovery period. Am Oper Room Nurse J 1997; 65: 777–785.
27. Stevens K. Patients perceptions of music during surgery. J Advan Nurs 1990; 15: 1045–1051.
28. Brandman M. The role of music in the development of the whole person. Online. Available: http://www.healey.com.au/~jazzem/art.html 15 Feb 2002.

Further reading

Bandolier. Evidence based health care. Oxford pain internet site. Available: http://www.jr2.ox.ac.uk/bandolier/

British Medical Association and The Royal Pharmaceutical Society of Great Britain. British National Formulary. London: British Medical Association; 2001.

Clancy J, McVicar AJ. Physiology and anatomy: a homeostatic approach. London: Edward Arnold; 1995.

Drain C. The post anaesthesia care unit: a critical care approach to post anaesthesia nursing, 3rd edn. Philadelphia: WB Saunders; 1994.

Hatfield A, Tronson M. The complete recovery room book. Oxford: OUP; 2001.

Litwack K. Post anaesthesia care nursing. St Louis: Mosby; 1995.

McQuay HJ, Moore RA. An evidence based resource for pain relief. Oxford: OUP; 2000.

Meeker MH, Rothrock JC. Alexander's care of the patient in surgery, 10th edn. St Louis: Mosby; 1995.

National Association of Theatre Nurses. Back to basics: perioperative practice principles. Harrogate: National Association of Theatre Nurses; 2001.

SECTION 3

Principles of care in different environments

Chapter 14

Day surgery

Roz McMillan

CHAPTER CONTENTS

Key points

- Background and current developments
- The day surgery process from preadmission to post discharge: adults and children
- Selection, assessment and preparation
- Admission, preparation and intraoperative care
- Recovery, discharge and home-readiness
- Organization, management and future developments

INTRODUCTION

This chapter emphasizes the key aspects relating to the needs and requirements of patients undergoing day surgery. The benefits of day surgery have been apparent for many years, with day surgery itself being one of the most rapidly growing trends in health care. The reasons for increased activity are not attributable solely to political and economic influences: surgical and anaesthetic developments have enabled an increase in day surgery activity in terms of volume and complexity. Procedures that were previously performed in day surgery are now being undertaken on an outpatient basis, such as hysteroscopy and cystoscopy. Social influences and organizational change have also made an enormous impact but, most importantly, it is widely documented that patients do prefer this service. Patients need to be carefully selected and prepared prior to admission, and a successful outcome is dependent on multiprofessional teamwork. Routine inpatient methods of nursing, anaesthetic and surgical management are not suitable for achieving a quality day surgery service. Regular evaluation of patient outcome, service delivery, and education and training programmes is a vital component of quality improvement. The NHS plan[1] indicated that 75% of elective operations are expected to be performed on a day case basis. More expert teams are now successfully performing procedures such as laparoscopic cholecystectomy, arthroscopic shoulder surgery, anterior cruciate ligament repair and partial thyroidectomy on a day case basis. Although day surgery rates have improved in the UK over the last decade, there is opportunity for further growth. The future development of day surgery depends on effective management, improved utilization of resources and consultant commitment.

HISTORY AND CURRENT DEVELOPMENTS

Definition: 'A surgical day case is a patient who is admitted for investigation or operation on a planned non-resident basis and who none the less requires facilities for recovery.' Royal College of Surgeons (1992).[2]

At the beginning of the last century, day surgery was embraced by Nicholl,[3] a Glasgow-based surgeon who first reported on 9000 paediatric day cases. In 1955, Farquharson had further developed day surgery in Edinburgh but, even though these pioneers were keen to reduce waiting times, the further progression of day surgery has varied greatly throughout the UK and Europe. In the US, economic factors and financial incentives with the various healthcare systems propelled the expansion of day surgery. In the UK, over the past 20 years, various reports have identified the economic benefits, challenges, solutions and recommendations for further development of day surgery.[4-9] There were clearly political and fiscal drivers for change, but the report *Measuring Quality: the Patients' View of Day Surgery*[9] clearly showed that 80% of patients were satisfied with the service. The benefits and challenges of day surgery are noted in Box 14.1.

The Royal College of Surgeons of England in 1992[2] revised the 1985 report *Guidelines for Day-Case Surgery*, stating that 50% of all elective surgery should be considered on a day case basis. At that time 15% was the national average. The influence of these reports, with the assistance and enthusiasm of the British Association of Day Surgery (BADS)

Box 14.1 Benefits and challenges of day surgery
Benefits
Quality service provided
Home same day
Guaranteed bed
Streamlined care
Fosters partnership in care
Low rate of postoperative morbidity
Effective utilization of resources
Minimize risk of hospital-acquired infection
Reduce waiting times and lists
Staff resources not required overnight
Recruitment and retention
Challenges
Carer commitment required
Consultant commitment
Patient may feel rushed
Pressure of boarding patients
Postcode variations
Skill mix reflecting developments
Management commitment

council members, a multidisciplinary group founded in 1989, enabled the further progression of day surgery. Surgical advances, such as minimally invasive techniques, progressive use of endoscopes, improved anaesthesia with the use of shorter-acting drugs, improved pain management, and the use of regional and local anaesthesia, have greatly increased the complexity and volume of day surgery activity.

The report *A Shortcut to Better Services*[4] indicated that day surgery activity varied enormously between Trusts, and specific operations within individual Trusts. Although it had explored the issues surrounding this disparity, the situation remained the same in 2001.[7] Of the 300 day surgery units (DSUs) audited, it was alarming to note that the actual percentage of 'true day surgery' varied from 0 to 80% for certain procedures, such as inguinal hernia repair.[7] Further progress has been restricted by poor organization, management and staff attitudes.[7,10] The publication *Day Surgery: Operational Guide*, published by the Department of Health in 2002, aims to assist managers and clinicians in progressing this service.

As the majority of hospitals in the UK are designed to provide an acute-led service, there is inevitable conflict and pressure on the limited resources. In

2002, the government investment of £40 bn in the NHS over a 5-year period was aimed at key results areas, of which day surgery was targeted to increase activity by 25% to 75% of all elective surgery. As a result of the Modernisation Agency Day Surgery Programme launched in 2002, clinical champions and Day Surgery Leads from Strategic Health Authorities are working together to facilitate the further development of day surgery.

DAY SURGERY PROCESS

SELECTION

The day surgery process is a structured programme which aims to reduce risk and postoperative morbidity, and provide quality care from preadmission to the postdischarge period. Patient selection and preparation are essential for a successful outcome. Patients are not only selected by type of operation: the assessment of physical health, social circumstances and willingness to participate are key requirements. The majority of day surgery patients are classified as ASA (American Society of Anesthesiologists) 1, ASA 2 or stable ASA 3 category. ASA classification is discussed in more detail in Chapter 11. Although the ASA status is used in many areas, this assessment tool requires to be used in conjunction with more detailed patient assessment. After recovering from anaesthesia, patients require to be escorted home by a responsible adult who provides support at least overnight. Appropriate postdischarge care and support is crucial.

PROCEDURES

In 2001, the Audit Commission,[7] in consultation with BADS, introduced a new basket of 25 procedures which superseded the original basket of 20 identified 10 years earlier. These day case procedures, reflecting technological developments, provide a more realistic indication of day surgery activity and facilitate the evaluation of performance in a more appropriate way. Cystoscopy was excluded from the original basket and six new operations added to the list (numbers 20–25) (Box 14.2).

BADS[11] indicated other suitable procedures, such as hydrocoele excision, pilonidal sinus excision and closure, tonsillectomy in children, and bilateral varicose veins, and proposed the withdrawal of carpal tunnel decompression, dilatation

---

Box 14.2   Modified list of 25 procedures suitable for day cases. (Audit Commission 2001)[7]

1. Orchidopexy
2. Circumcision
3. Inguinal hernia repair
4. Excision of breast lump
5. Anal fissure dilatation or excision
6. Termination of pregnancy
7. Laparoscopy
8. Varicose vein stripping or ligation
9. Operation for bat ears
10. Excision of Dupuytren's contracture
11. Carpal tunnel decompression
12. Excision of ganglion
13. Arthroscopy
14. Reduction of nasal fracture
15. Submucous resection
16. Extraction of cataract with/without implant
17. Correction of squint
18. Myringotomy
19. Dilatation and curettage/hysteroscopy
20. Removal of metalware
21. Bunion operation
22. Transurethral resection of bladder tumour
23. Tonsillectomy
24. Laparoscopic cholecystectomy
25. Haemorrhoidectomy

---

and curettage and myringotomy. In keeping with the supermarket analogy, it was proposed that 50% of the trolley of procedures could be performed on a day case basis, depending on the skills and expertise of the multiprofessional team.[11] More progressive DSUs are already undertaking the additional procedures identified in Box 14.3.

Selected general surgical emergencies can be successfully managed on a day case basis.[12] With improved pain management and increase in minimally invasive surgery (MIS), more complex surgery is being undertaken on an ambulatory basis.[13] Expert clinicians are successfully undertaking certain day surgery procedures, such as laparoscopic cholecystectomy, tonsillectomy, anterior cruciate ligament repair, shoulder surgery, and innovative techniques such as microdiscectomy and awake craniotomy.[14] Recovery times are longer for patients requiring more invasive procedures, therefore these operations need to be scheduled early on the list.

> **Box 14.3   Cahill's more advanced standard for day surgery activity[11]**
>
> 1. Laparoscopic cholecystectomy
> 2. Laparoscopic herniorrhaphy
> 3. Haemorrhoidectomy
> 4. Partial thyroidectomy
> 5. Submandibular gland excision with axillary clearance
> 6. Rhinoplasty
> 7. Superficial parotidectomy
> 8. Laser prostatectomy
> 9. Urethrotomy
> 10. Bladder neck incision
> 11. Transcervical resection of endometrium
> 12. Hallux valgus operations
> 13. Arthroscopic meniscectomy
> 14. Arthroscopic shoulder surgery
> 15. Subcutaneous mastectomy
> 16. Wide excision of breast cancer
> 17. Eyelid surgery, including tarsorrhoplasty and/or blepharoplasty
> 18. Tympanoplasty
> 19. Dentoalveolar surgery
> 20. Thoracoscopic sympathectomy

In the initial development of the service and/or the adoption of new procedures, locally agreed protocols for selection and assessment facilitate the implementation, evaluation and further progression of the service.

THE PATIENT'S JOURNEY

The patient's journey (Fig. 14.1), describes the progression of the patient from GP referral through to postdischarge period.

The question that needs to be asked is 'Why is this patient not being considered for day surgery?'

EXAMPLE OF SELECTION CRITERIA

1. Procedure not lasting more than 1 hour, or if so, assess invasiveness
2. Surgery and anaesthesia providing minimal or no risk of postoperative complications, such as homeostatic imbalance, thrombosis, haemorrhage, cardiac incident, respiratory complications

3. Patient generally fit and ambulant
4. Social circumstances:
   - Patient and carer willing and keen to participate in the complete day surgery process
   - Appropriate support postdischarge, including responsible adult at least overnight
   - Safe and comfortable environment: minimal stairs, easy access to toilet and telephone
   - Within reasonable travelling distance to/from home.

PATIENTS REQUIRING FURTHER SCREENING

1. History of anaesthetic complications
2. Cervical spine or mandible problems
3. Pre-existing conditions indicative of comorbidity, for example:
   - Myocardial infarction, transient ischaemic attack or cerebrovascular accident within previous 6 months
   - Symptomatic respiratory disease and cardiac disease
   - Hypertension
   - Poorly controlled diabetic
   - Obesity
   - Patients taking certain medications, such as digoxin, steroids, anticoagulants, monoamine oxidase inhibitor.

ASSESSMENT

The selection criteria are not rigid. Each patient is assessed on his/her ability to return to the same state of health as on admission. In other words, the patient is expected to be 'home-ready' and not street-fit on discharge home. Reasons for preassessment are noted in Box 14.4. Day surgery has a low morbidity rate of 0.15% and the patient selection, assessment and preparation cannot be underestimated in terms of avoiding or reducing risks and complications.[15] Patient and carer participation, cooperation and collaboration with the day surgery team are essential. A discussion of issues related to patient assessment is also in Chapter 10.

Surgeons are notorious for their optimism in patient selection. Experienced practitioners specifically trained to preassess are key players in providing a quality service. The practitioner works in partnership with the medical team by identifying actual and/or potential problems prior to admission.[16]

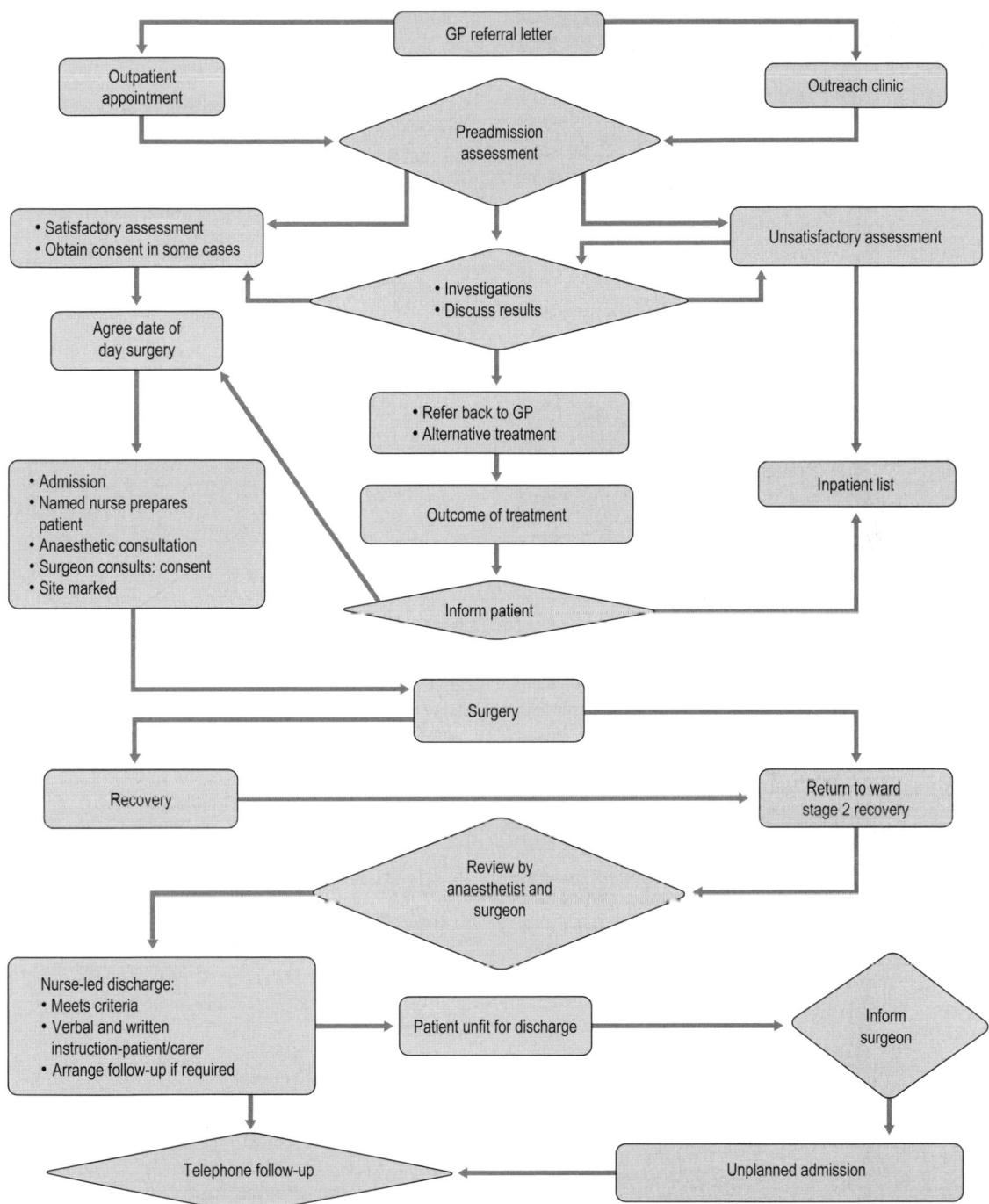

Figure 14.1 Day surgery process.

At this stage there is no need for the anaesthetist to see the patient, although it is vitally important to have anaesthetic support for advice and guidance when required.[17] The appropriately trained practitioner follows nationally and locally agreed policies and guidelines. In order to avoid conflict of expert opinions, it is prudent to seek advice and guidance from the appropriate anaesthetist, who ensures that the preanaesthetic assessment is satisfactory prior to admission.

Box 14.4   Reasons for preassessment

1. Identify actual or potential medical conditions and aim to minimize the risk
2. Arrange appropriate tests/investigations
3. Ability to plan perioperative care and discharge planning
4. Assess home circumstances
5. Encourage partnership in care and assess willingness to participate
6. Provide opportunity for patient to discuss concerns, anxieties
7. Provides opportunity for health promotion, such as smoking, alcohol, exercise, diet
8. Forewarn patient of possibility of overnight admission
9. Provide clear explanation of process, verbal and written, with the ability to offer date for surgery
10. Decreases cancellations
11. Improves efficiency of theatre utilization

Patients complete a questionnaire, and any concerns or issues regarding the medical condition and/or social circumstances are further explored by the trained preassessment nurse. Patients' baseline recordings, body mass index (BMI), past medical history and social and home circumstances are documented in the integrated care pathway or unitary records. Relevant comorbidities, such as diabetes, hypertension or respiratory conditions, are carefully assessed and any necessary investigations undertaken. Any variances in the assessment and/or results are discussed with the appropriate medical staff.

AGE

Age is not an impediment and the patient's biological rather than chronological age is far more relevant. Patients over 65 have a higher incidence of cardiovascular events and require appropriate intraoperative management, although age does not preclude day surgery.[18]

BODY MASS INDEX (BMI)

In England, nearly two-thirds of men and half of women are overweight or obese.[19,20] Considering the nationally increasing girth, attention to the relevance of obesity measurement is important. Obesity is defined as a BMI >30 and is linked to intraoperative and postoperative respiratory complications. Although the average limit in the UK is 32, depending on the type of procedure, patients may be selected with a BMI of 35[17] and for more peripheral operations BMI 37. Borderline patients with significant systemic disease or a history of sleep apnoea are not suitable.[17] BMI, which is measured as weight in kg divided by the height squared in metres, is at times not clearly indicative of a patient's suitability. Some patients who are muscle-bound, such as body builders, may have a high BMI but do not present with a relevant comorbidity. Distribution of fat is more relevant. Waist measurement is perhaps a clearer reflection of patient suitability in relation to perioperative complications[21,22] (Table 14.1). Procedures such as laparoscopy and hernia repair may prove difficult when there is increased abdominal fat. Therefore, 'pears' are better than 'apples'.[17]

PATIENTS WITH DIABETES

The anaesthetist assesses the appropriateness of administering a general anaesthetic and, if local anaesthesia is suitable, patients follow their normal regimen. Insulin-dependent diabetics need not be precluded unless they are poorly controlled.[17] Preadmission assessment by the anaesthetist or diabetologist is required, and clear instructions, both verbal and written, are vitally important. These patients are scheduled first on the list and guidelines are documented in the BADS handbook.[23,24] The additional stress of hospital admission and subsequent surgical trauma is also accounted for in the evaluation and management of these patients.

PATIENTS WITH ASTHMA

Well-controlled asthmatics who have good exercise tolerance need not be excluded from day surgery. If local anaesthesia is excluded, patients who have been recently hospitalized or require systemic steroids need more detailed preassessment, e.g. peak expiratory flow and spirometry, and referral to the appropriate anaesthetist. Non-steroidal anti-inflammatory drugs (NSAIDs) trigger bronchospasm in 5% of asthmatics, therefore aspirin and other NSAIDs should be avoided in these patients with known aspirin-sensitive asthma.

Table 14.1 BMI in relation to waist measurements

BMI	Waist measurement (cm)	
	Men	Women
>30	>102	>88
>35	>116	>98

Source: Lean[22]

Box 14.5 Outline of care for non–insulin dependent diabetics

Schedule first on list

1. Omit oral hypoglycaemics and breakfast
2. BM 6–10 mmol

Urinalysis – no ketones

3. As soon as able, oral hypoglycaemics and eat and drink

Insulin-dependent diabetics

1. Schedule first on list
2. Omit insulin and breakfast
3. BM 6–10 mmol
4. Minimize PONV
5. As soon as able, insulin and food or IV glucose if required until able to eat

---

PATIENTS WHO ARE HYPERTENSIVE

Hypertension needs to be controlled preoperatively because of the increased risk of complications and morbidity.[25] A blood pressure recording of ≤170/100 is acceptable, but ≥175/105 is a predictor of postoperative myocardial infarction[26] and such patients need to be referred to their GP for further assessment and/or treatment. Patients who are currently taking antihypertensives should not omit their medication on the day of surgery.

CURRENT MEDICATIONS

Patients taking certain drugs need to be carefully assessed in relation to anaesthetic, type of operation and past medical history, such as DVT or pulmonary embolism (PE). Examples are:

- Anticoagulant: require to be stopped and time period depends on procedure

- Monamine oxidase inhibitors (MAOI): if there is a need to continue with MAOI, then pethidine should be avoided
- Oestrogen: oral contraceptive – for lower limb surgery, stop 1 month preoperatively or give subcutaneous low molecular weight heparin[27]
- Hormone replacement therapy: review of use recommended by British National Formulary[28]
- Systemic steroids
- Digoxin.

INVESTIGATIONS

Selective preoperative tests need to be based on type of procedure, patient symptoms, interview, records, and physical examination for the purpose of improving perioperative management.[29] For example, urine testing undertaken in 30 000 patients identified only one with previously undiagnosed diabetes.[30] Routine tests are defined as 'tests ordered in the absence of a specific clinical indication or purpose'.[29] Some examples of reasons for investigation are given in Box 14.6.

SOCIAL CIRCUMSTANCES

Patients need to be escorted home by a responsible adult using private transport. The minimum recommended time for supervision is at least overnight, and for more invasive procedures this may be for the initial 24-hour period. Assessment of home circumstances is essential to identify the most appropriate discharge plan and postdischarge support. For a patient to return home to a household full of young children, or a frail elderly person who needs care, without suitable support, is unacceptable. If arrangements cannot be made, some units provide a hotel service. A hospital hotel may be available for patients who are technically discharged from the DSU but have no responsible carer at home. The demand for such facilities varies widely in the UK and its provision must reflect the needs and requirements of the local community. Patients should not require direct nursing care, and the hotel facility is staffed by a clinical support worker or healthcare assistant.

ANTIEMBOLISM PROPHYLAXIS

With the emphasis on early mobilization and discharge, patients may be inclined to become bedbound on their return home. Therefore, they must

Box 14.6   Some examples of reasons for investigations

ECG
1. Over 60 years
2. History of hypertension, chest pain
3. Heart murmur – check with anaesthetist regarding echo
4. Respiratory disease

U&E
1. Diuretic treatment
2. History of renal impairment

Full blood count
1. History of menorrhagia
2. Crohn's disease, ulcerative colitis, anaemia
3. Patients attending for termination or evacuation of uterus with history of anaemia

Sickle cell test
1. Afro-Caribbean parentage (check notes for previous test, trait acceptable)

Group and save
1. Termination and evacuation of uterus

Respiratory function test
1. Recent increased breathlessness

U&E/LFT
1. History of high alcohol consumption (>40 units per week) or jaundice (as adult)
2. Patients attending for cholecystectomy

Thyroid function tests
1. Thyroid surgery

Urinalysis[29]
1. If urinary tract symptoms present
2. Urological procedures

appropriate anaesthetist and/or surgeon. Unless the results of investigations are awaited, a mutually agreeable date for surgery is organized at the time of preassessment. Cooperation, coordination and collaboration with the multidisciplinary team is essential. At the preassessment clinic the physiotherapist assesses and educates patients who are scheduled for procedures such as anterior cruciate ligament repair and shoulder surgery. As day surgery teams provide care for patients with more complex needs, it is important to collaborate with appropriate clinicians. For example, patients attending for diagnostic interventions such as laparoscopic ultrasound or gastroscopy require sensitivity in relation to their information needs and those of their carers.[32] Therefore, the nurse specialists who coordinate these patients' care need to have strong communication links with the day surgery team.

WRITTEN INFORMATION

Written information must meet patients' needs in terms of confirming the information provided at the surgical consultation and preassessment. The information must be written in the appropriate language. Key points to be included are:

- Procedure-specific information
- Fasting guidelines
- Not to omit medications unless advised
- Women to inform unit if pregnant (unless this is the reason for admission)
- Date and time of admission
- Parking facilities and unit layout
- Admission process
- Wound and pain management
- Specific instructions regarding bathing, eating, drinking
- Follow-up if required
- Expected outcome; time off work and to resume normal activities
- Complications, risks, benefits (local agreement regarding amount of information)
- Emergency contact numbers and persons.

TIMING OF PREASSESSMENT

The importance of preassessment cannot be overemphasized. Certain DSUs are more progressive with regard to streamlining the patient's journey. As an example, the patient selection is initiated

be clearly informed about the risks involved and the importance of preventive methods such as mobilization, leg exercises and the use of TED (antithrombolytic) stockings. Any concerns regarding level of risk are discussed with the medical team and local unit guidelines/protocols for thromboprophylaxis consulted.[31]

TEAM APPROACH

Any actual or potential problems that might affect a successful outcome are discussed with the at GP consultation and followed up by telephone contact by the day surgery nurse prior to admission. At initial consultation, patients deemed suitable for day surgery can be offered nurse-led preadmission assessment. This service depends on waiting list times, patient preference, nursing resources and accommodation. Preassessment needs to be within an acceptable timeframe in order to optimize patients' physical state preoperatively and reduce anxieties. The acceptable period between preassessment and operation is indicated to be 2–4 weeks[33] or 3 months,[34] although there is no actual evidence. Test results obtained within a 6-month period are deemed acceptable unless there is a change in the patient's medical history or clinical need.[29] Further research is required to identify the optimum time for preassessment prior to the date for surgery with regard to patient preparation, information retention, and the acceptable interval between time of consent and surgery.

ADMISSION, PREPARATION AND INTRAOPERATIVE CARE

STAGGERED ADMISSIONS

Many DSUs have introduced a staggered admission programme which not only reduces waiting times for patients but reduces congestion within the DSU. The admission times need to be scheduled by addressing anaesthetic and surgical assessment time and minimizing any disruption during the morning or afternoon lists.

FASTING

The 12-hour fasting ritual for general and regional anaesthesia and sedation/analgesia has now been replaced with an evidence-based and more humane regimen,[35] as follows:

Six hours:

- Solids and milk
- No fried foods or meat
- Light meal tea/toast.

Two hours:

- Clear fluids
- Water, fruit juice without pulp
- Clear tea, black coffee
- Volume less important than type of fluid.

PREOPERATIVE CARE

The 'named nurse' concept ensures coordination of patient care from admission to discharge. A deputy/associate nurse is assigned to each patient to provide continuity of care in the absence of the named nurse. Good practice dictates that the anaesthetist visits the patient prior to transfer to theatre to undertake the final anaesthetic assessment and discuss it with the patient. The surgeon's visit provides an opportunity for further discussion and clarification, and patient consent is formalized, if not previously completed at the preadmission clinic. Where required, the wound site is clearly marked by the surgeon prior to theatre transfer. Preoperative preparation and the checklist are completed and, depending on the proximity and location of the theatre with respect to the ward, patients are encouraged to walk to theatre with their escort. Day surgery patients are well, and the majority prefer this approach[36] (see also Chs 10 and 11).

ANAESTHESIA

The development of anaesthetic drugs and the use of various agents and techniques have revolutionized day surgery.[37] Successful day case anaesthesia is based on minimizing dehydration and postoperative nausea and vomiting, and effective pain management. The concept of balanced anaesthesia is practised in day surgery with the use of NSAIDs, local anaesthesia, regional nerve blockade and short-acting opioids. Although there are fewer side effects with certain inhalational agents such as sevoflurane, the introduction of total intravenous anaesthesia (TIVA) using propofol for induction and maintenance has improved patient outcome by, for example, minimizing postoperative nausea and vomiting (PONV) and promoting early recovery. The use of local and regional anaesthesia is far greater in the USA, although many more anaesthetists in the UK are adopting this practice.

PREMEDICATION

Some examples of requirements for premedication in day surgery patients include:

- Anxious patients not responding to reassurance may require oral midazolam 7.5–15 mg or temazepam 10–20 mg, 30–60 minutes preoperatively.

- Patients at risk of gastric reflux are given ranitidine 150 mg 1 hour preoperatively, or for high-risk patients 150–300 mg the night before or on arrival.[38]
- Pre-emptive analgesia, such as NSAIDs, ibuprofen 600–800 mg or diclofenac 100 mg 1 hour preoperatively avoids the need for rescue opioids in recovery.[39] Rectal NSAIDs administered pre- or immediately postoperatively require patient permission. NSAIDs are avoided in operations associated with increased bleeding.
- Patients with needle phobia may be less stressed by having EMLA cream applied to the venepuncture site 1 hour preoperatively.
- Bronchodilators or nebulized salbutamol 1 hour preoperatively may be advised for asthmatics.

REGIONAL ANAESTHESIA

Regional anaesthesia decreases or avoids the side effects of general anaesthesia and effects good analgesia perioperatively. The choice of nerve block depends on not only the type of procedure, but also the anaesthetist's expertise and skill. Common nerve blocks used in day surgery are:

- Spinal/epidural
- Caudal
- Brachial plexus
- Interscalene
- Ilioinguinal
- Ankle
- Femoral nerve.

Adverse reactions and complications are documented in Chapter 11.

SEDATION WITH LOCAL AND REGIONAL ANAESTHESIA

Careful titration of sedation is important to avoid complications such as reduced airway control, respiratory depression and prolonged recovery. Target-controlled infusion (TCI) with propofol minimizes the risks compared to manual infusion devices. Baseline monitoring is required with IV access. With patients' understanding, cooperation and clear expectations, regional anaesthesia could be more widely adopted in day surgery.[40]

PAIN MANAGEMENT

Multimodal analgesia is clearly beneficial and minimizes side effects and risk. The visual analogue scale (VAS) is commonly used and, regardless of type of procedure or anaesthetic, the need for nurses to be sensitive to patients' pain perception and anxieties cannot be overemphasized. Paracetamol is useful for mild to moderate pain, and together with the action of NSAIDs is an effective combination. Fentanyl and alfentanil are commonly used intraoperatively. Opioids are not the drug of choice in the postoperative period because of dizziness and the side effects of PONV. An effective strategy depends on evaluation of each patient, the type of procedure, expectations, mental state and risk assessment.

LOCAL ANAESTHESIA

Local anaesthetics are more widely used for wound infiltration but have limited application to intermediate operations owing to the toxicity of large-volume doses, and it can be technically difficult to block relevant structures. Local anaesthetic regimens are used for many common day cases, in particular caudal, epidural or regional nerve blocks. Local anaesthetic techniques such as 0.5% bupivacaine injected in the mesosalpinx,[41] or 2% lidocaine (lignocaine) gel on the clip site following laparoscopic sterilization,[42] and the addition of morphine (1–2 mg) to bupivacaine for intra-articular infiltration, have proved effective.[43]

RECOVERY AND DISCHARGE

RECOVERY

The day surgery patient's recovery time is generally fairly rapid. This is due to a combination of anaesthetic techniques, the use of regional and/or local anaesthesia, pain management, and operations which tend to take an hour or less. The majority of patients are within ASA categories 1 or 2. Regardless of the type of procedure, the patient's vital signs need to be monitored in line with locally agreed policy. Some DSUs implement a fast-track recovery system which promotes selected patients to bypass first-stage recovery into the second stage or main ward.[44] Depending on the type of surgery, patients are encouraged to drink, eat and mobilize as soon as they are able. Even though well-designed day surgery trolleys are comfortable, patients are more inclined to mobilize more quickly. Patients can recover on reclining or high-backed

Box 14.7   Example of pain management for day surgery patients. Preassessment explanation of the process to the patient, including the patient's role in managing pain in the postdischarge period

Stage	Assess and evaluate	Assess appropriateness of
Preoperative	Type of procedure/duration Mental state Risk assessment Medical history and condition Surgeon's expertise Timing of theatre slot	Type of anaesthetic Premedication required Pre-emptive analgesia/antiemesis
Intraoperatively		IV opioids, e.g. fentanyl Regional, LA, sedation NSAIDs, antiemesis
Stage 1 recovery	Pain assessment	NSAIDs Rescue opioids, e.g. fentanyl
Stage 2 recovery	Pain assessment	NSAIDs Paracetamol Codeine-based drugs
Discharge packs	Verbal and written instructions	Take-home analgesia NSAIDs, paracetamol, co-codamol
Postdischarge follow-up	Telephone assessment	Reassure, reinforce instructions, pain score, advice

chairs. Beds are used for selected patients, such as post laparoscopic cholecystectomy, partial thyroidectomy or ACL repair, who require a longer recovery period. There is no mandatory minimum stay for these patients before discharge home[45] (see also Ch. 13)

DISCHARGE SCORING SYSTEMS (DSS)

A discharge scoring tool, the modified Aldrete Scoring System,[46] is used extensively in Canada and the USA. Although the Post-Anaesthesia Discharge Scoring System (PADSS) (Box 14.8)[47] aims to standardize patient discharge after day surgery, as with any tool it requires to be used in conjunction with the judgement of nurses and clinicians, and taking into account the patients' and carers' willingness and confidence in returning home.

The maximum score is 10, and patients scoring 9 or above are fit for discharge. Good communication between the patient/carers and the multidisciplinary team is essential for a safe and successful discharge.[48] The DSS provides an assessment tool for staff who are developing the day surgery service but it must be used with caution as it can be time consuming and may detract from nursing expertise.

DISCHARGE CRITERIA

Box 14.9 lists discharge criteria which are tailored to the patient's care pathway. Judgement regarding the appropriateness of these criteria may vary in relation to the particular patient's care pathway and the decision of the clinician. Variances must be recorded.

Some of the discharge criteria in Box 14.9 are in contrast to the American Society of Anesthesiologists' guidelines.[45] For example, drinking clear fluid used to be a prerequisite for discharge home, but is now only applicable in specific situations such as when patients are diabetic or nauseated.

Patients and carers are informed of postdischarge issues at preassessment.[49] It is important to ensure that appropriate information regarding pain management, wound care, ability to resume 'normal' activities, awareness of potential complications and contact numbers for advice and help are clearly communicated, both verbally and in writing. With the patient's permission, carers are encouraged to participate in the predischarge counselling. Appropriate follow-up arrangements are organized prior to discharge. With respect to certain gynaecological procedures, such as termination of pregnancy, the dilemma of ensuring patient safety on return home and respecting and safeguarding

Box 14.8   Post-anaesthesia Discharge Scoring System (PADSS)[47]

Category		Score
Vital signs	Vital signs must be stable and consistent with age and preoperative baseline	
	Able to move 4 extremities voluntarily or on command	2
	Able to move 2 extremities voluntarily or on command	1
	Unable to move extremities voluntarily or on command	0
Activity level	Patient must be able to ambulate at preoperative level	
	Steady gait, no dizziness (or meets preoperative level)	2
	Requires assistance	1
	Unable to ambulate	0
Nausea and vomiting	Patient should have minimal nausea and vomiting prior to discharge	
	Minimal: successfully treated with oral medication	2
	Moderate: successfully treated with intramuscular medication	1
	Severe: continues after repeated treatment	0
Pain	Patient should have minimal or no pain prior to discharge. Level of pain that the patient has should be acceptable to the patient. Pain should be controllable by oral analgesics. Location, type and intensity of pain should be consistent with the anticipated postoperative discomfort	
	Acceptability: Yes	2
	No	0
Surgical	Postoperative bleeding should be consistent with expected blood loss for the procedure	
	Minimal: does not require dressing change	2
	Moderate: up to two dressing changes required	1
	Severe: more than three dressing changes required	0

Box 14.9   Discharge criteria

- Stable vital signs for at least 1 hour
- Well orientated (or same level of orientation as on admission)
- Pain controlled
- No excessive bleeding/oozing from wound site
- Able to tolerate at least fluids
- Ability to pass urine, depending on type of procedure, e.g. inguinal hernia repair, postcaudal blocks
- Able to mobilize as expected in relation to type of surgery
- Responsible adult escorting patient home in private transport. Carer available at least

overnight and, where appropriate, over 24-hour period
- Home facilities adequate, i.e. telephone, easy access to toilet
- No sign of adverse reactions, complications
- Patient and carer have a clear understanding of postdischarge instructions and expectations
- Take-home analgesia pack supplied with full verbal and written instructions and information
- Emergency contact numbers supplied
- Follow-up arrangement if required

their wish for privacy, continually fires the moral and ethical debate. Patients who have had a general anaesthetic are advised not to drive, operate machinery, cook, sign documents or make important decisions for 24 hours. Advice regarding driving depends on the type of surgery undergone, and patients may be advised to contact their insurance company. Patients should have written information, e.g. a copy of the discharge letter stating operation, anaesthetic, take-home medication and any complications. This may be faxed to the GP, or the patient can retain a copy in case they need to contact their GP within the initial 24–48 hours.

TAKE-HOME ANALGESIA

Patients need verbal and written instructions and a clear understanding of side effects and management strategies if problems arise.

COMPLICATIONS

Studies have shown that there is a low incidence of major morbidity following day surgery.[18,50–52] Minor morbidity is more prevalent, such as pain, PONV, dizziness, minor bleeding, sore throat, headache and minor anaesthetic complications. Minor complications are not life-threatening but are not perceived as minor by the patient.

POSTOPERATIVE NAUSEA AND VOMITING (PONV)

PONV is the most commonly occurring postanaesthesia complication and causes distress, delayed discharge and unplanned overnight admission. PONV is multifactorial, and patients who are predisposed to travel sickness or previous problems incurred at surgery, need to be identified at preassessment. Factors that increase the incidence of PONV are procedures such as laparoscopy, otolaryngology, and the use of opioids and ketamine.[53] Combined treatment with ondansetron, droperidol or steroids is more effective than ondansetron alone.[43] PONV is minimized by ensuring the patient is adequately hydrated, and it is therefore important to avoid aggressive and inappropriate fasting regimens. IV fluids should be administered during longer procedures.

UNPLANNED OVERNIGHT ADMISSION

Unplanned overnight admission is attributed to postoperative anaesthetic and/or surgical complications and not solely to patient fitness. Some of these complications can be minimized by assessing risks related to the nature and extent of the operation and the type of anaesthetic.[54] The type and duration of certain procedures, such as laparoscopy or orthopaedic procedures, increase the risk of developing persistent symptoms. Twenty-five percent of 300 DSUs identified unanticipated admission rates of $\geqslant 3\%$.[7] At preassessment, patients are clearly informed of the possibility of an overnight stay. Unplanned overnight admission[17] can be a result of:

- Poor pain management
- Late return from theatre and inadequate recovery time
- PONV
- Bleeding
- Surgery more extensive than anticipated.

Therefore, it is important to recognize that day surgery patients need suitable methods and techniques to reduce or avoid postoperative complications. Good pain management, pre-emptive antiemesis where indicated, TIVA using propofol, and the commitment and skills of consultant surgeons ensure patients receive the optimum care.

POST DISCHARGE SUPPORT

Patient care does not terminate on discharge from the DSU. It is vitally important to ensure that both patients and carers are well informed of postdischarge support systems. Some patients may return for hospital-based follow-up. Although studies[55,56] indicate that there is minimal impact on the primary care team in this phase, the day surgery team must provide a suitable support system. Selected patients can be offered postdischarge telephone follow-up within the initial 24-hour period. This service reinforces instructions, provides reassurance, identifies actual or potential problems and reduces the impact on GPs.[57] It must be emphasized that the telephone service is offered to patients, and that their wishes must be respected if it is perceived as an intrusion on their privacy. With the increased expansion and development of day surgery in terms of complexity and activity, it is important that the day surgery team tailors the most appropriate system for their patients,[58] including factors such as those outlined in Box 14.10.

As the primary care team have the initial and, for some patients, the planned follow-up, it is important to develop a structured and integrated approach to communication between the DSU and GP centres.

CHILDREN'S DAY CARE

Children's needs and requirements are different from those of adults. The day surgery process already discussed is no different for children, but this section highlights key issues peculiar to this select group. The provision of paediatric day surgery service in settings other than a dedicated children's facility requires expert management to ensure optimum care. As advocated by the government report *Welfare of Children and Young People in Hospital*,[59] the distress caused by children's admission to hospital should be minimized by developing alternative approaches to care, such as day care, home care and outpatient treatment whenever possible. If a child is accommodated in the same adult day surgery area, their care must not be compromised and must meet the required standards as set out in *Just for the Day* (Box 14.11).[60] If this is not possible, 'childrens' days', such as one day a week, may suit their needs. Chapter 18 contains further discussion on the perioperative care of children.

PREOPERATIVE SELECTION AND ASSESSMENT

Selection and preparation include physical fitness, age and weight, psychosocial and psychological considerations and family circumstances.[61] Exclusions are premature babies under 60 weeks (respiratory risk), those over 60 weeks with a history of respiratory problems (bronchopulmonary dysplasia), and children under 5 kg (risk of hypothermia and hypoglycaemia).

Preoperative assessment is undertaken at the first consultation and/or the preadmission clinic. One to two weeks before the procedure the parent and child are invited to a preadmission club or

---

Box 14.10   Postdischarge follow-up

- Telephone follow-up 24–48 hours (structured questionnaire for audit)
- Day surgery community nurse
- Community liaison nurse
- District nurse
- Walk-in centre
- Mobile telephone contact overnight

Box 14.11   Quality standards recommended in *Just for the Day*[60]

Whenever and wherever a child (0–16 years) is admitted as a day case we suggest that the concept of a planned package of care is adopted. We recommend that such a package should contain the following standards, which might be used as quality standards in NHS contracts:

1. The admission is planned in an integrated way to include preadmission, day of admission and postadmission care, and to incorporate the concept of a planned transfer of care to primary and/or community services.
2. The child and parent are offered preparation both before and during the day of admission.
3. Specific written information is provided to ensure that parents understand their responsibilities throughout the episode.
4. The child is admitted to an area designated for day cases and not mixed with acutely ill inpatients.
5. The child is neither admitted nor treated alongside adults.
6. The child is cared for by identified staff specifically designated to the day case area.
7. Medical, nursing and all other staff are trained for, and skilled in, work with children and their families, in addition to the expertise needed for day case work.
8. The organization and delivery of patient care are planned specifically for day cases, so that every child is likely to be discharged within the day.
9. The building, equipment and furnishings comply with safety standards for children.
10. The environment is homely and includes areas for play and other activities designed for children and young people.
11. Essential documentation, including communication with the primary and/or community services, is completed before each child goes home so that aftercare and follow-up consultations are not delayed.
12. Once care has been transferred to the home, nursing support is provided, at a doctor's request, by nurses trained in the care of sick children.

Box 14.12   Most common paediatric day surgery procedures

Lymph node biopsy
Herniotomy
Hydrocoele excision
Ingrowing toenail treatment
EUA anal stretch
Circumcision
Orchidopexy
Myringotomy/grommets
Tonsillectomy
Adenoidectomy
Correction of strabismus
Prominent ear surgery
Arthroscopy
Dental extractions

'Saturday club', where the child has the opportunity to familiarize him/herself with the nurses, play specialist and DSU, and can participate in role play, donning masks, playing with stethoscopes, face masks, reservoir bags, etc. As previously indicated, the preassessment process is vital to ensure appropriate selection and preparation of both patient and carer. The information provided can be supported by written information and videos.

SURGICAL PROCEDURES

Appropriate operations are noted in the basket/trolley of procedures, and Box 14.12 lists the most common. Day case tonsillectomy is not widely accepted as suitable owing to the risk of primary bleeding. This risk is minimized by observing the patient for 8 hours,[62] and a further study indicated that a 5–6-hour period was safe practice.[63]

FASTING GUIDELINES

Clear fluids can be safely taken until 2 hours before the anaesthetic and solids until 6 hours,[64] and breast milk until 4 hours before anaesthesia.[29]

PREMEDICATION

Premedication is not usually recommended for paediatric day cases. However, a study has shown that although the presence of a 'relaxed' and well-informed parent in the anaesthetic room can reduce a child's (>4 years) anxiety, the inclusion of a premedication, such as midazolam, can be more effective.[65] Examples are chloral hydrate 30–50 mg/kg or oral midazolam (0.5 mg/kg), which has the advantage of a reduced postoperative sedative effect but tastes disgusting to most children.

Children wishing intravenous induction of anaesthesia have tetracaine or EMLA cream applied to two different sites which have been tested as the most suitable veins for cannulation.

POSTOPERATIVE NAUSEA AND VOMITING

Postoperative nausea and vomiting are one of the main indicators for children requiring overnight admission.[66] The same principles of prophylaxis and treatment as in adults apply to children. Children prone to PONV, or having procedures associated with an increased incidence of PONV, are administered an appropriate anaesthetic involving the following principles: balanced anaesthesia, avoiding opioids, use of TIVA with propofol, and use of ondansetron (0.1 mg/kg) or low-dose droperidol (20 μg/kg).[67] As noted, the same day surgery principles and processes apply to children as to adults, but it is important to meet the child's different needs and requirements and to ensure that the parents are fully informed and encouraged to participate in the child's care, from preadmission to postdischarge period. The standards in Box 14.11 provide a framework for the team to provide a safe and comfortable and positive experience for both child and parents.

ORGANIZATION AND DELIVERY

The design of a day surgery facility affects the management and delivery of the service. Each hospital needs to determine its individual needs based upon environment and structure in order to meet the changing needs and requirements of patients. There are currently various designs and approaches to providing a day surgery service. Easy access to the unit for patients and carers is crucial. Parking facilities are essential, with drop-off and pick-up points at the entrance.

TYPES OF FACILITY

1. Dedicated DSU ward with clearly identified day surgery theatres. This facility is designed to provide the optimal day surgery service. The systems, staffing, skills, structure and shared values are incorporated into the unit. Patient care is streamlined from GP referral to discharge.

2. Dedicated DSU ward with DSU theatre and inpatient theatres.

3. Dedicated DS ward providing care for patients attending inpatient theatres. Patients rely on portering support for transfer to other theatres. There is less control of theatre lists, as surgeons operating in other theatres may be more inclined to operate on more major cases rather than the day surgery patients. Communication and negotiation are required from all parties.

4. Inpatient ward providing care for patients in a variety of theatres. This is a poor use of resources and leads to cancellation of day surgery patients in times of bed crisis. This facility is not geared towards providing a day surgery service. It lacks strategy and leads to cancellations, delays, and increased frustration for patients and day surgery clinicians.

5. Free-standing units with appropriate facilities, such as those stated in (1) above.

6. Diagnostic and treatment centres (DTC)/ambulatory care and diagnostic units (ACAD). The continual pressures and impact of providing care within an acute-led service prompted the development of DTC and ACADs. This design is focused on patient care and outcome.[1]

Free-standing units which are separate from the hospital base and/or without appropriate medical cover can hinder the further development and expansion of day surgery. Patient selection needs to be rigid and the range of procedures may be limited.

MANAGEMENT

Senior management commitment is vital in developing and expanding this service. The multidisciplinary team needs a systematic integrated approach which encourages cooperation and collaboration to develop a successful and effective day surgery service. To function effectively, cooperative structures, both formal and informal, have to exist between the unit and the other services involved in patient care.

A lead clinician, consultant anaesthetist or surgeon, requires the skills to direct and liaise with a diverse multiprofessional group. Regular multidisciplinary group meetings need to involve medical, nursing, physiotherapy and pharmacy staff, and dissemination of information to all team members and encouragement of feedback ensures a healthy and live unit. Poor day surgery management reduces surgical and anaesthetic interest and confidence in considering any potential increase in day surgery activity.[5]

SKILL MIX

Multidisciplinarity and skill mix are essential in providing excellent patient care. Owing to the variation in design and organization of day surgery services throughout the UK, the skill mix must reflect patient needs.

Because of the changing face of day surgery and variations in activity and complexity, a regular review and evaluation of patients' needs and requirements from preassessment to postdischarge forms part of the clinical risk assessment programme. Integration and collaboration of theatre and ward staff is extremely beneficial to patient care. Day surgery staff recognize the importance of ensuring that there is a core team of specialist staff in preassessment clinics, anaesthetic, operating room, recovery and ward areas. Many day surgery staff are competent in many areas but expert in only a few. This leads to the definition of multiskilling. To avoid the 'Jack-of-all-trades, master of none', an appropriate skill mix ensures quality care and harmonious integration within the DSU. The study of a self-managing day surgery nursing team effectively integrated the expanded roles, management and caring roles to the benefit of the patients and staff, with increased activity and cost efficiency.[70]

NURSE SPECIALISTS

As noted, some patients, for example urology, upper gastrointestinal and orthopaedic, may require more specialist nursing care. Previous debate regarding the creation of an ambulatory nurse specialist role has been overtaken by the clear recognition of the need for expertise in each of the specialist areas. Increasingly, the day surgery staff liaise with the nurse specialists who, working in conjunction with the multidisciplinary team, can

Table 14.2 Staff allocation per shift or per day, depending on shift patterns[68]

	Perioperative practitioner	Ward nurse	Patients
Preassessment		1	20 (average interview takes 20 minutes of nursing time)
Ward		1*	7
Anaesthetics	1 per session or operating room		
Operating room	3 per session or operating room		
Recovery		1	2 (paediatrics 1:1)
Nurse-in-charge			1 per shift
Outpatient cover			

* Attention to the more complex procedures and patients with more complex conditions need to be reflected in the skill mix and staffing levels. One method of identifying skill mix and appropriate staffing levels is to record the activity, volume and complexity throughout the week.[69]

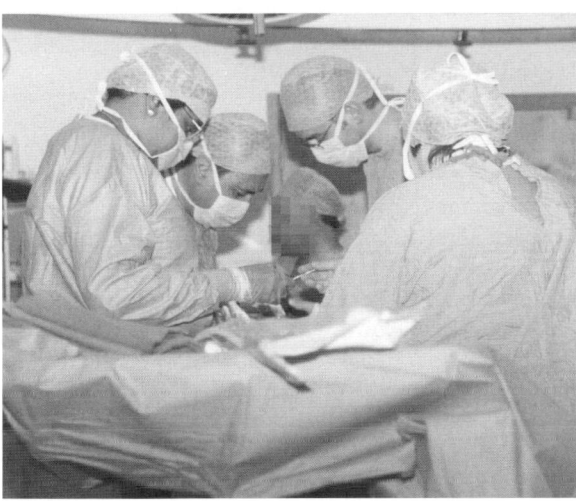

Figure 14.2 Teamwork in day surgery.

advise, support, provide care and enhance the patient experience.

WHAT CAN PERIOPERATIVE PRACTITIONERS OFFER DAY SURGERY PATIENTS?

Day surgery provides an invaluable opportunity to fully develop perioperative practice. Day surgery is not the environment to transfer into if it is perceived as a place to slow down. It is a fast-paced, dynamic and exciting area to work in, and an example of the diverse skills and knowledge required is given in Box 14.13.

Perioperative practitioners have a knowledge and understanding of anaesthesia, pain management, recovery, pathophysiology, interventions and the

Box 14.13   Sample of specific knowledge and skills required in day surgery. Communication verbal/non-verbal and written

Preassessment skills
Teaching and education patients/carers counselling
Record 12-lead ECG
Venepuncture
Specific interventions, pathophysiology
Principles of homoeostasis

Preoperative preparation
Assessment, planning, implementation, evaluation

Anaesthetic assistance

Theatre
Infection control
Scrubbing/circulating

Recovery
Risk management
IV therapy
Resource management
Pain management
Postoperative care
Infusion devices
Leadership
Management

Postdischarge
Research and development
Good verbal and written communication skills/flexibility
Ability to build relationships with patients and carers over a short period

implications of inappropriate day case selection. Patients benefit from educated practitioners who are familiar with all aspects of their journey. By sharing knowledge and expertise, the development and further progression of day surgery could be enhanced by the integration of ward and operating room-based practitioners. It is prudent for perioperative practitioners to review and reassess areas that require direct nursing care and to identify the right skill mix.

A structured integrated programme is required, and consultation with relevant staff members is essential to ensure continuity and harmony.

STAFF DEVELOPMENT AND TRAINING

Education and training are fundamental for the provision and continual development of the service. The unit requires written plans for education and training, and for continuing professional development, based on the recommendations of the relevant colleges and regulatory bodies. All permanent nursing or medical staff complete and agree, in consultation, a personal development plan. The day surgery manager reviews and assesses personal development plans and staff performance, at least annually. The importance of a structured education and training programme in preassessment cannot be overemphasized so as to provide a high standard of care, uniformity in information giving and safe practice. Preassessment programmes provide the foundation for developing confident and competent practitioners. Education and training programmes are based on skills assessment and needs analysis. In-house training programmes and learning packs provide a structured framework for learning and assessment. In conjunction with the facilitators in practice, research and development and education

---

Box 14.14   CPD opportunities available at diploma, degree or postgraduate levels

Operating department practice
Theatre skills
Perioperative practice
Critical care courses
Counselling
Teaching and assessment
Preassessment

---

coordinators, the most suitable courses and professional development programmes will be identified for each member of staff.

At the time of writing, ENB courses are being replaced by programmes developed by higher education institutions. Information regarding access is available.[71,72]

QUALITY IMPROVEMENT PROGRAMMES (QIPs)

A quality improvement programme incorporates risk management and clinical effectiveness. Clinical effectiveness, encompassing safety, efficiency and cost-effectiveness, is evaluated through clinical audit and the development of clinical outcome indicators.

MEASURING PERFORMANCE

Patient services

The quality assurance organizations, such as Quality Improvement Scotland, the Northern Ireland Practice and Education Council and the Healthcare Commission (England and Wales)[73] provide a framework for action. In 1998, The King's Fund Organizational Audit was relaunched as the Health Quality Service (HQS), providing an accreditation programme for the NHS and the independent sector. In collaboration with the HQS, BADS has developed a set of day surgery standards which, at the time of writing, are being piloted in four Trusts in England. This assessment tool aims to evaluate performance and, on successful completion, HQS accreditation will be valid for 3 years.[74]

Clinical outcome is measured by patient satisfaction, complications, and a reporting system which includes day surgery activity, for example reasons for cancellations, non-attendance, unplanned overnight admissions. Regular monitoring and effecting appropriate corrective action is a major part of the reporting system and quality improvement programme. Creating a framework to evaluate both clinical and non-clinical aspects of care is essential. An evidence-based approach is required, and set standards of practice are related to structure, resources and organization, processes, policies, protocols, practices, interventions and outcomes. Performance review is a valuable process to use as a means of planning and implementing appropriate objectives. Regular monitoring and control by the day surgery team is paramount to success.

INTEGRATED CARE PATHWAYS (ICPs)

An ICP determines locally agreed, individual health practice, based on guidelines and evidence – where available – for a specific user group.[75]

An ICP, as opposed to a unitary patient record, provides a user-friendly and evidence-based approach for an episode of care or treatment. It facilitates the auditing of care by analysis of variations from the agreed pathway. As part of the clinical governance framework, an ICP forms part of the QIP: monitoring care, clinical audit and evidence-based practice.[76] Good-quality information needs to be evidence based, clearly communicated, and involve patients. Information is the cornerstone of a successful day surgery service, and examination of the service will ensure a proactive approach to meeting patient needs and increasing public expectations.

- **Hospital performance indicators** – Hospitals subscribe to various services, such as CHKS Ltd, Newchurch, which maintain comparative databases
- **National performance indicators** – The Audit Commission for England and Wales[7] and Audit Scotland follow the recommendation that Trusts compare performance by specialty and procedure against Management Executive recommendations.

FUTURE DEVELOPMENTS

PREADMISSION ASSESSMENT

The National Booked Admissions programme has facilitated a more integrated approach to patient care. With improved communication in primary care, GPs identify fit and healthy patients who are offered telephone assessment by the day surgery team rather than requiring another hospital visit. Preassessment at this initial consultation depends on waiting times for surgery. If this is more than 3 months, the hospital-based preassessment nurse telephones the patient 1 week beforehand to ascertain any changes in their medical or social circumstances. Practice nurses, trained in preassessment and following local guidelines, are likely to undertake more assessments at the health centre/surgery. As previously noted, further research is required to explore the most suitable period between preassessment and day of operation. More hospitals may adopt the preassessment programmes and apply day surgery principles to inpatient care, providing a more patient-centred service.

EXPANSION OF DAY SURGERY

Political pressures to reduce waiting lists and times and the continual reduction of surgical beds influence the need to change existing practice. Improved techniques in anaesthesia and surgery will provide a continual increase in the types of procedure undertaken as day cases, with subsequent impact on inpatient and outpatient activity. The development of DTC and ACADs aims to improve patient care and outcome. The provision of appropriate services for outpatient treatments would facilitate the further development and expansion of true day surgery. More units extending opening times facilitate extended recovery. By 'extending the day' from the parameters of 12-hour to 23-hour stay, the scope for developing and expanding the service is far-reaching. Twenty-three-hour Recovery Care Centres were developed in North America for reasons of insurance reimbursement. Patients who would have been cared for on an inpatient ward are provided with a streamlined service from preassessment to discharge. Prior to adopting more complex procedures as day cases, it is prudent to provide an appropriate monitoring system for these patients within the initial 24 hours, which could be within the hospital setting[38] or by customizing postdischarge support. Pushing the boundaries in relation to patient selection requires common sense and caution. Notwithstanding the implications of developing such a service, maintaining the day surgery ethos requires strong clinical leadership, managerial commitment, and appropriate nursing and medical expertise. Regular evaluation and reporting are essential. Further research and audit are required, and the key challenge in developing modern day surgery is maintaining and improving the quality of patient care.

COMMITMENT

Day surgery lends itself to audit. It is, however, at specialty and directorate level where indicators become more meaningful, by allowing comparison with peers and addressing the agenda for change through tools such as benchmarking. Although set national targets are beneficial, collaboration between Trusts' clinicians and managers, with the appropriate involvement of purchasing teams, cannot be under-estimated in the further development and expansion of day surgery. The continual variation in day surgery activity and the reluctance of many surgeons to adopt best practice has indicated a need for either a change in culture and/or more effective use and management of DSUs.

Hospitals identified as 'effective and efficient' performers will be targeted as the epitome of best practice within specific areas of day surgery practice. Therefore, comparing like with like, the units will be magnet sites and a source of information and inspiration for other units.

References

1. Department of Health. The NHS plan: creating a 21st century NHS. London: HMSO; 2000.
2. Royal College of Surgeons of England (Commission on the Provision of Surgical Services). Report of the Working Party Guidelines Day Surgery. London: Royal College of Surgeons of England; 1992.
3. Nicholl JH. The surgery of infancy. BMJ 1909; 2: 753–754.
4. Audit Commission. A shortcut to better services: day surgery in England and Wales. London: HMSO; 1990.
5. NHS Management Executive. Value for money (VFM) unit day surgery – making it happen. London: HMSO; 1991.
6. NHS Management Executive. Report on the Day Surgery Taskforce. London: HMSO; 1993.
7. Audit Commission. Day surgery: review of national findings. London: HMSO; 2001.
8. Audit Commission. Day surgery follow-up: progress against indicators from a short cut to better services. London: HMSO; 1998.
9. Audit Commission. Measuring quality: the patients' view of day surgery. Day surgery in England and Wales. London: HMSO; 1991.
10. Watts G. Day surgery in a day's work. Health Serv J 2001; 111: 830–833.
11. Cahill CJ. Basket cases and trolleys. Day surgery proposals for the millennium. J One-day Surg 1999; 9: 11–12.
12. Conaghan PJ, Figueira E, Griffin MAS, et al. Randomised clinical trial of effectiveness of emergency day surgery against standard in-patient treatment. Br J Surg 2002; 89: 423–427.
13. Wilmore DW, Kehlet H. Management of patients in fast-track surgery. BMJ 2001; 322: 473–476.
14. Blanshard HJ, Chung F, Manninen PH, et al. Awake craniotomy for removal of intracranial tumour: considerations for early discharge. Anaesth Analges 2001; 92: 89–94.
15. Gabor M, Chung F. Return hospital visits and hospital readmission after ambulatory surgery. Ann Surg 1999; 230: 721–727.
16. Association of Anaesthetists of Great Britain and Ireland. Preoperative assessment. The role of the anaesthetist. London: Association of Anaesthetists of Great Britain and Ireland; 2001.
17. Millar J. Patient selection and investigation of adult day cases. In: Smith I, ed. Day care anaesthesia. London: BMJ Books; 2000: 2–18.
18. Chung F, Mezei R, Tong D. Adverse events in ambulatory surgery. A comparison between elderly and younger patients. Can J Anaesthesiol 1999; 46: 309–321.
19. White C. News roundup. BMJ 2001; 322: 450.
20. National Audit Office. Online. Available: http://www.nao.gov.uk 23 Apr 2003.
21. Hans TS, van Leer EM, Seidell JC, et al. Waist circumference action levels in the identification of cardiovascular risk factors: prevalence study in a random sample. BMJ 1995; 311: 1401–1405.
22. Lean ME, Hans TS, Morrison CE. Waist circumference as a measure for indicating need for weight management. BMJ 1995; 311: 61.
23. British Association of Day Surgery. Care of the diabetic patient. Handbook 2002 (unpublished at the time of writing).
24. King TA, Bending JJ, Higgins TM. Diabetic management of patient undergoing day surgery. L One-day Surg 2001; 11: 18–19.
25. Chung F, Mezei G, Tong D. Pre-existing medical conditions as predictors of adverse events in day case surgery. Br J Anaesth 1999; 83: 262–270.
26. Allman KG, Muir A, Howell SJ, et al. Resistent hypertension and preoperative silent myocardial infarction in surgical patients. Br J Anaesth 1994; 73: 574–578.
27. British Medical Association and the Royal Pharmaceutical Society of Great Britain. Combined oral contraceptives: surgery. BNF 1996; 32: 37.
28. British Medical Association and the Royal Pharmaceutical Society of Great Britain. Hormone replacement therapy. BNF 1999; 37: 323.
29. American Society of Anesthesiologists. Practice advisory for preanesthesia evaluation. Anesthesiol 2002; 96: 492.
30. Millar J, Rudkin GE, Hitchcock M. Selection and investigation of adult day cases: practical anaesthesia and analgesia for day surgery. Oxford: Bios Scientific; 1997: 5–18.
31. ENOXACAN Study Group. [Working party report.]. Br J Surg 1997; 84: 1099–1103.
32. Drew A, Fawcett TN. Responding to the information needs of patients with cancer. Prof Nurse 2002; 17: 443–446.
33. Hodge D. Day surgery, a nursing approach. Preparation for procedures. Edinburgh: Churchill Livingstone; 1999: 27–39.
34. Solly J. National booked admissions programme. J One-day Surg 2000; 10: 20–21.

35. American Society of Anesthesiologists Task Force on Preoperative Fasting. Anesthesiol 1999; 90: 896–905.

36. Porteous A, Tyndall J. Yes I want to walk to the OR. Can Oper Room Nurs J 1994; May/June: 15–25.

37. Philip BK. Problems in anesthesia. Acceptable agents for ambulatory general anesthesia. Ambul Anesthesia 1999; 11: 43–53.

38. Millar J. Assessment and preparation for adult day cases. In: Smith I, ed. Day care anaesthesia. London: BMJ Books; 2000: 19–29.

39. Rosenblum M, Weller RS, Conrad PL, et al. Ibuprofen provides longer lasting analgesia than fentanyl after laparoscopy. Anesth Analgesia 1991; 73: 255, 259.

40. Raeder J. Regional anaesthesia. In: Smith I, ed. Day care anaesthesia. London: BMJ Books; 2000: 97–126.

41. Alexander CD, Wetchler BV, Thompson RG. Bupivacaine infiltration of mesosalpinx in ambulatory surgical laparoscopic tubal sterilization. Can J Anaesthesiol 1987; 34: 362–365.

42. Ezeh VO, Shoulder VS, Martin JL, et al. Local anaesthetic on Filshie clips for pain relief after tubal sterilisation. Lancet 1995; 346: 82–85.

43. Jakobsson J. Postoperative pain and emesis: a systematic approach. In: Smith I, ed. Day care anaesthesia. London: BMJ Books; 2000: 155–179.

44. Mamaril M. Fast-tracking the post-anaesthesia patient: the pros and cons. J Perianaesth Nurs 2000; 15: 89–93.

45. American Society of Anesthesiologists. Practice guidelines for post-anesthesia care. Approved by the House of Delegates American Society of Anesthesiologists, Washington DC; 2001.

46. Aldrete JA. The post-anaesthesia recovery score J Clin Anaesth 1995; 7: 89–91.

47. Marshall S, Chung F. Discharge criteria and complications after ambulatory surgery. Anaesth Analgesia 1999; 88: 508–517.

48. Marshall S, Chung F. Assessment of home-readiness: discharge criteria and post-discharge complications. Curr Opin Anaesth 1997; 10: 445–450.

49. Cahill H, Jackson I, McWhinnie D. BADS handbook. Ready to go home? Norwich: Colman Print; 2000.

50. Warner MA, Shields SE, Chute CG. Major morbidity and mortality within 1 month of ambulatory surgery and anesthesia. JAMA 1993; 270: 1437–1441.

51. Duncan PG, Cohen MM, Tweed WA, et al. The Canadian four-centre study of anaesthetic outcomes: III. Are anaesthetic complications predictable in day surgical practice? Can J Anaesthesiol 1992; 39: 440–448.

52. Natof HE. Complications associated with ambulatory surgery. JAMA 1980; 244: 116–118.

53. Weinstein MS, Nicholson SC, Schreiner MS. A single dose of morphine sulphate increases the incidence of vomiting after outpatient inguinal surgery in children. Anethesiol 1994; 81: 572–577.

54. Hitchcock M. Postoperative morbidity following day surgery. In: Smith I, ed. Day care anaesthesia. London: BMJ Books; 2000: 205–211.

55. Wedderburn AW, Dodds SR, Morris GE. Survey of postoperative care after day surgery. Ann R Coll Surg Engl 1996; 78: 70–71.

56. Roddam P, Iredale J, Lewis I, et al. More expansion of day surgery? J One-day Surg 1997; 7(1): 11–16.

57. Kleinpell RM. Improving telephone follow-up after ambulatory surgery. J Perianaesth Nurs 1997; 12: 336–340.

58. McMillan R. Is there a need for a day surgery community nurse? J One-day Surg 2001; 10: 9.

59. Department of Health. Welfare of children and young people in hospital. London: HMSO; 1991.

60. Thornes R. Just for the day. London: National Association for the Welfare of Children in Hospital (NAWCH); 1991.

61. Scaife JM, Johnstone JM. Psychological aspects of day care surgery for children. In: Healy TE, ed. Anaesthesia for day case surgery. London: Baillière Tindall; 1990: 759–779.

62. Moralee SJ, Murray JAM. Would day-case adult tonsillectomy be safe? J Laryngol Otol 1995; 109: 1166–1763.

63. Gabalshi EC, Mattucci KF, Moleski P. Ambulatory tonsillectomy and adenoidectomy. Laryngoscope 1996; 106: 77–80.

64. Phillips S, Daborn AK, Hatch DJ. Preoperative fasting for paediatric anaesthesia. Br J Anaesth 1994; 43: 529–536.

65. Kaine ZN, Mayes LC, Caramico LA, et al. Parental presence during induction of anaesthesia. A randomised controlled trial. Anaesthesiol 1996; 84: 1060–1067.

66. Patel RI. Postoperative morbidity and discharge criteria. In: White PF, ed. Ambulatory anesthesia and surgery. London: WB Saunders; 1996: 617–631.

67. Morton NS, Camu F, Dorman T, et al. Ondansetron reduces nausea and vomiting after paediatric adenotonsillectomy. Paed Anaesth 1997; 7: 37–45.

68. Solly J. Management in day surgery. In: Hodge D, ed. Day surgery. A nursing approach. Edinburgh: Churchill Livingstone; 1999: 213–229.

69. Greenhalgh C. Using information in managing the nursing resource workload. Macclesfield: Greenhalgh; 1991.

70. MacDonald M, Bodzak W. The performance of a self-managing day surgery team. J Adv Nurs 1999; 29: 859–868.

71. NHS Careers England and Wales. Online. Available: http://www.nhs.uk/careers 23 Apr 2003.

72. NHS Education for Scotland. Online. Available: http://www.nes.scot.nhs.uk 23 Apr 2003.

73. The Centre for Health Information Quality (Online) Available: http://www.hfht.org/chiq/index.htm 23 Apr 2003.

74. Health Quality Service. Online. Available: http://www.hqs.org.uk 23 Apr 2003.

75. National Pathways Association 2000 FAQS. Online. Available: http://www.the-npaorg.uk

76. Department of Health. A first class service: quality in the new NHS. London: Stationery Office; 1998.

Recommended reading

Smith I. Day care anaesthesia. London: BMJ Books; 2000.

Hodge I. Day surgery. A nursing approach. Edinburgh: Churchill Livingstone; 1999.

Cahill H, Jackson I. Day surgery: principles and nursing practice. London: Baillière Tindall; 1997.

Millar J, Rudkin G, Hitchcock M. Practical anaesthesia and analgesia for day surgery. Oxford: Bios Scientific; 1998.

Websites

British Association of Day Surgery. www.bads.co.uk

NHS Careers www.nhs.uk/careers

NHS Education for Scotland www.nes.scot.nhs.uk

Chapter **15**

Surgery in the community

Judy Mewburn

Key points

- The development of community surgery
- Setting up a minor surgery room and sterilization facilities
- Aspects of clinical procedures

HISTORICAL PERSPECTIVE

Minor surgery has historically been performed in GP surgeries. Before the advent of the National Health Service in 1948 most doctors undertook minor surgery, and some had contracts with the local hospitals. Patients expected their doctors to be able to perform minor surgery, sometimes to deliver babies at home, and even to undertake tonsillectomies on the kitchen table. The rigid structure of the new service separated the GP from the hospitals. Payment by capitation to GPs was an active discouragement to do anything more than the bare minimum, as extra work lost the practice money. A study in 1951 by the British Medical Association showed that 96% of GPs believed that the NHS had reduced minor surgery in general practice. In 1955 a study by Hunt in London found that in 87 practices none provided minor surgery, although all the GPs had been trained. Specialist consultants, to whom the patients were referred, gradually replaced family doctors in hospitals; consequently, the general practitioner carried out less and less minor surgery. This led to an increase in surgery in the hospital setting, and inevitably to an increase in the hospital surgical waiting list.

It was not until the Charter for the Family Doctor Service in 1965, with improvements in terms and conditions of service, that general practice minor surgery began to increase.

In recent years there has been a renewed interest on behalf of the GP in performing minor surgery in the practice setting. This has coincided with the building of purpose-built surgeries, with treatment rooms where minor surgery can be carried out with the help of the practice nurse, and with the added assistance of postoperative care from the community nurse.

Patients have welcomed this. An opinion can be sought from the GP and the surgery performed in an environment that is familiar to the patient, without recourse to waiting lists. The added bonus of having surgery performed by a doctor who is known and trusted and having all aftercare from the practice nurse cannot be overestimated. Fears of the unknown are greatly reduced, and psychologically the patient feels at home in the familiar environment of the GP surgery. The surgery is usually closer to the patient's home than the local hospital. This means that the relative or escort bringing the patient to the surgery, and taking them home, does not have to travel so far. Parking is usually much easier than in the hospital setting. In-house patient satisfaction surveys show that patients and their relatives all appreciate these relevant facts. As all operations carried out by the GP are under local anaesthetic, a speedy return home is usual.

The government has been active in encouraging GPs to perform minor surgery. Even with the advent of day surgery units in many of the large teaching and independent hospitals in the 1990s, the capacity to carry out minor surgery has not been adequate to deal with the waiting lists. Patients have had prolonged waits for surgery for non-urgent lesions.

Some GPs hold a Fellowship of the Royal College of Surgeons or Gynaecologists. This qualification means that further training in surgical skills is not necessary. Other criteria for accreditation include a 6-month surgical hospital post, evidence of having performed minor surgery for 3–5 years, evidence of update and approval, and having performed a minimum of 15 operations per year. For the greater proportion of GPs training in minor surgery is essential.

GENERAL PRACTITIONER MINOR SURGERY TRAINING

The Royal College of General Practitioners (RCGP) has been proactive in setting up a minor surgery course. The main instigator has been Roger Kneebone, a GP from Trowbridge in Wiltshire. The course was held at the RCGP Headquarters in Hyde Park, and after the initial course, further courses were run in order to train doctors who wanted to take the course to their locality and further train GPs. This has proved invaluable, as courses are now held in many different locations in England, and GPs do not have to travel to London.

There are several elements to the minor surgery course, and it is essential to ensure that all procedures on the list of interventions that a GP may obtain payment for are covered.

Topics include:

- Anatomical hazards and pitfalls, Langer's lines
- Basic surgical technique; lecture and practical
- Excision of cysts, lipomas and abscesses; lecture and practical
- Dermatological surgery pigmented lesion; lecture and practical
- Rheumatology, anatomy and physiology, injection of joints; practical
- Ingrowing toenails; lecture and practical
- Medicolegal aspects of minor surgery
- Administration, facilities and audit
- Infection control and decontamination
- Setting up a minor surgery room: equipment needed.

This course covers all aspects of minor surgery and takes place over 2 days. The practical experience is gained using facsimile skin pads, cysts and lipomas, and ingrowing toenails. Dermatological surgery is taught also using pads with seborrhoeic keratosis, shave excisions, and lesions for cautery and cryotherapy. Rheumatology and injection and aspiration of joints are taught using models of shoulders, elbows, knees and wrists.

The medicolegal side of minor surgery is very important, and this lecture is given by a representative of the Medical Defence Union. Litigation in general practice is increasing, as it is in the hospital setting, and doctors need to have the pitfalls illustrated in order to try and avoid them. Most complaints are from patients who have not had an adequate explanation of the proposed procedure, and because of obvious mistakes, e.g. using diathermy after cleansing the skin with spirit before the spirit has had time to dry.

Consent to operation is a contentious issue and is dealt with elsewhere in this book. However, it must be stressed that each procedure, its side effects, and any scarring expected, possible nerve damage and average healing time, must be fully explained to the patient and the facts and the explanation documented. At present it is not legally necessary to get the patient to sign a consent form, but many GPs feel that it is in their best interest to do so as this gives them absolute proof of what was explained should the situation become litigious.

Most Primary Care Trusts (PCTs) insist that a GP undergoes this course before commencing minor surgery. Nurses who assist GPs during minor surgery should also have specific training: indeed, many PCTs also insist on this. The courses for nurses cover much of the same ground but are orientated towards setting up the minor surgery room, all aspects of the equipment needed, infection control, nurses' responsibilities for patient information, informed consent, timing of the operating list, aftercare and medicolegal aspects. A suturing module is also included. This course normally lasts for 2 days.

Advanced suturing courses are available for practice nurses, and are arranged by the PCT. In-depth cardiopulmonary resuscitation courses are also provided. These courses can be run in the GP surgery and are an excellent way to update all the surgery staff.

Courses for GPs in more intricate surgery, e.g. vasectomy and carpal tunnel release, are also available, arranged either by the PCT or by a company specializing in such courses.

PROCEDURES FOR WHICH A GP MAY CLAIM PAYMENT

A list of procedures that may be performed by a GP under Paragraph 42 schedule 1 of the statement of Fees and Allowances [2] (The Red Book) and for which payment will be made is shown in Box 15.1.

The procedures for which a payment may be made vary from the simple to the more complicated. A GP may claim for five procedures per month. This applies to all GPs. However, if a doctor in a practice does not want to operate, he can delegate

---

Box 15.1   Procedures that may be performed by a GP

- Injections (intra-articular, periarticular)
- Varicose veins
- Haemorrhoids
- Aspirations
- Joints
- Cysts
- Bursae
- Hydrocoele
- Incisions
- Abscesses
- Cysts
- Thrombosed haemorrhoids
- Excisions
- Sebaceous cysts
- Lipoma
- Skin lesions for histology
- Intradermal naevi, papillomas, dermatofibromas and similar conditions
- Warts
- Removal of toenail, partial and complete
- Curette cautery and cryocautery
- Warts and verrucae
- Other skin lesions, e.g. molluscum contagiosum
- Pathology

- Blood counts
- Tests for liver function and electrolytes
- Ophthalmology
- Chalazion operations
- Operations for obstruction of the nasolacrimal duct
- Ear, nose and throat
- Puncture of the maxillary antrum with washout
- Fibreoptic pharyngoscopy
- Fibreoptic laryngoscopy
- General surgery
- Endoscopy of the upper gastrointestinal tract
- Sigmoidoscopy
- Genitourinary surgery
- Diagnostic flexible cystoscopy
- Vasectomy
- Gynaecology
- Colposcopy
- Marsupialization of Bartholin's cyst
- Orthopaedics
- Excision of ganglion
- Carpal tunnel release
- Other
- Diagnostic ultrasound, not obstetric

his allowance to a fellow GP. In a 10-doctor practice this would mean that 50 procedures could be carried out per month. Payments per procedure do vary, but the government is seeking to put this on a much clearer footing. In fact, the latest government ruling for GP minor surgery sets out a system which will remunerate the GP properly and also take cognisance of his or her advanced skills. With the use of the Red Book and FP10, which govern what sutures, dressings, swabs, etc. a GP may claim for, consumables can be claimed for and reimbursed, thereby increasing the income from each procedure.

SETTING UP A MINOR SURGERY ROOM

The ideal size for the room is $13\,m^2$ or $140\,ft^2$. The walls must be washable. This is easily achieved in a new building, but in converted buildings walls may have to be faced with a laminate or, if the surface is good, a washable paint may be used. The floor should be easily cleaned and the edges must run up to the skirting board, leaving a rounded surface at the edge of the room. There should be at least one window – and preferably more – in order to provide a good natural light. Artificial lighting should be to daylight standard, with a dedicated operating light.

In the clean area, cupboards with doors provide dust-free storage for instruments, packs, sutures and other consumables. Small square trolleys are ideal for minor surgery.

DECONTAMINATION AND STERILIZING FACILITIES

It is of paramount importance that there are clean and dirty areas in the room for clean preparation and the disposal and processing of used equipment. Each of these two areas must have a sink: in the clean area a sink with elbow or remote control taps for scrubbing up, and in the dirty area for decontamination and sterilization. It is no longer acceptable to ask a practice nurse to scrub used instruments, as the risk of aerosol contamination is too high. An ultrasonic washer provides an ideal method of cleansing and decontaminating instruments and can be used for all speculae and other instruments used in the practice.

Many surgeries currently have their own autoclaves. It is convenient to be able to sterilize instruments used in the daily running of the surgery, as well as instruments used during minor surgery.

Tracking and traceability is obviously a problem, and many surgeries are grappling with this. Some surgeries obtain prepared packs of instruments from the local hospital's sterile services department. This works well if a good ordering system is in place, but is less reliable for obtaining the specialized instruments for chalazion surgery and vasectomy. The other problem is the quality of instruments and sharpness of scissors. Many GPs would rather buy and maintain their own instruments in order to circumvent this problem.

There is a question as to the use of autoclaves in general practice because of the difficulty of assuring the quality of the cycle. Any autoclave must be tested on a daily basis to ensure that it reaches the required temperature, holds that temperature for the required time, and that the cycle is complete and the test recorded in a register.[6–8] All autoclaves are required to meet strict validation requirements (see Ch. 8). There should be a contract with the manufacturer to carry out 3-monthly tests and maintenance.[9]

As product liability and European Directives and standards for decontamination and sterilization require that all sterilization of instruments is recorded, it is necessary to have an autoclave that gives a printed record of its cycle. This can be annotated in the patient's notes.

With the advent of variant Creutzfeld-Jakob disease, tracking of instruments has become a priority.[10] At the time of writing, this is mainly for instruments that have been used on brain, spinal cord, tonsil and appendix, as the prion has been found in these tissues. As further knowledge of the science of the prion emerges, it will no doubt become mandatory for all instruments to be tracked.

If the autoclave does not have a drying cycle,[11] the instruments must be used immediately after sterilization and not stored. If the autoclave does have a vacuum assisted drying cycle the instruments can be prepacked in two steam-permeable bags and used as needed. They should be stored in a dry cupboard and used within 1 year of sterilization (EN868 series).

An alternative to using instruments and sterile packs owned by the PCT is to obtain them from the local hospital sterile services department. This may prove a problem if the unit does not have the CE (Communauté Européen) mark. This guarantees that the facilities used to produce the packs have been inspected and have achieved a specific standard of manufacture. The CE mark allows users to be assured that all decontamination and sterilization processes are validated and meet the strict guidance enshrined in the European Directives. In producing packs for use by the GP, the sterile service unit has become a manufacturer and, as such, is responsible for any defect in the pack and its sterility. The Consumer Protection Act 1987 covers the liability of the legal manufacturer of sterile items. Advice may be sought from the local sterile service manager or the community infection control team.

Clinical waste must be bagged in yellow bags for incineration and disposed of at the end of every day. All GPs have a waste contract with local waste disposal contractors.

Ideally the minor surgery lists should be held on the same day each week, which allows for forward planning. Whereas some surgeries have a dedicated minor surgery room, others will use the room for dressing changes, suture removal and other non-sterile procedures. In this instance the room must be cleaned and left for an appropriate time for the airborne pathogens to settle. Although air conditioning with 20 changes per hour is recommended by many local infection control teams, many surgeries will have less efficient air conditioning, and in some cases none at all. It is very difficult to lay down hard and fast rules for filtration and ventilation, as differences in standards of building and equipment exist. NHS Estates has produced building notes for general practice. Standards are often dictated by local infection control policies. As some surgeries have been carrying out minor surgery for some years and have not had to apply for approval from the local PCT, standards are very hard to police.

The simplest and most economical way to ensure a good outcome for the patient undergoing minor surgery is to provide an environment in which the most complicated procedure may be safely carried out.

INSTRUMENTS AND PROCEDURE PACKS

Because of personal preference many GPs will opt to purchase their own instruments for minor surgery. The basic set of instruments comprises:

- No 3 Bard Parker handle
- Gillies toothed dissecting forceps
- McIndoe non-toothed dissecting forceps
- 5 in curved strabismus scissors
- 5 in Crilewood needle holder
- Blunt-ended scissors
- 5 in curved mosquito forceps

- Gillies skin hook
- Kilner catspaw retractor
- Other instruments that may be included:
  - Volkmans spoon
  - Miebomian cyst clamp and curette
  - Jobson Horne probe
  - Nail separator
  - Nail chisel
  - Thwaites nail nippers.

Sterile procedure packs are manufactured by several companies and are nearly identical in content. There is an outer wrapper that acts as a trolley cover and sterile field, cleansing sponges, a rigid container for cleansing fluid, sterile swabs, disposal bag and an aperture drape. Some companies will make up sterile packs to order, which is a cost-effective option.

CONSUMABLES

Consumables are items used during surgery. They include sutures, swabs, cleansing fluid, blades, Steristrips, dressings, injections, etc. These can all be obtained by the GP using the Red Book, utilizing paragraph 44.13 to obtain indirect reimbursement.

- The doctor personally purchases all injections, anaesthetics, sutures, coils and skin closure strips.
- For each patient where any of the above are used, and which the doctor or nurse personally administers, the doctor writes the items on a standard FP10 prescription form.
- The patient pays no prescription charge, irrespective of age or exemption category.

Once a month all prescriptions are sent to the Central Prescription Pricing Bureau, together with a claim form FP34, duly signed. The doctor is subsequently refunded as follows:

- The basic price of the item used
- An on-cost allowance
- A container allowance
- A dispensing fee.

This results in a very small profit on each item prescribed.

The list of sutures available to the GP on FP10 has recently been brought up to date. Catgut is no longer on the list, having been substituted by Vicryl. Black silk is no longer the suture of choice for anything other than scalp lesions. Prolene and Ethilon of varying thicknesses and with a choice of needles are available and now commonly used.

When the doctor buys local anaesthetic to be used on patients he in essence becomes a supplier. Under the Consumer Protection Act 1987, it is essential that the doctor knows what he gave to whom and when. To this end, a detailed record must be kept of the batch number and the expiry date, and the source of supply of the local anaesthetic used. This also applies to any drugs administered and to all suture materials.

It is recommended that this be annotated either in the register of operations performed or in the patient's notes.

A further important aspect of minor surgery is histology. All lesions removed should be sent for histology. This must be documented either in the patient's notes or in the operation register. It is also essential that the results of the histology are annotated, and paramount that the patient be informed. With the increase of skin cancer, patients are understandably worried about the nature of their skin lesions. Increasing litigation points to the fact that this essential task is sometimes forgotten.

RESUSCITATION

It is important that all the components for resuscitation are checked regularly, that they are in date, and that personnel are trained to use them. A resuscitation workshop for all staff in the practice should be held once a year to provide updates on new practice and to ensure that all staff are competent to carry out resuscitation. As supermarkets now carry full resuscitation equipment it is unacceptable for a GP surgery not to do the same.

A comprehensive selection of resuscitation equipment is vital when operative procedures are being performed under local anaesthesia. Adverse reactions to any of the elements of the anaesthetic agent used can be life threatening and need to be dealt with immediately. Most PCTs will have a list of minimal requirements for resuscitation. The following are guidelines:

- Oxygen
- Suction
- Ambubag and face mask
- Four sizes of Guedel airway
- Laryngoscope
- Endotracheal tubes and laryngeal mask airway
- Syringes and needles
- Intravenous cannulae (various sizes)
- Tourniquet

- Giving sets
- Intravenous fluids
- Plasma expander
- Atropine
- Adrenaline (epinephrine)
- Defibrillator.

Resuscitation equipment should be kept in the minor surgery room so that any adverse reactions can be dealt with swiftly.

PATIENT INFORMATION

This is one area where the practice nurse can be truly creative. Information leaflets on the operations performed by the GP can be prepared and given to patients preoperatively. The practice nurse can be instrumental in explaining the procedure to the patient, thereby allaying their fears, and postoperative care can be simplified with the aid of detailed leaflets for the patient to take home. A leaflet describing anticipated pain, its level and methods of control can be used for all operations. Specific leaflets for individual operations should have details of the procedure performed, the postoperative wound care regimen, when sutures should be removed, and any anticipated postoperative complications. Events that necessitate telephoning the surgery should be detailed.

LOCAL ANAESTHESIA

It is very important that the action of the local anaesthetic used and the extent of the duration of anaesthesia are explained to the patient; also, warnings about walking, if nerve blocks are being used for operations on the feet. The most commonly used local anaesthetics are lidocaine (lignocaine), Xylocaine and bupivacaine (Marcain). These are classified as amides and are metabolized by the liver. Clearance rate is fastest with lidocaine (lignocaine), followed by bupivacaine. Bupivacaine is a vasodilator, but lidocaine (lignocaine) appears to have no effect on blood vessels. Adrenaline (epinephrine) is added to some local anaesthetics and acts as a vasoconstrictor. When using an anaesthetic agent containing adrenaline (epinephrine), the action will be prolonged and a larger dose may be administered because the local vasoconstriction stops the spread of the agent. Local anaesthesia containing adrenaline (epinephrine) should never be used on end arteries, e.g. in the toes, fingers, nose or penis.

Local anaesthetic should be warmed before use and sufficient time should lapse between administration and the operation being carried out for the agent to take effect (a minimum of 5 minutes) – there should be no need to prod the patient with a needle asking if they can feel it! It is much better to gently go ahead with the incision, telling the patient that they should say if anything hurts. This approach will win the patient's confidence and ensure a smoother procedure. Local blocks are not currently used for postoperative pain control, but as the procedures carried out by GPs become more sophisticated this may well change.

MEDICOLEGAL ASPECTS

In these days of increasing litigation the GP must be proactive in explaining fully all the aspects of the procedure about to be performed and documenting this explanation. With some lesions, especially on the face, preoperative photographs will provide evidence should a patient not be satisfied with the cosmetic outcome. The Medical Defence Union and the Medical Protection Society provide very good booklets detailing the kinds of cases that have been brought. This is invaluable information for the GP, and will increase awareness of potential troublesome situations.

KINDS OF SURGERY PERFORMED

As can be seen from the list, the procedures a GP can carry out are extensive.

Some doctors perform many types of surgery and some prefer to perform one operation or a reduced number. This obviously varies with the individual (Table 15.1).

Table 15.1 Procedures performed 1/2/99–1/12/00 (Courtesy of Dr R. Gabriel)

Procedure	Number
Dermoid cyst removal	2
Sebaceous cyst removal	11
Mole removal	29
Skin tag removal	9
Hormone implant	5
Ingrowing toenail removal	11
Papilloma removal	2
Lipoma removal	5
Wart removal	7
Chalazion removal	2
Abscess drainage	1
Solar keratosis removal	2
Telangiectasia removal	2
Granuloma removal	2
Seborrhoeic wart removal	12
Joint injection	44

CONCLUSION

Performing minor surgery in the GP practice has never been a profitable endeavour. However, many GPs take great pride and pleasure in providing a community-based service for their patients. The patients in turn are very grateful for a service that directly answers their needs and is within easy travelling distance.

Most doctors who perform minor surgery do so because it offers their patients a personalized and convenient way of having their operations without having to visit the hospital, and also because it gives them a great sense of fulfilment and satisfaction. The very obvious advantages to patients have been described already.

References

1. Brown JS. Minor surgery. A text and atlas, 4th edn. London: Chapman & Hall; 2003.
2. Schoefield J, Kneebone R. Skin lesions. A practical guide to diagnosis, management and minor surgery. London: Chapman & Hall; 1996.
3. Wall DW. A review of minor surgery in general practice in the United Kingdom. Fam Pract 1987; 4: 322–329.
4. Department of Health/The Welsh Office. Statement of fees and allowances payable to general medical practitioners in England and Wales. London: HMSO; 1990.
5. Department of Health. Terms of service for doctors in general practice. London: HMSO; 1989.
6. Medical Devices Agency. The purchase, operation and maintenance of benchtop steam sterilizers. DB 9605.
7. Medical Devices Agency. The validation and periodic testing of benchtop vacuum steam sterilizers. DB 9605.
8. Medical Devices Agency. Guidance on the purchase, operation and maintenance of vacuum benchtop steam sterilizers. DB 2000.
9. Health Technical Memorandum 2010. Part 1 Management policy. Sterilization. NHS Estates.
10. Health Service Circular 1999/178. Variant Creutzfeldt-Jakob disease (vCJD): minimizing the risk of transmission.
11. Health Services Circular (2000) 178. Variant Creutzfeldt Jakob Disease.

Chapter 16

Surgery outside the operating department

Mark Radford

CHAPTER CONTENTS

Key points

- Care of the trauma patient in the prehospital environment
- Care of the critically ill requiring intensive care
- Care of the critically ill patient during inter- and intrahospital transfer
- Care of the patient requiring diagnostic and interventional radiological procedures
- Care of the patient undergoing an endoscopic procedure

CARE OF THE TRAUMA PATIENT IN THE PREHOSPITAL ENVIRONMENT

BACKGROUND

Trauma is an epidemic that causes 10% of deaths worldwide, and is the leading cause of death in the young.[1] Trauma may cause significant injury that leads to lifelong disability, with significant whole health costs, and is secondary to growing populations, demographic changes, continued urbanization and drug and alcohol use, which affect the patterns of injury seen. The developed world has three distinct patterns of injury: road traffic accidents (RTA), intentional injuries such as murder and suicide, and domestic injury/death.[1] In the UK, RTAs cause 3000 deaths, 40 000 serious injuries and 320 000 injuries per year,[2] with approximately one-third being preventable.[3] Suicide is more difficult to quantify, as many cases go unreported, but estimates suggest that 15/100 000 men and 5/100 000 women commit suicide each year, with 20 times more attempts being made.[4]

THE NATIONAL ORGANIZATION OF TRAUMA/PREHOSPITAL CARE IN THE UK

Prehospital care in the UK has for many years remained an underdeveloped specialty and largely organized by the ambulance service.[5] This traditional system aimed to move injured patients, with little or no restorative treatment, to hospital as fast as possible, where it was felt that hospital staff were better placed to provide thorough assessment and treatment. The development of trauma centres and prehospital care in the USA provided lessons on the organization of trauma care in the UK, including the introduction of paramedic ambulance staff, and trials of centralized trauma centres in urbanized areas, notably Birmingham, Stoke on Trent and London, which have significantly improved outcomes. The British Orthopaedic Association Report.[6] *The Care of Severely Injured Patients in the United Kingdom* advocates 30 centralized tertiary trauma units with 24-hour consultant cover, serving a population of 2–3 million. Each centre would act as a hub to other hospitals, with developed trauma teams of senior clinicians and on-site facilities including A&E, anaesthesia, surgery, operating theatres and intensive care. Three tertiary units would be supported by a helicopter emergency service (HEMS). Greater involvement of hospital clinicians in prehospital care planning and training would serve to provide a seamless service from point of injury to hospital. Although this organization may be realized in the future, the adaptation of a US-based trauma system may not be as successful here in the UK.[7]

THE ROLE OF THE PERIOPERATIVE PRACTITIONER IN PREHOSPITAL CARE

Perioperative practitioners may be involved in prehospital care in many ways: arriving first at the scene of an accident or major incident, as part of a dedicated mobile medical unit (land based or aeromedical), or as part of a local major incident plan for a hospital. The guidance given in this chapter is generic, although clinical expertise and support may vary at the scene.

Any practitioner can find themselves attending an incident as a bystander. The clinical care that can be provided is often limited, and stopping to attend can often be a disorientating and frightening experience. It is reasonable to expect any practitioner to provide care that is appropriate to their experience and competence, and not beyond. The safety of the attendee is paramount, and hazards such as electrical, water or chemical should be checked before entering a scene. The emergency services should be called, and provided with accurate information about the site and potential casualties. Containment of the scene is important, preventing other bystanders from injury, and moving walking wounded to safety. Unless trained in prehospital care, prioritizing casualties for the untrained is problematic, although basic assessment of the casualties via the ABC methodology (Box 16.1) would be deemed appropriate. Casualties should not be moved unless they are in immediate danger of further injury. If the practitioner is trained in basic life support, these skills may be used. When emergency services arrive at the scene, the practitioner should identify him- or herself and provide a succinct hand-over. The emergency services will make a repeat assessment and in most cases end the practitioner's participation.

Prehospital systems in the UK involving mobile medical teams, with doctors, nurses and paramedics, are few in number, but the use of hospital-based practitioners – primarily nurses in prehospital care – is common in the European Union.[8] The role these teams play is important in providing additional skill and experience at the scene, in incident

---

Box 16.1   ABC methodology for basic assessment of casualty

- Safety first – Is the environment safe to approach?
- Airway – Control the airway: jaw thrust or chin lift
  - 'Little c' – Cervical spine – Is there potential cervical spine injury?
- Breathing
- Circulation – Control bleeding by direct pressure

Box 16.2   Threat profile of major incidents

- Air accidents
- Civil contingencies, riots and civil unrest
- Severe weather and floods
- Fire (rural and urban)
- Train accidents
- Chemical, biological and nuclear accidents/attacks
- Terrorist activity
- Large-number spectator events

management, prioritization and triage, in treatment in specific circumstances and in safe transfer of casualties to hospital.[9] For practitioners particiating in mobile medical teams it is suggested that Battlefield Advanced Trauma Life Support, Advanced Trauma Life Support or Prehospital Trauma Life Support courses are useful preparation.

The threat profile of a major incident has changed considerably over the last few years (Box 16.2). Mass casualty situations such as the Paddington and Selby train accidents and the World Trade Centre attacks on 11 September 2001 have caused a rethink of major incident planning. National plans in the UK for dealing with such events are coordinated by the Civil Contingency Secretariat, recognizing that major incidents require sophisticated organization across a broad range of intergovernmental agencies.

ARRIVAL AT AND MANAGEMENT OF THE TRAUMA SCENE

The next part of this chapter will focus on care delivered as part of a mobile medical unit. As with all scenarios the safety of the team, bystanders and patients remains paramount. Such scene assessment is made together with other emergency services. Regular reassessments must be made, together with identification of visible and invisible hazards. Those attending must be appropriately dressed in protective gear, including high-visibility clothing with clear identification, hard hat and protective gloves.

CAUSE AND DISTRIBUTION OF DEATH DURING A TRAUMA SCENE

Understanding the accident scene is vital to an assessment of the potential for loss of life and serious injury (Fig. 16.1). Evidence[3,10] suggests that deaths following trauma are distributed along a continuum (Fig. 16.2). Differences in the distribution between the US and UK are attributable to modality of trauma and subsequent management. An initial peak of

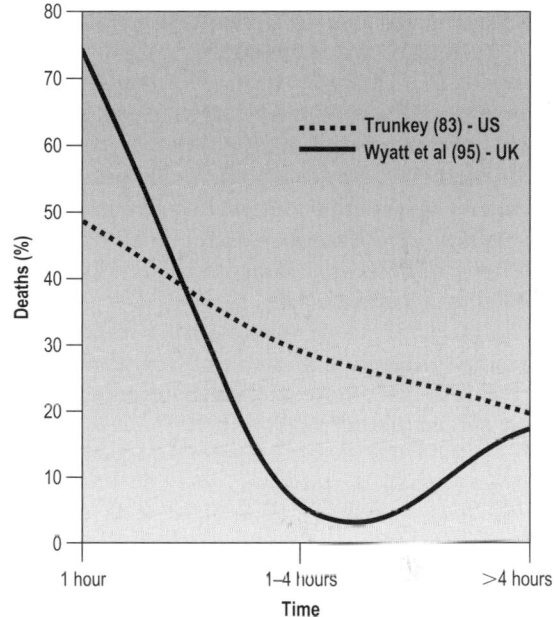

Figure 16.2   Distributions of deaths (%) following in US and UK.

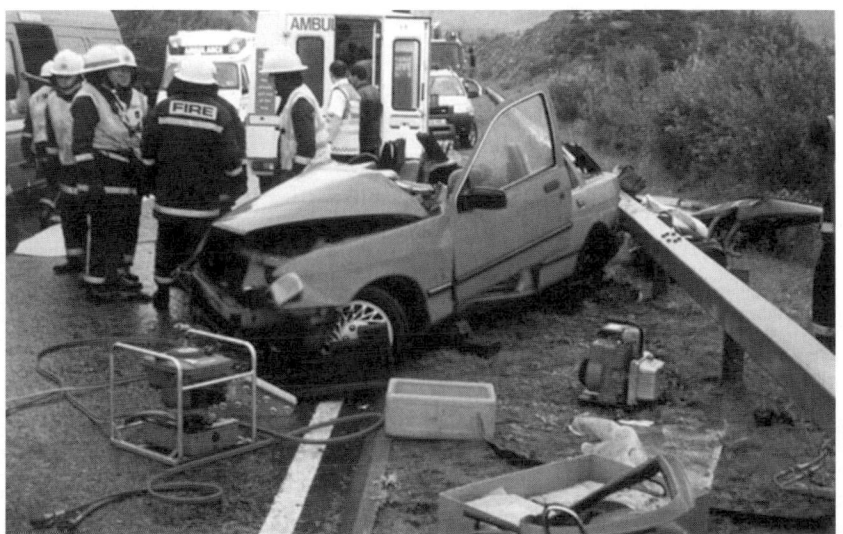

Figure 16.1   Accident scene safety and management. (With permission from Surgeon Lt Cdr Paul Rees RN, Intensive Care Unit, Ministry of Defence Hospital Unit Portsmouth, UK).

Box 16.3   Mechanisms predictive of serious injury[1]

- Fall greater than 6 m (20 ft)
- Pedestrian or cyclist hit by a car
- Death of other occupant in same vehicle
- Ejection from vehicle or bike
- Major vehicular deformity or significant intrusion into passenger space
- Extraction time greater than 20 minutes
- Vehicular rollover
- Penetrating injury to head or torso
- All shotgun wounds

Box 16.4   ABCD trauma assessment methodology

- Safety first – Is the environment safe to approach?
- A – Airway
  - 'Little c' – Cervical spine – Is there potential cervical spine injury?
  - Is there a risk of aspiration?
  - Is a defined airway required? – ET tube, Combitube via RSI (see Ch. 17)
- B – Breathing
  - Is the rate abnormal <9–>25
  - Is adequate ventilation being achieved?
  - Are there any obvious external chest injuries?
  - Is there a potential pneumothorax? (deviated trachea, high RR, hyper-resonant percussion and reduced breath sounds)
- C – Circulation
  - Is there obvious bleeding?
  - Is the patient haemodynamically stable?
  - Ideally rapid transfer to hospital and cannulate en route
  - Trapped patients – cannulate, restorative blood pressure for clot formation and cerebral perfusion only – not to aim for normotension.
- D – Dysfunction
  - Central neurological function intact? (GCS)
  - Peripheral neurological function intact? Spinal injury?
- E – Exposure
  - Assess for hypothermia
  - Treat symptoms (warm IV fluids, cover, protect from elements)

---

deaths occurs at the point of trauma or shortly afterwards, leading to the term 'golden hour', where good management will improve patient outcome.

Therefore, the issue of entrapment during an RTA has promoted a rethink on the role of mobile medical teams and HEMS.

The mechanisms of injury during trauma have been universally categorized as blunt, penetrating, thermal and blast; however, mechanisms of serious injury can be predicted (Box 16.3).[1]

ASSESSING THE PATIENT

Patient assessment is best facilitated by the ABCDE methodology (Box 16.4).

PRIMARY TRANSFER AND HANDOVER TO THE TRAUMA TEAM

Transfer modality from the accident scene will be decided by patients' clinical condition and the locality. Stabilization and safety of the patient prior to transfer are vital, and likewise for secondary transfer.

Clear and concise documentation will aid the hospital team to evaluate and treat the patient. On arrival, the questions asked by the trauma team will be dictated by the primary and secondary survey system.

CARE AND TRANSPORTATION OF THE CRITICALLY ILL PATIENT

BACKGROUND

Perioperative practitioners will often be involved in the management of the critically ill, both inside and outside the operating theatre.

Policy initiatives by the UK government[11–13] have afforded perioperative practice a real opportunity by providing a framework to extend the skills of practitioners into areas that can truly challenge the care delivery system. Theatre units have provided the key as flexible extensions to critical care when there have been increased demands on ITU beds[14] – a recognition of the skills of perioperative staff. Evidence also suggests that there is an increasing need for critical care skills on the wards,[15,16] and the development of critical care outreach teams, which may include theatre practitioners, to prevent intensive care admissions is one strategy that has been advocated.[17,18]

The reasons for referral of a critically ill patient can be many:

- Stabilization of patients from ward/A&E departments
- Lack of intensive care beds within the hospital
- Transfer of critically ill patients from theatre, wards, A&E to radiology and diagnostic units
- Transfer to specialist hospitals, such as neurosurgical, cardiac and paediatric units
- Postsurgical patients, not previously identified as requiring critical care.

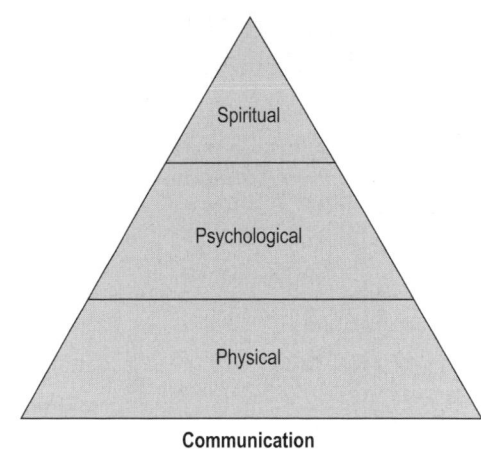

Figure 16.3   Components of care.

NATIONAL AND LOCAL ORGANIZATION OF CRITICAL CARE

In the UK intensive care beds comprise 1–2% of total bed numbers, costing the NHS £0.7 billion per year, with a yearly cost increase of 5–10%.[18] During periods of peak demand, access can be problematic and other hospitals' critical care units are needed to take patients. Critical care organization in the UK is on a national basis. Hospitals, including those in the private sector, have been organized on a regional basis into dependant critical care groups. The aim is for interdependence of hospitals in the demands placed upon them by the critically ill, including safe and effective transfer of patients to available critical care beds and specialist units. Central to the concept of 'critical care without walls' is the role and function of nurses and allied health professionals in the care of these patients.[17]

Intensive care units are staffed with anaesthetists and physicians with a special interest in intensive care, in most cases providing 24-hour cover with junior medical staff. The patient is supported by a specialist nursing team on a one-to-one basis, although for those not requiring ventilatory support, as on high-dependency units, this ratio is 1:2. If patients are ventilated in the operating room or elsewhere in the hospital this ratio must remain at 1:1 with senior anaesthetic support. Supporting this are critical care outreach teams, preventing ITU admissions and training and educating medical and nursing staff on the practicalities of critical care management at ward level. Physiotherapists and other allied health professionals are also involved in the care of these patients.

PRINCIPLES OF NURSING THE CRITICAL CARE PATIENT

The fundamentals of care for all patients remain the same (Fig. 16.3), but the tools and knowledge may vary.

Central to the role of managing physical, psychological and spiritual care are the communication needs of the patients and their families. The critical care patient may require a dynamic care process where needs are addressed at different levels during treatment. These patients often require significant support owing to the range of clinical conditions that they present with. In most cases these patients have dysfunction or failure of one or more organs, requiring intensive monitoring, mechanical and pharmacological support, in addition to complex psychological and spiritual needs.

PHYSICAL CARE AND MONITORING

Monitoring may vary according to the patient's individual needs and system dysfunction. Typically the following systems may be monitored:

- Cardiac and haemodynamic:
  - Non-invasive blood pressure (NIBP)
  - Invasive blood pressure monitoring via arterial line
  - Central venous pressure monitoring
  - Cardiac function via Swann-Ganz catheter and oesophageal Doppler
  - ECG (3-, 5- and 12-lead)

- Respiratory:
  - Respiratory rate (both on and off ventilatory support)
  - Oxygen level
  - Oxygen saturations via pulse oximetry
  - Tidal volume, minute volume and airway pressure
  - Ventilatory mode
  - Arterial blood gas analysis
- Renal and fluid balance:
  - Fluid input
  - Output from urinary catheter, nasogastric tube and wound drains
  - Biochemical testing
- Neurological:
  - Sedation level
  - Neurological activity
  - Cerebral perfusion pressure and intracranial pressure monitoring in specialized circumstances.

All monitoring information is recorded and documented on specialist observation charts: these will show trends and allow further treatment decisions to be made.

As well as mechanical and pharmacological support, other interventions are required to support organ function, including good respiratory care to prevent long-term problems due to tracheal intubation and mechanical ventilation. Complications such as barotrauma from high inflation pressure and tidal volumes, or retention of secretions may cause collapse/consolidation of the lung. This may lead to ventilation-perfusion mismatching of the whole or part of the lung. Therefore, during ventilation tracheal suction, monitoring of secretions for colour and purulency, humidification and warming of gases will combat these effects. Access to physiotherapy support is also vital in maintaining good respiratory function.

Nutritional support of the critical care patient is vital, because of their inability to maintain adequate nutritional input. Nasogastric or enteral feeding should be considered for those patients ventilated for more than 48 hours, with specialist input from pharmacy for those with bowel injury/insufficiency, who may require intravenous nutrition (total parental nutrition).

Immobility produces effects upon the respiratory, cardiovascular and renal systems, as well as causing muscle wasting and reduction in bone density. It also reduces peripheral perfusion owing to the action of vasoactive drugs and the clinical condition, increasing the risk of pressure sores. Pressure sores can be prevented by identifying at-risk patients and obtaining specialist tissue viability advice regarding bed type, repositioning the patient, and regular inspection of susceptible areas every 4 hours.

Eye care can often be missed in the immediate management of the critical care patient; however, when the patient is sedated the lack of corneal reflex and inability to close the eye can lead to corneal drying, infection and keratosis. These conditions can lead to long-term problems, including permanent visual field loss. Artificial tears, lubricating ointments and non-adherent occlusive dressings can all be employed to reduce the level of complications.

PSYCHOLOGICAL AND SPIRITUAL CARE

Care of the critically ill is a complete holistic process, focusing on the needs of the patient and their family, and it is important that the patient's psychological and spiritual needs are addressed. Psychological disturbances associated with critical care are common. 'Intensive care psychosis' or acute anxiety disorder may arise from the disorientating environment of the ITU, causing agitation, anxiety, confusion and hallucinations. Clinical conditions such as sepsis or head injury, and concurrent drug therapy, may also contribute. These effects can continue long after discharge from critical care.[19] Effective management should concentrate on controlling normal circadian rhythms with the use of natural and artificial light, surrounding the patient with familiar objects and stimuli, and constant support and explanation of the environment and care being delivered. Family and cultural issues should also be addressed to ensure continuity with their normal lives, feelings and beliefs.

DEALING WITH COMPLEX CLINICAL, ETHICAL AND MORAL DILEMMAS

The development of intensive care has allowed many patients to have more complex treatment. With this innovation there is an extension to the ethical and moral dilemmas faced when caring for these patients. Intensive care is a process of supporting organ systems that does not necessarily offer a cure, and in many cases can prolong the process of dying.[20] Issues such as withdrawal of treatment and organ donation are commonly faced in critical care.[21] Specialist advice and management are required when dealing with relatives if the decision is made to withdraw treatment, the timing of such withdrawal, and the actual process of withdrawal. Support must be made available to those caring for patients in such cases.

PRINCIPLES OF SAFE SECONDARY TRANSFER OF THE CRITICAL CARE PATIENT

The level of interhospital transfers in the UK has been estimated at 11 000 per year[22] and will continue to rise because of the continued centralization of specialist services. Transport between theatre, intensive care unit, imaging departments for MRI and CT, and secondary interhospital transfers is an area of practice where perioperative practitioners are often involved. The principles of transfer of any critical care patient are broadly similar (Box 16.5). All acute hospitals must have systems to resuscitate, optimize and transport these patients. The organization of transportation between hospitals is subject to the dependant networks described earlier, so that unless clinically indicated otherwise (i.e. paediatric or neurosurgical transfer), transfer distances are kept to a minimum.

Both types of transfer have been associated with increased morbidity and mortality,[23,24] and have often been performed by staff with little or no experience of these complex clinical situations. In recent years the management of these patients has been heavily scrutinized and comprehensive standards and guidelines produced by the Intensive Care Society,[25] guidelines for paediatric transfers[26] and neurosurgical/head injuries are also available.[27]

Box 16.5   Principles of safe transfer of critical care patients[28]

- Experienced staff
- Appropriate equipment and vehicle
- Full assessment and investigation
- Extensive monitoring
- Careful stabilization of patient
- Reassessment
- Continuing care during transfer
- Direct handover
- Documentation and audit

MODALITY OF TRANSPORT

The UK experience of interhospital transfer primarily involves a land-based ambulance, with either paramedic or technician crews supported by a doctor (anaesthetist) and theatre practitioner, ITU or A&E nurse. However, because of the large numbers of transfers, dedicated transfer ambulances, where particular attention is paid to equipment specification and design, with reference to the safety and comfort of patients and staff, have been identified as ideal (Fig. 16.4).

The use of aeromedical transport is common in Europe, Australia and the United States, but has only been introduced into the UK over the last decade. The majority of UK aeromedical units are funded by charitable donations, or more recently joint police and emergency air support units have been created (Fig. 16.5).

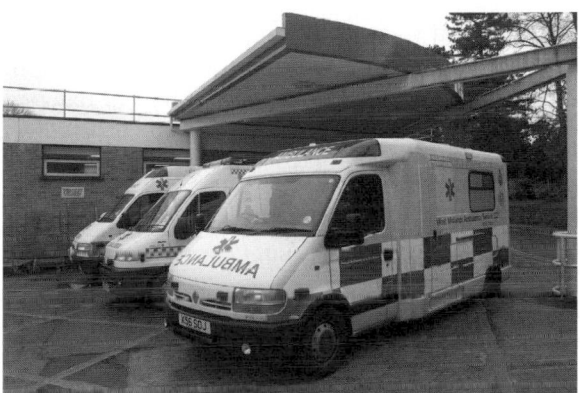

Figure 16.4   Dedicated transfer ambulance.

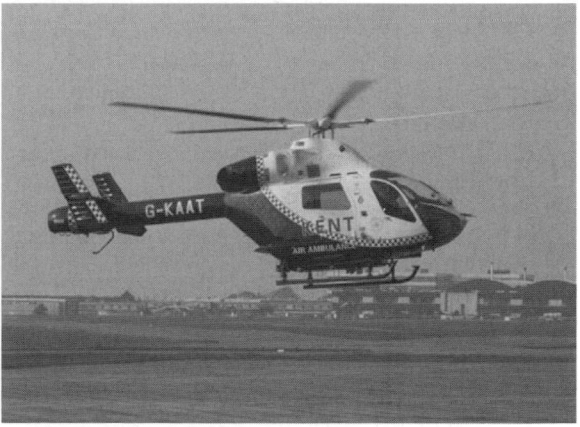

Figure 16.5   Joint police/aeromedical helicopter. (Reproduced with permission from Medical Aviation Services Ltd, Gloucester)

Aeromedical transport can be via helicopter or fixed-wing aircraft. Helicopters are favoured for short transfers (<250 miles), remote locations without airstrips, and built-up areas. Fixed-wing aircraft are more suited to long-distance transfers (>250 miles) with airstrip support. There are several advantages of this mode of transport:

- Speed: modern helicopters routinely used in medical emergencies are capable of speeds in excess of 150 mph, combined with the ability to move point to point.
- Accessibility: vertical take-off and landing capabilities permit evacuation of patients from areas inaccessible to other vehicles.
- Specialized personnel and technology: aeromedical services are for the most part based at tertiary care centres and are staffed with highly skilled and trained personnel, such as the London-based HEMS service.

Aeromedical transfer of patients requires detailed knowledge of aviation medicine and the implications for care, in particular attention to oxygenation and changes in partial pressure of gases at altitude, deceleration and acceleration, noise, vibration, and the potential for hypothermia. Practical consideration must be given to managing care in the confined environment of an aircraft cabin (Fig. 16.6).

STAFF AND RESOURCES

Guidelines from the Intensive Care Society[25] state that in addition to the emergency medical team crew (either ambulance or aeromedical unit) critical care patients should be accompanied by two transfer staff, one of whom should be a medical practitioner with experience in transfer care or intensive care/anaesthesia. The second should be a suitably experienced nurse (ITU, theatre or A&E) or paramedic. Both should be fully versed in equipment use and procedures to manage resuscitation, airway management, ventilation and organ support, and hold Advanced Cardiac Life Support qualification.

EQUIPMENT AND MONITORING

Ideally all equipment used should be standardized between hospitals and the ambulance service. The equipment should be light, compact, user friendly and easy to clean and disinfect. Battery-powered equipment should allow 2 hours of continuous use, with spare batteries being carried by the team. The equipment should be stored and maintained for transfer purposes only and be accessible in an emergency. The following equipment is vital (Fig. 16.7):

- Portable monitor – a clear backlit display (for low-light situations), able to monitor electrocardiogram, non-invasive blood pressure, saturations, arterial invasive blood pressure, central venous pressure and temperature. capnography for monitoring end-tidal CO_2 is vital for head-injured patients. The monitor should have an alarm system.

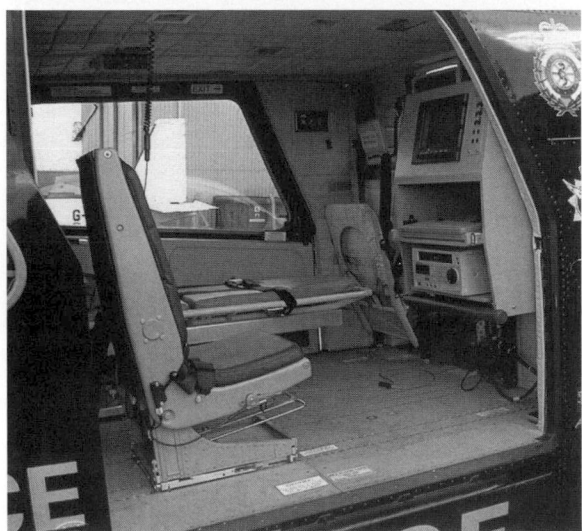

Figure 16.6 Cabin of emergency air ambulance. (Reproduced with permission from Medical Aviation Services Ltd, Gloucester)

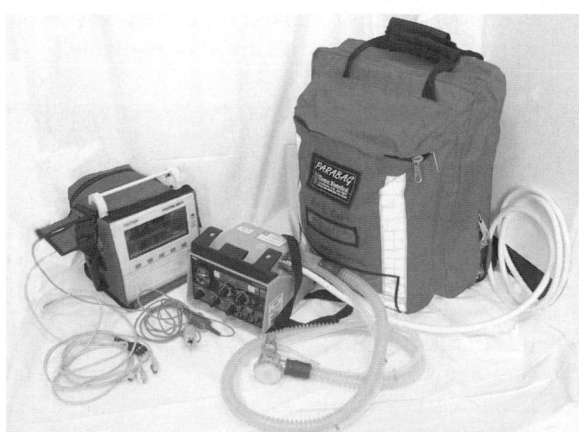

Figure 16.7 Equipment used during transfer of critical care patients.

- Syringe drivers for drug administration.
- Portable ventilator, often gas driven from a portable oxygen cylinder, that allows changes to be made to oxygen concentration, inspiratory: expiratory (I:E) ratio, respiratory rate and tidal volume. The ventilator should allow positive end-expiratory pressure (PEEP) to be added, and also monitor respiratory function, including high airway pressures.
- Transfer equipment bag, which includes a variety of airway equipment, cannulation, IV equipment, and emergency and transfer drugs.
- Mobile phone for transfer team to maintain contact with admitting hospital.
- Warm and comfortable clothing for the transfer team.

TRANSFER CARE

It is important that the decision to transport a critically ill patient is made with a full understanding of the clinical condition, its urgency, the timing of when it should take place, and the availability of staff and equipment. In many cases staff will have to be relocated from other duties, which may often affect inpatient work.

The decision to transfer will often be made at consultant level, depending on the clinical specialty. It is important that the appropriate specialist in the receiving hospital has had adequate clinical information regarding the patient and that a team is available to take over the care of the patient; for example, an intubated post cardiac arrest patient will need not only intensive care referral, but also physician referral. These details should be clearly written in the transfer notes.

PRETRANSFER PREPARATION

Detailed preparation prior to transfer is vital to prevent complications. In many cases the transfer team may not have been directly involved with the clinical situation and should take time to familiarize themselves with the patient's condition, drug therapy, investigations performed and the results, social and family issues, and the details of the receiving hospital. All of these checks must be made during a thorough assessment of the patient. Prior to any transfer, clinical optimization must be achieved: a modified trauma protocol ABCDE is a useful guide for assessing condition. The questions asked will vary according to clinical condition and the reason for transfer:

- A – Airway maintenance, with care and control of a possible injury to the cervical spine
  - Is the airway controlled?
  - What method has been used?
  - Is the airway likely to deteriorate during transfer?
  - Is the cervical spine stable?
- B – Breathing control or support
  - Is there good gas exchange?
  - Have PaO_2, $PaCO_2$ been measured via arterial blood gas?
  - What oxygen level is needed to support the above?
  - Does the patient need sedation, ventilation or paralysis?
  - What type of ventilation/pressure support is required?
- C – Circulation control and support
  - Is the patient haemodynamically stable?
  - Perfusion status assessed (urine output)?
  - Blood loss vs. fluid replaced?
  - Inotropes utilized?
- D – Disability
  - Neurologically stable (AVPU scale, Glasgow Coma Scores)?
  - Other injuries (chest, long bones, etc.)?
  - Comorbid condition prior to injury/illness?
  - Mode of analgesia?
- E – Exposure
  - Is the patient hypothermic?
  - Will this be exacerbated during transfer?

Immediately prior to transfer the practical considerations of transfer should be addressed:

- Ambulance transfer team sent for?
  - Land support required, such as police escort?
- Equipment checked?
  - Oxygen?
  - Drugs?
  - Batteries?
- Case notes, investigations (chest X-ray, MRI, etc.) collated?
- Transfer arrangements confirmed? Including:
  - Hospital?
  - Admitting ITU/ward/theatre?
  - Admitting consultants?
  - Directions to the above?
  - Time of departure?

– Estimated transfer time?
– Telephone numbers?
• Team members familiar with above?
• Family and relatives informed of transfer arrangements?
– Advise of admitting hospital, ward?
– Contact telephone numbers?
– Estimated transfer time?
– Update on clinical condition?
• Clinical condition reassessed?
• Transfer documentation started?

TRANSFER AND HANDOVER

The transfer conditions should aim to maintain the optimized condition of the patient and protect their safety. Monitoring of the patients' condition and documenting the information is vital, as this will highlight changes in clinical condition and allow remedial action to be taken. The patient should be secured in the vehicle or aircraft, and all equipment be secure and accessible. Equipment should not be rested on the patient's extremities and a check should be made to ensure cables and IV lines are not trapped against their skin. If the clinical condition of the patient deteriorates during transfer, the admitting hospital should be informed via phone or radio and alternative arrangements made, such as diverting to a closer hospital. If an immediate emergency occurs, then the ambulance may be stopped so that corrective measures can be taken and then driven directly to the nearest hospital.

It is important that on arrival at the admitting hospital, immediate access to the ITU/ward or theatre is given. The admitting team should be present and an immediate clinical assessment made to identify any changes that have taken place since departure. The transfer team should give a comprehensive history of the presenting condition, past medical history, drug history and current drug therapy, optimization that has taken place, clinical procedures performed, results of any investigations, and details of relatives' transport arrangements.

GENERIC CARE FOR PATIENTS REQUIRING SURGICAL TREATMENT OUTSIDE THE OPERATING THEATRE

The next section will focus on the delivery of care to patients who require surgery outside the operating theatre, but within the acute hospital. In these circumstances generic principles of perioperative care, such as preassessment (see Ch. 10), selection for day procedures (see Ch. 14), and information and consent (see Chs 1 and 3), are described in this book. However, more specific care for those patients having diagnostic and interventional radiological and endoscopic procedures will be detailed in this chapter.

SEDATION AND ANALGESIA OUTSIDE THE OPERATING THEATRE

Endoscopy and interventional radiological procedures can be uncomfortable, and it is routine to use sedation and analgesia to control anxiety and pain during the examination. The 1990s saw a re-examination of the efficacy and safety of sedation in adults, and more specifically with endoscopic procedures, where a high mortality rate was highlighted,[29] and recommendations have been made to improve the safety of sedation techniques.[30–32]

Sedation in any clinical scenario carries with it the risk of loss of consciousness. Sedation has been defined as a technique in which the use of a drug or drugs produces a state of depression of the central nervous system, enabling treatment to be carried out, but during which communication is maintained such that the patient will respond to commands.[30]

It is important to be aware that sedatives and anxiolytics such as benzodiazepines do not have any analgesic qualities, and should not be given as such. Benzodiazepines have long half-lives and so should be administered orally or intravenously, titrated to the patient, which will produce the required level of sedation. The use of polypharmacy, with adjunct analgesics, which work synergistically on the cardiovascular and respiratory systems,[33] can cause a significant reduction in safety between sedation and anaesthesia, where the patient will lose consciousness. A strategy should be developed to control pain as it occurs during the procedure, or in those cases where pain may be inevitable then the opioid is administered first and time given for it to take effect, and then a sedative administered.

Patient safety remains the paramount concern with sedation, and the reversal agent for benzodiazepines – flumazenil – must be available. The half-life of flumazenil is shorter than that of benzodiazepines, which means that further incremental doses may be administered. The patient should remain fully monitored throughout this period.

In the case of paediatric patients requiring sedation for endoscopic and radiological procedures, it is advocated that a general anaesthetic is given to ensure that full cardiorespiratory assessment and monitoring can be maintained. Complications are unpredictable in this patient group and do not appear to be predictable on age, weight or tolerance of the procedure.[34]

MONITORING

Consistent evidence has promoted better standards of monitoring during sedation, as predominately cardiorespiratory complications can occur. Monitoring will not prevent complications occurring during the procedure, but it will alert practitioners to potentially life-threatening problems, earlier. There are risk factors that predispose patients to hypoxaemia, such as old age, obesity, emergency procedures and previous cardiovascular (CVS) and respiratory (RS) comorbidity.[35] However, circulatory changes are largely unpredictable and therefore better standards of monitoring will improve safety for patients.

Established clinical guidelines for standards of monitoring during anaesthesia and recovery[36] stipulate that during sedation techniques the following are mandatory:

- Pulse oximetry
- Non-invasive blood pressure monitoring
- ECG.

Further recommendations are made to ensure that monitoring is continued into the recovery period, until the patient is sufficiently recovered from the effects of the drugs.

CARE OF THE PATIENT DURING SURGERY

The patient may be brought to the department either on a trolley or walking. As with all surgery, preprocedure checks (see Chs 11, 12) should be made prior to the delivery of any sedation or analgesic drug. The patient is then made comfortable on the trolley or X-ray table. Monitoring equipment is set up and baseline observations are taken. If required, the patient is then cannulated with a narrow-gauge cannula (20 G) or butterfly needle; in an emergency,

or in a patient with a significant risk of large blood loss, two large-bore cannulae (16 G) for rapid infusion of intravenous fluid should be inserted. The patient is then positioned to start the procedure; for most endoscopic procedures this will be in the lateral position. The perioperative practitioner positions themselves at the head end of the trolley, where they will be able to support the patient, maintain the airway and administer oxygen via a nasal cannula, assist in the delivery of drugs and monitor clinical condition. The care of the patient is the responsibility of the team, although the interventionist (physician, surgeon, radiologist or nurse endoscopist) remains responsible for the direction of the team during the procedure.

The ancillary or support practitioner supports the team, documenting care, providing technical support with radiological and imaging equipment, and recording and labelling any specimens taken during the procedure.

RECOVERY AND DISCHARGE

Following completion of the procedure the patient is moved to the recovery area, which in many units will also be the preprocedure area (Fig. 16.8). The trolley bays require monitoring points, oxygen and suction. The privacy and dignity of patients recovering from sedation should be maintained, with immediate access to trained recovery practitioners.

Criteria for those patients who may be managed and discharged as a day procedure are detailed in Chapter 14. In terms of discharge from specialized areas the following are useful in assessing readiness for discharge:

- Stable observations for at least 1 hour since procedure, in line with age, comorbid condition and preprocedure observations.
- The patient must be able to orientate themselves in person, place and time; keep down oral fluids; dress themselves; walk without assistance, at or near preoperative level.
- The patient must not have more than minimal nausea and vomiting, that cannot be controlled with oral antiemetics; excessive pain; bleeding, from catheter site, oesophagus or rectum following the procedure.

An organizational criterion for discharge also examines postprocedure information, and any follow-up arrangements that need to be made before leaving the unit.

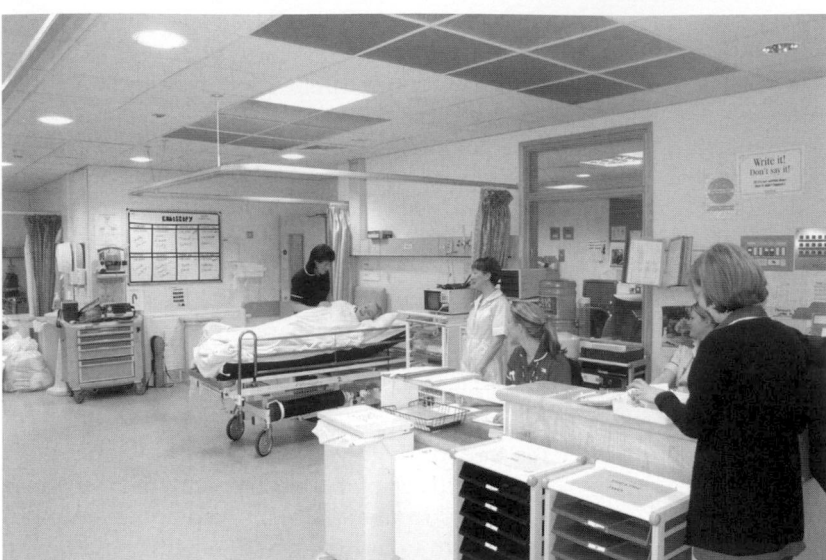

Figure 16.8 The recovery area.

CARE OF THE PATIENT IN THE RADIOLOGY DEPARTMENT

BACKGROUND

Radiology has seen many recent advances in both interventional and diagnostic techniques.[37] In terms of interventional work, these procedures have allowed patients previously denied surgery, because of the risks, to have access to treatment. Procedures are often completed under sedation or local anaesthetic and utilize percutaneous techniques that involve a minimal surgical insult to the patient. Diagnostic procedures such as computed tomography (CT) and magnetic resonance imaging (MRI) are now performed as routine on a wide range of patients, both acutely and critically ill.

Many radiology departments may not have been designed specifically for anaesthesia and interventional procedures, and so such equipment competes with large radiological gantries, providing less than optimal conditions. Equipment can be used infrequently or differ greatly from that in the operating theatre, and particular attention must be paid to its maintenance and patient safety. In departments with a large interventional workload, purpose-designed suites are commonplace, the organization of such units being similar to those of the theatre department. The radiology practitioners will be dedicated to the unit, providing pre-, intra- and postoperative care for patients.

Room design for both diagnostic and interventional radiology must maintain safe standards of care for all patients, whether they require sedation or not. It is essential that the rooms have direct access to the following:

- Piped oxygen
- High-pressure suction
- Intercom and telephone
- Emergency alert system
- Monitoring (ECG, SpO_2 and NIBP)
- Emergency resuscitation equipment
- Airway management equipment.

It is important that access to the patient is not limited, including head and chest for emergency situations.

DIAGNOSTIC RADIOLOGY

Computed tomography (CT)

The CT scan is a widely used radiological procedure for examination of the entire body. The introduction of spiral CT scanning has reduced scan times and radiation exposure.[38] The advent of digital technology allows processing for three-dimensional imaging, giving greater diagnostic flexibility. Radiation levels that a patient may be exposed to during CT can be high, particularly with multiple scans – a typical dose with abdominal CT is 10 mS-1, or the equivalent of 500 chest X-rays or 3.3 years of background radiation.

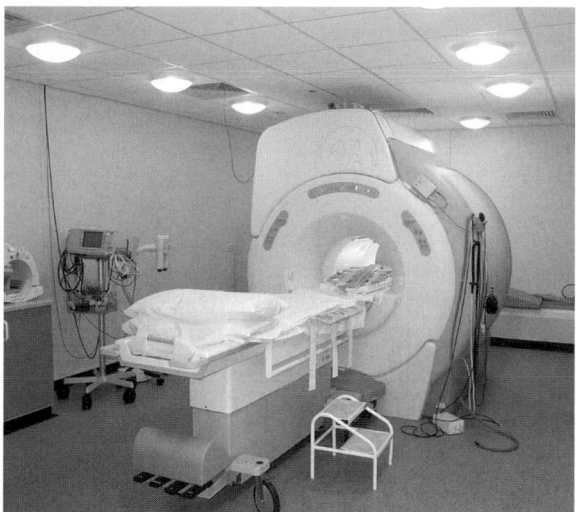

Figure 16.9   MRI scanner.

Managing a patient having a CT scan can be problematic because of the poor access: the scanning cylinder can be as small as 55 cm wide, causing feelings of claustrophobia for awake patients, and where patients are sedated or anaesthetized the confined space will pose problems for airway access and monitoring. Although the procedures are invariably short (<20 minutes) the radiation risk to the anaesthetic team can be high, and remote monitoring is advisable. The CT scan may be far from other support within the hospital, and those in attendance should be familiar with emergency equipment and its location.

Magnetic resonance imaging (MRI)

MRI uses magnetic energy and radio waves to create cross-sectional images of the body or organ under examination. The main component of most MR systems is a large cylindrical magnet (Fig. 16.9); more recent developments have seen C-shaped magnets and other types of open design. The strength of the system's magnetic field is measured in metric units called Tesla. Most of the cylindrical magnets have strengths between 0.5 and 1.5 Tesla, and open or C-shaped magnets have a magnetic strength between 0.01 and 0.35 Tesla. The development in technology and software design for MRI has seen a significant increase in its use, both diagnostically and therapeutically. Breath-hold scanning techniques, with both static and moving images, have allowed detailed examination of patients with structural heart disease and other previously difficult imaging scenarios, allowing a greater degree of clinical impact.

The practical considerations of managing a patient in an MRI scanner are similar to those for CT scanning. However, because of the large magnetic force generated by the MR unit, special consideration must be given to the type of support equipment needed.

Monitoring equipment is prone to electromagnetic interference, and the insulation of the ECG leads must be checked, leads being placed close together and in the same plane as the magnet to prevent voltage being induced into the cable, potentially causing burns. Pulse oximeters can be affected in the same way, and parts (e.g. the spring clip) should be non-ferrous and moved as far away as possible from the site of investigation. Blood pressure can be managed from an automated inflation cuff system, although invasive blood pressure monitoring is relatively unaffected.

Anaesthetic machines should be non-ferrous, with particular attention paid to mechanical ventilators. Although technologically challenging, this is achievable.[39] The noise generated by the MR machine can be a risk for both patients and staff, and protection should be given to both.

Metallic implants can be subjected to magnetic forces that can disturb their position, therefore identification of implants during preassessment is vital (Box 16.6).

Although metallic cardiac valve replacements are placed under magnetic forces during MR scanning, these are not significant enough to cause physiological effects.[40]

Managing claustrophobia during scanning

Five to ten percent of patients may suffer claustrophobic feelings during MR and CT scanning.[40] The cause is multifactorial, for example the restrictive dimensions of the scanner, the duration of the scan (MR can take more than 40 minutes), the noise generated by the machine, and the ambient conditions, including temperature and light. A plan of care should aim to minimize conditions of isolation and control ambient conditions, including:

- Preprocedure explanation
- Communication (physical or verbal contact during scan)
- Headphones and music
- Prone position, looking ahead and through scanner
- Mirrors to maintain eye contact with radiology practitioners
- Creative use of light, in room and through scanner
- Use of C-shaped or open design MR scanners.

INTERVENTIONAL RADIOLOGY

Interventional radiology is an expanding field of practice which can be useful for both diagnosis and treatment of a broad range of clinical conditions. Interventional radiology suites should be specifically designed for the purpose, with space for both operative equipment and the radiological fluoroscopy gantry (Fig. 16.10).

The principles of sterility as applied to the operating theatre must be maintained and emergency equipment should be available and accessible.

Clinical applications of interventional vascular radiology

The availability of smaller luminal and transluminal devices has broadened the range of disorders treatable using this method, and there has therefore been an increase in the use of interventional vascular radiology over the last 20 years.

Diagnostic angiography

Angiography is performed specifically to image and diagnose diseases of the blood vessels, including coronary, hepatic, pulmonary, renal and visceral arteries. Following an injection of local anaesthetic into the tissue surrounding the femoral or brachial region, using a Seldinger technique a catheter is inserted into the vein or artery. The catheter is moved by the radiologist into position so that a contrast medium can be injected into the blood, and X-ray interpretation of the flow carried out. This is usually performed under fluoroscopy, but more recently newer technologies, such as digital subtraction, MR and CT, have been used to enhance imaging.

Percutaneous transluminal angioplasty and stent procedures

The use of diagnostic angiography has allowed greater flexibility in the treatment of vascular disease. Coronary artery interventions such as balloon dilatation (percutaneous transluminal coronary angioplasty (PTCA)) of atheromatous plaques and stenosis are commonplace. With extensive or recurrent lesions, stents can be placed to maintain vessel patency. Similar techniques are utilized for other arterial lesions, including the renal artery, aortoiliac, femoral, popliteal and distal vessels in lower limb ischaemia.

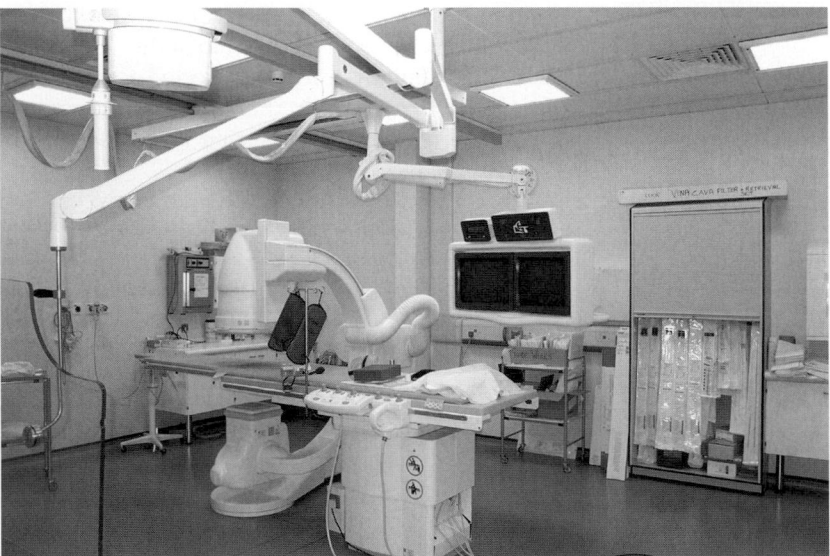

Figure 16.10   Interventional radiology suite.

Embolization and thrombolysis

The access permitted by angiography to the greater and lesser vessels has seen an increased interest in embolization techniques that aim to reduce or occlude blood flow to one or more vessels. This can be a permanent or an intermittent treatment that controls or prevents abnormal bleeding via a catheter and agent (gelatin foams, polyvinyl alcohol, metal coils and sclerosing agents) injected into the vessel. Thrombolysis involves a thrombolytic substance (streptokinase or urokinase) being administered directly into the obstructed part of the vessel. This provides a high local concentration and a reduced systemic load of the thrombolytic agent.

Clinical applications of non–vascular interventional radiology

Percutaneous transhepatic cholangiography (PTC)
Percutaneous transhepatic cholangiography is performed via a midaxillary puncture just above the inferolateral edge of the liver. The biliary tract is then filled, through a needle or a catheter introduced into the liver. This method can visualize any stenosis, compression, obstruction or other filling defect, and can also be used for papillectomy or drain placement.

Nephrostomy and percutaneous nephrolithotomy Obstructive uropathy, caused by small kidney stones, can be treated by nephrostomy, where a thin needle is placed into the obstructed renal pelvis under ultrasound or fluoroscopic guidance. When urine backflow is obtained, indicating correct needle position, contrast medium is injected to indicate the size and location of the obstruction. A guide wire can then be advanced into the ureter and a drainage tube advanced into the obstructed system over the wire. The tube is either advanced into the bladder past the stone or left in place above the obstruction, so the urine flows out into a collection bag.

Percutaneous nephrolithotomy is used to extract larger kidney stones. The patient usually requires a general anaesthetic, and is placed in the prone position. An incision is made below the rib line on the affected side and the stone removed with a minimally invasive technique, using a rigid endoscope and stone extraction forceps. In most cases fibreoptic endoscopic examination of the renal pelvis is completed after stone extraction.

Contrast medium

Contrast medium is an essential tool to many imaging procedures, as it increases the image contrast of anatomical structures; media can be grouped as positive or negative. In general, positive contrast media are those with an increased absorption of X-rays and show up as white or light grey; negative media, which have less absorption, show up as dark grey. Contrast medium can be injected into veins and arteries for vascular and renal imaging, or absorbed orally for enhanced abdominal/bowel images.

Intravascular contrast media are subdivided into low and high osmolar iodinated compounds. The level of toxicity for both is low, although both have known interactions and complications, but low osmolar compounds have reduced local and systemic reactions. The effect on organ systems is widely reported and can be summarized as follows:

Cardiovascular

- Venous injection can cause arm pain, erythema and swelling
- Arterial injection can cause irritation, spasm and endothelial damage
- Soft tissue extravasation, leading to cellulites
- Cardiovascular effect resulting in action upon myocardium, conduction tissue, pulmonary and peripheral vasculature
- Vasodilatation, hypotension, bradycardia and electrophysiological changes, including VF, VT and asystole. Reduced LV function on direct intracardiac injection.

Renal

- Contrast media are almost entirely eliminated by glomerular filtration
- Change in renal blood flow occurs, initially a small transitory increase, followed by several hours of reduced flow
- Contrast-induced renal injury can occur, damaging glomerular and tubular structures via hypoxia and toxicity.

Neurological, haematological and endocrine reactions have also been reported. Preassessment is vital to identify those patients at risk from complications. In particular, careful consideration must be given to the following:

- Renal insufficiency
- Diabetes – possible peripheral vascular and renal conditions
- Dehydration
- Drug idiosyncrasies – particularly cardiac and nephrotoxic

- Cardiac dysfunction, including arrhythmias, angina, recent myocardial infarction and pulmonary hypertension
- Patients who are generally debilitated, critically ill and haemodynamically unstable
- Previous contrast reactions
- Those undergoing multiple contrast injections.

The contrast medium used for MR scanning is primarily gadopentate dimeglumine (Gd-DTPA); this provides better imaging than iodinated compounds, with a reduced level of complications. As with most contrast media, reactions usually occur within 1 hour of delivery of the drug. With Gd-DTPA reactions such as headache, nausea and vomiting, local injection site burning and rash can be seen; these symptoms usually resolve within a few hours. Extravasation of Gd-DPTA causes pain, erythema and swelling at the injection site, with symptoms resolving within 1 week. Anaphylactic reactions are rare.

CARE OF THE PATIENT REQUIRING AN ENDOSCOPIC PROCEDURE

BACKGROUND AND DEVELOPMENTS IN ENDOSCOPY SERVICES

The UK has seen significant progress in the management of gastrointestinal disease in the last decade.[41] Central to this is the role of the endoscopy unit in diagnosing and treating gastrointestinal disease, where new technology coupled with increased knowledge has revolutionized care of this patient group. Over 800 000 endoscopic procedures are performed each year in the NHS, accounting for 12% of day case procedures at an annual cost of £50 million.[42,43]

Endoscopy services are seen as a central diagnostic and treatment tool for the management of a range of cancers.[12,44] Endoscopy will also play a crucial role in the development of treatment centres[12] providing open-access treatment for many patients.

Many endoscopy units are centralized within hospitals, complementing both inpatient and day unit services, with clinicians from both medicine and surgery utilizing the highly specialized facilities and trained practitioners. It is recognized that there is a need for expansion of specialized medical and nursing staff in endoscopy to fulfil future demands for this service.[45]

CLINICAL APPLICATIONS FOR ENDOSCOPY SERVICES

A diverse range of clinical procedures are performed in the endoscopy unit. Patients present from several sources, including primary care, outpatients and inpatient urgent, and emergencies. The common procedures and their indications are described below.

Oesophagogastroduodenoscopy (OGD)

An upper GI examination using a flexible endoscopic system is more commonly known as an oesophagogastroduodenoscopy, or OGD. This procedure is used as a diagnostic and treatment aid for problems found within the oesophagus, stomach, gastric sphincters and duodenum.

Indications:

- Evaluation of symptoms of persistent upper GI pain (dyspepsia), nausea and vomiting, difficulty in swallowing
- Upper GI bleeding
- Detection and diagnosis of peptic ulceration and carcinoma of the upper gastrointestinal tract
- Removal of ingested foreign bodies.

Colonoscopy and flexible sigmoidoscopy

Utilizing a longer endoscope, the flexible colonoscope allows visualization of the colonic lining, including examination of the sigmoid, descending, transverse and ascending colon. The colon, at approximately 150 cm in length, terminates at the ileocaecal junction.

Flexible sigmoidoscopy involves an examination of the rectum and distal sigmoid colon. The technique is similar to that of colonoscopy, although utilizing a shorter endoscope; it can also be called a limited colonoscopy. Indications for both examinations are:

- Change in bowel habit, including the addition of blood, mucus in the stool, diarrhoea and constipation
- Screening for patients with a significant family history of polyps and adenoma
- Abnormalities found during other imaging modalities (barium enema, CT and MRI)
- Follow-up examination after surgical treatment of known malignant disease
- Evaluation of diverticular disease

- Assessment and follow-up of inflammatory bowel disease
- Emergency investigation and treatment of obstruction, sigmoid volvulus.

Endoscopic retrograde cholangiopancreatography (ERCP)

ERCP is a specialized investigation using a side-viewing flexible endoscope under radiological image intensification. Injection of contrast medium is also used to visualize the ampulla of Vater to identify disorders of the pancreas, biliary tree, and ducts of the gallbladder.

Indications:

- Severe and persistent dyspepsia consistent with biliary or pancreatic disease
- To detect the cause of jaundice, such as structural disease of the biliary tree, gallstones, and carcinoma
- Therapeutic ERCP is used in stent placement, endoscopic papillotomy, and extraction of stones impacted in the cystic duct.

Endoscopic ultrasound

Endoscopic ultrasound is increasingly being used for high-resolution imaging of gastrointestinal pathology, and its role is advocated in both local and nodal staging of cancers of the oesophagus and stomach.[46,47] The technical development has relied upon imaging and radiology improvements, so that the ultrasound device can be placed in the tip of the endoscope. Endoscopic ultrasound can be performed in two planes, radial 360° or linear 20° and is used to examine mucosal and submucosal carcinomas.

ORGANIZATION OF ENDOSCOPIC SERVICES IN THE HOSPITAL

MANAGING PATIENT FLOW AND ACCURATE SCHEDULING

Increasing demands are being placed on endoscopy units, leading to significant delays in treatment. Modernization of endoscopy services to improve the patient's journey time may require a fundamental review of how resources are allocated and services organized. Such a review needs to examine the whole patient journey, from point of referral to discharge. Modernising Endoscopy Services, an NHS Modernisation Agency initiative, has examined many areas to improve the flow of patients through endoscopy units. It is recognized that endoscopy services are under-resourced, although key processes, such as homogeneous waiting lists (grouped by case complexity or type rather than by consultant), electronic referral systems and reduced care handovers, have been shown to improve patient flow in a timely and patient-centred way.[48]

Information technology can also play a major role in managing, scheduling and improving a patient's journey. Common data sets that work across the health community, such as electronic health records, reduce workload when gathering health-related information, reduce risk in managing patients' clinical information, integrate care, and improve clinical and operational outcomes.[49]

THE RECEPTION AREA

It is recognized that endoscopy facilities should be solely dedicated to the purpose, although many units will have been developed within existing hospital areas. In many cases endoscopy and day unit facilities have been combined, because of the similarities of patient flow.

It has been identified that the patient's experience of endoscopy can be very distressing.[50] Therefore it is important that the design of the facility reflects an emphasis on promoting a pleasant and comfortable environment for both patients and their relatives.

In addition to the clinical facilities are non-clinical areas such as reception. Reception areas should be open, friendly, and utilize as much natural light and space as possible. There should be open access to administrative staff to gain information, but also screened areas for confidential consultations. The administrative staff should have access to IT terminals, scheduling systems and electronic health record (EHR) information. Toilet facilities, including those with disabled access and for families, are important. A clear and distinct separation should be maintained from clinical areas, as these are often busy and disorientating for many patients prior to their procedure. If possible, staff and delivery access should be separate from the public entrance.

THE ENDOSCOPY ROOM

The facilities within the endoscopy room itself should provide the team with all the instrumentation, equipment and drugs that could be required during the procedure. Preparation of the room and equipment by the endoscopy practitioners and ancillary staff prior to the procedure is fundamental to maintaining a safe environment. Preprocedure checks should be made of the following equipment:

- Tilting trolley
- Emergency drugs and resuscitation equipment
- Patient suction
- Oxygen delivery system
- Endoscopy trolley system, including light source, video processor, monitors and suction equipment
- Staff and environmental hazard equipment should be available, e.g. gloves, X-ray badges
- The endoscope
- Endoscopic accessories pertinent to the procedure.

The position of equipment in the endoscopy room should always be conducive to safety for both staff and patient, to allow full viewing of the patient, monitoring equipment and video information during the procedure. A typical set-up is shown in Figure 16.11.

THE MANAGEMENT OF ENDOSCOPY EQUIPMENT

Diagnostic and interventional endoscopy is an expensive hospital resource. It is important that such equipment is maintained and cared for in the appropriate environment.

CHANGES IN ENDOSCOPIC TECHNOLOGY

Traditional endoscopic technology has relied upon fibreoptics, which uses bundles of thin glass fibres to transmit light to and from the area under examination. These fibres use the principle of total internal reflection to transmit almost 100% of the visible light entering one end to the other. The orientation of fibres used in endoscopy has to be coherent, so that the spatial orientation of each one of the fibres is constant, thereby producing an accurate image. A traditional endoscope has one set of fibres to transmit light via a halogen or xenon light source, and another set to transmit reflected light out to the eye of the operator.

The addition of video links to high-definition monitors has allowed the endoscope to be developed as a teaching tool and improved operator comfort. The development of digital technology has vastly improved imaging for endoscopic examinations. The introduction of charge coupled devices (CCDs), placed at the tip of the endoscope and replacing the fibreoptic viewing bundle, can produce images of 450–850 000 pixels. CCD video allows digital storage, printing and manipulation of diagnostic and treatment information during the endoscopic examination, and has reduced the overall diameter of endoscopes.

Many manufacturers produce endoscopes, although the technical requirements of each are similar. Most endoscopic equipment, either CCD (Fig. 16.12) or direct-vision fibreoptic, has common features:

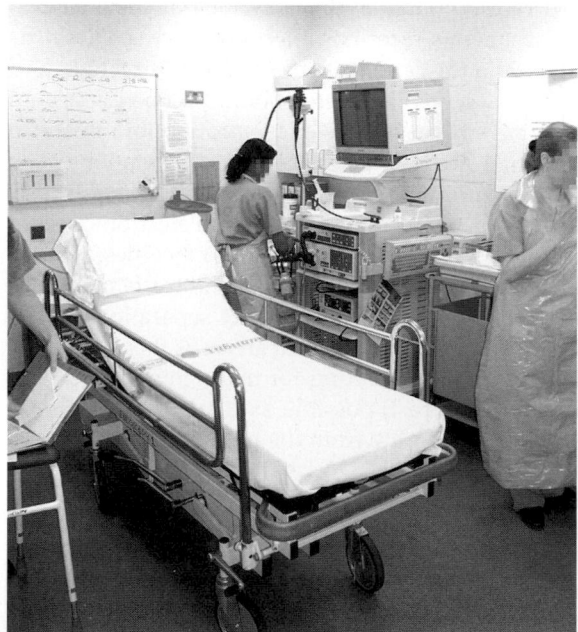

Figure 16.11   Organization of the endoscopy room.

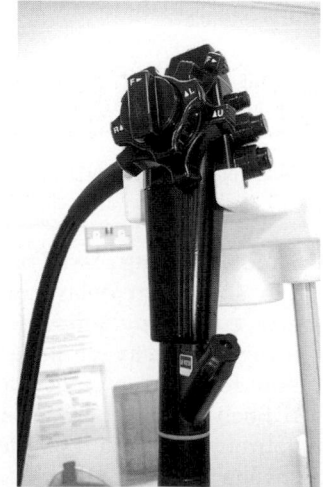

Figure 16.12   CCD endoscopic unit.

- Flexion and lateral angulation of the flexible tip through manipulation of wheels at the operator end
- Light feed, video or direct-viewing feed fibreoptics (Fig. 16.13)
- Combined air/water/suction channel
- Instrument channel for endodiagnostic and treatment accessories (e.g. brushes, biopsy forceps, stone baskets, snares).

Table 16.1 gives the technical specifications for each type of instrument.

Storage of endoscopes in a locked vertical cupboard ensures that the fibreoptic or electronic components are not damaged (Fig. 16.13). Appropriate policy and procedures must be established for the maintenance of endoscopy equipment through medical engineering departments and equipment manufacturers.

THE CLEANING AND DISINFECTION PROCESS

Gastrointestinal procedures carry the potential risk of pathogen transfer from patient to patient, unless adequate cleaning and disinfection procedures have been put in place. Bacterial and viral transfer can be eliminated through a thorough cleaning, disinfection and basic maintenance programme (Fig. 16.14). The first stage following an endoscopic procedure is the manual removal of organic debris, both externally and from the instrument and water/suction channels. This process should be used even when the endoscope is cleaned and disinfected with an automated scope washer, and also applies to endoscopic accessories.[51]

The use of automated scope washers (Fig. 16.15) has revolutionized the cleaning and disinfection process for endoscopes by reducing the risk of exposure to harmful disinfection solutions. The withdrawal of glutaraldehyde in May 2002 saw a rethink on the type of chemical disinfection process and preparation used. Current guidance from the British Society of Gastroenterologists (BSG) advocates the use of alternatives such as para-acetic acid, chlorine dioxide and superoxidized water. Chemical disinfection remains the only route available for flexible endoscopes, which are not suitable for steam or heat sterilization.

Automated scope washers are not without problems, and the Hospital Infection Society Working Party Report[51] identified the following issues that must be taken into account with their use:

- Availability of systems and compatibility problems with chemical disinfection products
- Training and education of staff to ensure endoscopes are cleaned and disinfected correctly
- Adequate policy exists for maintenance of equipment in line with manufacturers' recommendations
- Adequate rinse water filtration or sterilization takes place to ensure no recontamination of scopes after disinfection cycle
- Monitoring systems and records for disinfection process, rinse water and maintenance are in place.

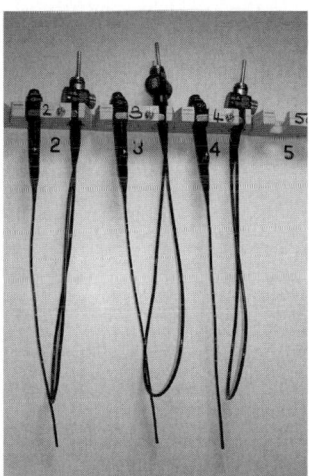

Figure 16.13   Storage of fibre optic and video endoscopes.

Table 16.1   Technical specifications of endoscopic instruments

Instrument	Field of view (°)	Angle of view (°)	Working length (cm)	Outer diameter (mm)
Gastroscope	120	0	90–105	5–11
Sigmoidoscope	140	0	70–80	13
Colonoscope	140	0	100–120	13
Choledocoscope	90	0	160–180	12
ERCP	80	5° Backward oblique	110–120	12
Ultrasound endoscope	20° linear 360° radial			

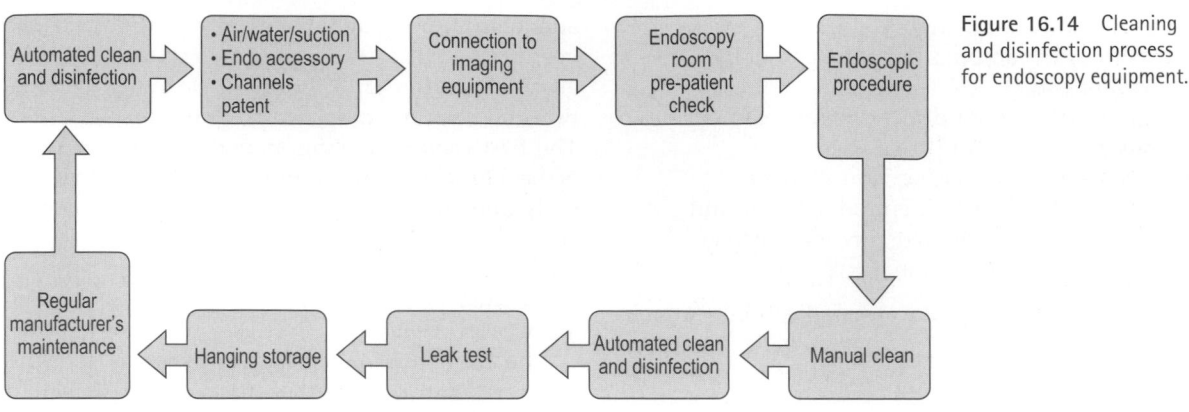

Figure 16.14   Cleaning and disinfection process for endoscopy equipment.

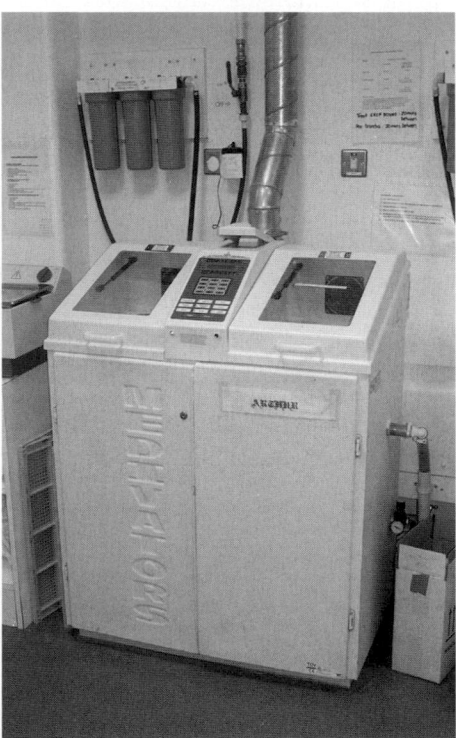

Figure 16.15   An automated endoscope washer.

DEVELOPING THE ROLE OF ENDOSCOPY PRACTITIONERS

THE NON-PHYSICIAN ENDOSCOPIST

There is a great deal of interest in developing the role of endoscopy practitioners to perform endoscopic examinations,[52] and such initiatives have been supported by both medical and nursing organizations. The BSG guidelines on nurse endoscopy are clear: that nurse endoscopists are to be trained to the same criteria and standards as medically trained endoscopists;[53] specifically, the ENB D05 Nurse Endoscopist Practitioner course has been designed to fulfil the needs of this developing role, and requires over 600 hours of study, including in-depth anatomy and physiology, with 150 supervised endoscopic examinations assessed by a lead medical clinician. Clinically the results of nurse endoscopy have been positive: published research has found that nurse endoscopists successfully identified all 'significant' pathology during sigmoidoscopy, and similar results have been found with colorectal screening.[54, 55]

CONCLUSION

This chapter demonstrates two important principles in perioperative practice. First is the diversity of skills required in caring for patients who may present in a variety of complex clinical situations, and this chapter provides a guide for the principles of care. Further study and experience would be required to care for patients in such specialized settings outside the operating room environment; a list of further reading is included to enhance understanding.

Second is the leading role that perioperative practitioners can have in the innovative delivery of care in a modern health economy. The transferability of skills from the perioperative environment to these specialist areas is clear and produces great clinical benefits, and coincides with a time when pressures are high to improve efficiency and productivity in health care.

References

1. Greaves I, Porter K, Ryan J. Trauma care manual. London: Arnold; 2001.
2. Coats T, Davies G. Prehospital care for road traffic casualties. BMJ 2002; 324: 1135–1138.
3. Wyatt J, Beard D, Gray A, et al. The time of death after trauma. BMJ 1995; 310: 1502.
4. Jenkins R, Griffiths S, Wylie I, et al. The prevention of suicide. BMJ 1994; 309: 886.
5. Thakore S, McGugan E, Morrison W. Emergency ambulance dispatch. Is there a case for triage? J R Soc Med 2002; 95: 126–129.
6. British Orthopaedic Association. The care of the severely injured patient in the United Kingdom – an urgent need for improvement. London: Br Ortho Assoc; 1997.
7. McGeehan D. Pre-hospital implications of the British Association and the Royal College of Surgeons trauma reports 1997: an alternative view. Pre-Hosp Immediate Care 1999; 3: 108–112.
8. Crouch R, Hodgetts T. Involvement of nurses in UK ambulance services. A national survey. Pre-Hosp Immediate Care 2000; 4: 64–67.
9. Moakes S, Kilner T. Nurses' understanding of their role as part of the mobile medical team and nursing team during a major incident. Pre-Hosp Immediate Care 2000; 5: 34–37.
10. Trinkey D. Trauma. Scientific American 1983; 249: 28–35.
11. Department of Health. Making a difference – strengthening the nursing, midwifery and health visiting contribution to health and healthcare. London: HMSO; 2000.
12. Department of Health. The NHS plan. London: HMSO; 2000.
13. Department of Health. Comprehensive critical care – a review of adult critical care. London: HMSO; 2000.
14. Ziser A, Alkobi M, Markovits R, et al. The postanaesthesia unit as a temporary admission location due to intensive care and ward overflow. Br J Anaesth 2002; 88: 577–579.
15. Smith GB, Poplett N. Knowledge of aspects of acute care in trainee doctors. Postgrad Med J 2002; 78: 335–338.
16. McQuillan P, Pilkington S, Allan A, et al. Confidential inquiry into quality of care before admission to intensive care. BMJ 1998; 316: 1853–1858.
17. Department of Health. The nursing contribution to the provision of comprehensive critical care for adults: a strategic programme for action. London: HMSO; 2002.
18. Audit Commission. Critical to success. London: Audit Commission; 1999.
19. Griffiths R, Jones C. Recovery from intensive care. BMJ 1999; 319: 427–429.
20. Winter B, Cohen S. Withdrawal of treatment. BMJ 1999; 319: 306–308.
21. Radford M. Unexpected perioperative death. Br J Anaesth Recover Nurs 2001; 2: 3.
22. MacKenzie P, Smith E, Wallace P. Transfer of adults between intensive care units in the United Kingdom: postal survey. BMJ 1997; 314: 1455.
23. Britto J, Nadel S, Maconochie I, et al. Morbidity and severity of illness during interhospital transfer: impact of a specialised paediatric retrieval team. BMJ 1995; 311: 836–839.
24. Cooper RM. Transfers within hospitals can be as risky as those between hospitals. BMJ 1996; 312: 120.
25. Intensive Care Society. Guidelines for the transport of the critically ill adult. London: ICS; 2002.
26. Paediatric Intensive Care Society. Standards for paediatric intensive care, including standards of practice for the transport of the critically ill child. Bishops Stortford: Salatore; 1996.
27. Neuroanaesthesia Society of Great Britain and Ireland and Association of Anaesthetists of Great Britain and Ireland. Recommendations for the transfer of patients with acute head injuries to neurosurgical units. London: AAGBI; 1996.
28. Wallace P, Ridley S. Transport of critically ill patients. BMJ 1999; 319: 368–371.
29. Quine MA, Bell GD, McCloy RF, et al. Prospective audit of upper gastrointestinal endoscopy in two regions of England: safety, staffing and sedation methods. Gut 1995; 36: 462–467.
30. British Society of Gastroenterologists. Guidelines for informed consent for endoscopic procedures. London: BSG; 1999.
31. Royal College of Surgeons of England. Commission on the provision of surgical services. Report of the working party on guidelines for sedation by non-anaesthetists. London, Royal College of Surgeons; 1993.
32. Royal College of Anaesthetists. Implementing and ensuring safe sedation practice for health care procedures in adults: report of an intercollegiate working party. London: Royal College of Anaesthetists; 2001.
33. Charlton JE. Monitoring and supplemental oxygen during endoscopy. BMJ 1995; 310: 886–887.
34. Stringer MD, McHugh PJ. Paediatric endoscopy should be carried out under general anaesthesia. BMJ 1995; 311: 452–453.
35. Yen D, Hu SC, Chen LS. Arterial oxygen desaturation during emergency non sedated upper gastrointestinal endoscopy in the emergency department. Am J Emerg Med 1997; 15: 644–647.
36. Association of Anaesthetists of Great Britain and Ireland. Guidelines for monitoring during anaesthesia and recovery. London: AAGBI; 2000.
37. Hannaur J. Diagnostic radiology. BMJ 1999; 319: 18–171.
38. Garvey C, Hanlon R. Computed tomography in clinical practice. BMJ 2002; 324: 1077–1080.
39. Williams EJ, Jones NS, Carpenter TA, et al. Testing of adult and paediatric ventilators for use in a magnetic resonance imaging unit. Anaesth 1999; 54: 969–974.
40. Ansell G, Bettman M, Kaufmann J, et al. Complications in diagnostic imaging and interventional radiology. Oxford: Blackwell Science; 1996.
41. Barrison IG, Bramble MG, Wilkinson M, et al. Working party report: Provision of endoscopy related services in district general hospitals. London: British Society of Gastroenterology; 2001.

42. Loft D. BSG summer newsletter. BSG Newsletter 2002; 10(24).
43. Williams B, Whatmore P, Mcgill J, et al. Impact of private funding on access to elective hospital treatment in the regions of England and Wales. National records survey. Europ J Public Health 2001; 11: 402–406.
44. Department of Health. The cancer plan. London: HMSO; 2001.
45. MacFarlane B, Leicester R, Romaya C, et al. Colonoscopy services in the UK. Endoscopy 1999; 31: 409–411.
46. Vickers J, Alderson D. Oesophageal cancer staging using endoscopic ultrasound. Br J Surg 1998; 85: 994–998.
47. Shen EF, Arnott IDR, Plevris J, et al. Endoscopic ultrasonography in the diagnosis and management of upper gastrointestinal submucosal tumours. Br J Surg 2002; 89: 231.
48. NHS Modernisation Agency. Improvement leaders: guide to matching capacity and demand. London: HMSO; 2002.
49. Department of Health. Information for health: an information strategy for a modern NHS 1998–2005. London: HMSO; 1998.
50. Samuels A. A patient's view: endoscopy. BMJ 1995; 311: 1625.
51. Hospital Infection Society. Rinse water for heat labile endoscopy equipment. A report from a Joint Working Group of the Hospital Infection Society and the Public Health Laboratory Service. London: Hospital Infection Society; 2001.
52. Royal College of Physicians Joint Advisory Group. Recommendations for the training of gastrointestinal endoscopy. London: Royal College of Physicians; 1999.
53. Duthie GS, Drew PJ, Hughes MA, et al. A UK training programme for nurse practitioner flexible sigmoidoscopy and a prospective evaluation of the practice of the first UK trained nurse flexible sigmoidoscopist. Gut 1999; 43: 711–714.
54. Basnyat PS, Gomez KF, West J, et al. Nurse-led direct access endoscopy clinics: the future? Surg Endoscopy 2002; 16: 166–169.
55. Eisemon N, Stucky-Marshall L, Talamonti MS. Screening for colorectal cancer: developing a preventive healthcare program utilizing nurse endoscopists. Gastroenterol Nurs 2001; 24: 1219.

Further reading

Aitkenhead A, Smith G. Textbook of anaesthesia, 3rd edn. London: Churchill Livingstone; 1996.

Bernard K, Young A, eds. The new Aird's companion in surgical studies, 2nd edn. London: Churchill Livingstone; 1998.

Greaves I, Porter K, Ryan J. Trauma care manual. London: Arnold; 2001.

Knightingale K. Understanding perioperative nursing. London: Arnold; 1999.

Meeker M, Rothrock J. Alexander's care of the patient in surgery, 11th edn. London: Mosby; 1999.

Pinnock C, Lin T, Smith T, eds. Fundamentals of anaesthesia. London: GMM; 1999.

Whitwam JG, ed. Day-case anaesthesia and sedation. Oxford: Blackwell Scientific; 1994.

Whitwam JG, McCloy RF, eds. Principles and practice of sedation, 2nd edn. Oxford: Blackwell Scientific; 1998.

Internet resources

The Royal College of Anaesthetists
www.rcoa.ac.uk

Association of Anaesthetists of Great Britain and Ireland
www.aagbi.org.uk

British Society of Gastroenterologists
www.bsg.org.uk

Royal College of Physicians
www.rcplondon.ac.uk

The National Health Service
www.nhs.uk

NHS Modernisation Agency
www.modernnhs.nhs.uk

Hospital Infection Society
www.his.org.uk

Civil Contingency Secretariat
www.ukresilience.info

Royal College of Radiologists
www.rcr.ac.uk

Royal College of Surgeons (England)
www.rcseng.ac.uk

Royal College of Surgeons (Edinburgh)
www.rcsed.ac.uk

British Association of Accident and Emergency Medicine
www.baem.org.uk

British Association for Immediate Care and the Royal College of Surgeons of Edinburgh Faculty of Pre-hospital Care
//www.basics.freewire.co.uk/

Acknowledgement

The authors wish to thank the following for advice and assistance: Dr S Walker (GP), Dr E Walker (SpR Anaesthesia), Mr I Wharton (SpR Surgery), Dr A Williamson (Consultant Anaesthetist).

Chapter 17

Emergency surgery

Caroline MacDonald

Key points

- Theatre scheduling and utilization
- Preparation of the patient for surgery
- Intraoperative complications
- Intensive therapy unit (ITU) transfer
- Major incident planning

Emergency surgery is a challenging specialty. The surgery covers many disciplines, ranging from general surgery through to vascular, gynaecology and neurosurgery. Procedures can be minor, such as upper gastrointestinal endoscopy, or major-life saving surgery such as repair of a ruptured abdominal aortic aneurysm.

The principles of emergency surgery therefore differ from those of elective surgery. Most significantly, the patient preparation time is dramatically reduced and the condition of the patient can change rapidly. However, the same high standards of patient care are still essential, even with a reduced time window.

By its nature the work is unpredictable and the perioperative practitioner has to be prepared for any eventuality. Whatever the surgery or the condition of the patient, the practitioner must be adaptable and able to work under pressure.

THE EMERGENCY PERIOPERATIVE TEAM

Perioperative practitioners must be multiskilled in order to support and care for the patient to ensure a safe and efficient experience of surgery and anaes-thesia. High-quality care is a priority, and working together as a team is essential to achieve this. During a quiet period all staff may be sitting together having coffee in the rest room, but when an emergency comes in the team must work together as one cohesive unit to ensure that the patient receives safe and effective care. Nurses, operating department practitioners (ODPs), medical staff and support workers all work together towards a com-mon goal of quality perioperative patient care. The importance of working together to improve clinical standards and ultimately the quality of patient care is emphasized in the NHS plan[1] and supported by a clinical governance framework.

A rapid response is often necessary, and prepar-ation of the anaesthetic room and operating theatre for the arrival of a patient is a team effort. In emer-gency surgery a patient's condition can change rap-idly, and it is vital that practitioners are familiar with their own role and have an insight into the role of other team members to allow fluid working and pooling of resources in critical situations.

Practitioners should not be constrained by job titles,[2] and the most appropriately skilled and knowledgeable person should provide care. It may be necessary for a practitioner to assist in the anaes-thetic room before scrubbing for surgery, or an anaesthetic practitioner may be required to assist the circulating practitioner during surgery. There are many possible combinations of role, but most importantly staff must work together and comple-ment each other's skills.

EMERGENCY SURGICAL PROVISION

NATIONAL CONFIDENTIAL ENQUIRY INTO PERIOPERATIVE DEATHS

Emergency surgery is carried out in designated emergency theatres as well as in elective theatres with specific emergency operating time. The waiting time for emergency procedures does vary depend-ing on the patient's condition and the urgency of the surgical requirement. For example, one patient may require immediate life-saving surgery and the next may wait up to 24 hours for surgery. The avail-ability of a staffed operating theatre is an important consideration in this decision making.

The past 10 years have seen marked changes in the provision of emergency surgery, largely as a result of recommendations by the National Confidential Enquiry into Perioperative Deaths (NCEPOD). NCEPOD is a registered charity whose aim is 'to review clinical practice and identify potentially remediable factors in the practice of anaesthesia, surgery and other invasive medical procedures. The aim is to look at the quality of the delivery of care and not specifically the causation of death'.[3] NCEPOD continues to produce reports to improve the quality of the service provided which can be accessed via the NCEPOD website.

One of the most significant recommendations affecting emergency surgery is included in the 1995/1996 report.[4] This recommends that all hos-pitals admitting patients for emergency surgery should have a designated 24-hour emergency sur-gery list and a fully equipped and staffed 24-hour operating theatre. The service should be continuous throughout the year, including weekends and pub-lic holidays.

In response, many hospitals have complied with this recommendation and have established specific emergency theatres, often referred to as CEPOD theatres. The implementation of such facilities will increase the number of emergency operations per-formed during daytime hours and thus reduce the number of out-of-hours operations performed by junior medical staff due to the unavailability of daytime theatre space, two of the points identified by NCEPOD in the 1995/1996 report.[4]

SCHEDULING AND THEATRE UTILIZATION

Scheduling of emergency cases is a complex task, coordinated by a senior perioperative practitioner in consultation with senior medical staff. Whether the emergency list is performed in an elective thea-tre or a designated emergency theatre, several spe-cialties will be entitled to emergency operating time, and more than one team may have an emer-gency case requiring immediate theatre access. Ultimately, the urgency of the required surgery and the condition of the patient will dictate the order of the operating list, with priority being given to the most urgent case.

Communication is the key to efficient use of the service, and it is important that a designated person is responsible for scheduling cases to avoid unneces-sary delays and double booking. Changes to the order of the operating list are common in emer-gency surgery when an unscheduled urgent case requires immediate surgical intervention, and should be made only by the practitioner responsible for scheduling cases. Good communication between teams is essential to ensure relevant personnel are kept informed of changes to the schedule, thereby avoiding confusion and conflict.

Inevitably, there will be times when minor emergency surgical cases are delayed to allow access to more urgent cases. Close liaison with ward staff is necessary to keep patients and relatives informed when this occurs.

Operating department facilities are often under-utilized. Reasons for this include the need for essential preoperative preparation of the patient, the unavailability of surgical or anaesthetic staff, portering delays, and overrunning of elective lists. This applies equally to emergency surgery. An effective way to combat this problem is the introduction of a specialist practitioner in emergency surgery whose role is to coordinate the workload. This role involves preoperative assessment, coordination of emergency cases, and essential redistribution of minor surgical emergencies to elective theatres. There is evidence that this type of role has been successful in improving theatre utilization and efficiency by redistributing workload and reducing delays. In one hospital, the employment of a nurse specialist has reduced out-of-hours operating time and the number of patients operated on outside these hours by 30%.[5]

PATIENT PREPARATION FOR EMERGENCY SURGERY

CONSENT

Consent is covered in detail in Chapters 1 and 3. However, in emergency surgery there are exceptions to the general rules regarding informed consent. It is not always possible to obtain written or even verbal consent from an emergency patient, and in some cases it may be necessary to proceed with life-saving surgery in the absence of their expressed consent. Examples may include life-saving surgery on an unconscious patient, or even life-saving surgery where a patient may have intentionally attempted suicide.

In such cases, medical staff must document in the patient's records the reason for proceeding with surgery without express consent. The Department of Health[6] recommends the use of a specifically designed form for individuals who are unable to

consent to investigation or treatment, detailing the reasons why surgery was essential. It is good practice to obtain consent from the next of kin where possible, although this should not be allowed to delay surgery.

In the absence of the patient's expressed consent, the surgeon must only carry out surgery required to save life. The patient must be woken prior to any further non-urgent treatment in order to obtain their informed consent before surgery can proceed.

There are often limitations in emergency surgery, including time, owing to the seriousness of the patient's condition and the immediacy of the surgical requirement. This does not reduce the patient's need for sufficient information about the impending anaesthetic and surgery, and informed consent must still be obtained whenever possible.

All forms of consent are acceptable, although written is preferred as it is the most reliable form of evidence that consent has been obtained. The Department of Health[6] provides guidance on obtaining consent and sample consent forms are available online in several languages. In certain situations it may be appropriate to record the patient's consent and any related discussion in the medical notes, rather than using a form.[6]

It is acknowledged that the urgency of the patient's situation may limit the quantity of information that can be given, but it should not affect its quality.[6] It is also important to understand that the patient may actively withdraw consent, effectively preventing further life-saving treatment. Under these circumstances, multiprofessional decision making, with an appreciation of the wishes of the patient and his or her relatives, must be considered.

The perioperative practitioner is often the last person to whom the patient can voice concerns before surgery begins. If there is any doubt about the validity of the consent, the practitioner, acting as an advocate for the patient, should inform medical staff before further treatment is given.

INFECTION STATUS

It is not always possible to know the infection status of every emergency patient. A patient may be unconscious on admission, or may present with limited medical information, reinforcing the need to implement standard infection control precautions for all cases in line with hospital policy. Practitioners must be ready to respond to an increased risk of contamination, such as during major haemorrhage, which may necessitate changes in protective measures taken by staff. The principles of risk assessment are important to consider, but in the emergency situation equally important is the ability to constantly update the assessment of the risk of contamination by blood or body fluids.

Following a procedure that has generated a great deal of contamination, thorough decontamination of the emergency operating theatre environment is necessary before the operating list can continue. If the delay is significant another theatre may have to be made available for any other pending emergency procedures.

RISK ASSESSMENT

All surgical patients are exposed to a variety of risks during the perioperative period, including, for example, surgical positioning, anaesthesia-induced immobility, diathermy burns, inadvertent hypothermia, the formation of pressure sores, reactions to medication, etc. In emergency cases, perioperative risks are compounded by reduced time for preoperative preparation, owing to factors such as the urgency of the surgery and the poor physical condition of the patient.

It is essential for safe patient care that an effective risk management strategy is in place. The principles of risk management are covered in depth in Chapter 3.

Risk management itself, however, is the responsibility of individuals, and many risk assessment tools have been developed both locally and nationally that address specific issues: the Waterlow Risk Assessment Tool for pressure areas is a typical example. Where available, these tools should be used as part of an overall approach to risk management and the delivery of safe and effective perioperative care.

Three areas of risk with elements particularly associated with the emergency situation will be considered: patient transfer and positioning, pressure sore development, and the formation of deep vein thrombosis (DVT).

Moving and handling

It is often necessary to transfer the patient quickly from a trolley/bed on to the operating table. The transfer is planned using sufficient numbers of staff and transfer equipment to ensure safety and to prevent injury to both staff and patient. Correct moving and handling techniques must be employed at all times as per hospital policy, and regular staff training provided. Inaccurate or inefficient moving and handling of a patient can cause further delay to surgery if the patient or a member of staff is injured in the process.

The critically ill patient may have intravenous (IV) infusion pumps or drains in situ, and it is important that these do not become disconnected during the transfer. One practitioner should coordinate the move to ensure a team effort. Specific equipment identified from a risk assessment to assist the transfer, such as a glide sheet or Easy Slide, must be readily available, and staff must be knowledgeable and competent in its use.

Risk assessment is a continual process and should be undertaken for all subsequent transfers, for example if a position change is requested during surgery by the anaesthetist or surgeon, or when transferring the patient from the operating table on to a bed after surgery.

Practitioners must also ensure that they use correct moving and handling techniques when moving equipment, such as large instrument trays and equipment used when transferring the patient back to the ward. In an emergency it may appear quicker to lift instrument trays rather than use a trolley to transport them, but this is dangerous practice and can cause further delay to surgery if an injury is sustained or equipment damaged.

Deep vein thrombosis and pulmonary embolism

Common measures for DVT prophylaxis are discussed in Chapter 12. In an emergency, when there is limited time for DVT risk assessment using a recognized tool, clinical judgement should be relied upon. Following a risk assessment, prophylactic measures are applied in the anaesthetic room and clearly documented in the patient's notes. For most patients, graduated compression stockings and intermittent pneumatic compression cuffs are used. Effective risk assessment at this time, followed by the appropriate use of available resources, even when time is limited, will help to prevent further complications.

Observation of the patient and equipment and continual assessment are an integral part of the practitioner's role in providing individualized patient care. It is important to remember that DVT risk assessment is ongoing, especially for the emergency patient, as their risk status may have changed from the time of initial assessment owing to changes in their surgical condition.

Pressure sore prevention

Pressure sore risk assessment is ongoing throughout the perioperative journey, and as the emergency patient's condition or position changes, reassessment is necessary. An initial assessment is carried out prior to or on arrival at the operating department. A recognized tool (such as the Waterlow Pressure Sore Assessment Tool) is used to provide the relevant score. Subsequent preventative care is documented in the notes.

Pressure-relieving aids such as overlay mattresses (Pre Vent mattresses) and gel-filled pads are used to protect the patient and prevent pressure sore development. It is important that stocks of such equipment are maintained to prevent delay in application. The use of appropriate moving and handling techniques and equipment during patient transfer is essential to prevent friction and prevent pressure sores. In an emergency, lack of time should not reduce the preventative measures essential for good pressure area care.

PREPARATION FOR SURGERY

In many emergency situations rapid preparation of the operating theatre and the team is imperative. Each team member must be clear about their role in the patient's care, that is, who will be the anaesthetic, scrub and circulating practitioners for the procedure.

Communication with medical staff and the ward is a key factor at this time, and is usually the responsibility of the practitioner in charge.

ANAESTHESIA

The anaesthetic room remains set up to receive emergency cases. Specific equipment is organized when the nature of the procedure and the condition of the patient are identified. Preoperative resuscitation of the patient will be started prior to arrival in the anaesthetic room, and equipment to continue this made available and ready for use. For example, a patient with substantial preoperative blood loss is likely to require a rapid infusion of fluid, and therefore a warming device and a pressure/rapid infuser will be required.

In emergency surgery, preoperative preparation is reduced and preparation for anaesthesia can take some time, especially if the patient's condition is unstable. Support for the patient during this period in the anaesthetic room is important, and it may therefore be necessary for a second perioperative practitioner to stay with the patient. Patients who are critically ill or in shock may be agitated, enforcing the need for extra personnel to provide support and maintain patient safety.

Critically ill patients require invasive monitoring during surgery, and this will begin in the anaesthetic room. Two peripheral intravenous lines for venous access and fluid infusion are normally required. Blood and fluids are warmed and infused through a rapid infuser (level 1).

An arterial line for continued blood pressure monitoring is normally inserted. When the patient is hypovolaemic rapid infusion of fluids is indicated, and a central venous catheter may be inserted to monitor the central venous pressure, which gives a more accurate indication of reduced blood volume.[7] Urinary catheterization enables accurate monitoring of urine output. This is commonly done in the anaesthetic room when the patient is anaesthetized.

If the patient has not fasted for the recommended length of time prior to surgery, a rapid-sequence induction is necessary to prevent regurgitation of stomach contents. Cricoid pressure is applied and maintained while the anaesthetist places the endotracheal tube, and only released when the tube is in the correct position. The application of cricoid pressure is only undertaken following specific training[7] (see Chapter 19 for more information on cricoid pressure).

OPERATING ROOM PREPARATION

The operating room normally remains set up to receive emergency cases. Specific sterile instrument trays can be ordered when the nature of the case is known. At times when the exact nature of the surgery is unknown, for example an exploratory laparotomy, extra instruments are ordered just in case they are needed, for example long instruments and gastrointestinal instruments in case the bowel is involved. This also applies to supplementary instruments and perishable equipment such as abdominal packs.

The anaesthetic practitioner will give a handover to the scrub practitioner detailing the patient's name, date of birth and any known allergies. This will help the scrub practitioner to prepare the correct environment for the patient.

The scrub practitioner will ensure that all the instruments and equipment necessary to commence surgery are available and set out ready for use. Generally, operating departments have reference cards detailing common operations and the sterile trays, instruments and supplementary equipment required for each. In emergency cases it is not always easy to be so prescriptive, and the scrub practitioner will have to use initiative and anticipate what might be needed as surgery progresses. The circulating practitioner also needs to be experienced in major emergency surgery and be able to follow the surgery, anticipating the scrub practitioner's needs.

Swab and instrument checks are undertaken as per hospital policy before surgery begins. However, there may be situations when it is necessary to use instruments from the tray before an instrument check has been undertaken, for example if it is necessary for surgeons to begin operating immediately after induction of anaesthesia in the operating theatre (for example repair of a ruptured abdominal aortic aneurysm). In this instance the scrub practitioner will have little time to prepare, and so minimum instrumentation is used initially – for example drapes and sponges – until a check can be undertaken. The instrument tray is then checked thoroughly when time and circumstances permit.

Circulating practitioners need to be able to anticipate which supplementary instruments and extra supplies will be required for surgery. Pre-emptive ordering of these may prevent unnecessary delay and save crucial time during the operation. For example, if a patient has a ruptured abdominal aortic aneurysm, significant blood loss is to be expected, and therefore extra swabs, abdominal packs and suction supplies will be necessary and must be available without delay.

Support workers are an integral part of the perioperative team and have an important role to play in the smooth running of the theatre. Among other duties, the support worker undertakes the circulating role in theatre and is involved in its setting up. In emergency cases the scrub practitioner needs experienced personnel to support them in their role and, with training, the support worker can fulfil this requirement.

The scrub practitioner needs to be experienced in the role to deal with the potentially rapidly changing condition of the patient. Although the surgery may be exploratory in the first instance, it may evolve into major emergency surgery requiring considerable skill from the scrub practitioner and circulating team members.

INTRAOPERATIVE PROBLEMS

HAEMORRHAGE

Control of haemorrhage is vital in order to prevent deterioration of a patient's condition and to provide a clear operating field for the surgical team.

A patient's condition (for example a stab wound) may be the cause of bleeding prior to arrival in the operating theatre, or the surgical procedure itself may be the cause of bleeding. Whatever the reason, immediate control is necessary to prevent further blood loss.

Haemorrhage can be controlled using a number of methods:

- Direct pressure to the bleeding site
- Suture/ligation of vessels
- Diathermy.

The choice of method will depend on the patient's medical condition. For example, pressure may be applied to an open wound until the patient is anaesthetized and ready for surgery. During surgery, diathermy or ligatures may be the method of choice for haemostasis.

Suture and ligation is recommended for large bleeding vessels. A selection of vascular clamps will be available on the surgical tray and the scrub practitioner will have a selection of suture materials and ligatures ready for use.

Direct pressure can be applied to stem the blood flow. A supply of swabs will be necessary, and these must be counted and recorded before use. It requires skill and concentration to keep account of swabs during severe haemorrhage. There may be upwards of 40 swabs in use and several surgeons working and handling them, trying to stem the bleeding and maintain a clear operative field. Swabs should always be counted off as soon as possible to avoid having a large number on the operating table at any one time and to minimize the risk of losing one or more in the patient.

Abdominal packs are used for severe haemorrhage as they absorb more blood than smaller swabs. Fewer are needed, therefore, and it is easier to monitor and count them.

Weighing of swabs and recording blood loss is an ongoing process throughout the operation and requires diligence from circulating staff to maintain accuracy.

If capillary oozing is evident before closure of the cavity, an absorbent cellulose gauze such as Surgicel can be applied. If the surgery is complete and the patient is still oozing blood, the surgeons may decide to leave an abdominal pack in the cavity. The exact location of the abdominal pack must be recorded in the patient record and operating book. The patient will return to theatre, usually within 48 hours, for surgical removal of the pack(s). This must also be documented in the patient record and operating book.

Suction is a vital aid to remove blood from the operating field. Additional suction units are available in the emergency theatre and can be set up quickly for use in cases of major haemorrhage. Extra suction supplies may be necessary to meet the demand.

It is important for the surgical and anaesthetic teams to have a continual estimate of the total blood loss to assist with accurate fluid replacement. Swabs must be weighed and recorded on a visible board, and blood in the suction receptacles measured and recorded at regular intervals to provide an accurate total blood loss volume. Blood transfusion may be required depending on the blood loss during surgery.

A surgical drain may be inserted before closure of the wound to remove fluid from the operative site and assist with accurate fluid recording. Careful handling of the drain is necessary when moving the patient after surgery. Fluid recording will continue in recovery.

In common with other body fluids, blood also presents an infection risk to perioperative staff. A working knowledge of the hospital standard precaution policy is essential in emergency surgery, and protective clothing must be readily available so that staff are adequately protected from contamination.

BLOOD TRANSFUSION

Blood transfusion is an essential life-saving treatment commonly used during emergency surgery. However, it is important to remember that blood transfusion poses potentially fatal risks to a patient from reactions to incompatible blood and potential infection from donor blood. Transfusion of the wrong blood type remains the main cause of transfusion reaction.[8]

The 2000/2001 SHOT[8] report identified the operating theatre, including recovery, to be the site of 11.9% of the incidents of incorrect blood components being transfused. It is vital that hospital policy for the administration of blood products is strictly observed to ensure the quality of care and safeguard the patient against potentially fatal complications.

The decision to transfuse a patient within the emergency perioperative environment is made following careful consideration of their clinical condition.[9] In most cases the patient will have suffered acute blood loss and is at risk of further bleeding during surgery.

A blood sample is collected preoperatively and sent to the hospital transfusion service for grouping and cross-matching. In emergency cases, when blood is required urgently, the transfusion service must be notified of the quantity required and the urgency. ABO- and rhesus-compatible blood can normally be supplied within 15 minutes of receiving a blood sample.[10] Cross-matched blood will take longer.

In extreme emergencies, when a blood transfusion is required, O-negative (universal donor) blood can be used from emergency supplies. O-negative blood is normally in short supply and should only be used when the patient's life is at risk.

The blood is delivered to the department and a trained member of staff must check that the correct blood has been sent,[10] ensuring that it is stored correctly. The storage guidelines below must be followed to ensure the vitality of the blood:[11]

- Blood must be stored at 4°C to prevent cell damage
- Blood must always be stored in a blood transfusion refrigerator to maintain the correct temperature
- Blood must be used within 30 minutes from the time it was removed from the blood fridge
- If a unit of blood has been out of the blood fridge for more than 30 minutes, the hospital blood bank must be notified and the blood returned to the transfusion services department for disposal
- Empty blood packs must be kept for 24 hours so that they can be examined and tested if a transfusion reaction occurs.

When blood is collected from the fridge it must be checked against the patient prescription sheet, ensuring that it is within the expiry date and there is no evidence of leakage.

The guidelines for the administration of blood and blood components recommend that only one unit of blood is removed from the blood transfusion refrigerator at a time, unless large quantities are required for rapid infusion in an emergency.[12] The transfusion should be commenced within 30 minutes of removing the blood from the fridge, and if there is going to be a delay the blood should be returned to the fridge and the time of return recorded.

Blood and blood products are viewed as medicines and must only be administered by a doctor or a nurse holding current registration. It is recommended that 'one member of staff should be responsible for carrying out the identity check of the patient and the unit of blood'.[12]

The patient must be positively identified using full name, hospital unit number and date of birth. All patients in the perioperative department must wear an identification wristband. However, during emergency surgery problems of identification may arise, such as gaining access to the wristband. This may be because of the position of the arm or the need to ensure the maintenance of a sterile field. It may be that the wristband has been removed to gain arterial access, in which case the removed wristband may be secured to the patient's shoulder or forehead using a clear film dressing to ensure correct identification.

The perioperative practitioner will be involved in the checking of blood for transfusion. It is imperative that adequate time is taken to carry out all steps of the checking procedure as per hospital policy to ensure that the patient receives the correct blood. The bedside check is the last opportunity to prevent a mistransfusion.[8] There is no excuse for not following the correct procedure: even in emergency situations when blood is required immediately, all procedural steps must be followed. Blood is administered using a sterile giving set designed for transfusion, and aseptic technique must be followed to prevent contamination.

Blood warming devices are commonly used during emergency surgery. The British Committee for Standards in Haematology[10] advocates the use of a blood warmer for adults receiving an infusion of blood greater than 50 ml/kg/h. Blood Transfusion Services of the UK (1996)[12] specifies that blood should be warmed using a specially designed device with a thermometer and audible alarm system. Blood should never be warmed using improvisations, such as placing the blood in a warming cabinet or on a radiator, as it is impossible to ensure a safe temperature. After use, the blood warmer must be thoroughly cleaned in preparation for the next patient, to prevent cross-infection.

Transfusion reactions can be fatal, and once the transfusion is commenced close observation of the patient is necessary to ensure early recognition of complications. Severe reactions are likely to occur within the first 15 minutes of transfusion.

During emergency surgery the patient is continually monitored and signs of complications should be noticed quickly. However, signs of transfusion reactions are more difficult to detect in the unconscious patient, as they are unable to complain of pain, restlessness and dyspnoea. Signs of an acute haemolytic reaction, including hypotension, uncontrolled bleeding or oliguria, may be attributed to the patient's deteriorating clinical condition and not the transfusion. Careful monitoring of vital signs is necessary to prevent ongoing problems.

In the event of an adverse reaction the transfusion must be stopped immediately, the cause assessed and remedial action taken. If further transfusion is required, the blood giving set must be changed.

SHOCK

Shock is a life-threatening condition characterized by an inability of the circulatory system to supply sufficient oxygen and nutrients to the body tissues.[13] Emergency patients are susceptible to shock as their condition is often critical on admission to the emergency operating theatre and their condition can change rapidly.

There are three types of shock:

- Hypovolaemic
- Cardiogenic
- Distributive – neurogenic, septic and anaphylactic.

Only hypovolaemic shock will be discussed with relevance to emergency surgery. This is the most common type and is due to a reduction in circulating blood volume, causing reduced cardiac output and inadequate tissue perfusion. It is important to remember that an adult can tolerate 700 ml of blood loss without demonstrating signs of shock.

Rapid detection of shock necessitates immediate action to prevent irreversible damage to the body and subsequent death. The key to managing hypovolaemic shock is to restore the circulating blood volume.

The cause of haemorrhage and subsequent shock may be obvious on admission to the emergency theatre, for example a stab injury. Practitioners must be vigilant for signs of shock caused by an internal injury. Careful observation of the patient is essential in all situations.

In most cases, arresting the haemorrhage and replacing circulatory volume will reverse the signs and symptoms of shock. However, if a patient reaches what is known as the refractory stage, shock is irreversible and death inevitable.

Invasive monitoring of the central venous and arterial pressures is required for accurate assessment of the patient and rapid fluid replacement. A urinary catheter is inserted to monitor the patient's renal function. The perioperative practitioner assists anaesthetic staff in the preparation of the patient and equipment.

Anaesthetic staff will dictate the fluid replacement regimen using a combination of colloid and crystalloid solutions. The replacement of blood and blood products may be indicated and blood transfusion necessary. If blood is to be transfused rapidly a level 1 rapid infuser/blood warming device should be used to prevent excessive cooling of the patient.

RAPIDLY CHANGING CONDITION

The patient's condition can change rapidly due to complications related to both anaesthesia – for example uncontrolled airway – and surgery, for example unexpected haemorrhage.

Problems with anaesthesia may require extra perioperative and anaesthetic assistance. The anaesthetic practitioner will be working closely with the anaesthetist and be unable to leave the patient, and will rely on other members of the team to obtain any other items of equipment or drugs that are required.

All perioperative staff should be familiar with the storage of equipment and extra supplies in all areas of the theatre, so that they can assist each other when problems or complications arise – another reason for effective team working.

A relatively simple but urgent investigative procedure, such as an upper GI endoscopy, may diagnose an underlying serious illness and necessitate immediate major surgery. Any of the above intraoperative complications may cause a rapid deterioration in the patient's condition. The team must be alert to possible complications and react rapidly when they occur.

When extra surgical/anaesthetic assistance is required during surgery, practitioners need to be familiar with the paging system to contact senior staff such as a consultant or specialist registrar for assistance. Circulating practitioners will organize any extra equipment that may be necessary, such as rapid fluid infuser or long instruments.

Good practitioner–patient communication is essential. The patient is a vital source of information in emergency surgery, when little is known about his or her preoperative condition, and can assist in detecting deterioration in their condition, for example verbalizing a change in pain level, increasing anxiety or change in sensation/temperature. It is possible during an emergency to become distracted with the urgency of the situation and forget to communicate with the patient.

Changes in level and type of pain may indicate a change in condition. Perioperative practitioners should be aware of the implications of this and alert medical staff. For example, cramping abdominal pain that progresses into continuous severe pain may indicate bowel ischaemia.

Alteration to conscious level, temperature elevation and reduced urine output can all be indicators of a deterioration in the patient's condition. Close observation in the anaesthetic room and recovery area is vital.

INTENSIVE THERAPY UNIT TRANSFER

Following emergency surgery a number of patients will require to be transferred to the intensive therapy unit (ITU) or to another hospital. Perioperative practitioners play a vital role in the transfer of patients to ensure their safety. Considerable planning by the team is necessary pre- and postoperatively.

PREOPERATIVE PREPARATION

Prior to surgery, senior anaesthetic and surgical staff will decide whether a patient requires postoperative admission to ITU for continued intensive therapy, and a bed in the unit is reserved before surgery is commenced. The patient's condition and the type, duration and expected outcome of surgery will be the basis for this decision. However, if during surgery a patient's condition deteriorates, admission to the ITU may be deemed necessary. The anaesthetist will then communicate with the ITU team to organize a bed, and liaise with ITU staff during the preparation for transfer.

Preparation for transfer is ongoing during surgery. Communication between ITU and operating theatre staff may be delegated to a perioperative practitioner. Patient and transfer details must be clear and accurate. Anticipated arrival time and any subsequent delays are communicated to both perioperative and ITU staff. The patient's relatives should be informed of the transfer and the estimated time the patient is expected to arrive in ITU.

Alterations to the transfer plan are communicated to all staff involved to avoid any unnecessary confusion.

ORGANIZATION OF THE TEAM

An anaesthetist leads the team during transfer, which will include a perioperative practitioner. In most instances a second perioperative practitioner will be involved to go ahead of the team to ensure corridors are clear and lifts available and empty, thereby avoiding unnecessary delays.

PREPARATION OF THE PATIENT

A bed is brought from the ITU to the operating theatre before surgery is finished. The patient is carefully transferred on to the bed using correct moving and handling techniques according to local policy.

To allow for continued monitoring of a patient's condition during transfer, specialized equipment is assembled and checked beforehand. Some equipment may be carried by accompanying staff, although some items may be carefully attached to the bed. It is essential that no equipment is resting on the bed, to avoid injury to the patient. All nursing and medical notes and X-rays must accompany the patient, who must be kept warm and completely covered during transfer to ensure privacy and dignity.

EQUIPMENT

The equipment used for transfer should be used solely for that purpose. Most equipment will be stored in specifically designed bags that unzip for easy access. Controlled drugs will probably not be kept in the bag, and so before transfer a check should be made that a sufficient quantity has been loaded. Battery-operated pumps and monitors must be kept fully charged and oxygen cylinders checked to ensure they are full before transfer.

Equipment required for transfer will include:

- Transport ventilator
- Emergency equipment – defibrillator, emergency drugs, Ambubag, IV fluids
- Battery-operated syringe pumps
- Portable ECG monitor and blood pressure monitor
- Oxygen
- Suction equipment.

When accompanying a patient on a transfer to ITU, it is imperative that practitioners are fully trained in emergency procedures and familiar with the patient's clinical condition and all the transport equipment.[14]

Regular training should take place to update knowledge about equipment and emergency procedures – for example if the lift were to fail and the patient's condition deteriorate rapidly. All practitioners should be confident that in any given emergency situation they would be able to assist the anaesthetist competently using all the equipment.

PERIOPERATIVE DEATH

A death related to anaesthesia or surgery must be referred to the Coroner or Procurator Fiscal for investigation. A postmortem may be carried out to establish the cause of death and an inquest held at a later date to ascertain the exact cause. Advice should be sought from the Coroner or Procurator Fiscal before last offices are undertaken, to ensure that potential evidence is not disturbed. In accordance with this, local hospital policy is followed.

Guidelines regarding the removal of technical equipment from the patient's body after death may vary locally. In most instances, the points below will apply.[15]

- Breathing tubes (ET tubes/tracheostomy tubes) removed
- Catheters and cannulae sealed using a spigot
- Drains and packs left in position
- Wounds covered with a clean dressing.

In most cases, perioperative practitioners undertake last offices. However, there may be instances when it is necessary or more appropriate for ward staff to undertake this important nursing duty when, for example:

- The next case requires immediate entry to the operating theatre
- Insufficient time or space is available within the operating theatre to undertake last offices
- The patient is well known to the ward staff and they specifically request to carry out last offices.

The decision as to who undertakes this procedure will be made following discussion with both teams.

Routine last offices are not always appropriate: the patient's cultural and religious beliefs may dictate a particular pattern of care. It is always advisable to ascertain the patient's – or their family's – cultural or religious beliefs in order to avoid transgressing their right and dignity to be treated according to their wishes. However, in general circumstances, the body is straightened, the eyes are closed and limited cleansing is undertaken. If the patient is soiled with blood or iodine solution, for example, further cleansing may be warranted so that patient dignity is maintained.

Members of the patient's family may wish to be involved in last offices, and this should be facilitated where possible. They may also wish to see the deceased before transfer to the mortuary. A private room where relatives can wait before viewing the body may be appreciated.

The theatre manager should be informed of a perioperative death and the event recorded in the patient's notes. It is important that perioperative care is documented accurately and not simply memorized, as this information may be required for legal purposes at a later date.

It is essential that practitioners are supported following a perioperative death. A team or individual debriefing session is often helpful to facilitate appreciation and understanding of the event.

MAJOR INCIDENTS

A major incident is defined as 'any emergency that requires the implementation of special arrangements by one or more of the emergency services, the NHS or the local authority'.[16] Many hospitals in the United Kingdom have had to contend with major incidents. In a recent statement, the Department of Health[17] reinforces the need for preparation for a major incident. In today's society, it is unacceptable to think it will not happen in one's own hospital.

Depending on the cause of the major incident and the injuries sustained, operating theatres will play a vital role in the care of casualties. A theatre controller (consultant surgeon) is identified who will liaise closely with the theatre manager to coordinate the theatre response. Effective communication between all professionals is paramount.

The emergency operating team is alerted and the operating theatres prepared for surgery. In cases where there are numerous critical casualties requiring emergency surgery, elective surgical procedures may be postponed and operating theatres and perioperative teams utilized.

It is essential to remember the sterile services department in the communication loop, as they need to be aware of the potential for an increased demand for instruments and sterile perishable goods.

Knowing the cause of the major incident is important for perioperative practitioners. The set-up of the theatre and the ordering of instruments and consumable goods will depend on the nature of the incident and the number of casualties. Preparation and equipment for casualties of a major fire with burn injuries will differ from those required for casualties with trauma and orthopaedic injuries, for example from a bus crash. Extra supplies of swabs, fluids, blood and drugs can be ordered in advance and extra equipment obtained from other theatres to prepare for surgery.

Triage is vital to ensure that casualties receive appropriate care and facilities are used to the greatest effect. This takes place at the scene of the incident, on arrival at hospital, and at regular intervals thereafter.

Major incident triage categories are as follows:

- Priority 1 – in need of immediate intervention
- Priority 2 – in need of admission and early intervention
- Priority 3 – can wait for treatment. Usually the 'walking wounded'.[18]

The theatre controller and theatre manager will normally schedule triaged cases and organize staff resources.

The assistance of on-call teams and volunteer off-duty practitioners may be required to cope with the workload. Off-duty staff may not be needed immediately but may be required to relieve staff if surgical time is prolonged beyond scheduled working hours. The major incident plan will identify the procedure for volunteer staff to contact the hospital. Perioperative staff must be familiar with this guidance to avoid blocking essential communication lines. Equally importantly, staff contact details must be accurate to ensure a quick response should it be necessary to enlist off-duty staff.

Receiving hospitals have a Major Incident Plan and perioperative practitioners must be familiar with it. The Department of Health[18] specifies that each hospital department likely to be involved in treating casualties of a major incident must have action cards, detailing key activities for staff. It is important that action cards are accessible in the operating department to allow practitioners to familiarize themselves with their roles and requirements well in advance of a crisis, so that they are used as a referral aid in the event of a major incident.

In any emergency situation panic can be avoided by efficient and effective preparation and communication. The emergency operating theatre provides an environment that stimulates the development of these skills and provides an excellent basis for future professional development in any field of patient care.

Case studies

Holly (25) is admitted for the incision and drainage of a pilonidal sinus that is causing her pain and discomfort. She is added to the emergency operating list, and because of the current emergency caseload it is anticipated that she will have surgery within the next 2 hours. An hour later Holly is told her surgery is delayed by a more urgent case requiring emergency theatre access. Perioperative staff keep the ward and Holly informed of the progress of the emergency list. The urgent priority case is taking longer than initially anticipated, and to prevent Holly waiting any longer she is added to the end of the elective general operating list. Holly has her surgery and is admitted to the recovery unit after 45 minutes in theatre.

John (78) is admitted to A&E with a suspected ruptured abdominal aortic aneurysm. The emergency operating theatre team is alerted to his imminent arrival and the operating theatre set up for the emergency surgery. John is admitted to theatre directly from A&E and anaesthesia is induced. Surgery begins immediately after induction of anaesthesia. John is haemorrhaging severely and blood transfusion is necessary. A level 1 rapid infuser is used for transfusion and accurate identity checks are undertaken prior to the administration of each unit. Two suction units are in use to assist with the maintenance of a clear operating field. The circulating practitioner maintains an accurate record of the blood loss on a visible board and in the patient record. An ITU bed is arranged for John following surgery, and close liaison with ITU is continuous. Transfer equipment is checked and an ITU bed delivered to the operating theatre for transfer. John is carefully transferred on to the ITU bed using the correct moving and handling technique and equipment. A perioperative practitioner accompanies John and provides a handover to the ITU nursing staff.

Paul (20) is admitted to A&E following an accident at work, where he has been crushed by a piece of machinery. He requires an urgent exploratory laparotomy for serious abdominal injuries. Paul is assessed by the anaesthetic and surgical teams and the emergency theatre team is notified of his urgent surgical requirement. There is an appendicectomy currently in the emergency theatre and only minor cases on the list thereafter, which are subsequently postponed.

Paul is admitted to the receiving surgical ward and 30 minutes later to the emergency operating theatre. He is transferred on to the operating table using a patslide and four members of the perioperative team. A Pre Vent mattress and gel pads are used to reduce pressure area risk, and a forced air warming device to combat inadvertent hypothermia. An arterial line is inserted prior to a rapid-sequence induction of general anaesthesia. Paul is catheterized, and graduated compression stockings and intermittent pneumatic compression cuffs are applied before transfer to the operating theatre.

A laparotomy, splenectomy and repair of a tear to the liver are performed.

References

1. DOH 2000. Online. Available: http://www.doh.gov.uk/cancer/cancerplanch8.htm 10 July 2003.
2. National Association of Theatre Nurses. Future ways of working: unleashing the potential of perioperative practice. Harrogate: NATN, 2001.
3. NCEPOD. What is National CEPOD? Online. Available: http://www.ncepod.org.uk/index.htm 10 July 2003.
4. NCEPOD. Summary of the 1995/1996 report 'Who operates when?' Sep 1997. Online. Available: http://www.ncepod.org.uk/index.htm 10 Jul 2003.
5. Radford M, Johnson P, Williamson A, et al. Co-ordination of the emergency surgical workload by a specialist nurse pre-assessment: the effect on emergency theatre operating patterns. Br J Surg 2001; 88(Suppl. 1): 28.
6. Department of Health. Good practice in consent: implementation guide. London: HMSO; 2001. Online. Available: http://www.doh.gov.uk/consent/implementationguide.pdf
7. Simpson PJ, Popat M. Understanding anaesthesia, 4th edn. Oxford: Butterworth-Heinemann, 2002.
8. SHOT. Annual Report 2000/2001. Serious Hazards of Transfusion Steering Group; 2002. Online. Available: http://www.shot.demon.co.uk/Report%2000-01.doc
9. British Committee for Standards in Haematology. Guidelines for the clinical use of red cell transfusions. Br J Haematology 2001; 113: 24–31.
10. McClelland DBL. Handbook of transfusion medicine, 3rd edn. London: The Stationery Office; 2001.
11. Burkitt G, Quick CRG. Essential surgery problems, diagnosis and management, 3rd edn. Edinburgh: Churchill Livingstone; 2002.
12. British Committee for Standards in Haematology, Blood Transfusion Task Force. The administration of blood and blood components and the management of transfused patients transfusion medicine. Oxford: Blackwell Science; 1999. Online. Available: http://www.bcshguidelines.com/pdf/tme203.pdf
13. Hand H. Shock. Nurs Standard 2001; 15: 45–52, 54–55.
14. Driscoll P, Macartney I, Mackway-Jones K, et al. Safe transfer and retrieval: the practical approach. London: BMJ Books; 2002; 7–12.
15. National Association of Theatre Nurses. Principles of perioperative practice in the perioperative environment. Harrogate: NATN, 1998.
16. Controller and Auditor General. Report. Facing the challenge – NHS emergency planning in England. London: Controller and Auditor General; 2002. Online. Available: http://www.nao.gov.uk/publications/nao_reports/02-03/020336pts1-5.pdf 15 Jul 2003.
17. Doran A. Planning for major incidents: process over next 3 months. London: DOH; 2003. Online. Available: http://www.doh.gov.uk/epcu/refdocs/alandoran14jano3.doc 15 Jul 2003.
18. Department of Health. Planning for major incidents: the NHS guidance. London: DOH; 1998. Online. Available: http://www.doh.gov.uk/epcu/nhsguidance.htm 15 Jul 2003.

SECTION 4

Principles of care for specific patient groups

SECTION CONTENTS

Chapter 18

Care of children and adolescents

Jane Donnelly

Key points

- The emotional needs of the child
- The need for trained children's staff
- Preparation of children for surgery
- The management of pain
- The child in the perioperative environment
- Discharge home

INTRODUCTION

During the last 40 years major changes have been witnessed in the role and sociological status of children in society. Increased awareness of children's vulnerability and developmental needs has served to change the public's attitude towards them, and has motivated professionals to work towards the provision of high-quality childcare services.

With that understanding has come an awareness of the emotional vulnerability of the young child and the effect early experience can have on later development. This has influenced how perioperative practitioners should care for the sick child.

Children are no longer regarded as 'little adults', and this is now reflected in health, education, government and the law.[1,2]

BRIEF HISTORY OF RECOGNITION OF CHILDREN'S NEEDS

The first major change in hospital care for children grew out of a study in 1945 on emotional deprivation in institutionalized children.[3] Realization of the child's need for close, affectionate human contact eventually led to relaxation of the visiting rules.

A crucial step forward in addressing the needs of children in hospital was identified by psychologist James Robertson, who was influenced by Bowlby's work[4] on child/parent separation. In his harrowing 1953 film 'A Two Year Old Goes To Hospital' Robertson showed that the most distressing part of hospitalization was not pain or illness, but separation from mother.[5]

The Health Ministry set up a committee to investigate arrangements made by hospitals for the welfare of children. Their report, *The Welfare of Children in Hospital* 1959, known as the Platt Report,[6] recognized the importance of parental involvement and of understanding the emotional needs of children.

Harry Platt, a young orthopaedic surgeon, was greatly influenced by Robertson's findings on the effects of child/parent separation. He stated: 'We are unanimous in our opinion that the emotional needs of the child in hospital require constant consideration. Changes of environment and separation from familiar people are upsetting and frequently lead to emotional disturbances, which vary in degree and may sometimes last well into adult life. The risk that any child will be disturbed by hospital admission can be reduced by suitable preparation of both parents and children.'[6]

Following the Platt Report, groups of parents and professionals came together and in 1961 formed the National Association for the Welfare of Children in Hospital (now Action for Sick Children).

In 1991, the government launched the Patients' Charter[8] outlining the rights, standards and expectations of all patients in the health service. The Patients' Charter also included for the first time *Services for Children and Young People,*[9] regarded as the bible for all who care for children in hospital and the community.

On 14 October 1991 The Children Act 1989[10] became law and is the most comprehensive piece of government legislation involving children. The Act stresses that the welfare of the child is paramount, and attaches great importance to the feelings and wishes of the child.

In 1991 an international agreement was drawn up by the United Nations to protect children's rights.[11] The standards apply to all children and young people up to 18 years of age. The convention includes four key principles:

- Non-discrimination: All rights apply to all children equally, no matter what their race, sex, religion, language, disability, opinion or family background.
- Best interests: When adults or organizations make decisions affecting children they must always think first about what would be best for the child.

Box 18.1   Millennium charter for children's health services

1. All children shall have equal access to the best clinical care within a network of services that collaborate with each other.
2. Health services for children and young people should be provided in a child-centred environment separately from adults, so that they are made to feel welcome, safe and secure at all times.
3. Parents should be empowered to participate in decisions regarding the treatment and care of their child through a process of clear communication and adequate support.
4. Children should be informed and involved to an extent appropriate to their development and understanding.
5. Children should be cared for at home with the support and practical assistance of community children's nursing services, unless the care they require can only be provided in hospital.
6. All staff caring for children shall be specifically trained to understand and respond to their clinical, emotional, developmental and cultural needs.
7. Every hospital admitting children should provide overnight accommodation for parents, free of charge.
8. Parents should be encouraged and supported to participate in the care of their child when they are sick.
9. Every child in hospital should have full opportunity for play, recreation and education.
10. Adolescents will be recognized as having different needs from those of younger children and adults. Health services should therefore be readily available to meet their particular needs. (reproduced with the permission of Action For Sick Children).[13]

• Right to life: All children have the right to life and the greatest possible opportunities to develop fully.

• The child's views: Children have the right to say what they think about anything that affects them. When courts or official bodies are making decisions affecting children they must listen to what children want and feel.[11]

In 2002, the Children's' National Service Framework[12] was launched to address some of the key challenges facing children's health services, placing children at the centre of care and building services around their needs.

THE EMOTIONAL NEEDS OF CHILDREN

The greatest single factor in the prevention of damaging emotional stress in children between 0 and 5 years is the continued presence of the mother/familiar adult. A young child's emotional development is immature, and separation during any stage of hospitalization only serves to increase their anxiety and sense of abandonment.

Unlike adult patients, young children are unable to rationalize or to draw on experience of life in order to gain comfort during the absence of their parents. The bond between parent and child can be damaged, and this is very upsetting for both.

Hospital policies must reflect and include the needs of the child and family unit, acknowledging that a parent's natural feelings of tenderness and protectiveness are increased when their child is ill or requiring hospital treatment.

MacCarthy[14] states that 'separation anxiety is responsible for great stress and an ordeal over and above the child's medical or surgical condition'. He described behavioural signs that hospitalization had been a harmful experience for the child. These include:

• Sleep disorders, insomnia, nightmares, sleep walking
• Anorexia or polyphagia
• Loss of recently acquired bladder/bowel control
• Regressional behaviour
• Child unable to tolerate mother being out of sight
• Panic when reminded of hospital, doctors, nurses, instruments
• Hypochondriac reactions, overprotectiveness of self

• Specific phobias, e.g. needles
• Tempers more frequent or severe than expected for age.

The severest form of disturbance is when the child shows complete indifference towards his/her parents and has no interest in play or other children.

Such behavioural difficulties should be a rare occurrence. However, community health professionals continue to meet a variety of childhood behavioural disturbances in the post-hospitalization period, and a major part of the health practitioner's role must be to help minimize these.

Today, parental participation in a child's hospital care is encouraged, with health professionals demonstrating a greater awareness of children's physical, intellectual, emotional and social needs.

PREPARATION OF CHILDREN FOR HOSPITAL ADMISSION

Going into hospital can be a particularly traumatic experience for children. Parents need information in order to be able to help, inform and support their child. Information also helps reduce a child's anxiety, enabling them to feel more in control of what is happening. The hospital admission should always be child centred, based on a partnership between the family and the healthcare team. Children's books and videos about going into hospital for surgery can help to prepare the child psychologically.

A hospital 'colouring book' is ideal in helping prepare the young child for a hospital experience. The child could be given the book during a clinic appointment or preadmission visit, thereby providing an opportunity for parent and child to work together on preparation for surgery.

By maximizing the information available, parents and children are given the opportunity to make informed decisions about their hospital stay, thus enhancing individualized quality patient care.

Information for families should include:

• List of items to bring in to hospital, including the child's favourite toy/comforter
• Parents' sleeping accommodation available
• Ward education/play facilities/visiting arrangements
• Information about the various health professionals who will be involved in the child's care
• Hospital mission statement

- Health and Safety policies, e.g. no smoking, no alcohol
- Information about going home and follow-up care and services.

Useful ward information should include:

- Leaflets on the child's particular condition
- Advice on role of the parent and how to best help their child
- Information about the multidisciplinary team who will be caring for their child
- Ward procedures and routine
- Preparation for operation
- Methods of pain relief and aftercare.

A child's special needs should ideally be discussed in the outpatient department or preassessment clinic prior to the date of admission, for example:

- The need for an interpreter and provision of audiovisual tapes in local minority languages for patients who do not easily understand English
- Religious/cultural requirements
- Special dietary needs
- Medical needs
- Operation fears.

The provision of adequate information facilitates the efficient delivery of care, avoiding unnecessary parental anxiety that is often quickly perceived by the child. Service provision is improved when information and expectations are shared.

THE HOSPITAL ENVIRONMENT

When a child comes into hospital it is important that the environment is set up to be as supportive as possible. The child is used to a bright, warm, safe place. The hospital environment can easily replicate this by providing bright, colourful surroundings to avoid a cold and clinical appearance. If a parent/carer remains with the child during the hospital stay the child's sense of security is maintained, and this helps to normalize the situation.

The hospital environment can be improved by:

- Painted murals along corridors
- User-friendly signposts to wards and departments
- Artificial plants
- Framed wall paintings
- Children's paintings on the walls

> **Box 18.2   Children's comments about the hospital environment**
>
> 'The school room made me feel normal, it was brilliant – it has posters and is bright and OK.'
> 'Its good to have my own television.'
> 'The things that made me feel better were the bright pictures.'
> 'It would have helped if there was something to look at, not just a depressing wall.'
> 'All those awful pale green corridors. ...'
> 'The hospital does not look cheery.'
> 'I hate the dark room.'
> (RCN Clinical Practice Guidelines 1999)[15]

- Play areas in outpatient departments, wards, perioperative waiting area, A&E
- Children's patterned curtains and screens
- Patterned pyjamas
- Patterned disposable nappies
- Patterned sheets, quilt covers
- Patterned tabards worn by staff
- Coloured hats, masks
- Patterned cushioned trolley sides
- Coloured staff name badges
- Books, toys and games for all age groups
- Mobiles, painted ceiling/floor designs
- Music, TV and video games
- Toy cars/bikes to ride to the operating department
- Child-sized furniture and bathroom facilities
- Parents' overnight stay facilities.

The provision of a welcoming environment enhances the child's sense of comfort and security.

THE NEED FOR TRAINED CHILDREN'S STAFF

In 1990, the CEPOD Report[16] identified that children under the age of 5 developed a higher rate of complications and that the outcome of surgery was dependent on the skill and experience of both the surgeon and the anaesthetist. Recommendations followed that every hospital offering a surgical service for children should have a designated consultant surgeon and consultant anaesthetist responsible for paediatric surgery.

Department of Health guidelines stipulate that there should be two nurses qualified to nurse sick children (RSCN or Project 2000 child branch) per shift on children's wards. Perioperative practitioners should also have training and experience in the needs of children and parents.

Qualified paediatric nurses, paediatricians, anaesthetists and those experienced in child care must be available to provide a professional service with an understanding and recognition of the child and family needs.

Those who work with children are subject to a police check and should be aware of both local and national child protection guidelines.

Appointments should be subject to a satisfactory (Criminal Records Bureau) disclosure check. There are two levels of such checks, standard and enhanced. Standard disclosure is for positions that involve regular contact with those aged 18 or under, or people of all ages who may be vulnerable for other reasons. The check contains details of all convictions, including any cautions, reprimands or warnings held on the Police National Computer.

Enhanced disclosure is for posts involving greater contact with children or vulnerable adults. Such work involves regularly caring for, supervising, training or being in sole charge of such people. Enhanced disclosures may also contain information that is held by police locally.

PREADMISSION VISIT

Invitations for preadmission visits may be sent to each child/family with information about the hospital. 'Saturday clubs' or their equivalent can be arranged when workload is less demanding and quality time can be given to preparing children for surgery.

The hospital visit can be made fun and an adventure, giving children and parents the opportunity to ask questions and resolve uncertainties. A visit to the ward to meet staff helps children to actually look forward to coming into hospital. Therefore, a child-friendly environment is most important. Play specialists and nursing staff can tailor the visit to be appropriate for specific age groups. A perioperative practitioner would also be a valuable member of the preadmission team. A visit to operating department and the recovery area may be possible, but such visits should be carefully planned and conducted when the theatre is fairly quiet.

The provision of a positive hospital experience for children on their first admission will be of great benefit to the child, family and health professionals, particularly if further treatment is required.

THE IMPORTANCE OF PLAY

Play services are essential to the quality management of children. Play is generally considered to be an intrinsic part of childhood, instrumental in how we grow to understand the world around us.[17] It is the primary medium through which children learn from birth to make sense of their environment. As an integral part of a child's life, it plays a major role in child development and the acquisition of skills. All children who come to hospital, whether as patients or 'accompanying' patients, need normal play. In hospital, children do not play naturally. Before children can relax sufficiently they need to be familiar with the hospital setting, and the hospital should be as friendly and as normal as possible.

Play gives the child or adolescent some outlet and a means of adjusting to a potentially frightening environment, removing some of the tension from the formality of medical routines and thereby providing a normal experience in an otherwise abnormal environment.

The games that children play tend to reflect aspects of their experiences in real life. When children

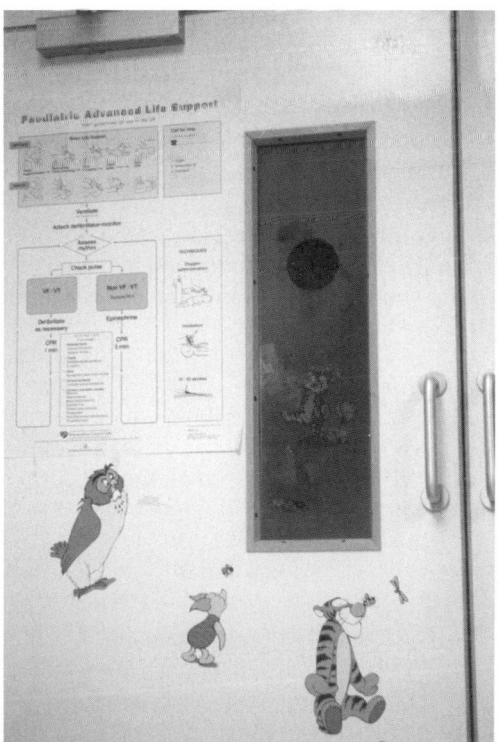

Figure 18.1 Focussing on the needs of children in the anaesthetic room.

find it difficult to communicate their perceptions of events in other ways, observation of their play can provide clues to these perceptions.[18,19]

Children and adolescents have differing play needs according to their age, length of stay, symptoms and previous clinical history. Play services should be led by hospital play specialists, whose major responsibility is the social/emotional welfare of the child and family.

Hogg[20] described play services involving many activities that demand different levels of competence from staff. This can be illustrated as a pyramid (Fig. 18.2).

Play can thus be seen as a therapeutic tool:

- Many children need help in coming to terms with their experiences of hospital and this can best be done by directed play
- Those undergoing surgery or clinical procedures need preparation play
- Children who face particular difficulties need individual therapeutic play
- Play is used effectively as a diversion therapy to distract the child while treatment is being given.

Play therapy using dolls or medical puppets is an effective means of preparing children for the appearance of cannulae, catheters, special wound dressings, etc., and can be adapted to any surgical specialty. 'Because the patient puppet has the same illness as the child, it can act as a role model to demonstrate procedures which the child will be experiencing'.[21]

Photograph albums are also useful for preparation. In 1991 it was recommended[20] that a play specialist should be available on all wards where children are being nursed.

As the benefits of play have become increasingly recognized, hospitals are beginning to employ play specialists to work in:

- Accident and emergency departments
- Radiography departments
- Neonatal and intensive care units
- Operating departments
- Outpatient departments.

The Save the Children Fund[22] outlined the benefits of play as follows:

- To provide a normalizing experience in stressful environment to prevent developmental regression
- To promote normal development and the meeting of specific developmental goals
- To reduce stress and anxiety for both children and parents
- To facilitate communication between staff and children
- To aid diagnosis, improve recovery rates and encourage children to cooperate with hospital procedures.

Lansdown[23] identified that 'play needs to be a fully integrated part of family-centred care, and is recognized and valued as a potentially cost-effective strategy in helping to speed the recovery process'.

THE ADOLESCENT

Adolescents have particular needs that are completely different from the care needs of the child or the adult. The need for dedicated hospital facilities for teenagers was formally recognized in the Platt Report (1959). Adolescence is an age of increased

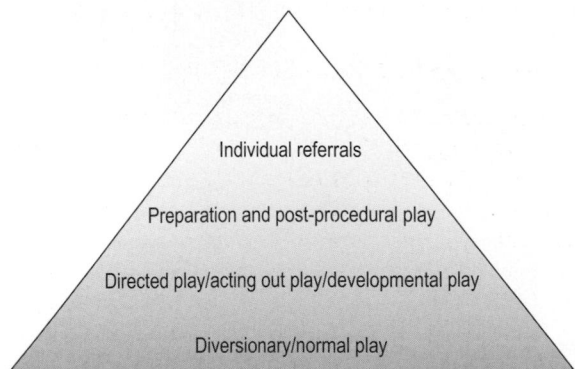

Figure 18.2   A pyramid of play services.

Individual referrals

Preparation and post-procedural play

Directed play/acting out play/developmental play

Diversionary/normal play

Box 18.3   The views of an adolescent

'When I was in hospital I learnt how important it is to ask and not to assume you will be offered choices. For example, I have a great fear of needles. I asked if I could therefore take drugs orally, and in many cases this was possible. I also had to ask if I could go to the adolescent ward, as otherwise I would have been admitted to the children's ward. The idea of early lights out, Postman Pat videos and screaming kids did not appeal to me!'
Robert, aged 16.
(Setting Standards for Children Undergoing Surgery 1994)[24]

awareness and concern about body integrity, which makes hospitalization and surgery a special threat. Children mature at different rates, so adolescence may start as early as 10 or as late as 14 years.[25]

When placed on a children's ward the adolescent will not appreciate being surrounded by children's articles, and may be too embarrassed to want to invite his friends. The teenager does not easily share space with a younger child who is a threat to his maturity,[26] yet the adolescent in hospital particularly needs the comfort and support of his peer group just as much as he needs his family. A special environment should be designated for adolescent patients and reflecting teenage tastes. A room should be available for reading, watching TV and seeing visitors in private if they wish. Adolescents need space for noisy pastimes where they will not disturb other patients. A CD player with headphones, a private telephone, and recreational facilities such as pool or table tennis could be provided.

The most appropriate place to care for adolescents is a self-contained unit, which may be attached to or entirely separate from the general paediatric unit. Viner[27] offers evidence-based guidelines for setting up and operating adolescent inpatient units, and a foundation on which clinical governance for young people can be based.

Education is also of great importance, as some adolescents may be preparing for examinations. Facilities should be provided to teach patients while they are in hospital.

The adolescent's privacy and dignity should be maintained at all times and bathroom facilities should be designed to include patients with disabilities, encouraging independence. Good facilities for shaving, hair-washing and make-up should be included.

Adolescents are snack eaters, and the provision of kitchen facilities will offer flexibility while a choice of menu will offer some measure of control.

Adolescents are in a constant state of developmental, physical and psychological change. They have special requirements that should be met by people who have the appropriate skills, knowledge and understanding to work with this age group.[28]

CONFIDENTIALITY

Older children should always have the opportunity to be interviewed without their parents. There may be factors that affect the operation, such as smoking, medicine/drug taking or pregnancy that parents do not know about.

Children's confidentiality should be respected. Under the Access to Health Records Act 1990[29] children can refuse access to their records by parents, as long as, in the view of the health professional, they understand what the application to see the records involves.[24]

PREPARATION OF CHILDREN FOR SURGERY

It is the responsibility of the parents to inform the child that they will be going into hospital to have an operation.

Older children should be involved in making the decision about the operation. It should be openly discussed and the child should participate in the planning, if this is what they want. To avoid unnecessary anxiety, the younger child should be informed of the date of admission between 4 and 7 days in advance. This gives opportunity for the child to think about it and to ask questions. Very young children (aged 2–3) should be told 2–3 days beforehand, and again on the morning of admission.[24]

Good use of preadmission time and preparation play in the form of children's videos/books about hospital will enhance the child's ability to accept the forthcoming admission without undue worry.

THE DAY OF ADMISSION

On the day of admission (assuming that the child is attending for elective day surgery), the child/parent should bring into hospital:

- A favourite toy, comforter, quiet game or book
- Nightdress/pyjamas, dressing gown and slippers if possible
- Loose comfortable clothing for the journey home
- Medication that the child is taking.

A member of the surgical team and the anaesthetist will examine the child to assess fitness for surgery and answer any questions that the child or parent may have. The surgeon should assess the child, as their condition may have changed since the last clinic appointment. In some instances the condition will have improved and surgery will no longer be required. The operative procedure should be explained, giving time for parent and child to ask questions before the consent form is signed.

The anaesthetist should discuss all aspects of the anaesthetic, including preparation, starvation time, the type of anaesthesia to be given, and problems of nausea and vomiting after surgery. Parents and children should be involved in the discussion about the type of anaesthesia that may be given.[24] An interpreter should be available for children and families from ethnic minorities who have difficulty in understanding the English language.

PREOPERATIVE VISITING

The benefits of giving preoperative information to patients have long been recognized.[30–33] Children and parents worry about many aspects of the planned surgery or anaesthetic procedure and can be afraid to ask questions. The removal of items such as children's underwear, spectacles or hearing aid while they are still awake is a common fear.

The perioperative practitioner can provide information, education and the continuum of patient care, to help alleviate unnecessary fear and anxiety, thereby promoting a smooth postoperative recovery.[30,34] If patients are not visited preoperatively little or no information can be obtained on which to plan and deliver individualized care in theatre.[35]

STARVATION TIMES

The rationale behind a preoperative fast is to minimize the risk, in the absence of the gag reflex, of the patient inhaling gastric contents while under anaesthetic.[36] It was reported[37] that 71% of 233 anaesthetists in a New Zealand study had experienced at least one case of gastro-oesophageal reflux in their career. In the interest of patient safety it seems that there is good reason to believe that preoperative fasting is desirable. Current US guidelines specify a minimum fluid fast of 2 hours.[38]

Children should be starved for the minimum time necessary before surgery. In general, the following starvation times are a guide:[24]

- Two hours for clear fluids
- Three hours for babies on breast milk
- Six hours for food and solid drinks (such as milk).

Children starved for longer periods may become distressed and try to obtain food by other methods. When fasted for long periods the body will draw on its own reserves and enter into a period of catabolism, which might leave the patient with insufficient strength and energy to negotiate postoperative recovery. Hypoglycaemia and ketosis might also result.[39]

Clear instructions should be given to parents on the scheduled time of the operation, the reason why starvation is necessary, and the types of food that would be regarded as 'light', 'solid' or 'fluids'. For example, parents may consider milk to be a drink, and a 'light breakfast' may be interpreted differently from one family to the next.

A timely and well planned starvation regime will facilitate a more comfortable preoperative experience for both patient and family, reducing the risk of operation delay because of a full stomach.

Good perioperative planning will ensure that younger children are placed first on the operating list to avoid prolonged starvation and unnecessary discomfort. Ward staff should also monitor the child's period of starvation, adjusting accordingly should any delays arise due to unforeseen difficulties.

CONSENT FOR SURGERY

See Chapters 1 and 3 for a full discussion of all aspects of consent. For the hospital to treat a child, consent must be obtained from either the patient, if he or she is considered mature enough to consent on his/her own behalf, or a person who has parental responsibility for the child.[10] Young people aged 16 and 17 are presumed by English law to have the competence to give consent for themselves.

Asking for consent is about giving children choice and control over what is happening to them. Children need to be consulted and involved according to their age and understanding. They may not be able to share in the overall decisions, but may have strong views on how things are done, for example how they would like to travel to the operating department, who they would like to have with them during induction of anaesthesia, method of anaesthesia, and choice of pain relief.[24] By assessing each child's maturity level and wishes, staff can provide the level of information appropriate to them.

To ensure 'informed consent' doctors must respect both the child's and the parents' capacity to receive and evaluate information, and give time to explain, listen and sort out any misunderstandings. For example, although parents are often the best advocates for their children, decision making for major surgery or in an emergency can be difficult. Parents may feel unsure, especially when they are making a decision on behalf of someone who is dependent on them. In such cases, where possible, consent should be obtained from both parents.

According to the Children Act 1989, where parents are separated, staff should find out who has parental responsibility.

- A mother automatically has parental responsibility. When parents are married at the time of the child's birth, both mother and father have parental responsibility
- If a child's mother and father were married at the time of the child's birth, even though they may subsequently separate or be divorced, both parents retain parental responsibility
- An unmarried father can obtain parental responsibility for his child by:
  - Agreement with the child's mother, which must be confirmed by the court
  - Obtaining a court order granting him parental responsibility.

Step-parents (unless they have legally adopted the child), grandparents, aunts, uncles or other relatives do not automatically have parental responsibility, even if the child lives permanently with them. However, they may obtain a Residence Order from the court, which will grant them parental responsibility for the child.

Foster parents do not automatically have parental responsibility. However, if the local authority has obtained a Care Order for the child, they may delegate parental responsibility to the foster parents. It is sufficient for consent to be obtained from one person who has parental responsibility.

URGENT TREATMENT

In cases where urgent treatment is required and there is no one available with parental authority who could give consent, if possible – and given the age and understanding of the child – the hospital should endeavour to obtain the child's consent. If the child is too young or unable to consent on their own behalf, the decision to give or withhold treatment should be made in the best interests of the child.

ACCESS TO RECORDS

Only a child who is considered to be mature enough to consent on their own behalf, or a person who has parental responsibility for the child, may give permission for access to their medical records made on or after 1 November 1991.[29]

THE MANAGEMENT OF PAIN

In 1990, the Royal College of Surgeons of England and the College of Anaesthetists published a report[40] confirming that 'pain experiences in children, although different from the adult experience, are no less severe'.

It was recommended that Acute Pain Services be established in hospitals to address the problem of inappropriate and ineffective postoperative pain management.[41] A widely held belief was that children did not experience pain with the same intensity as adults because of their immature nervous system. Misconceptions about children's pain have only recently begun to be dispelled.[42] Until comparatively recently there were too many myths clouding the issue of pain in children. Some people believed that an active child could not possibly be in pain, whereas it is now known that increased activity is recognized as a possible sign of pain. Some believed pain to be character building, though many children – often those with chronic illness – carry the psychological scars of past episodes of poorly managed pain and the ill effects of a bad hospital experience. Some children have become acutely phobic, taking hours – even days – to begin to regain the trust and confidence they had prior to receiving treatment.

It was a common belief that infants do not feel or remember pain, but Anand[43] identified that pain is felt even by the fetus. Research on the long-term effects of pain in neonates and infants[44] indicates that early experience of pain in the human newborn could alter the development of the nociceptive system and hence affect behaviour in adulthood.

Nociceptors are neurons that respond to noxious thermal, mechanical or chemical stimulation.[45] It is now a well established fact that neuroanatomical and neurophysical functions, in regard to nociception, are present as early as the 24th week of gestation.[46]

Early pain interventions have been shown to affect behaviour and pain later in life.

Therefore, it is most important to minimize pain and the number of painful stimuli, particularly in small children.

Pain comprises several different components:

- Physiological
- Psychological
- Social

- Ethnic
- Cultural.

These factors will contribute not only to how the child interprets and displays pain, but also the response of the carers.[47] During one interview with a 5-year-old boy, a doctor visited and said, 'How are you today, alright'? The boy answered: 'I'm fine thank you' (although he was actually crying in pain at the time). On being asked why he said he was fine, he answered: 'You must, its polite'.[15]

THE PAIN SERVICES TEAM

There is an increasing body of evidence supporting effective paediatric pain management.[48] Acute pain services have become established in many hospitals, comprising a multidisciplinary team led by a designated consultant anaesthetist and including the pain nurse specialist. The team operate a daily 'pain round', ensuring that patients have the analgesia they need while being offered a policy of balanced multimodal analgesia tailored to meet their individual needs.

In 1999, guidelines[49] were published to help recognize and assess acute pain in children. The document recommends the need to develop pain protocols to facilitate a standardized approach to pain assessment and pain management strategies.

A major factor influencing pain assessment in children is the nurses' characteristics. For example, experience, knowledge, attitudes and beliefs will affect decision making when assessing pain.[50]

PAIN ASSESSMENT

Pain in children can be assessed using a variety of behavioural or self-report tools, depending on the age of the child.

Good pain relief relies on accurate assessment of the pain that the child experiences. A pain history is important for baselines to be established. As 50% of children in hospital are under 5 years of age they have difficulty in communicating their level of pain. It is therefore essential to work in partnership with parents when assessing and controlling pain in children.

Pain symptoms in babies and children are expressed in a variety of ways that can be observed, measured or audibly assessed. Pain assessment tools have proved useful in helping to assess children's pain.[51]

Many children like to use 'pain thermometers' – simple pictures of a thermometer, one end marked '0' where there is no pain, whereas at the other end a '10' indicates the most pain possible. The child draws a cross on the line according to how much pain is being experienced.

Face scales are popular, based on a row of simply drawn faces ranging from a big smile to tears and a downturned mouth. The child places a mark against the face that most represents their pain. These assessment tools depend upon the child's level of understanding.

The Liverpool Pain Score Chart (Fig. 18.3) includes a visual analogue scale, the face scales for children between the ages of 5 and 10, and two useful scoring systems to help assess pain in children under the age of 5.

METHODS OF PAIN RELIEF

The choice of drugs and other techniques used for pain relief should be tailored to the severity of the child's pain.

A major preoccupation when a child first presents for surgery is the fear of needles. This can also stem from a phobia about being restrained or 'held down' from a previous traumatic hospital experience. 'Clinical holding policies' are already being developed in some hospitals.

Topical anaesthetic

The routine use of topical anaesthetics (magic cream), such as lidocaine (lignocaine)-prilocaine (EMLA) or tetracaine gel (Ametop), has proved very effective in reducing pain on venepuncture. The 'magic cream' can be applied directly in casualty or admissions department, so providing maximum effect for those children arriving for immediate elective/emergency surgery or treatment requiring injection. EMLA cream needs to be applied at least 1 hour before the procedure, whereas Ametop only needs to be applied 30 minutes beforehand. Premedication can also be given to relax a child before anaesthesia.

Oral analgesics

For mild pain, children are regularly prescribed paracetamol. The introduction of sublingual piroxicam (Feldene Melt) has been successful in treating moderate preoperative and postoperative pain. It is acceptable to children because it tastes like sherbet

ROYAL LIVERPOOL CHILDREN'S HOSPITAL PAIN SERVICE-PATIENT SCORING SYSTEMS PATIENTS UNDER ONE YEAR OF AGE – MODIFIED CRIES

PARAMETER	SCORES 0	SCORES 1	SCORES 2
Crying	None	Crying <20 sec; consolable	Crying >20 sec; inconsolable
Facial expression	Neutral	Grimace * <30 sec	Grimace * >30 sec
Movement/sleep	Normal; awake <30%	Reduced movement; awake >30% <50%	Immobile or restless; awake >50%
Physiology	+ or −10 % of baseline ***	>10% <20% change in HR or BP	>20% change in HR or BP
Requires O₂ to keep SaO₂ >95	No	Needing oxygen but <30%	Needing oxygen but >30%

Grimace = open mouth, lips pulled back at corners; creased/furrowed forehead and/or between eyebrow; eyes half closed, wrinkled laterally. (****REM** = rapid eye movement.) No REM = 0, REM = 1, REM + restlessness = 2.
** **Baseline** = measurements taken pre op. Parental and nurse pain score use VAS below

PATIENTS BETWEEN THE AGES OF ONE AND FIVE YEARS - MODIFIED TPPS

PARAMETER	SCORES 0	SCORES 1	SCORES 2
Verbal expression	None	Verbal complaint or cry <20 sec; consolable	Crying >20 sec; inconsolable
Facial expression	Normal	Grimacing * <20 sec	Grimacing * >20 sec
Posture	Normal	Touching/protecting/rubbing painful area	Defensive, tense, curled up
Movement	Normal	Reduced movement or restlessness	Immobile or thrashing, flailing
Physiology	+ or −10 % of baseline ***	>10% or <20% change in HR, SaO₂ or RR	>20% change in HR, SaO₂ or RR

*Grimace = open mouth, lips pulled back at corners; creased/furrowed forehead and/or between eyebrows; eyes closed, wrinkled at corners. N.B. must be awake. *** **Baseline** = measurements taken pre-op. **Parent pain score:** use VAS

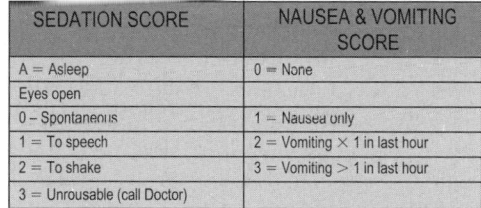

SEDATION SCORE	NAUSEA & VOMITING SCORE
A = Asleep	0 = None
Eyes open	
0 – Spontaneous	1 = Nausea only
1 = To speech	2 = Vomiting × 1 in last hour
2 = To shake	3 = Vomiting > 1 in last hour
3 = Unrousable (call Doctor)	

PAIN MEASUREMENT SCALE

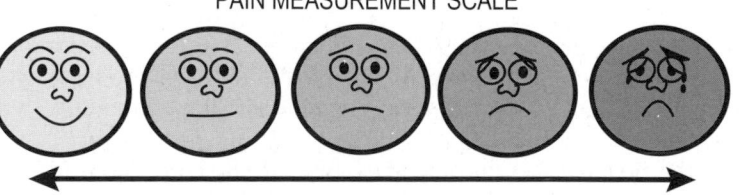

no pain 0   10 worst possible pain

Visual Analogue scale

Figure 18.3   The Liverpool Pain Score Chart. (Reproduced by kind permission of the Royal Liverpool Children's Hospital)

and is simple to administer. It can be given in the anaesthetic room just prior to induction.

Non-steroidal drugs such as piroxicam, ibuprofen and diclofenac (Voltarol) are very effective but should be used with caution in children with clotting deficiencies, gastric ulceration or renal problems. In a small percentage of asthmatic children they may cause bronchospasm. Codeine phosphate can be prescribed as an alternative.

Suppositories

Codeine, diclofenac or paracetamol can be given in suppository form during surgery under general anaesthetic, providing effective postoperative pain relief for several hours. It is important to remember that the absorption of paracetamol by this route can be very slow (i.e. 1 hour).

Local anaesthetic blocks

Levobupivacaine local blocks are commonly used in conjunction with prescribed oral medications to provide comfort during the initial postoperative period.

In day surgery, a local anaesthetic block is often given following induction of anaesthesia (e.g. in circumcision, orchidopexy or hernia repair), or at completion of many other surgical procedures, thereby providing additional pain relief.

Intermediate and major surgery may require other forms of pain relief, for example:

- Morphine infusion
- Patient-controlled analgesia
- Nurse-controlled analgesia
- Epidural
- Local anaesthetic block.

PREPARATION FOR THE OPERATING ROOM

Good communication between ward and perioperative staff will facilitate the development of a well-planned regimen for the child's arrival and return from the operating department.

It is important that the hospital has an agreed policy that parents can accompany their child into the anaesthetic room, provided the anaesthetist is in agreement and there are no clinical implications for them not to be present.

Parents should not feel pressurized to accompany their child to the anaesthetic room, but should be encouraged and welcomed. When children were

asked what helped them most when they were in pain, 99% stated the presence of their parents.[52]

Children from ethnic minorities may wear specific items of jewellery that are of religious significance. If possible, these should be taped to the body. In instances where jewellery has to be removed the family should be asked to do this and an explanation given.

A presurgery checklist should be completed to show the preparation and information that have been given to the child/parents.

TRAVEL TO OPERATING DEPARTMENT

Children without premedication should have the option to choose how they would like to travel to the operating department. They may wish to:

- Walk
- Be carried by a parent/carer
- Ride a toy car or bike
- Sit in their own bed
- Ride on an operating department trolley.

Children should be allowed to wear their own clothing when going for surgery. Ideally, clothing should be loose-fitting cotton with no metal fasteners, and easy to remove when the child is unconscious. If special surgical gowns/pyjamas need to be worn they should have bright patterns/designs.

The child should be able to take their favourite toy or comforter to the operating department. Parents should be told not to worry if the child's favourite blanket or soother looks a bit worn or old: it will provide comfort and allow the child to settle more easily.

Privacy and dignity must be respected at all times and, where necessary, children's underwear should not be removed until they are unconscious. The named nurse should accompany the child and parent to the operating department, introducing them to the staff receiving the child. Ideally the child should be received by the practitioner who conducted the preoperative visit.

PERIOPERATIVE INFORMATION LEAFLET

A patient information leaflet about going to the operating department is reassuring, particularly for parents whose children are admitted directly for emergency surgery and with limited preparation time. Information about the multidisciplinary team who will be caring for their child, collecting their child from recovery, and hospital facilities available will be useful.

A waiting area should be available, providing a quiet place where parents may wish to sit while their child is in the operating room.

THE PERIOPERATIVE ENVIRONMENT

On arrival in the operative department, parents and children should be made welcome in a non-threatening environment. The presence of the carer will provide reassurance and help to maintain the child's sense of security.[53–55] Children should never feel that they have been handed over to strangers, or suddenly feel abandoned by their carer, in whom they have complete trust.[56]

The perioperative environment should be colourful and interesting, creating distraction for the child and providing a calm, relaxed atmosphere, for example:

- Pictures in anaesthetic rooms/recovery room
- Ceiling or floor designs, such as butterflies/footprints that children can follow along the corridor
- Mobiles
- Soft toys
- Music
- User-friendly signposts.

Research-based evidence demonstrates that the wearing of gowns, overshoes, hats and masks by parents in the anaesthetic room is unnecessary in normal circumstances[57–60] and only serves to alienate the child. However, if specific infection control precautions do need to be taken and the parent is required to change into special clothing, the child should never be left alone.

THE CHILD IN THE ANAESTHETIC ROOM

Children should be welcomed into the anaesthetic room and greeted according to age and level of maturity. Anaesthetic staff should introduce themselves if they have not previously visited the ward. The anaesthetic room should be quiet, with minimal disturbances. Unnecessary medical and surgical equipment should be removed from the room prior to the child's arrival.

During the handover from ward nurse to perioperative practitioner, the identity of the child should be thoroughly checked along with consent for surgery.

Unlike the adult patient, who is able to confirm personal details and understands the surgical plan, young patients rely totally upon the advocacy of parents or professionals responsible for their care.

The child's privacy and dignity should be maintained at all times. The unnecessary removal of clothing should be avoided until the child is unconscious, although the patient's safety is paramount. For example, clothing may be restrictive and attempts to remove it after the induction of anaesthesia may compromise the child's airway and intravenous lines. Additionally, once the child is anaesthetized, the natural range of movement is less defined and overextension of limbs could result in nerve damage or joint injury. Children need to be dressed appropriately for their operative procedure.

It is important that the parent's role is discussed before coming to the operating department so that maximum support can be given to the child, on the understanding that the parent must leave the room when asked to do so.

The ward nurse or other specifically identified member of staff plays an important role in guiding the parent and helping to keep the child occupied and distracted while the 'magic cream' is being removed. In some instances the child may be more settled sitting on the parent's knee and can be distracted by playing with a toy, looking at pictures, or even blowing bubbles. This latter is a fun way to encourage a child to slow down their breathing and relax.[61]

Once the child is asleep, the nurse should be available to escort the parent out of the operating department and safely back to the ward. It is quite normal for parents to feel upset as they leave the anaesthetic room, and they often require some reassurance and support.

The parent of a neonate should be welcomed to accompany their baby into the anaesthetic room. Once the handover between ward nurse and anaesthetic staff is completed, the neonate will be transported into the operating room for induction of anaesthesia on the operating table. A neonatal anaesthetic trolley must be available, carrying a full range of appropriately sized equipment.

THE CHILD IN THE OPERATING ROOM

As with all patients, the environment should be suitably prepared with all necessary equipment, reflecting the child's specific needs.[56]

The normal operating room temperature should be at a minimum 24–25°C. This will need to be much higher for smaller premature babies or children with extensive tissue damage, following burns injuries for example. If a Bair Hugger is able to be used then the theatre temperature could remain constant for perioperative personnel. Alternatively, a warm-air blanket or warming mattress placed on the operating table prior to surgery will reduce the risk of hypothermic development. The child should be safely positioned on the operating table with potential pressure areas protected, using:

- Pressure relief mattresses such as KCI or a gel mattress
- Gel pads, foam rings, foam wedges
- Soft gauze, cotton wool or gamgee as appropriate.

The child's privacy and dignity should always be maintained and a warm blanket should be used to cover the child until surgery commences. For patient safety, appropriately sized equipment should be used at all times, e.g.:

- Paediatric-sized operating table
- Arm boards/specific paediatric table attachments for positioning
- Tourniquets
- Blood pressure cuffs
- Oxygen masks
- Diathermy plates.

Good planning, including provision of an adequate staff skill mix, avoids unnecessary delays, which could lead to complaints and unnecessary parental distress.

Effective communication between ward and departments and the operating department is a continual process promoting:

- Adequate and timely preparation of patients
- Shared information regarding adjustments to the operating list
- Reducing parental anxiety by offering reassurance and a progress report for children undergoing prolonged operative procedures
- Liaison between all members of the multidisciplinary team.

An intraoperative document should be completed to provide an accurate record of the total care the child has received in the operating department.

PROCEDURES UNDER LOCAL ANAESTHETIC

For some minor and short operative procedures children may choose or be encouraged to have surgery under local anaesthetic. The anaesthetist will preassess the emotional maturity of the child with regard to his/her ability to cope with the procedure.

The operating room should be suitably prepared for the admission of a conscious patient. Confidentiality must be protected regarding patient information displayed in the operating department.

A designated perioperative practitioner should greet the child on arrival and develop a rapport while remaining with the child to provide support throughout the procedure. The anaesthetist should remain within the vicinity just in case a general anaesthetic becomes necessary.

Following transfer into the operating room the child can be made comfortable on the table and quietly entertained in conversation while the surgical procedure is performed. Background music is effective in providing a calm, relaxed atmosphere.

The child should never be left alone, and personal contact, e.g. holding the child's hand if this is required, will help to maintain their sense of security. Once the procedure is completed, the child should be offered a cold drink prior to returning to the ward.

THE CHILD IN RECOVERY

Effective communication/handover between the theatre and recovery practitioners, including all information regarding the child's operative procedure, will enhance the quality of care in the postoperative period.

Some children may have special needs: for example, recovery practitioners will need to be aware of a child's physical disabilities, behavioural, hearing or language difficulties. Relevant previous history, including the child's social circumstances and family situation, will be important. The presence of an interpreter or parent may be required as soon as the child begins to wake.

All recovery rooms should have a designated area for children. A child must never be nursed alongside adult patients, as this could be highly disturbing to the child.

Privacy, dignity and warmth should be maintained, with curtains or screens being available during invasive procedures.

The recovery room environment should be non-threatening. Coloured walls, pictures, toys, mobiles, patterned curtains are important, and the atmosphere should be peaceful and quiet, with limited numbers of people and few telephone disturbances.[24]

A full range of paediatric resuscitation equipment must be available at all times.

Children should be allowed to find their own comfortable position where medically possible, and the use of padded trolley sides will reduce the risk of injury. For safety's sake a child should never be left alone.

Recovery practitioners should be trained in caring for children and have the ability to recognize when a child is in pain. It is important to have a knowledge of:

- Airway management
- Resuscitation
- Pain assessment
- Monitoring and equipment
- Wound management
- Fluid balance
- Health and safety
- Accurate record keeping.

Qualified recovery practitioners must have knowledge of the paediatric dosage of medications, and medical staff should be readily available to prescribe adequate analgesia.

Parents should not be pressurized to visit their children in recovery, but be given information about what to expect and guidelines on their role.[65]

Departmental policy should include the welcoming of a parent into the recovery room where possible, and the opportunity should be offered for a parent to accompany the ward nurse to collect their child.[62–64]

To minimize distress all children should be returned to their parents as soon as medically possible.[10,24,25]

Before returning to the ward, it is important that children are pain free and suffering minimal discomfort. All documentation and prescription sheets should be completed to facilitate a smooth recovery and handover to the ward nurse.

DISCHARGE HOME

When the child is ready for discharge, carers should be given both verbal and written information about aftercare, including pain relief and any potential signs or symptoms of which they need to be aware.

A 3-day 'take-home analgesia pack' may be prepared for the child. The medication should be given regularly or as prescribed, whether or not the child complains of pain. This will ensure comfort and continuity of pain relief. A hospital helpline could be available for parents who may require additional advice or support at home.

The primary/named nurse is responsible for the discharge planning based on assessment and information from all members of the multidisciplinary team.

The patient discharge plan should be discussed with the carers and arrangements made for continuing care.

In the UK:

- Children under the age of 5 are referred to the health visitor
- Children over the age of 5 are referred to the school nurse
- Community nurse referrals are generated as a result of needs assessment.

Agreed guidelines and protocol between hospitals, GPs and community nursing staff ensure a seamless transition of care between the hospital and the community.

References

1. Department of Health. A first class service: quality in the new NHS. London: DOH; 1998.
2. The Human Rights Act 1998. London: HMSO.
3. Spitz RA. Hospitalism: an inquiry into the genesis of psychiatric conditions in early childhood: the psychoanalytic study of the child. New York: International Universities Press; 1945: 53–74.
4. Bowlby J, Ainsworth M, Boston M, et al. The effects of mother–child separation: a follow-up study. Br J Med Psychol 1956; 29: 211.
5. Robertson J. Film. A two year old goes to hospital. 16 mm. English or French. London: Tavistock Clinic; New York Film Library; 1953.
6. Ministry of Health. The report of the Committee on the Welfare of Children in Hospital. Platt Report. London: HMSO; 1959.
7. The National Association for the Welfare of Children in Hospital. Final report: preparing children for hospital. London: HMSO; 1980.
8. Department of Health. The patient's charter. London: HMSO; 1991.

9. Department of Health. The patient's charter. Services for children and young people. London: HMSO; 1996.

10. Children Act 1989. London: HMSO.

11. Department of Health. The United Nations Convention on the Rights of the Child. London: HMSO; 1999.

12. Department of Health. The national service framework acute services document. London: HMSO; 2000. Online. Available: http://www.doh.gov.uk/childrens task-force 2000

13. Action for Sick Children. The millennium charter for children's health services. 2000.

14. MacCarthy D. The under fives in hospital. London: NAWCH; 1979.

15. RCN. Clinical practice guidelines. Ouch! Sort it out. Children's experience of pain. London: RCN; 1999.

16. CEPOD. The report of the National Confidential Enquiry into Perioperative Deaths. London: HMSO; 1990.

17. Webster A. The facilitating role of the play specialist. Paed Nurs 2000; 12: 14–27.

18. Goldman LR. Child's play, myth, mimesis and make-believe. Oxford: Berg; 1998.

19. Pellegrini AD, Bjorklund DF. Applied child study. A developmental approach. London: Lawrence Erlbaum Associates; 1998.

20. Hogg C. Quality management for children. Play in hospital. London: NAWCH; 1991.

21. Chakrabati A. Patient puppets. Cascade, Action for Sick Children; Jan 1993.

22. Save the Children. Hospital. A deprived environment for children? London: Save the Children Fund; 1989.

23. Lansdown R. Children in hospital. Oxford: Oxford Medical; 1996.

24. Action for Sick Children. Setting standards for children undergoing surgery. Quality review series. London: Action for Sick Children; 1994.

25. National Association for the Welfare of Children in Hospital. Setting standards for adolescents in hospital. London: NAWCH; 1990.

26. Kenny TJ. The hospitalized child. Symposium on behavioral pediatrics. Ped Clin Nth Am 1975; 22: 583–591.

27. Viner R. Youth matters: evidence-based best practice for the care of young people in hospital. London: Action for Sick Children; 1998.

28. Mortimer G. Children and young people in adult wards. Paed Nurs 2001; 13: 39–42.

29. Access to Health Records Act 1990. London: HMSO.

30. Hayward J. Information – a prescription against pain. London: RCN; 1975.

31. Boore J. Prescription for recovery. London: RCN; 1978.

32. Booth K. Preoperative visiting. A step by step guide Part 1. Br J Theatre Nurs 1991; 1(7): 30–31.

33. Booth K. Preoperative visiting. A step by step guide Part 2. Br J Theatre Nurs 1991; 1(8): 6–7.

34. Kalideen D. The case for preoperative visiting. Br J Theatre Nurs 1991; 1(5): 19–22.

35. Carter L, Evans T. Preoperative visiting: a role for theatre nurses. Br J Nurs 1996; 5: 204–207.

36. Rodgers S. The patient facing surgery. In: Alexander M, Fawcett J, Runciman P, et al, eds. Nursing practice. Hospital and home. The adult. London: Churchill Livingstone; 2000.

37. Kluger M, Willemson G. Anti-aspiration prophylaxis in New Zealand 1. A national survey. Anaesth Intens Care 1998; 26: 70–77.

38. Dean A, Fawcett T. Nurses' use of evidence in preoperative fasting. Nurs Standard 2002; 17: 33–37.

39. Rowe J. Preoperative fasting: is it time for change? NT 2000; 96: 14–15.

40. Royal College of Surgeons and College of Anaesthetists. Pain after surgery. London: RCS; 1990.

41. Llewellyn N. A headache all over my body. Paed Nurs 1991; September: 14–16.

42. Coffman S, Alvarez Y, Pyngolil M, et al. Nursing assessment and management of pain in critically ill children. Heart Lung 1997; 26: 221–228.

43. Anand KJS, Hickey P. Pain and its effect in the human neonate and fetus. N Engl J Med 1987; 317: 1321–1329.

44. Anand KJS. Long term effects of pain in neonates and infants. Eighth World Congress on Pain, August 1996. Vancouver: IASP Press; 1996.

45. Basbaum A. Basic mechanisms: anatomy and physiology of nociception. In: Kanner R, ed. Pain management secrets. Philadelphia: Hanley and Belfus Medical; 1997.

46. Anand KJS, Carr DB. The neuroanatomy, neurophysiology and neurochemistry of pain, stress and analgesia in newborns, infants and children. Ped Clin Nth Am 1989; 36: 795–822.

47. Seers K. Factors affecting pain assessment. Prof Nurs 1988; 3: 201–206.

48. Gibson F, Llewellyn N. Learning about paediatric pain. Paed Nurs 1997; 9: 20–23.

49. Royal College of Nursing Institute. Clinical practice guidelines: the recognition and assessment of acute pain in children. London: RCN; 1999.

50. Abu-Saad H, Hamers M. Decision making and paediatric pain: a review. J Advan Nurs 1997; 26: 946–952.

51. Lansdown R, Sokel B. Commissioned review. Approaches to pain management in children. ACPP Review and Newsletter 1993; 15: 105–111.

52. Ross DM, Ross SA. Childhood pain: the school aged child's viewpoint. Pain 1984; 20: 179–191.

53. Day A. Can Mummy come too? NT 1987; 83: 51–52.

54. Donnelly J. A question of parents in the anaesthetic room. Br J Theatre Nurs 1991; 28: 4–8.

55. Glasper A, Powell C. First do no harm: parental exclusion from anaesthetic rooms. Paed Nurs 2000; 12: 14–17.

56. National Association of Theatre Nurses. Principles of safe practice in the operating theatre. A resource book. Harrogate: NATN; 1993.

57. Orr N. Is a mask necessary in the operating theatre? Ann R Coll Surg 1981; 63: 390–392.

58. Mitchell N, Hunt S. Surgical face masks in the modern operating room – a costly and necessary ritual? J Hosp Infect 1991; 18: 238–242.

59. Hubble MJ, Weale AE, Perez JV, et al. Clothing in laminar flow operating theatres. J Hosp Infect 1996; 32: 1–7.

60. Belkin N. Evolution of the surgical mask. Infect Control Hosp Epidemiol 1997; 18: 49–56.

61. Scobie N. Bubbles can make pain float away. NZ Pract Nurse 1995; November: 31–34.

62. Diniaco MJ, Ingolsby BB. Parental presence in the recovery room. AORN J 1983; 38: 685–693.
63. Brown V. Parents in recovery: parental and staff attitudes. Paed Nurs 1995; 7: 17–19.
64. McGinty SE. Parental presence in the recovery room: help or hindrance? Who benefits? Anaesth Recov Nurse 1999; 5: 12–17.
65. Perthen C. Involving the parents. Nursing 1990; 4: 12–16.

Further reading

Adams M. A hospital play program. Helping children with serious illness. Am J Orthopsych 1976; 46: 3.

Alderston P. Children's consent to surgery. Oxford: OUP; 1993.

Audit Commission. Children first. A study of hospital services by the Audit Commission for local authorities and the NHS. London: HMSO; 1993.

Ball A, Ferguson S. Analgesia and analgesic drugs in paediatrics. Br J Hosp Med 1996; 55: 586–590.

Barnett L. Young children's resolution of distress through play. J Child Psychol Psychiatry 1984; 25: 477–483.

Baxter R, Long A, Sines D, et al. The legal and ethical status of children in health care in the UK. Nurs Ethics 1998; 5: 189–199.

Becker RDC. Illness and hospitalization in adolescence. A developmental perspective. Paediatrician 1980; 9: 242–260.

Bevan P. The management and utilization of operating departments. London: HMSO; 1989.

Bird C. No need to starve. Nurs Standard 2000; 14: 20.

Blunden R. An artificial state. Arguments in favour of adolescent units in hospitals. Paed Nurs 1989; 2: 12–13.

Chan JM. Preparation for procedures and surgery through play. Paediatrician 1980; 9: 210–219.

Cox FN. Young children in a situation with and without their mothers. Child Develop 1968; 39: 123–131.

Department of Health. A first class service: quality in the new NHS. London: HMSO; 1998. Online. Available: http://www.doh.gov.uk/newnhs/quality.htm

Dimond B. Patient's rights, responsibilities and the nurse. Dinton: Quay; 1995.

Gauntlett I. Analgesia in the neonate. Br J Hosp Med 1987; 36: 518–519.

Glasper EA, Powell C. The challenge of the children's charter. Rhetoric vs reality. Br J Nurs 1996; 5: 26–29.

Glasper EA. Parental presence during anaesthesia induction in children. Children in hospital. J Ass Welfare Child Health 1993; 19: 1–4.

Hannallah RS, Rosales JK. Experience with parents' presence during anaesthesia induction. Can Anaesth Soc J 1983; 30: 886–889.

Howard V, Thurbar F. The interpretation of infant pain. Physiological behavioural indicators used by NICU nurses. J Paed Nurs 1998; 13: 164–173.

Kuykendall J. Teenage trauma. NT 1989; 86: 26–28.

McGinty SE. Parental presence in the recovery room. Anaesth Recov Nurse 1999; 5: 12–17.

McGrath PA. The multi-dimensional assessment, management and research of pain syndromes in children. Behav Res Therapy 1987; 25: 251–262.

Millar S. The psychology of play. London: Penguin; 1996.

National Association for the Welfare of Children in Hospital. Caring for children in the health services. Just for the day. London: NAWCH; 1991.

National Association of Theatre Nurses. Nursing the paediatric patient in the adult perioperative environment. Harrogate: NATN; 1996.

O'Brien S, Konsler G. Alleviating children's postoperative pain. Am J Maternal Child Nurs 1988; 13: 183–186.

Phillips S, Hutchinson S, Davidson T, et al. Preoperative drinking does not affect gastric contents. Br J Anaesth 1993; 70: 6–9.

Price S. The special needs of children. J Advan Nurs 1994; 20: 227–232.

Roberts D. Adolescence. Overview of adolescents' development and how this affects health care. Nursing 1987; 24: 914–919.

Simons J. Growing pains. Paed Nurs 1999; 11: 10–11.

Townsend P, Monartey A, Bagshaw O, et al. Pain control on the paediatric intensive care unit. Br J Intens Care 1998; 8: 186–193.

Wilson K. Management of paediatric pain. Br J Nurs 1993; 2: 524–526.

Wolf A. Pain, nociception and the developing infant. Paed Anaesth 1999; 9: 7–17.

Useful website/reference addresses

Action for Sick Children c/o National Children's Bureau
8, Wakely Street, London EC1V 7QE
www.actionforsickchildren.org
Children's Taskforce
www.doh.gov.uk/children's taskforce

National Association of Theatre Nurses
Daisy Ayris House, 6 Grove Park Court, Harrogate, North Yorkshire
HG1 4DP
www.natn.org.uk

National Service Framework for Children
http.www.doh.gov.uk/nsf/children.htm

Royal College of Nursing Institute
20 Cavendish Square, London W1M 0AB
The NHS Plan (July 2000)
www.nhs.uk/nationalplan

Chapter 19

Care of the obstetric patient

Brian Smith, Tom Williams and Josie Williams

Key points

- The safe care of the perioperative obstetric patient, the partner and the baby
- The role of the perioperative practitioner in the birthing process
- The care of the patient undergoing caesarean section
- The emergency situation

There are a variety of conditions affecting pregnant women that may lead to surgical intervention, including pre-eclampsia and placenta praevia.

Pre-eclampsia is a condition that occurs in the late stages of pregnancy. If untreated, pre-eclampsia will develop into full eclampsia, causing fits, seizures and possible other system failures affecting, for example, the kidneys, liver or brain.

Placenta praevia occurs in 1 in 250 births.[1] The condition involves the partial growth of the placenta in the lower section of the uterus, either near to or actually covering the internal os.

CAESAREAN SECTION

According to legend, Julius Caesar was born by what we now term caesarean section or, more literally, abdominal delivery. However, alternative theories suggest that the origins of the procedure and its title may relate to an ancient Roman law or dictate, ratified by Caesar, declaring that any woman dying in labour must be cut open in the hope of saving the child. Whichever explanation applies today is somewhat academic, and of more importance to perioperative practitioners is what the procedure involves, i.e. the surgical opening of the abdominal wall during the later stages of pregnancy in an attempt to deliver the baby safely.

Almost universally – but technically incorrectly – the operative procedure is referred to as lower uterine segment caesarean section (LUSCS). This description is somewhat misleading, as it refers to a specific anatomically lower approach as opposed to upper segment or classic approach using a midline incision. The lower approach actually utilizes a transverse or Pfannenstiel incision. However, it is understandable why in hospital jargon the operation is usually referred to as caesarean section or section. Likewise, in written form the procedure is also often recorded as C/S or C/section.

Elective sections are usually conducted about 1 week before the estimated date of delivery. Patient-focused care is important, as the procedure can be very stressful for all involved.

Elective surgery has advantages and disadvantages for the mother.

Advantages:

- The mother is fully aware of the date for surgical delivery and can plan around that date
- There is an absence of fetal stress and a comfortable birth for the child.

Disadvantages:

- Surgical intervention includes incision through a variety of muscular tissues, which will need time to repair; therefore the mother's hospital stay will be longer than with vaginal delivery
- Often the postoperative care for the mother will be dependent on others in terms of mobility for the first couple of days
- There will be tenderness to the abdominal incision area, which may make breastfeeding difficult
- There are associated infection risks
- There may be rupture or trauma to associated structures, i.e. bladder or ureter
- There is potential postoperative haemorrhaging and clotting. According to Miller[2] the blood loss is commonly between 500 and 1000 ml because of the vascular nature of the anatomical region.

PREGNANCY

Throughout the pregnancy there will have been significant changes in blood composition, but not necessarily in blood pressure. During a normal pregnancy the output volume of the heart is crucial to nourish the baby within the uterus. According to Redman,[3] blood volume and heart rate increase by 30%, thereby increasing cardiac output. The result would normally be an increase in blood pressure because of the reactive constriction of the arteries. However, hormones associated with pregnancy, such as prolactin and progesterone, could have the opposite effect and cause the arteries to relax and dilate. This results in a demand on the mother's other vital organs. The increased volume in the circulation and the collection of waste products from the mother and baby will require the kidneys to play a greater role. The function of the kidney is to produce urine (which contains urea, creatinine and uric acid) and deposit it in the bladder. From the filtering stage of the kidney, some water is reabsorbed in the glomerulus along with glucose and amino acids. An increased presence of protein in the urine indicates that there might be a source of infection in the kidney, or signs of kidney failure. The latter would be a good reason to bring the pregnant mother to theatre for a caesarean section.

Caesarean sections present several considerations for the practitioner in relation to patient support. First, the chance of natural birth has been excluded for many mothers. Some may have preferred to give birth by themselves in surroundings that are more natural, while experiencing the natural pain and stresses of childbirth. In theatre, the absence of the factors surrounding natural childbirth, such as the pain of delivery, may have a significant effect on the parents.

Theatres can be a cold and clinical environment and may not result in the 'special moment' that an expectant mother and partner may wish for. However, practitioners should still aspire to maintain the special feeling of giving birth, even in the theatre environment.

PREPARING THE THEATRE ENVIRONMENT

It is standard practice and desirable for caesarean sections to be carried out in a dedicated theatre sited within an obstetric unit, staffed by practitioners who are free of other theatre commitments. The expectation, therefore, is that those personnel responsible for or involved in staffing obstetric theatres should be continually available and have the operative environment prepared and ready for surgery at all times. It is also of paramount importance that these practitioners are familiar with the unique physical and psychological needs of mother and baby throughout the entire period of surgical intervention.

The same meticulous preparation and commitment are required for both elective and emergency caesareans, which although non-scheduled by nature can and do present with their own differing and inherent problems, which practitioners should be prepared for and trained to deal with. Likewise, whether general (GA), regional or local anaesthesia is involved, the same high standards and attention to detail apply. The skills of communication are of added importance when the mother is awake and conscious during procedures under local anaesthetic. This aspect should be awarded even greater emphasis when the partner is present during surgery, as is the current practice in most centres.

Use of a regional technique also has the advantage of immediate mother and baby bonding, as opposed to later introducing the baby as a potential 'stranger' to the mother, as may be the case with a general anaesthetic.

Further considerations for the perioperative practitioner involve all the usual factors concerned with surgery. For example, unnecessary equipment should be removed from sight but not put out of mind: it should be nearby, with all the team aware of its location.

Noise and people pollution must be kept to a minimum when the mother is being anaesthetized in theatre. Otherwise, her anxiety could increase and cause reactions, such as a vasovagal attack.

Resuscitators should be unobtrusive but within easy reach to give the paediatricians and midwives sufficient space and time to look after the baby when born.

Perioperative practitioners should deliberate on how their theatre looks and should adopt a 'through the patient's eyes' approach, drawing on their knowledge and skills of risk management and health and safety. For example, the ambience of the operating room should be considered when decorating, and appropriate and soothing colours chosen.

GETTING THE MOTHER AND PARTNER READY FOR THEATRE

A major factor to consider is that there are two patients to consider – the mother and the baby. This is different from most other procedures. Also, because the mother is not necessarily 'ill' as such, and the

caesarean section does not 'cure' her, the end result is more than just curing a condition, it is introducing a life.

Mothers coming to theatre need to be well informed of the procedures and be reassured they still have an involvement in the birth. There should be adequate medical and ward preparation, ensuring that factors such as blood taken and identified for blood grouping or group and save, along with blood results and 2 units of blood cross-matched ready for use, ultrasound scans and patient notes are available. In relation to intravenous (IV) infusion, it should be mentioned that all obstetric units will have a protocol for major bleeding and which will involve the availability of group O-negative blood for non-cross-matched transfusion.

Scans are very different from X-ray images. Ultrasound (Fig. 19.1) works by a series of sound waves emitted at a high frequency passing through water and bouncing off solid objects, in this case the fetus. The bouncing effect creates echoes, which are then picked up by the machinery and computed electronically into the image.

It is worth noting that the reason for using ultrasound is to determine fetal activity, growth rate and abnormalities.[4] X-rays are contraindicated in pregnancy because the fetus is particularly susceptible to tissue damage from irradiation. Perioperative practitioners do not have to be trained specialists in ultrasound, but must appreciate the reasons for care in the use of X-rays. Normally there will be two images of the unborn, at approximately 16 weeks' and (if necessary) 32 weeks' gestation. These are also useful in helping practitioners develop skills for interpreting images in general, for example during vascular (e.g. venography) or neurosurgery (e.g. computed tomography (CT) scans).

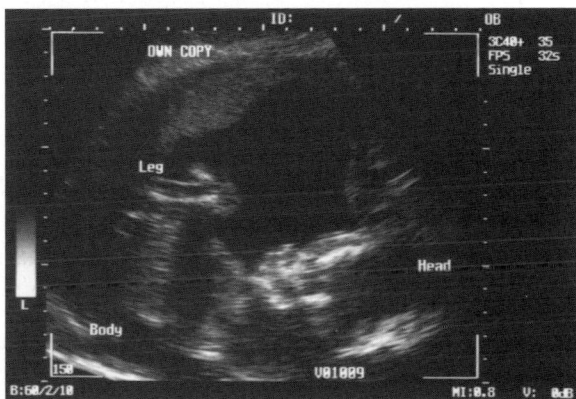

Figure 19.1 Ultrasound scan.

Perioperative practitioners also need to consider the accompanying partner, as they are often entering a theatre for the first time and can find the experience very frightening. There will be those who may freely express how they feel, whereas others try to hide their feelings in support of the mother's needs. The experience of accompanying their pregnant partner can be overwhelming, and on occasion may result in their requiring treatment themselves. For example, the stress of the situation could produce vagal stimulation, causing a change in pallor and lowering the heart rate, with the possibility of fainting. Therefore, it is essential to ensure that the holistic needs of the mother and partner are considered simultaneously.

Many practitioners experience feelings of satisfaction and achievement as they reflect on the birth, and also on the achievement of teamwork as a reality and not simply a cliché. Discussion between qualified staff and students who are witnessing their first caesarean section confirm this and reveal the full range of human emotions.

Related to these reasons, practitioners often have a feeling of involvement rather than just being a deliverer of service, especially if it is a planned procedure and pre- and postoperative visiting has been involved. The peace of mind, not to mention elation, following the safe and satisfactory outcome of emergency caesarean gives most perioperative practitioners both personal and professional satisfaction.

Possibly, with this surgical procedure, more so than with any other, the perioperative practitioner touches on the full spectrum of aspects from technician through to practitioner, as the full range of equipment, practices and personal responsibilities are brought into play.

To some extent the practitioner experiences a reversal of circumstances when dealing with caesarean, in that a relatively healthy patient enters their domain as opposed to the usual surgical situation. However, during the entire perioperative period there is the potential for this to be adversely affected, with some outcomes being within their control and dependent on their ability, training and professionalism. Probably no other activity that the practitioner encounters creates such a situation. Added to this potential dichotomy are the issues surrounding the two lives of mother and baby.

The practitioner's feelings and desires for the mother to exit the situation in good health, which are further enhanced by the addition of a healthy baby, involves the perioperative practitioner in a unique experience.

CARE OF THE MOTHER WHILE IN THEATRE

The document *Guidelines for Obstetric and Anaesthetic Services* recommends that the 'person assisting the anaesthetist during anaesthesia should have no other duties at that time'.[5] The role of anaesthetic practitioner is not an isolated technical one because of the ever-increasing awareness of patient empowerment. The anaesthetic practitioner has a key role as advocate to ensure that the patient's rights are maintained, as well as the previously mentioned special situation. Kneedler[6] encourages practitioners to adopt a 'personable and friendly' approach helps the practitioner to convey a supportive and caring attitude.

As part of their role the anaesthetic practitioner will be expected to have planned the anaesthetic requirements. This will include the checking of anaesthetic machines in accordance with the manufacturers' recommendations, as well as the requirements set by the Association of Anaesthetists. Increased vigilance is required, especially in the light of events such as the tragic death of 9-year-old Tony Clowes (Box 19.1).[7,8]

The controversial argument about reusing disposable equipment is being highlighted to make the public more aware of this questionable practice. It is worth remembering professional codes of practice for practitioners in respect of promoting and protecting the rights of the patient.

Operation Orcadium, led by Essex police, investigated the death of Tony Clowes along with 12 other incidents involving blocked anaesthetic tubing. The Department of Health, the Medical Devices Agency and the Health and Safety Executive later concluded, in a report which was supported by Essex police, that 'a lengthy and detailed investigation has produced no evidence to show that the series of blockages was the result of criminal conduct'.[10]

Box 19.1 Tony Clowes
'Doctors have been warned to check oxygen tubes before use after a series of mystery blockages, one leading to the death of a boy.
Youngster Tony Clowes, from Dagenham, died on 18 July in the preoperation room after being admitted to Broomfield Hospital to have the top of his finger sewn back on following a bike accident.' BBC, Friday 10 August 2001, 12:24 GMT 13:24 UK[9]

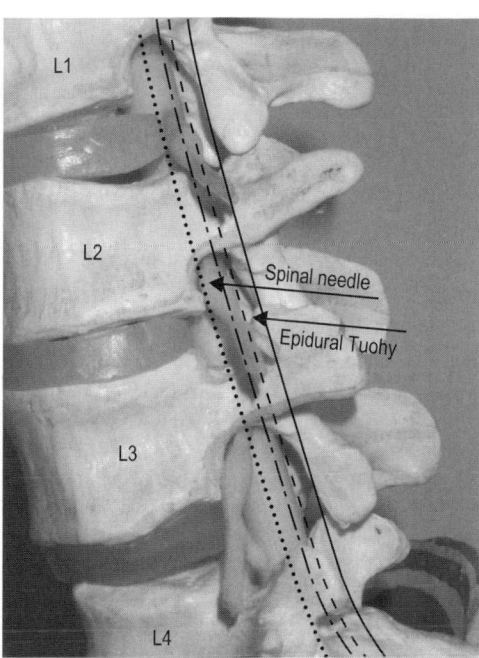

Figure 19.2 Representation of insertion point for spinal and epidural needles. — Ligament, – – – Dura, – – – Arachnoid, ······· Pia.

The practitioner must continue to consider the delivery of perioperative care to all patients, including the unborn child, who develops sensitivity to sound even in the early stages of pregnancy.

EPIDURAL AND SPINAL ROUTES OF ANAESTHESIA

Local anaesthesia has become the most popular choice of pain relief during birth because of the associated lower risks compared to those of general anaesthesia. Epidurals are performed where there is sufficient time to prepare the mother. A Tuohy needle is inserted into the epidural space (Fig. 19.2), followed by the introduction of a fine catheter. Once in situ the catheter can then be secured to the mother's back with adhesive tape. Epidurals are very successful for offering controlled pain relief after surgical intervention.

However, time does not always allow the opportunity to offer an epidural because of the urgency of the impending delivery, therefore a spinal anaesthetic is often given.

The major differences with a spinal anaesthetic are the anatomical positioning of the needle and the drugs used to create the blocking effect. A spinal needle (usually much finer and longer than an epidural needle) is carefully placed into the subarachnoid space of the meninges. This is where the cerebrospinal fluid circulates around the outer surface of the brain and spinal cord. A flashback of cerebrospinal fluid (CSF) will be seen at the syringe end of the needle. Once it is clear that this is indeed CSF, infiltration of 3–4 ml of heavy Marcaine 0.5% containing glucose will commence. The weight of glucose encourages the Marcaine to remain in the lower end of the spinal canal, allowing the anaesthetic block to act at the correct dermatome and thus reducing the risk of respiratory problems.

The main advantage of local over general anaesthesia is that the mother maintains spontaneous respiration, provided the anaesthetic block does not rise too high. The regional approach helps the patient to play a significant part in the delivery of their child. Above dermatome T8 a greater risk of diaphragmatic relaxation and respiratory depression may occur.

GENERAL ANAESTHESIA

General anaesthesia presents increased risks with obstetric patients, partly because in the pregnant mother there is a large weight from the child pressing on the organs in the abdominal region.

Common risks associated with general anaesthesia in obstetric patients include occlusion of the inferior vena cava, leading to reduced blood return to the heart. This may lead to hypotension, especially when the patient is in the supine position.

To avoid this, the weight of the child can be displaced to the left by inserting a 'wedge' or tipping the table to one side, thereby reducing caval obstruction. This should be done as early as possible.

Further consideration must be given to the pressure placed on the stomach, the diaphragm and, consequently, the airway.

The insertion of an endotracheal tube can become problematic owing to the temporary altered anatomy of the mother. Hormones during pregnancy cause enlargement of the breasts, limiting access into the oral cavity for insertion of the laryngoscope. Polio and McCoy's blades can be used to assist in difficult intubations. The McCoy blade has a manipulable epiglottis end, which has had a significant impact on the successful and safe access to the patient's airway. However, there are still some risks from the altered anatomy of the patient that can only be addressed through tried and tested techniques. Sellick's manoeuvre, more commonly known as

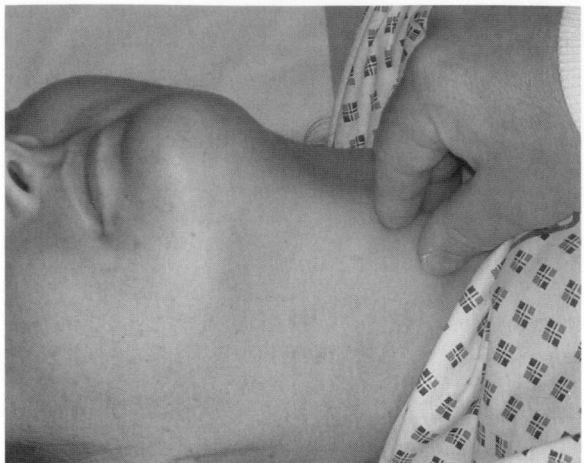

Figure 19.3   Cricoid pressure.

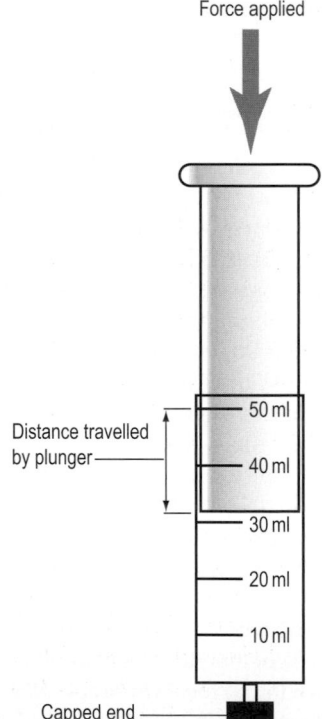

Figure 19.4   Representation of force applied to a Plastipak syringe.

Table 19.1   Syringe plunger travel. Data shown are mean (SD) in ml, n = 40[13]

	20 N	30 N	40 N
Plastipak (B–D)	37.4 (0.5)	32.9 (0.1)	30.0 (0.2)
Omnifix (Braun)	38.0 (0.1)	33.5 (0.5)	30.4 (0.5)
OPS (Braun)	38.4 (0.5)	33.8 (0.4)	30.9 (0.4)
Sherwood	37.9 (0.6)	33.6 (0.5)	30.3 (0.5)

the effective application of cricoid pressure has been difficult to perfect, but new training techniques support the realistic practice of such a skilful procedure. Ruth and Griffiths[13] offer a 'training aid using a capped air-filled 50 ml syringe' which is capable of producing the required force of 30 N (Fig. 19.4). Their results (Table 19.1) show the distance the syringe would need to travel to exert a force of 20, 30 and 40 N.

Practice in a skills laboratory will offer greater awareness of the correct force required and the method offers a safer solution to regurgitation in anaesthesia.[14]

MENDELSON'S SYNDROME

Named after a US obstetrician, Mendelson's syndrome is the condition that occurs when stomach contents are inhaled into the lungs while the patient is anaesthetized. The patient could suffer extensive lung damage and has the potential for severe bronchospasm. Ultimately, death could occur as a result of oxygen starvation or lack of availability of oxygen to the body tissues.

Whether caesarean section is elective or an emergency there are many standard aspects to preparation of the mother prior to surgery. Preoperative fasting is of course desirable, but not always possible. However, even if the mother has been fasted the accumulation of acid in the stomach is an ever-present danger, and therefore a 'rapid-sequence' or 'crash induction' is standard for both emergency and elective sections in order to prevent passive regurgitation. Gastric emptying is delayed in pregnancy and labour, and further enhanced by the action of many narcotics, and so creates the potential for an increased residue of stomach acidity. Additionally, during pregnancy the actual acidity of stomach contents is higher than usual, and so further increases the potential for lung damage should aspiration occur.

cricoid pressure, is applied to the cricoid cartilage to prevent reflux of gastric contents into the trachea and subsequently the lungs. Sellick[11] promoted the effective application of cricoid pressure (Fig. 19.3). It has been recommended by Vanner[12] that a force of 30 N (3 kg) should replace the traditional method of applying blind pressure. For many practitioners

The situation is worsened by incompetence of the gastro-oesophageal sphincter due to hormonal changes. Patients for caesarean section are usually given a preoperative antiemetic combined with an H_2 blocker and an alkali such as sodium citrate in an effort to reduce passive regurgitation. These drugs help to neutralize acid and improve gastric emptying in an attempt to reduce risk in the event of aspiration.

FAILED INTUBATION

In the event of a failed intubation, for whatever clinical reason, it is imperative that cricoid pressure is maintained. The situation is usually managed by immediately placing the patient in the left lateral position, with 100% oxygen being given directly via a face mask.

Occasionally the patient may need assistance with respiration: this should be carefully applied until she resumes spontaneous respiration. As a note of caution, cricoid pressure should not be removed until the anaesthetist is confident that the airway is patent and under the direct control of the patient's own respiratory system.

REPORTED AWARENESS UNDER GENERAL ANAESTHESIA

Awareness under anaesthesia may occur in obstetric patients. 'Light anaesthetics' are often given to reduce the risk of drugs crossing the placenta. In 1985 and 1989, two women who were aware of pain during caesarean section were awarded sums of £13 000 and £18 000 respectively.[15] Devina Ludlow was a 28-year-old mother who was admitted to Princess Margaret Hospital, Swindon, on 19 September 1983 and gave birth to her second child via caesarean section. A general anaesthetic was given. In 1985 she claimed in court that she had felt a 'searing pain across her stomach' and recollected hearing noises of machinery and a baby crying in the distance. It was also inferred that there may have been communication difficulties between the ward staff and the anaesthetist with regard to Mrs Ludlow's request for an epidural.[15] Studies conducted between 1982 and 1989[16] regarding 3076 patients undergoing caesarean section showed that '28 patients (0.9%) were able to recall something about their operation'. Lyons and McDonald[16] continues to show that 189 (6.1%) of patients reported having experienced intraoperative dreams.

Studies by Lyons and McDonald[16] show a change in anaesthetic protocols for caesarean section. Until 1985, their department followed the most acceptable method for endotracheal intubation, created in the 1970s by Moir:[17] the delivery of thiopental sodium in a 3–4 mg/kg solution followed by suxamethonium 100 mg. Ongoing maintenance of anaesthesia was then produced by a therapeutic dose of non-depolarizing muscle relaxant with 50% oxygen/nitrous oxide to provide a vehicle for the 0.5% halothane.[16] Following delivery of the baby their gas ratio was changed to '30% oxygen in nitrous oxide', and 0.3 mg/kg of papaveretum was given. No halothane was used following delivery of the baby.

In 1986, Lyons and McDonald[16] changed their protocol after finding that the number of reported awareness incidents reached 1.3%, which is 0.3% above the accepted level using the Moir technique. Studies by Rosenberg and Alila[18] found inaccuracies in the measurement of the concentration of halothane delivered by vapourizers. There were differing output values from the vapourizer, some showing a range between '0.34% and 1.06%' despite being set at 0.5% on the dial. Because of this, the induction dose of thiopental was increased to 5–7 mg/kg. Isoflurane 1% replaced halothane 0.5% and was frequently continued until the end of the operation at a lower concentration. As a result, awareness under general anaesthesia fell to 0.4%.

Obstetric anaesthesia is a very delicate and skilful process, and although these cases occurred almost 20 years ago they underline the fact that human error or mechanical failure cannot be ruled out.

Increasingly sophisticated technology brings more opportunities for accurate measurements of individual needs during anaesthesia. To prevent awareness under anaesthesia, the Bispectral Index was introduced in American anaesthesiology to reduce mortality rates and awareness. The Bispectral Index, also referred to as the BIS (pronounced BIZ), provides electronic readouts on the electrical activity in the brain. The measurement of the direct effects of anaesthesia give a real sense of being able to control the depth of anaesthesia, thus offering patients a more rapid recovery. Cynthia Anderson, Chairman of the Department of Anaesthesia at UCI Medical Centre,[19] reports that 'The BIS monitor is a highly sophisticated electroencephalogram (EEG) machine designed specifically for operating rooms. Because it monitors brain waves on a continuous basis, it is now possible to administer up to 30% less anaesthetic than before, while ensuring that the patient remains in a state of deep sleep'.[19]

TRANSFERRING THE PATIENT ON TO THE OPERATING TABLE

Pethidine remains popular in the control of maternal pain, despite its potential to cross the placental barrier and exert a detrimental effect on the baby's vital signs, particularly respiration. Mothers should be transported to theatre as soon as possible after the decision to operate has been made. In order to avoid venal occlusion and subsequent blood pressure problems, a left-lateral tilt should be initiated even at this stage, combined with the delivery of oxygen. Venal occlusion is also referred to as aortocaval occlusion and supine hypotension, although both can refer to an alternative set of causes and effect.

It is usual practice to take the mother directly into theatre and position her on the operating table, where left-lateral tilt is created either by placing a wedge under the right hip or by tilting the table approximately 15° to the left. Care should be taken that a member of staff is positioned on the patient's left side to prevent her slipping or falling, which is an ever-present possibility. This situation can also be worsened by the mother's physical condition, or if a regional technique is being used, when she may not have full control of her movements and senses.

An arm board positioned on the left side is usual and good practice, not only because most patients have a cannula in the non-dominant left arm, but also as this arrangement helps provide some stabilization and balance for the patient in what can be a precarious position. Irrespective of the site of an infusion, such use of an arm board has never been reported as a hindrance, and alternative positioning of the right arm – for example bent at the elbow across the chest – has access benefits while creating no obstacles to the surgical field.

Throughout the period of transfer to the operating table both fetal monitoring and oxygen delivery to the mother are essential and should be interrupted for no longer than necessary.

The practitioner should also consider any religious or cultural aspects, remembering that the patient is female and in a vulnerable dependant situation, possibly involving a preponderance of male staff. Therefore, factors such as female escorts, family attendance, dress codes, etc. should be considered, while also keeping the patient informed of all that is happening and expected to happen. Because

of the nature of an emergency caesarean there will be much unavoidable activity and noise due to theatre preparation and the assembling of various staff, and the patient should be prewarned of this and reassured that all is normal.

Keeping the patient informed should be an ongoing process that runs concurrently with preparation. Once the patient is positioned suitably and safely on the tilted operating table and receiving oxygen, procedures such as pubic shaving and bladder catheterization can be performed. Depending on policy, these can be carried out either at this stage or after the patient has been anaesthetized. However, there is opinion that carrying out these tasks after the induction of anaesthesia can waste valuable time by delaying the onset of surgery. In practice, the decision lies with fetal condition, local policy, and/or whether an elective or an emergency caesarean is involved.

Box 19.2 lists the items contained in a caesarean section tray.

Box 19.2   Caesarean section tray

- Rampley sponge-holding forceps × 5
- Spencer Wells artery forceps 20 cm × 10
- Spencer Wells artery forceps 12.5 cm (straight) × 5
- Spencer Wells artery forceps 12.5 cm (curved) × 5
- Green Armitage forceps 20 cm × 5
- Littlewoods tissue forceps × 2
- Mayo scissors 17 cm (curved) × 2
- Mayo scissors 17 cm (straight) × 1
- Thompson Walker needle holder × 2
- Bonney's toothed dissecting forceps × 1
- Bonney's non-toothed dissecting forceps × 2
- Jean's toothed dissecting forceps 17 cm × 1
- Doyens retractor 11.5 (large) × 1
- Doyens retractor 8 cm (small) × 1
- Morris retractor 5 cm × 2
- Wrigley's forceps (pair) × 1
- Bachaus towel clips × 5
- BP no. 4 handle × 2
- Payr intestinal clamp 10 cm blade × 1
- Mayo pin 11.5 cm × 1
- Mayo pin 15 cm × 2
- Gallipots × 2
- Receivers (1 small and 1 large) × 2

THE SURGICAL 'SCRUB' PRACTITIONER

In order to operate within the safest and most suitable conditions, obstetric surgeons rely on the provision of a quality service from the entire perioperative team, combined with meticulous preparation of the operative environment.

Although they are usually accompanied by a junior member of the medical staff acting as first assistant, supervision of the direct surgical area and the provision of instrumentation is the responsibility of the scrub assistant. This role is increasingly undertaken by a variety of different staff disciplines; depending on geographical location, local policy or necessity, this could include midwife, registered nurse or operating department practitioner. More recently, it has been reported at some UK centres that care workers who have undertaken further specialist training also act as scrub assistants.

Irrespective of grade or discipline, the role of the scrub practitioner is to provide a quality service and a safe environment in which surgery can be carried out. The delivery of this service should adhere to accepted and safe practice, thereby enhancing patient care throughout the entire perioperative period.

Although a designated midwife is in attendance at all stages of the procedure, as specialists in this environment, perioperative practitioners should never feel that their position and responsibility as patient advocate are diminished or reduced to any degree.

The reasons for surgical intervention have already been stated, but generally involve conditions that heighten the possibility of both fetal and maternal risk compared to continuing with vaginal delivery.

The procedure of caesarean section is, of course, not without risk, and still carries higher mortality and morbidity rates than vaginal delivery. Common among these risks include gastric regurgitation, difficult intubation, awareness under anaesthesia, fetal CNS depression, postoperative bleeding and, of overall paramount significance, the 'two lives' syndrome. However, improvements in surgical and anaesthetic technique, combined with monitoring of both maternal and fetal condition and physiological parameters, have reduced perioperative complications.

Percentage rates of caesarean section versus normal births differ from centre to centre and indeed from country to country, but in more recent times rates have become dependent somewhat on vogue. Indeed, there is evidence that many women,

predominantly in western cultures, are now requesting caesarean section by choice and for a variety of reasons not always related to a medical condition or the advice of their physician. There is also evidence that parental choice for caesarean section can at times be influenced by cultural and/or religious leanings.

It will be interesting to see if choice is further influenced by the current findings that caesarean section birth reduces the HIV transmission risk from mother to child by up to 80% compared to vaginal delivery.[20]

Approximately 25–30% of caesareans currently performed are carried out because the woman has had a previous caesarean birth. At one time this was fairly standard practice, with repeat caesarean birth rates in excess of 80%, but now women who have undergone caesarean are encouraged to attempt vaginal delivery with any subsequent pregnancy.

This consideration of repeat section versus vaginal delivery is referred to as 'trial of labour' or 'trial of scar'. When planning the approach to delivery, obstetricians also take into consideration the added hazard of adhesions due to previous caesarean and pelvic surgery.

As anaesthetic staff are settling the anaesthetized patient, scrub personnel should be ready with skin cleansing agents and drapes. By this time all instruments, swabs, needles etc. will be laid out, checked and counted (see Box 19.2). At this stage, time is at a premium and all efforts to prevent delays could be significant. Preferences for skin cleansing agents vary, but common preparations include iodine, alcohols and Hibitane, according to department policy, surgeon preference and, importantly, patient allergies. The area to prepare usually covers from pubis to under the breasts, extending around to the lateral aspect of the iliac crests. It is important to take care to avoid pooling under the thighs and buttocks, and avoid the use of alcohol-based solutions on sensitive areas. Draping is fairly standard and should conform to accepted practices of asepsis.

By this stage, all instruments will be ready as well as equipment such as suction and diathermy.

In synchrony with these activities, the attending midwife will have checked and prepared the resuscitaire (Fig. 19.5) and be scrubbed and ready to receive the baby.

It is desirable at this stage for the paediatrician to be present. However, presence and availability are dependent on local policy and, to some extent, anticipated outcomes.

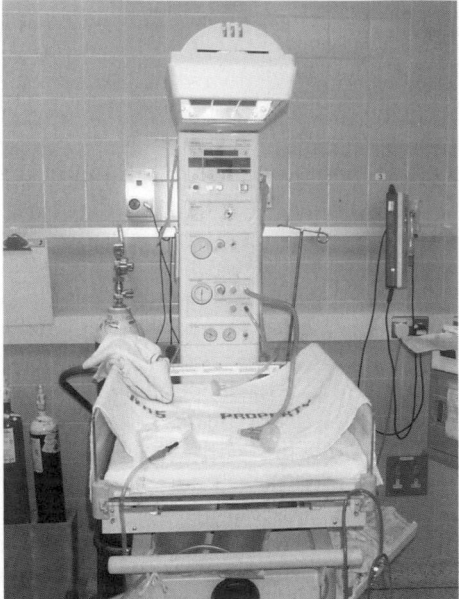

Figure 19.5   Resuscitaire.

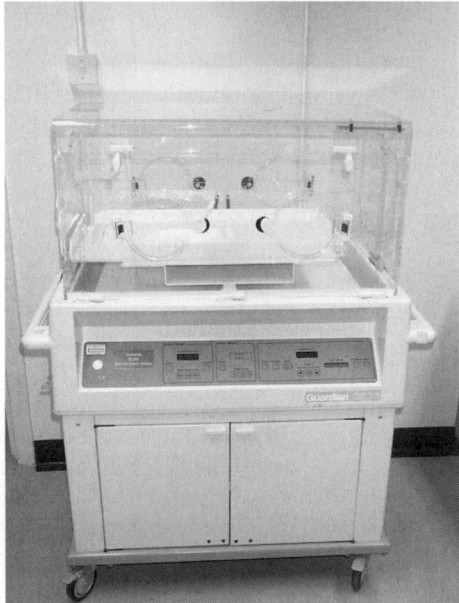

Figure 19.6   Incubator.

Safety checks of the resuscitaire concentrate on oxygen availability and delivery, suction, heating, as well as intravenous equipment and drugs. It is also common for the midwife to take responsibility for checking the transport incubator, which is yet another standard piece of equipment required for this procedure (Fig. 19.6).

> **Box 19.3   Simplified procedure for lower uterine segment caesarean section**
>
> - Incision: through skin and fat using, for example, a 23 blade
> - Incising muscle fascia, using inside knife
> - Digital muscle splitting
> - Insertion of a Doyens retractor on the pubic side of the wound
> - Dissect bladder from pelvic peritoneum, using scissors and forceps
> - Grasp peritoneum with two artery forceps, enter with scissors and extend digitally
> - Displace bladder inferiorly
> - Lower segment incised with, for example, number 10 blade and extended digitally
> - Rupture of membranes and suction
> - Attempt to position and extract fetus with assistant applying external pressure on fundus
> - Surgeon delivers the head, maintaining head-down position for free drainage
> - Two clamps on cord; cut with cord scissors
> - Transfer baby to midwife
> - Deliver placenta and membranes
> - Grasp angles of uterus using two Green Armitage forceps
> - Swab out uterus
> - Close uterus in two layers*
> - Pelvic peritoneum reconstituted
> - Abdomen closed in layers
>
> *Clips commonly used on skin; sutures vary according to personal preference*

Following skin preparation and draping the surgeon will await the anaesthetist's assent before proceeding to make the incision.

Although an acute situation, surgery for caesarean section is a rather routine procedure and easier dealt with in a step-by-step manner, although this varies depending on surgeon, centre policy, etc. For lower uterine segment caesarean section (LUSCS) see Box 19.3.

There are several important interventions by the anaesthetist throughout this sequence. For example, at the stage where the baby is delivered, an oxytoxic (e.g. ergometrine) or similarly acting drug is injected to help contract the uterus and assist in controlling bleeding. In addition, at this stage the anaesthetic is deepened with the addition of a narcotic, and

Table 19.2   The Apgar scoring system

Sign	0	1	2
Heart rate	Absent	Slow (<100)	>100
Respiratory effort	Absent	Slow, irregular	Good, crying
Muscle tone	Flaccid	Some flexion of extremities	Active motion
Reflex irritability	No response	Grimace	Vigorous cry
Colour	Blue, pale	Body pink, extremities blue	Completely pink

possibly increases of the inhalation agent. This is also an opportune time for the table, or the patient, to be levelled out.

Sometimes an infusion of Syntocinon or similar, is set up should the uterus appear to be lacking tone, and this may be continued into the immediate postoperative period. This involves, for example, the use of 30–40 IU Syntocinon in 500 ml normal saline.

Antibiotic regimens are common but not standard, and can involve antibiotics in combination with an antimicrobial such as metronidazole. Once the baby is delivered the midwife or member of the surgical staff will assess the need for oral suction, usually prior to the baby being handed to the midwife, who at this stage may use a mucus extractor for the purpose. The baby is usually accepted by the midwife using a padded preheated tray and from here is transferred to the resuscitaire. Visual and audible assessment of colour, whether crying or not, need for stimulation and so on, will determine the sequence of interventions such as suction, oxygen, intubation, narcotic antagonist, vitamin K. It is standard for the midwife to make reference to Apgar rating, taken twice at 1-minute intervals (Table 19.2), which provides a numerical value to appearance, colour, pulse, heart rate, respiration and muscle tone reflexes. A low score may warn that urgent attention is needed.

Once all is settled with the baby, the midwife will take responsibility for checking the placenta for completeness and take a sample of cord blood for haemoglobin and bilirubin checking.

After skin closure the scrub practitioner will clean and dress the wound. The urinary catheter can be removed at this stage, and the surgeon will clean out the vaginal vault while checking for fresh bleeding. Sometimes, due to policy or circumstances, urinary catheters are left in situ into the postoperative period, and in this event a Foley-type catheter will probably be used.

Once all surgically related procedures are complete the anaesthetist can commence reversal. It is common practice to transfer patients to their beds and into the lateral position for extubation. Postoperative oxygen is commenced and, if possible, the baby is introduced to the mother if there are no indications for incubator transfer to the special care baby unit (SCBU).

Unlike general theatre procedures, where all patients are kept in recovery in the immediate postoperative period, in an obstetric unit it may be possible, in the absence of complications, to return the mother directly to the postnatal ward together with the baby.

Even in the absence of a dedicated recovery unit, postoperative observations include attention to the usual vital signs and pain relief. There is an ever-present danger of reactionary haemorrhage, and continued vigilance as regards abdominal/pelvic girth and the vagina, combined with pain relief, is standard practice.

Postoperative pain relief may involve intramuscular (IM) injection as and when required, or patient controlled analgesia (PCA). Of course, the patient would have been introduced to this before surgery, especially if the case is elective.

The intravenous infusion will be maintained until the patient is able to take oral fluids – usually 24 hours – and mobility is encouraged approximately 6–8 hours postoperatively. Physiotherapy involving leg movement, deep breathing, coughing and, later, abdominal exercises is common, but not standard in all centres.

Immediate postoperative complications for the mother are mainly anaesthetic related and postoperative haemorrhage. However, subsequent complications can also include infection, thromboembolism, bladder injury, wound and urinary tract infection.

Caesarean section is a monumental event for parents as well as an emotional one for even seasoned operating department staff. However, the sudden cessation of contact with their patients (mother and baby) leaves some staff feeling somewhat robbed and unrewarded, as the midwives and ward staff take over and are able to share in parents' joy and witness the realization of what has occurred once the trauma of events has passed. It has been reported anecdotally that theatre staff find some reward in centres where it is the practice for them to collect the mother from the ward preoperatively, and possibly more so when they assist in returning and settling mother and baby in the postnatal area.

DEVELOPMENTS IN THE PERIOPERATIVE FIELD

The NHS[21] stated: 'Throughout the NHS the old hierarchical ways of working are giving way to more flexible team working between different clinical professionals'. It is recognized that midwives are having a larger involvement in childbirth services. Irrespective of who is on the perioperative team in the obstetric theatre it is acknowledged that they must be trained to offer a truly effective obstetric service.[18] There is greater collaboration between staff – surgeon, anaesthetist, perioperative practitioners and midwives – to provide a patient-centred approach.

CONCLUSION

Over the last two decades, new practices have been introduced into the clinical workplace which offer very distinctive advantages for the patient. Evidence-based practice in medicine and health care have offered the very best in treatment, and for the practitioner opportunities to continually advance their contribution to care.

Some of these practices include the early monitoring of the mother and baby prior to delivery. This provides greater opportunities for the early detection of potential risks, and stages of distress or disorders can be identified and responsive timescales of treatment commenced. Evidence suggests that early identification of warning signs can minimize the morbidity and mortality risk to both mother and baby. Furthermore, it can be suggested that this important level of monitoring supports the practitioner by giving more time to ensure best theatre practice is applied.

Changes and advances in anaesthesia have also contributed to the overall risk assessment of a caesarean section. Epidural and spinal anaesthesia is predominantly used to avoid intubation hazards. There are also clearer guidelines and recommendations for having trained anaesthetic assistance.

Most mothers and partners engaging in the birth process in the theatre environment will openly express their emotional response to the event and to the environment. Practitioners who have undergone similar experiences themselves may well be able to empathize with these feelings. For parents, caesarean section can be a traumatic intervention in the birth process, whereas for the perioperative practitioner it is an opportunity to exercise all aspects of training and experience. All practitioners can of course find it an emotional event, while at the same time, from a somewhat detached standpoint, providing opportunities for learning and development. Students find it challenging, and those recently qualified have the opportunity to consolidate skills. Experienced staff also continually have the reward of witnessing what can be instant success, as mother and baby exit the theatre environment in a healthy and improved state. This situation may be somewhat different from normal theatre work, when their input constitutes just one aspect of the treatment pathway. This example of holistic involvement may lend itself to further development of models for continuing professional development (CPD).

Obstetric experience is truly remarkable for all those who either visit or practise in theatre, and offers the opportunity for the development of transferable skills for the practitioner.

References

1. Tortora G, Grabowski S. Principle of anatomy and physiology, 7th edn. New York: HarperCollins; 1993.
2. Miller A, Callander R. Obstetrics illustrated. London: Churchill Livingstone; 1989.
3. Redman C, Walker I. Pre-eclampsia: the facts. Oxford: OUP; 1992.
4. Proud J. Ultrasound for midwives: a guide for midwives and other health professionals. Hale: Books for Midwives; 1994.
5. Association of Anaesthetists of Great Britain and Ireland and Obstetric Anaesthetists Association. Guidelines for obstetric and anaesthetic services. London: AAGBI and OAA; 1998.
6. Kneedler JA, Dodge GH. Perioperative patient care: the nursing perspective. Boston: Jones and Bartlett; 1994.
7. Medical Devices Agency. HN 2001(02) anaesthetic breathing system components: risk of blockages. London: Medical Devices Agency; 2001. Online.

Available: http://www. medical-devices.gov.uk 3 Apr 2002.

8. Hutton P. President's statement. Bulletin 10. London: Royal College of Anaesthetists; 2001: 451–453.

9. BBC News. Warning after 'blocked pipe' death. Online. Available: http://news.bbc.co.uk/hi/english/health/newsid_1484000/14844709.stm 24 Jan 2002.

10. Department of Health. Chief medical Officer announces action on blocked breathing tubing. 2002. Online. Available: http://tap.ukwebhost.eds.com/doh/interpress.nsf/page/2002-0320?OpenDocument 19 Aug 2002.

11. Selick BA. Cricoid pressure to control regurgitation of gastric contents during induction of anaesthesia: preliminary communication. Lancet 1961; 2: 404–406.

12. Vanner RG, Asai I. Safe use of cricoid pressure. Anaesthesia 1999; 54: 1–3.

13. Ruth MJ, Griffiths R. Assessment of 50 ml syringe as a simple training aid in the application of cricoid pressure. Br J Anaesth 1998; 81: 292.

14. Meek T, Gittins N, Diggan JE. Cricoid pressure: knowledge and performance amongst anaesthetic assistance. Anaesthesia 1999; 54: 59–62.

15. Aitkenhead A. Awareness during anaesthesia: what should the patient be told? Anaesthesia 1990; 45: 351–352.

16. Lyons G, McDonald R. Awareness during caesarean section. Anaesthesia 1991; 46: 62–64.

17. Moir DD. Anaesthesia for caesarean section. An evaluation of a method using low concentration halothane and 50 percent oxygen. Br J Anaesth 1970; 42: 136–142.

18. Rosenberg PH, Alila A. Accumulation of thymol in halothane vaporisers. Anaesthesia 1984; 39: 581–583.

19. Anderson C. New monitor revolutionizes anaesthesia delivery. South Orange, California: University of California; 2002. Online. Available: http://www.uci-health.com/News/UCI%20Health/anaesthesia.htm 9 Sep 2002.

20. Hofmeyr F. Elective caesarean section delivery reduced the HIV-1 mother to child transmission rate by 80%. Evidence Based Obstetrics and Gynaecology 2000; 2(1): 9.

21. Department of Health. The NHS plan. Norwich: HMSO; 2000.

Further reading

Aitkenhead A, Smith C. Textbook of anaesthesia, 3rd edn. Edinburgh: Churchill Livingstone; 1996.

Bonnar J. Recent advances in obstetrics and gynaecology. London: Churchill Livingstone; 1990.

Brahams D. Caesarean section: pain and awareness without negligence. Anaesthesia 1990; 45: 161–162.

Chadleigh P, Pearce JM. Obstetric ultrasound: how, why and when. Edinburgh: Churchill Livingstone; 1986.

Crawford J. Fetal well being and maternal awareness. Br J Anaesth 1988; 61: 247–248.

Human Rights Act 1998. Norwich: HMSO.

Davey A, Ince C. Fundamentals of operating department practice. London: Greenwich Medical Media; 2000.

Fortunato N. Operating room technique, 9th edn. St. Louis: Mosby; 2000.

Gray H. Anatomy of the human body. Philadelphia: Lea & Febiger; 1918. Online. Available: http://www.bartleby.com/107/illus1213.html 12 May 2002.

Heath S. Perioperative care of the child. Salisbury: Wiltshire Quay Books (a division of Mark Allen Publishing); 1998.

Hind M, Wicker P. Principles of perioperative practice. Edinburgh: Churchill Livingstone; 2000.

Klaus MH, Kennell JH. Bonding: the beginning of parent-infant attachment. London: Mosby; 1983.

McCaughey W, Howe JP, Moore J, et al. Cimetidine in elective caesarean section. Effect on gastric acidity. Anaesthesia 1981; 36: 167–172.

Morgan B. Controversies in obstetric anaesthesia II. London: Hodder & Stoughton; 1993.

Moir D, Thorburn J. Obstetric anaesthesia and analgesia. London: Baillière Tindall; 1986.

Ponte J, Green DW. Handbook of anaesthesia and perioperative care. London: WB Saunders; 1994.

Symonds EM, Macpherson M. Colour atlas of obstetrics and ultrasound. London: Mosby-Wolfe; 1994.

Chapter 20

Care of the elderly in the operating department

Rita Hehir

'You can't help getting older, but you don't have to get old.'

American comedian George Burns

Key points

- Societal and demographic changes that influence perioperative care of elderly patients
- Physical, psychological, legal and ethical issues related to the care of the elderly perioperative patient

The requirement to understand the needs of the elderly patient is not new. There is a long history of neglect in the provision of appropriate care for elderly patients. It was not until the launch of the National Health Service (NHS) in 1948 that geriatric medicine became known as a specialty. Even then, nursing care of the elderly had a low status and was seen as the province of State Enrolled Nurses; not until 1977 did it become part of the General Nursing Council syllabus.[1] As a consequence of this development Registered General Nurses were educated in the care of the aged.

Traditionally, perioperative practitioners were predominantly nurses who had chosen this particular specialist area of practice after a minimum of 3 years' nurse training. Customarily, training was followed by a period practising in the various wards and departments of a hospital to consolidate the experience gained during training. Consequently, perioperative practitioners from this background brought with them to the operating department a knowledge of various disciplines of care. This included experience in delivering nursing care to elderly patients. Accordingly, these practitioners understood the complex nature of the needs of this patient group, subsequently integrating this education and knowledge into perioperative practice.

Current service demands and practice needs dictate that as a profession, operating department practitioners (ODPs) are recruited directly to the operating department to undertake their training; they do not necessarily have the experience of the care of the elderly that nurses gained during their preregistration training. It is essential, therefore, that practitioners from an ODP background understand that the care of the elderly in surgery is not just to focus on the sum of their patients' potentially infirm body parts.

There are many reasons why knowledge of the care of the elderly is important. The official recording of births and deaths, which began in the mid-1800s, showed that the percentage of the population over 65 in 1850 was approximately 5%. Current demographic trends indicate that the average life expectancy for males by 2021 will be 88.2 years and for females 90.0 years.[2]

Medical and surgical advances continue to generate greater expectations on the part of the public as consumers of health care. In tandem with these expectations is the ongoing debate on rationing of healthcare provision, and the possibility of measuring on a value-for-money basis which groups in our society are worthy of this investment.[3]

Much of the research into this subject suggests that the elderly as a category do not rate very highly in terms of priority. Research carried out by the organization Help the Aged points out that typically patients over 60 waited an average of over 5 hours in A&E departments, in contrast to an average wait of less than 3 hours experienced by patients under 40.[4]

A more comprehensive reading of this research shows that 51% of the British population consider that Britain behaves towards the elderly as if they were second-class citizens.[5]

The failure to continue the provision of mammography to screen for breast cancer in older women indicates the presence of age discrimination in healthcare services, and potentially reflects a deeper societal stance on the value of elderly individuals.[4]

There are many cultural differences in attitudes to old age. In modern societies older people tend to have lower status. However, in many non-western societies, for example China and India, old age is revered as an usher of wisdom, and the elders of the community are those designated to make and enforce the major decisions that impinge on the group.

Notwithstanding these cultural differences, older people in western societies do not accept the concept that old age is synonymous with decay and decline. Advances in social conditions, such as housing, changes in working hours and conditions, plus advances in medicine and nutrition, all mean that the historical, rather than biological, ravages of old age can be better countered or decelerated.[2]

There is much evidence of this shift in the attitude of older people aspiring to maintain a healthier and more productive life, despite the accumulation of years. Age Concern provides a national network of projects that encourage older people to engage in healthier lifestyles. These activities, which come under the sponsorship of their 'Ageing Well UK' initiative, encourage older people to be active in pursuit of at least minimally physically challenging disciplines such as walking, line dancing, and joining hobby and interest groups. Intellectually demanding activities, such as art projects and becoming Senior Health Mentors and Age Resource volunteers, are encouraged. Senior Health Mentors is a programme for older people that entails a core training programme and enables the participants to provide health promotion advice and support to peers and carers.

Age Resource is an enterprise, again under the umbrella of Age Concern, which encourages retired and older people to use their experience, skills and talents in any way that benefits their communities.[6]

'Grey power' is a comparatively recent idiom to be used regularly in reference to the political and social status of older people. It is now recognized that all the major political parties in the UK wish to court the votes of an estimated 11 million voters from this section of the population.[7]

This awareness of the potential to capitalize on the power of older voters is an international phenomenon. The 2002 mission statement of the Grey Power movement in New Zealand includes the following aims:

- To advance, support and protect the welfare and wellbeing of older people
- To promote recognition of the wide-ranging services provided by senior citizens of New Zealand
- To strive for the provision of a quality health care to all New Zealand residents regardless of income and location.[8]

Tinker,[9] who examines similar themes, i.e. the position of elderly people in society, begins by looking at the difficulty of finding a definition for this group, arguing that degrees of disability can be measured, individuals who commit crime can be categorized by the type or nature of the offence they have perpetrated, and members of ethnic minority communities can by subdivided in distinct fraternities based on country of origin, cultural heritage, and possibly religious beliefs.

By contrast, 'older people are the whole people of a generation who have survived to a certain age. They are not a deviant group or one small section of the population. They are ordinary people who happen to have reached a certain age. This cannot be emphasized too much, particularly to professionals who are, as a result of their training and experience at work, concerned primarily with the abnormal'.

While exploring these attitudes commonly held by professionals, i.e. that individuals automatically fall into convenient categories, the point is made that very few would assign identical distinguishing features to a 30-year-old and a 60-year-old. Yet it is not uncommon to have 60-year-olds and 90-year-olds classed as a homogeneous group. The question relevant to the perioperative practitioner that Tinker poses is: Would such factors as social class, absence of illness/disability, family structure, religion, contribution to society, career, and social supports, educational attainments, talents and skills be seen as similar amongst, say all 20–45-year-olds?[9]

If not – and surely the answer has to be no – why should older people not be acknowledged to be as diverse and individual as the rest of the population?

This notion of stereotyping old age as dependent, impoverished and grateful for any small acts of kindness is also challenged by Vincent.[10]

An anthropological stance on the social construction of old age states that age is one of a few truly universal criteria. However, how age is measured and subsequently valued differs widely. Western culture uses the Gregorian calendar to record age; in other cultures the occurrence of natural events such as floods and storms is used to chronicle lifespan. This results in a higher status for those that survive and contribute to their society. The use of various rites of passage designates social roles appropriate to the needs of the group, rather than a specific number having particular significance.[10]

It must be acknowledged that in western society the cult of body image reigns supreme. Being an unsuitable size, shape, or lacking the contemporary 'good looks' makes for a sense of failure.[11]

Given that this approach is taken as a legitimate currency for placing a value on the individual, it is little wonder that older people are often seen in negative terms.

It provokes no astonishment that being unable to control their body functions gives rise to feelings of shame in older people. The issues concerning body image and the inability to govern physical functioning, particularly during illness, can lead older people to perceive themselves as a burden to others and as having lost the property of adult status.[12]

It is possible, argues Vincent, that old people are considered unsightly on the basis of lacking power and property, rather than because of physical characteristics.

Victor[13] examines the theme of negative stereotyping of the elderly, looking at the depiction of the elderly in literature, most especially in children's books. This reveals a tendency to cast elderly characters as playing a supporting role, and furthermore as having lonely, insular lives with very little positive influence or contact with other people.[13]

In her seminal work *The Unpopular Patient*, Felicity Stockwell demonstrated that patients who had a history of frequent admissions were thought to 'moan and groan' needlessly. Those demanding what nursing staff read as excessive attention, those with mental health problems and those with physical defects invariably ended up in this category (i.e. unpopular patients).[14]

It is fairly clear how an elderly patient might fall into this group. Increasing age, failing health and chronic ill-health conditions requiring surgical intervention may easily necessitate frequent visits to the operating department, therefore perioperative practitioners need to be aware of, and avoid the temptation to make, these negative associations. Such prejudice would result in treating elderly patients in a discriminatory fashion.

The question of care of the aged anywhere within the healthcare system, including the operating department, gives rise to the question of rationing.

As Dauchot and Lina[15] state, financial constraints mean that rationing of health care is most probably taking place with regard to the elderly, but they go on to point out that chronological age is no longer a suitable criterion for the selection of patients for various interventions, as with the exception of cardiac and neurological patients, age per se can no longer be an independent indicator.[15]

Also on this theme, the concept of quality adjusted life years (QUALYS) was developed, a system that proposed to use a mathematical equation to determine the potential outcome of medical interventions.[15] Issues such as probable return to functional physical status and – controversially – 'quality of life' are concepts that are very subjective and difficult to quantify. An attempt was made in the state of Oregon, USA,[42] in the 1980s to 'produce explicit criteria for resource allocation based on a prioritized list derived from modified QUALYS'. The weightings for quality of life were derived from a telephone survey of local citizens. The experiment has not proven effective in practice. Some of the results were distinctly odd, with cosmetic breast surgery being rated as more important than the treatment of a compound fracture of the femur.

No account is taken of the individual response to illness and healing if this approach is followed. Frame of mind can be an influence, i.e. mental and physical robustness, as can be factors such as genetic makeup, which influences resistance to infection and healing.[16]

The skill of the surgical team and the availability of resources such as intensive care beds, if needed, have been attested to as further factors that may decide the outcome of medical/surgical intervention in the elderly. The contribution of the elderly to society, and the fact that some treatments will become cheaper not more expensive with the development of technology, all militate against the deliberate targeting of the elderly for rationing of scarce resources.[17]

THE ROLE OF THE PERIOPERATIVE PRACTITIONER IN PREPARING THE PATIENT FOR SURGERY

The previous section is intended to highlight the need to see the person and not merely a set of symptoms attached to an age when caring for the elderly in the operating department. As Gibson[18] argues, training of healthcare professionals needs to be frequently reviewed in order to respond to the needs of the 'new elderly', who differ greatly from previous generations in expectations and in the nature of their requirements from healthcare professionals and ODPs.

Bearing in mind the individuality and dignity of each human being, whether young or old, there are certain common factors that apply to elderly people. This being the case, there are certain basic principles that apply to the care of the elderly and which should be adhered to by the operating department practitioner. 'All physiological functions decline as ageing increases, and ageing increases susceptibility to stress and disease. Healing and recovery are much slower in the elderly. Normal elderly people have a physiology that is adequate for resting conditions but, compared to younger people, they show slower adjustment to environmental change and a diminished reserve capacity'.[19]

Elderly people are increasingly being exposed to surgery and anaesthesia for the following reasons:

- Improvement in health trends, which leads to longer life expectancy
- Advances in anaesthetic techniques that facilitate surgery on patients who would previously have been considered unfit for surgery.

Systemically a number of changes occur that can have a negative impact on the outcome of surgical intervention. The following conditions are frequently found to affect the elderly and need to be taken into account both prior to and during anaesthesia and surgery. Practitioners need to be familiar with these issues and have a working knowledge of how to manage them in order to provide the best standard of care.

RESPIRATORY SYSTEM

Changes that can occur in the respiratory system as a consequence of ageing are:

- A breakdown of the septa, giving rise to emphysema
- A reduction in vital capacity
- Airway narrowing, resulting in a decrease in arterial oxygen
- During surgery the patient is placed in the supine position, which can affect functional residual capacity, thereby creating hypoxia.

For the above reasons it is essential to oxygenate elderly patients ahead of surgery and to make certain that oxygen is administered postoperatively.

If a decision has to be made about whether or not to remove an elderly patient from a ventilator it is important to access the level of arterial oxygenation for a decreased response to CO_2, which is heightened by the use of opiates, anaesthetic agents, and incomplete reversal of muscle relaxants. There is also a greater potential for the aspiration of stomach contents.

Because of their slower circulation time very ill elderly patients are probably not suited to rapid-sequence induction or intubation. If the patient has a full stomach, consideration could be given to an awake induction.[20]

Some medical conditions may appear more commonly in certain sections of the elderly population. For instance, the incidence of chronic respiratory disease is disproportionately high in individuals who are ranked as being of lower economic status. Poor living conditions, coupled with poor nutrition, environmental pollution, low educational attainment, history of unemployment, family breakdown and lifestyles that include smoking and excessive use of alcohol, all contribute to a decreased health status.[21,22] The pre-existence of chronic medical conditions can create additional problems in the assessment of these patients for anaesthesia and surgery.

In parts of the country where chronic obstructive airways disease is endemic, asking the patient about their breathing difficulties is of little or no use. It is not that they will knowingly or deliberately provide misleading information, but being used to having restricted pulmonary function, and to having friends and peers whose condition is even worse, may cause the patient to dismiss their problem as not worthy of consideration.[23]

CARDIOVASCULAR SYSTEM

There are numerous problems relating to the cardiovascular system that generate risks during the administration of anaesthesia to the elderly.[24]

Hypertension is common in the elderly as a consequence of the thickening of arterial walls. Measurement of both diastolic and systolic blood pressure is necessary. Blood pressure should be controlled in the region of 140/90 prior to surgery. If the patient's blood pressure needs to be lowered this needs to be done slowly, as the elderly are susceptible to developing postural hypertension.

During anaesthesia elderly patients are likely to display sudden changes in blood pressure in response to stimulation and the effect of anaesthetic drugs. Because of their inability to automatically regulate the blood supply to their various body systems, due to decreased cardiac output, elderly patients are at increased risk of strokes – myocardial ischaemic episodes.

Decreased cardiac output also means that circulation time for drugs and anaesthetic agents used is longer, which in turn prolongs surgery.[25]

Mortality rates associated with patients in heart failure who require anaesthetic and surgical intervention are high. Therefore, unless the condition is life-threatening it is necessary to correct it prior to surgery. It is also recommended to continuously monitor central venous pressure, as this facilitates the safer management of the patients undergoing surgery.

The choice of anaesthetic drugs may also be influenced by cardiac functioning, as an ageing heart may not be able to respond to the increased oxygen demands created by the actions of drugs such as atropine and gallamine. The advice given by some authors on this subject is that all elderly patients ought to be regarded as and treated as having cardiac dysfunction.

NERVOUS SYSTEM

One unfortunate side effect on the nervous system of elderly patients is the occurrence of confusion and short-term memory loss.

THERMOREGULATION

The ability of the elderly patient to maintain a normal body temperature during surgery is much diminished. Aged patients, neonates, patients who are debilitated who lack energy at a cellular level, and those with an enfeebled metabolic or circulatory physiological structure are at very high risk to develop hypothermia. Circumstances that contribute to loss of body heat are lengthy surgical procedures, the administration of intravenous infusions which may be given at below normal body temperature, the use of fluid which is at room temperature for cavity irrigation, the environmental temperature in perioperative areas, and drugs that affect the patient's own temperature control functioning.[26]

The consequences of hypothermia include the following:

- Permanent ventricular fibrillation may occur
- Shivering on recovery from anaesthesia considerably increases the patient's need for oxygen
- 'Hypothermia can cause postoperative shivering, decreased drug metabolism and clearance, and a delay in wound healing'.[27]

Hypothermia can lead to a decreased blood supply to the skin, thereby increasing the risk of pressure sores and wound infection.[28]

A decrease in body temperature of 2°C triples the occurrence of wound infection and extends the patient's stay in hospital by 20%. Therefore, maintaining normal body temperature is vital.[29,30]

ENDOCRINE FUNCTION

Diabetes, in particular late-onset diabetes mellitus, is a medical condition to be aware of. In the UK there are in excess of 750 000 individuals diagnosed with diabetes,[31] but the association Diabetes UK claims that there may be as many as 1 million adults as yet undiagnosed with type 2 non-insulin dependent diabetes. Further, they suggest that the condition may exist for at least 7 years prior to diagnosis, so the patient may not be aware that they suffer from diabetes until admission to hospital.[32]

Accordingly, some of the long-term problems linked to this condition, e.g. vascular and renal disease, may already be manifest. As the prevalence of this condition increases with age it is prudent to be aware of its possible presence in aged patients. It is easily diagnosed on examination of a urine specimen, followed by blood tests if indicated.

It is also crucial not to allow hypothyroidism to go undetected, as the prognosis for the patient's wellbeing is reduced if surgery proceeds with this condition untreated.

SKELETAL CHANGES

Poor-quality and weak bones are common in the elderly. This condition can advance to fractures of the vertebral body, femoral neck and distal end of the radius. Such fractures can result from rough handling and not enough attention paid to positioning the patient on the operating table.

Arthritic changes can make intubation difficult owing to lack of flexibility and movement of the neck and head. Practitioners are responsible for ensuring that the practice of leaning on the body and limbs of the patient is avoided. It should not be necessary to make this point, but anecdotal evidence suggests that it is not uncommon to see surgical assistants using a part of the patient's body as a 'resting place' for their arms.

Some more facts concerning the quality of the bones of the elderly are that 1 in 3 women and 1 in 12 men will suffer from osteoporosis over the age of 50; and that every 3 minutes someone in the UK suffers a fracture due to osteoporosis.[33]

CONNECTIVE TISSUE

Many elderly patients have no teeth, which means endotracheal intubation can be easier, but it is also easy to damage the gums. Flaccid cheeks in a mouth without teeth can make ventilation using a mask easier said than done. Loose or decayed teeth can make laryngoscopy and intubation hazardous. If there is the likelihood of dislodging an unstable tooth it is wise to confer with the patient beforehand and make them aware of this possibility, and to record the conversation in the patient's notes.

ALTERED SENSITIVITY TO DRUGS

Many elderly patients are on prescribed medicines. Commonly in use are antihypertensive drugs, painkillers, diuretics, potassium supplements and digitalis.

Research has shown that age affects the distribution and effect of anaesthetic drugs.[34] For example, the half-life of diazepam is prolonged from 20 hours in a 20-year-old to 90 hours in an 80-year-old.[32–35]

PREPARATION OF THE PATIENT FOR SURGERY

To address these issues the key to good management of the elderly patient is thorough preassessment.

In centuries past, surgery was carried out in all sorts of places, some of the most popular being the barber's chair, the battlefield, and on the kitchen table. At the beginning of the 20th century it was not uncommon to find that surgeons used their offices or the patient's home as an operating room.[36]

Although this situation may have eliminated contemporary problems such as bed shortages, staff shortages, cancellations and operating lists that regularly overrun, it nevertheless resulted in very high mortality rates and possibly not the most positive experience for the patient.

Nowadays a more formal and extensive approach to surgery and patient preparation is adhered to, resulting in a more satisfactory outcome for the patient. A vital component of this development is the advent of a comprehensive preoperative assessment. Failure to undertake this activity places the patient at increased risk of perioperative morbidity or mortality. The overall aims of preoperative assessment should include the following:

- Confirm that the surgery proposed is realistic when comparing the likely benefit to the patient with the possible risks involved
- Anticipate potential problems and ensure that adequate facilities and trained staff are available to provide satisfactory preoperative care
- Ensure the patient is prepared correctly for the operation, improving where feasible any existing factors that might increase the risk of an adverse outcome
- Provide adequate information to the patient and obtain consent for the planned procedure
- Prescribe premedication and/or other specific prophylactic measures if required.[24]

The essential principles of preoperative assessment apply to all patients. They carry additional weight with elderly patients because, as mentioned earlier, a very high percentage may have a multiplicity of medical conditions, all of which could further complicate their surgery and recovery.

Research during the 1980s illustrated that the surgical mortality rates among the elderly began to decline by comparison with preceding decades. Despite this, rates were still seen to rise with age, continuing to be two or three times higher in older than in younger patients.[15]

A preoperative assessment should be well planned and organized. A cursory exchange with the patient will not achieve the desired result, i.e. to unearth the maximum amount of information.

The anaesthetist normally meets and examines the patient long before they arrive in the anaesthetic room. The opportunity to carry out this encounter is of benefit to both the patient and the doctor. It helps establish rapport with the patient, which will increase their confidence before they go for surgery, subsequently lessening their anxiety. It allows the patient to seek more information about what lies ahead if they wish to ask questions, and it assists the anaesthetist in making a thorough assessment of the patient's state of wellbeing. In addition, a decision can be made regarding the choice of anaesthetic and the most advantageous analgesia to employ to control and eliminate postoperative pain.[35]

Although it has been emphasized that the elderly as a group must not be stereotyped as suffering from physical disabilities, e.g. hearing or sight impaired, reduced mobility, or suffering from some degree of below-average intellectual functioning, it is worth bearing in mind that in some cases these conditions will exist, therefore sufficient time must be allowed to conduct an interview and physical examination.

The checklist for preparing the elderly patient for surgery should include the following.

COMPLETE PHYSICAL EXAMINATION

This includes an inspection for any scarring (possibly very faint), which may testify to previous surgery. For an elderly patient, for example aged over 80, the import of a medical/surgical intervention 60 or more years ago may seem irrelevant. Even one of 30 years ago may not seem very important to mention; if that episode involved an adverse reaction to the drugs used, however, it would of course be highly significant. Therefore, asking direct questions such as 'Have you had an anaesthetic or an operation in the past, and did everything go alright?' is good practice. It is well to bear in mind the number of times a patient makes a statement along the lines of ' I didn't want to bother anyone or take up the doctor's time talking about that', which results in vital information being missed which has a bearing on the management of their current condition. In the case of the elderly this tendency to believe they are unworthy of taking up the time of staff, especially medical staff, who 'always seem to be rushed off their feet', can be particularly marked.

EXAMINATION OF TEMPERATURE, BLOOD AND PULSE

These are elementary but highly effective investigative techniques the importance of which should never be ignored. Along with the fact that these basic tests permit a record to be taken of these vital signs, which are used intra- and postoperatively as a baseline for comparison to the patient's norm, these details provide information that is easily deciphered by all members of the surgical care team, and may be the first indicators that something is amiss with the patient.

URINALYSIS

Such an everyday procedure is frequently undervalued with regard to its significance as a diagnostic tool. The presence of glucose can, for example, alert the care team to the presence of undiagnosed diabetes mellitus; other diagnoses that results can reveal include renal disease or existing urinary tract infection.

FULL BLOOD COUNT

This reveals the status of the haemoglobin concentration, white cell count and platelet count. It is recommended to include a full blood count for all female patients and males over 50 years of age. When assessing elderly patients the issue of malnourishment is always a consideration, as it can lead to lower than normal haemoglobin levels. Malnourishment in the elderly can be a consequence of pecuniary difficulties if they are solely dependent on income from social welfare, or be due to lack of mobility, resulting in difficulty getting to the shops to bring home and cook nourishing food; or it can be a product of apathy in regard to self-care if living alone.

In the past, obesity was seen as a sign of prosperity and in many cultures it still is; however, obese elderly patients are more likely to be victims of an unhealthy, unbalanced diet, and a full blood count will detail these conditions.

BLOOD CHEMISTRY

These include serum concentration of urea, creatinine, electrolytes, blood glucose levels and liver function tests.

CHEST X-RAY

This is always indicated for patients over 60 years of age.

ADDITIONAL X-RAYS

The management of elderly patients may profit from X-ray of the cervical spine to determine the presence of vertebral unsteadiness. This takes on a singular consequence when the patient is presenting with any type of arthritis.

ELECTROCARDIOGRAM (ECG)

A 12-lead ECG can reveal many abnormalities, whether a recent or a chronic condition. In the event of discovery of an abnormality, corrective therapy may be initiated, and surgery may be cancelled or postponed to a later date. A preoperative ECG also helps by creating a baseline for comparison.

PULMONARY FUNCTION TESTS

Peak expiratory flow rate, forced vital capacity (FVC) and forced expiratory volume need to be calculated and recorded. This is another investigation that has added importance in the context of care of the elderly, owing to the increased probability of existing respiratory disorders.

COAGULATION STUDIES

Assessed here are partial thromboplastin time with kaolin (PTTK) and international normalized ratio (INR) times. Patients with a history of anticoagulant treatment and those with a history of bleeding disorders and/or liver disease require these tests urgently.

GROUP AND CROSS-MATCH BLOOD

This is carried out if a blood transfusion is anticipated during or following a major surgical intervention. If the patient does not wish to have a blood transfusion then the appropriate documentation is completed and recorded.

OBTAINING INFORMED CONSENT FOR SURGERY

When it comes to the matter of consent, legal and ethical considerations come into play. The paternalistic attitude of 'the professional knows best' are long gone. This applies equally in the case of elderly patients, many of whom may have a subservient attitude towards 'professional people', and doctors in particular. This in no way undermines their right to have an appropriate explanation of the planned procedure, the nature of the intervention and the expected outcome.

The history of the concept of informed consent can be traced to the USA in the late 1950s. In the UK the Patients' Charter sets out the patient's rights in this regard, stating that the patient has the right 'to be given a clear explanation of any treatment proposed, including any risks and any alternatives, before you decide whether you will agree to treatment'.[16]

For invasive procedures and surgery a written signed consent is required. Failure to procure this represents a trespass against the person and could allow for prosecution on the grounds of assault.

It behoves every practitioner to know and understand the law on consent in order to be able to function as a patient's advocate, to adhere to the principles of their Code of Conduct, and to act in response to the demands inherent in the concept of professional accountability.[37]

The law incorporates regulations that allow for the protection of individuals who may not be in a position to give consent for themselves. In the context of the care of the elderly, the next of kin may give consent if, for example, because of impaired intellectual functioning the elderly patient cannot comprehend the need for or the nature of the required surgical intervention.

Where a patient cannot give consent, for example an elderly patient suffering from dementia, the surgical intervention may proceed if it is the opinion of the doctor in charge that it is in the patient's best interest. Another doctor must bear witness to this.[38]

The perioperative practitioner needs to be familiar with local protocols on this subject, as many hospitals have a separate and distinct consent form for this purpose, i.e. two doctors acknowledging the need to proceed with surgery. The consent form used is identified by being different in colour and format from the most commonly used one to ensure the patient's best interests are always served.[25,34,39]

PLANNING FOR THE CARE OF THE ELDERLY PATIENT

In the previous section the accent on preparation of the patient for surgery was on what might be seen as the technical aspects of care, i.e. taking blood specimens for analysis, recording ECG readings and vital signs, etc. This may imply that this is the key to preoperative care and that a successful outcome is achieved singularly by attention to this criterion, in which case the perioperative practitioner would have very little input to the care of an elderly patient beyond checking that these standard procedures had been completed. This process would involve merely perusing the patient's medical notes and paperwork to check for errors and omissions, and finally their only role would be to furnish care in the capacity of an assistant to serve the needs of the surgeon.

This, fortunately, is now far from the truth. A look at the evolution of philosophy of care over the last four decades chronicles the transition of the perioperative practitioner from little more than a mechanically orientated assistant focused on equipment and procedural routines, to a dynamic knowledgeable provider of care, which shows the role of the practitioner in a new light. The development of study and research into the absolute concept of care, and its application for superior models of patient care, can be traced to nurse theorists and educationalists of the 1960s and 1970s. This period was an exciting time in the development of surgery too, an example being the advent of the cardiac transplant programme. This placed the emphasis for the perioperative practitioner on preparing for the reception of a patient in the operating department, in terms of having ready the necessary instrumentation and equipment in keeping with the surgeon's preferences. With this mindset the patient was relegated more to being an object of care than in any way being conceived of as a discrete, autonomous individual who had rights and needs beyond mere physical care.[40]

The move away from 'task-allocation care' to 'patient-centred care' in the 1970s provided the opportunity for perioperative practitioners to adopt a new value system, which incorporated an all-round view of the patient's needs. Following the initial negative response to the use of care plans as either paper exercises or 'empire building',[46,47] a change in interpretation took place. Care plans began to be seen as a method of identifying patient needs based on a holistic concept of care. These developments also laid the foundation for practitioners to continue researching, validating and providing solid proof of their contribution to care.[41,42]

To relate the role of the practitioner and the application of care strategies to the perioperative care of the elderly, three themes can be embraced: the principles contained in the application of care plans; communication; and assessing the specific needs of elderly patients.

PERIOPERATIVE CARE PLANS IN THE CARE OF THE ELDERLY

The previous section was titled 'Planning for the care of the elderly' to address a singular issue. Debate about the existence of care plans usually generates more heat than light. It is true that on hospital wards there exist separate and distinct documents on which to record a patient's care. The absence of a similar product in the perioperative environment does not negate the fact that for every patient there exists a plan of care or care plan based on their physical, social, intellectual and emotional needs.

APPLICATION OF CARE PLANS

What has the patient the right to expect when they come to the operating department for surgery? Most probably, if one were to pose this question in, for example, a lecture theatre full of perioperative practitioners, a chorus of all the correct responses and buzzwords would resonate throughout the room. This would include the principle that encapsulates the following beliefs. Based, perhaps, on Maslow's[49] classification of human needs, i.e. the need for physical safety and security, and intensifying to higher cognitive needs connected to feelings of self-esteem and intellectual proficiency, the following sentiments may be echoed:

- The patient has a right to considerate and respectful care
- The patient has the right to obtain from the physician information necessary to give informed consent prior to the start of any procedure and/or treatment
- The patient has the right to refuse treatment to the extent permitted by law, and to be informed of the medical consequences of his action
- The patient has the right to every consideration of privacy concerning his own medical care programme
- The patient has the right to expect that all communications and records pertaining to his care should be treated as confidential
- The patient has the right to expect reasonable continuity of care.[42]

These ideals apply to the delivery of care to all patients, and in particular to the care of the elderly.

The discussion of the delivery of care by healthcare professionals inspires reflection on Henderson's definition of nursing, in the context of which the word 'nurse' must be interpreted generically, i.e. someone 'trained to give assistance to the sick or injured' (Concise Oxford Dictionary).

Henderson defined nursing as follows: 'The unique function of the nurse is to assist the individual, sick or well, in the performance of those activities contributing to health or its recovery (or to a peaceful death) that he would perform unaided if he had the necessary strength, will or knowledge, and to do this in such a way as to help him gain independence as rapidly as possible'.[43]

As detailed earlier, the ageing population is the fastest-expanding segment of the overall population.

Increasing advances in surgery and anaesthesia suggest that these two elements will combine to guarantee that perioperative practitioners will see more and more elderly patients presenting for surgery. Therefore, the application of care plans for the aged will be very relevant, so that perioperative practitioners can identify and respond to their needs. Many older people suffer from depression caused, at least in part, by the loss of physical health, partners, siblings, peers and social status due to retirement. This frequently goes undiagnosed and ignored. 'Doctors say that the typical image of the "moaning old git" could be hindering attempts to deal with one of the most common ailments of old age, depression. It is estimated that up to 17% of elderly people living in the community suffer from depression – twice the number who have dementia, yet it mostly goes undetected and untreated'.[43]

Communication, although often used as a cliché, is actually a vital component of care. An important function of communication is to transmit messages from one person to another. The real purpose of communication is to create meaning. With this intent, senders choose certain words and gestures in a way they believe is congruent with their intended message.[44]

How often, when dealing with elderly patients, do practitioners use what Pratt and Norris[45] term 'motherese'? This is defined as a shallow, insincere verbal communication usually aimed at small children, who are perceived to have a rather limited vocabulary and comprehension skills. This is the sort of language used with not only very young children, but also adults with learning difficulties and when communicating with pets.[45]

This 'elderspeak' – i.e. requiring little effort, more direct and more controlling, examples of which include 'Let's turn over on our side, dearie' – is demeaning and associated with the stereotyping of older people as ineffectual, and is therefore a barrier to any meaningful social exchange. Such attitudes may, even if conveyed through thoughtlessness rather than an implicit lack of respect, trigger feelings of invisibility and worthlessness on the part of the elderly patient.

Meaningful communication in the operating department is not only limited to interactions between practitioner and patient: to deliver the optimum standard of care and construct a partnership between practitioner, patient and colleagues requires attention to recording details of the care of the patient in the operating department. The use of a care plan assists towards this end. The wise and watchful practitioner realizes that the elderly patient presents unique risks, and knows that planning for a team approach to perioperative care is the best method of eliminating these risks.

In order to assess the patient with a view to planning care, one source of information is the patient's case notes. This information is complemented by visual assessment of the patient. Skin integrity can be evaluated: in elderly patients physiological changes occur that make the skin more susceptible to breaking down, bruising and an increased risk of infection, and of course the creation of pressure sores.

The latter are one of the most unacceptable potential complications of hospital care. They can cause permanent tissue damage and penetrate through muscle to bone, resulting in a longer hospital stay, loss of mobility, or even death if a systemic infection takes hold.[46]

The use of the Waterlow risk assessment checklist plays a vital part in the evaluation of a patient's susceptibility to develop pressure sores. This rates the patient's risk factors – age, gender, smoking history, nutritional status, mobility, build, medication, incontinence, existing vascular diseases and proposed duration of the operation to be undergone; the higher the score the greater the danger of compromising the integrity of the skin, therefore preventative measures must be taken to protect the patient. Moving and positioning are carried out by lifting and sliding, thereby avoiding pulling the patient. Care is also called for in the application and removal of the diathermy pad if one is used, so as to avoid tears and breaks to the skin.[47]

In elderly patients the skin is often thin and easily damaged. The risk of pressure sores is very real in surgery, especially if the patient is undergoing a procedure that takes a number of hours. The skin must be protected by the use of appropriate materials. Care needs to be taken also with the use and removal of ECG leads, and any adhesive tape used to secure any such paraphernalia in place.[47]

The vulnerability of the elderly patient's musculoskeletal system requires particular attention, so that moving and positioning must be undertaken with great care. Documentation of the position the patient was placed in during surgery, and additional information regarding the use of support materials, can assist the ward staff in monitoring the patient's level of discomfort and mobility postoperatively.

Ageing patients are more susceptible to changes in temperature and less able to respond to them. The practitioner must therefore ensure that warm blankets, 'space' or reflective blankets or forced air warmers are used, together with careful monitoring of temperature and only uncovering the area of the body that needs to be exposed for surgery. Keeping the patient's body dry as much as possible during surgery will also aid the maintenance of normal body temperature.

Communication is helped by allowing patients to wear their hearing aids or spectacles in the anaesthetic room when explaining standard procedures, etc. Patients' anxiety will not be reduced if they can neither see nor hear properly. In keeping with improved communication techniques and maintaining the patient's sense of dignity, autonomy and self-esteem, patients can be permitted to wear their false teeth so that they can speak clearly. On the grand scale of things these 'minor' details may seem somewhat irrelevant, but they tend to matter greatly to the patient. Hearing aids (with a note as to which ear they fit), glasses and dentures are stored and kept safe according to local policy.[42]

Further topics for consideration in the care of the elderly patient are highlighted by the 1999 Report of the National Confidential Enquiry into Perioperative Deaths:

- Because fluid management is often poor it should be treated with the same seriousness as prescribing drugs, therefore a multidisciplinary team should review local custom and develop good practice[48]
- There should be enough fully staffed daytime and recovery facilities to ensure that older patients are not left more than 24 hours when needing surgery
- A team of senior surgeons and anaesthetists need to be engaged in the care of the elderly patient, especially those at risk because of coexisting medical conditions[42]
- Older patients need their pain management to be given by staff with suitable experience, so that they receive safe and efficient pain relief.

These recommendations could be seen as including the input of perioperative practitioners, as successful outcomes in surgery also depend on the expertise of non-medical staff. A thorough knowledge of instrumentation and proposed procedures, and not simply following routine but knowing what to do and why, enhances patient care.[47]

Box 20.1   The story of the wooden bowl

This is the often-told story of 'the wooden bowl'.[18] It concerns the life of three generations of one family living together. The young son asked his father why his grandfather had to drink and eat from a wooden bowl. His father told him that it was pointless using any other kind of crockery, as the old man would only break it.

One day not long afterwards, the father heard the little boy working and chipping away in the shed. Going in to investigate, he asked his young son what he was doing. The little boy showed him the piece of wood from which he was attempting to design a wooden bowl. 'This is for you when you're old,' replied the boy.

In conclusion, the elderly patient has specific and urgent perioperative needs as has every patient, and it behoves the practitioner not only to be aware of these needs but also to deliver them with the respect and dignity they themselves would wish to be accorded.

References

1. Faulkner A. Nursing: a creative approach. London: Baillière Tindall; 1985.
2. Giddens A. Sociology. Cambridge: Polity Press; 1997.
3. Seedhouse D. Ethics: the heart of health care. Chichester: Wiley; 1988.
4. Akid M. Age of contempt. NT 2002; 98: 12.
5. Help the Aged. Newsletter. Online. Available: http://www.helptheaged.org.uk/news 10 Mar 2002.
6. Age Concern Online. Available: http://www.ageconcern.org.uk/ageconcern/staying.htm 3 June 2002.
7. Assinder N. Parties bow to grey power. Online. Available: http://www.news.bbc.co.uk 3 June 2002.
8. Grey Power Online. Available: http://www.greypower.co.nz 3 June 2002.
9. Tinker A. Older people in modern society. London: Longman; 1997.
10. Vincent J. Politics, power and old age. Buckingham: Open University Press; 1999.
11. National Eating Disorders Association. Online. Available: http://www.edap.org
12. Ellis P, Ellis N. The trivializing process. Oxford: Blackwell; 1982.
13. Victor C. Old age in modern society. London: Croom Helm; 1987.
14. Stockwell F. The unpopular patient. London: RCN; 1972.
15. Dauchot P, Lina A. Geriatric anaesthesia. In: Brown D, ed. Risk and outcome in anaesthesia. Pennsylvania: JB Lippincott; 1992.
16. Allijfri AM, Kingsworth A. Fundamentals of surgical practice. London: Greenwich Medical Media; 1998.
17. Ravlin M. Protecting elderly patients: flaws in ageist arguments.: BMJ; Online. Available: http://www.bmj.com 5 May 2002.
18. Gibson H. The emotional and sexual lives of older people. London: Chapman and Hall; 1992.
19. Winwood RS, Smith JL. Sears' anatomy and physiology for nurses. London: Edward Arnold; 1985.
20. Waldman C. The safety of anaesthesia in old age. In: Taylor TH, Taylor E, eds. Hazards of anaesthesia. Edinburgh: Churchill Livingstone; 1987.
21. Trowler P. Investigating health, welfare and poverty. London: Collins Educational; 1989.
22. Townsend P, Phillimore P, Beattie A. Health and deprivation. Inequality and the north. London: Routledge; 1988.
23. Breech J, Harding L. Assessment of the elderly. Berkshire: NFER-Nelson; 1990.
24. Brown D. Risk and outcome in anaesthesia, 2nd edn. Philadelphia: JB Lippincott; 1992.
25. Ellis F, Campbell I. Essential anaesthesia. Oxford: Blackwell Scientific; 1986.
26. Fox J. Cited in: Bernthal E. Inadvertent hypothermia prevention: the nurse's role. Br J Nurs 1999; 1: 17–25. (Originally published in 1993.)
27. Keen M. A patient temperature audit within a theatre recovery unit. Br J Nurs 2000; 3: 150–156.
28. Giesbrecht GC, Ducharme MB, McGuire JP. 1994. Cited in: Bernthal E. Inadvertent hypothermia prevention: the nurse's role. Br J Nurs 1999; 1: 17–25. (Originally published in 1994.)
29. Schmied H, Kurtz A, Sessler D, et al. Cited in: Bernthal E. Inadvertent hypothermia prevention: the nurse's role. Br J Nurs 1999; 1: 17–25. (Originally published in 1996.)
30. Kurz A, Sessler D, Lenhardt R. Cited in: Bernthal E. Inadvertent hypothermia prevention: the nurse's role. Br J Nurs 1999; 1: 17–25. (Originally published in 1996.)
31. Day I, Benchley S, Redmond S. Living with non-insulin diabetes. Crowborough: Medikos; 1992.
32. Diabetes: missing millions. Online. Available: http://www.internurse.com 3 Mar 2003.

33. National Osteoporosis Society. Online. Available: http://www.nos.org.ok 3 June 2002.

34. Aitkenhead A, Rowbottom D, Smith G. Textbook of anaesthesia. Edinburgh: Churchill Livingstone; 2001.

35. Simpson P, Popat M. Understanding anaesthesia. Oxford: Butterworth-Heinemann; 2002.

36. Forest A, Carter D, MacLeod D. Principles and practice of surgery. Edinburgh: Churchill Livingstone; 1995.

37. Nightingale K. Understanding perioperative nursing. London: Arnold; 1999.

38. Davey A, Ince C. Fundamentals of operating department practice. London: Greenwich Medical Media; 2002.

39. Fortunato N. Operating technique. St Louis: Mosby; 2002.

40. Kalideen D. Delivering planned perioperative care. In: Nightingale K. Understanding perioperative nursing. London: Arnold; 1999.

41. Burn J, Michell J. Cited in: Kalideen D. Delivering planned preoperative care. In: Nightingale K. Understanding perioperative nursing. London: Arnold; 1999: 36.

42. Atkinson L. Berry and Kohn's operating room technique. St Louis: Mosby; 1992.

43. Tomey A, Alligood M. Nursing theorists and their work. St Louis: Mosby; 2002.

44. Riley J. Communication in nursing. St Louis: Mosby; 2000.

45. Pratt M, Norris J. Social psychology of ageing. Oxford: Blackwell; 1994.

46. Family Doctor. Online. Available: http://www.familydoctor.org 3 June 2002.

47. Waterlow Risk Assessment. Online. Available: http://www.aromacaring.co.uk 3 June 2002.

48. Department of Health. Extremes of age. The 1999 Report of the National Confidential Enquiry into Perioperative Deaths. London: HMSO; 2002. Online. Available: http://www.doh.gov.uk 3 June 2002.

49. Meleis A. Theoretical nursing: development and progress. Pennsylvania: JB Lippincott; 1991.

Chapter 21

Care of patients with serious or multisystem disease

Vicki Clark

Key points

- Optimize patient systems before surgery if possible
- Seriously ill patients may need input from several specialties
- Intensive care involvement should be considered early rather than late
- Holistic approach to care

PRINCIPLES OF CARE

Ideally, patients who have serious or multisystem disease should undergo surgery in as optimal a physical state as possible. Occasionally this is not practical if surgery is urgent, but if it is elective or semielective then every effort should be made to stabilize the patient physiologically before the stress of surgery. This is because in seriously ill patients there is much less room for error, and what would be tolerated in a healthier patient may end in serious morbidity or mortality in the sicker patient. If the seriously ill patient is made as physiologically 'normal' as possible, then there is some leeway and time to rectify the situation if untoward events occur.

To this end, thorough preoperative assessment and workup are vital. Inadequate preoperative investigations may result in the case being cancelled just before surgery, with obvious delay in treatment, disappointment for the patient, waste of resources and ever-lengthening waiting lists for surgery. Organized units will have preoperative protocols for laboratory investigations, cross-matching requirements, etc. to prevent this happening.

Most patients with multisystem disease will be on numerous medications, and these must be carefully checked and prescribed shortly after admission. Often the patient is unsure about the names of the drugs, the reason for the medication or the frequency of dosage, and a telephone call to the GP is wise.

Some drugs are contraindicated before surgery. Warfarin must be stopped at least 3 days beforehand, and the international normalized ratio (INR) checked daily – it should be less than 1.5 before surgery. Angiotensin-converting enzyme inhibitors (ACEI) must not be given on the morning of surgery as they interact with anaesthetic agents and can result in resistant hypotension. Monoamine oxidase inhibitors must be stopped at least 2 weeks before surgery as they affect the intraneuronal metabolism of sympathomimetic amines and can cause hypertensive crisis. They can also interact with pethidine.

Conversely, other drugs are vital before surgery despite the fasting restrictions. Stopping β-blockers abruptly will cause rebound hypertension. Prednisolone inhibits the pituitary-adrenal axis, and stopping it will result in a lack of sympathetic response and the ability to cope with the stress of surgery. Again, units should have protocols for drug administration prior to surgery, or the anaesthetist on their preoperative visit should clearly state which drugs should be withheld and which given.

Common sense dictates that any patient with serious or multisystem disorder should not be cared for in a small isolated unit. In larger hospitals a patient with multisystem illness may have several specialists involved in their care. Each may have contributions to management which are sometimes conflicting. For example, a renal physician may wish the patient well hydrated to maintain urine output, but the cardiologist may wish the patient relatively dehydrated if he or she is in cardiac failure. There must therefore always be an overall physican in charge who coordinates the different strategies. This is usually the admitting physician/surgeon, or in ITU, the anaesthetist.

If surgery is elective, it should be scheduled for a time when domestic carers are available to look after patients in the rehabilitation phase.

SUPPORT

Patients with serious or multisystem disease have greater perioperative morbidity and mortality. Whereas most will appreciate the potential complications during and after surgery, many will deny they exist or may not be fully aware of the gravity of their illness. Both patient and family must be made cognisant of the risks that surgery involves, and time must be set aside for discussion and decision-making. Senior staff members are usually involved in such discussions, but patients and family members often approach junior staff, who may be more familiar to them. Practitioners of all disciplines must ensure that a holistic approach is adopted, and both physical and psychological care must be undertaken with sensitivity and empathy.

In large specialist units procedures are well rehearsed and routine, so patients may feel as if they are on a production line. A personal and unhurried approach should be adopted and communication between staff and patients and their families encouraged. The support of a named nurse is often pivotal in this process, in order to maintain continuity of care during a time when the patient may face a seemingly endless procession of different professionals, each contributing a different aspect of care.

In the wards, patients may speak to postoperative patients and be encouraged by their progress. On the downside, they may know of fellow patients who have not done so well, although this may also bring a sense of realism.

In the event of extreme illness, intensive care may be necessary postoperatively. It is better for the physician in charge to be pessimistic and book a bed in ITU and then not have to use it, rather than being overly optimistic and then have to negotiate a bed in an already full ITU if the patient needs one. This may result in critically ill postoperative patients being looked after in wards which are not adequately staffed, or where the staff are not appropriately trained.

ITU admission is inevitable following cardiac, thoracic or neurosurgery. Medical and nursing ward staff should liaise with ITU staff to provide continuity of care. If time permits, a visit to ITU may be possible preoperatively so that the patient is made familiar with the environment, equipment and staff likely to be used in their care. Surgery may only be possible if the ITU bed is guaranteed, and with the shortage of ITU beds nationally it may be necessary to cancel surgery until a bed becomes available.

Patients may need sedation in ITU. This is done sometimes for humanitarian reasons, in order to make the ITU experience less traumatic, and also to facilitate necessary procedures, particularly tolerating the endotracheal tube and ventilation. Combinations of propofol, midazolam and opiates are commonly used. However, carers must always be aware that their patients may well be conscious and must therefore be treated with respect and dignity at all times. Talking to the patient as if he or she is awake is much appreciated by both family and patient.

If the patient is less seriously ill, then a high-dependency unit may be more appropriate for post-operative care. Again, a visit before surgery is much appreciated by both patient and family.

SPECIFIC CONDITIONS

CARDIOVASCULAR DISEASE

Surgery for cardiac disease may be necessary at all stages of life and is carried out in specialist centres. Paediatric cardiac surgery may be required following congenital heart disease, and there is often a huge emotional component as it may involve a neonate or toddler, and parental expectation of success is high. The presence of valvular heart disease is not as common in the UK as in the developing world, owing to the rarity of rheumatic fever. It tends to affect the elderly and its incidence may be on the wane. In contrast, ischaemic heart disease is on the increase, as is the need for coronary artery bypass surgery. Atherosclerosis often accompanies ischaemic heart disease and is responsible for hypertension as well as compromised vascular supply to several organs, resulting for instance in strokes and peripheral vascular disease. Vascular surgery aims to revascularize those areas where arterial supply is reduced, for example in the brain and legs.

By the time these patients arrive on the wards for their surgery, many will have had several complicated investigations such as angiography, echocardiography and lung function tests. Most will be aware of the gravity of their illness. On the day before surgery they may be introduced to the ITU and be seen by the anaesthetist, although in some centres there are preanaesthetic clinics so that the anaesthetist and patient meet weeks beforehand.

The anaesthetist will assess the patient's cardiac function by enquiring about angina, exercise tolerance, breathlessness, especially on lying flat, and palpitations. A previous history of myocardial infarction and cardiac failure is a poor prognostic feature, and only emergency surgery should be carried out within 6 months of a heart attack, or if the patient is in obvious failure.

The ECG is very informative. Arrhythmias are another sign of poor cardiac status and these should be controlled. Atrial fibrillation with a ventricular rate of over 100 may lead to cardiac failure, so once again surgery should be postponed until a lower rate is achieved, either by digoxin or by a β-blocker. If the rate is such that there is cardiac compromise, cardioversion may be indicated. Some types of second-degree and complete (third-degree) heart block require pacing before surgery.

The ECG will also identify axis deviation of the heart and hypertrophy of any of the heart chambers, indicating that there has been considerable heart strain already.

Uncontrolled hypertension, for example a systolic greater than 180 mmHg, or a diastolic greater than 100 mmHg, is associated with considerable perioperative morbidity and mortality, and attempts should be made to lower blood pressure before surgery. Beware, however, of the 'white coat' syndrome, where the patient is actually normotensive but the presence of a member of staff induces such anxiety that hypertension ensues. If, however, the BP is consistently elevated, all but the most urgent surgery should be postponed.

The agents used for anaesthesia of the critically ill cardiovascular patient vary from unit to unit and from anaesthetist to anaesthetist. There is no 'formula', but each technique is chosen such that the anaesthetist is aware of the agents' potential advantages and drawbacks, and each is tailored for the individual patient.

Premedication in a hypotensive patient may be contraindicated. On the other hand, anxiety will increase the endogenous catecholamines and may cause a tachycardia, which increases cardiac work. It is vitally important in this group to give all the usual cardiac medications the patient is taking, with the exception of angiotensin-converting enzyme inhibitors, which may cause hypotension.

If the patient is abnormally hypotensive, the anaesthetist will induce anaesthesia with etomidate rather than thiopental or propofol, as the latter two will worsen hypotension. However, it must be remembered that in cardiac patients, hypertension and tachycardia should also be avoided, as they will increase the work of the heart. Usually large doses of opiate are given prior to induction and laryngoscopy. Again, in the choice of muscle relaxants, those that cause tachycardia and hypertension, e.g. gallamine and pancuronium, are best avoided.

Patients with significant cardiovascular disease undergoing major surgery require arterial lines for real-time blood pressure monitoring. These are usually inserted before induction in the radial artery of the non-dominant hand, but arterial access may also be via the brachial, femoral and dorsalis pedis arteries. Blood samples are taken from these lines to avoid multiple venepunctures.

Central venous lines are used not only to monitor the central venous pressure (CVP), which guides fluid management, but also to permit the use of inotropic agents, which may be irritant to peripheral veins. The commonest central vein used is the internal jugular, but the subclavian and femoral veins may also be used. If the patient has left ventricular failure or sepsis, then a pulmonary artery flotation catheter (PAFC) may be necessary (Fig. 21.1). This facilitates cardiac output and systemic vascular resistance measurements.

Inotropic therapy, which improves cardiac output and blood pressure, may be required in the perioperative period. Each unit tends to have its favoured agents, but drugs such as adrenaline (epinephrine), noradrenaline (norepinephrine), dopamine and dobutamine are common. Their dosage is dictated by arterial, CVP and PAFC readings. They require extremely close monitoring and appropriately trained staff who can prevent and, if necessary, recognize and deal with complications. Strict aseptic techniques must be adhered to in looking after invasive lines, as sepsis introduced from lines may prove fatal. Air can be inadvertently introduced into any of the lines if care is not taken when using them. Air embolism into the CVP can be catastrophic if there is a coexisting patent foramen ovale. This will result in air bubbles in the systemic side of the circulation, with the potential for strokes or myocardial infarcts. Furthermore, if the balloon of the PAFC is accidentally left inflated for any length of time, then the lung distal to the balloon is deprived of its blood supply, with potential infarction. Because of the extended training required by ITU staff, critical care courses are promoted and practitioners undertake extensive 'shadowing' before being left on a one-to-one basis with their patients.

Pulmonary oedema reduces gas exchange and patients in cardiac failure may often require ventilation. Most seriously ill patients and those immediately postoperatively may require intermittent positive-pressure ventilation (IPPV), with or without positive end-expiratory pressure (PEEP) which, by preventing the alveoli collapsing at the end of expiration, promotes oxygen delivery to the blood. Turning patients prone may enhance gas exchange. As the patient improves, weaning modes can be employed, e.g. spontaneous intermittent mandatory ventilation (SIMV) or assisted spontaneous breathing (ASB).

The perioperative practitioner should liaise with the anaesthetist before the case, as he or she may request unusual equipment, for example a PEEP valve. Preparing the equipment in the anaesthetic room/theatre prior to the arrival of a seriously

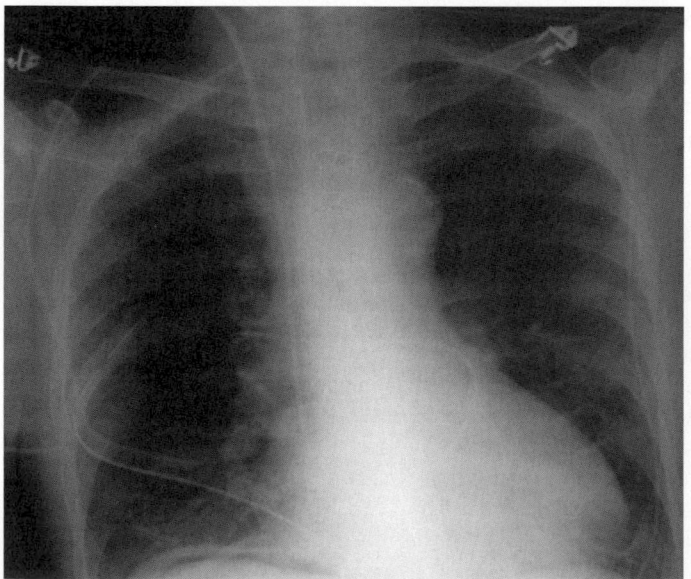

Figure 21.1   Chest X-ray of a patient following mitral valve replacement showing cardiomegaly, a pulmonary artery flotation catheter, sternal wires and chest drain.

compromised cardiac patient is good practice, so that all drugs and equipment are to hand should a crisis occur. This includes checking that all equipment is present and working, and that the resuscitation drugs are available, especially vasopressors, and running through the lines for invasive monitoring. Blood may be needed and should be checked before the case starts. The likely ward destination of the patient should be discussed, so that a bed and the appropriate monitors plus or minus ventilator can be prepared for transfer.

RESPIRATORY DISEASE

Persistent coughing, breathlessness, wheezing and purulent sputum are all signs of lung pathology. Occasionally the first two may occur in cardiac disease, but a good history and examination will differentiate between the two. With time, respiratory disease will cause right heart disease (cor pulmonale). If time permits, the function of the lungs should be optimized. Bronchodilators, nebulizers and chest physiotherapy, along with judicious use of antibiotics, are often required.

Patients with significant lung disease will require oxygen perioperatively. Occasionally if they have severe chronic obstructive pulmonary disease (COPD), the anaesthetist may insist on using a Venturi (fixed-performance) mask rather than a Hudson (variable-performance) mask. Venturi masks deliver a fixed amount of oxygen which is independent of the patient's breathing pattern. They come in a variety of inspired oxygen concentrations, including 24%, 28%, 35%, 40% and 60%, and these concentrations are obtained by altering the flow rates as indicated on the mask. All operating rooms should have a selection of these available.

If severe lung disease is detected, the patient must have a chest X-ray, lung function tests (Table 21.1) and arterial blood gas measurements (Table 21.2), especially if the planned procedure is extensive and lengthy.

Patients with respiratory disease are disadvantaged if they have a general anaesthetic (GA), and if at all possible, regional anaesthesia should be employed. However, if the surgery is above the umbilicus or prolonged this may be impractical, and a general anaesthetic is indicated.

Regional techniques vary according to the proposed surgery. Spinals provide rapid, dense anaesthesia but are of limited duration. Epidurals are more difficult to site, but have the advantage of being able to be topped up, so that the anaesthesia can be adjusted to suit the duration of the surgery. Some anaesthetists will carry out a combined spinal and epidural, achieving a fast onset of block with the spinal and using the epidural if the surgery is prolonged, or for postoperative analgesia. A drip must be sited before the initiation of any central block, and vasopressors should be prepared beforehand.

Should GA be necessary the anaesthetist must avoid a 'light' patient, as patients with irritable airways will cough at the slightest stimulus and develop bronchospasm readily. Some anaesthetists spray the cords with lidocaine (lignocaine) so that

Table 21.2 Arterial blood gases on air

pH	7.38–7.44
H+ (mmol/l)	36–43
PaO_2 (kPa)	12–13
PCO_2 (kPa)	4–6
HCO_3 (mmol/l)	21–25

Table 21.1 Lung function tests

	Normal (male, 40 years)	Chronic pulmonary airways disease (COPD)	Restrictive airways disease
FEV_1 in litres	3.1–4.2	<2	<2
FVC in litres	3.8–5.4	3.0–4.0	<2
PEFR in litres/min	500–600	100–200	200–300
FEV_1/FVC %	>75	<50	>60

FEV_1 = forced expiratory volume in 1 s, the volume of air expired forcibly in 1 second;
FVC = forced vital capacity, the volume expired at the end of maximum expiration;
PEFR = peak expiratory flow rate.

the stimulus of the tube is removed. The patients must also be given an adequate dose of induction agent and volatile maintenance. If patients are anaesthetized too deeply their blood pressure will fall, and so the best technique is 'balanced anaesthesia', which involves paralysing the patient to prevent coughing and bronchospasm while maintaining unconsciousness with lighter and less hypotensive volatile concentrations.

Even if a GA is necessary, regional anaesthesia can still be employed for postoperative analgesia. The classic example of this is following laparotomy in a patient with COPD. An epidural used postoperatively will reduce opiate requirements and the accompanying respiratory depression. Good analgesia will also improve oxygenation, as abdominal pain prevents adequate lung expansion.

Most patients with COPD can be managed in a high-dependancy unit (HDU), particularly if there is an appropriate analgesia regimen. However, if gas exchange is poor as indicated by arterial blood gases ($PaO_2 < 8\,kPa$ on air, or $PaCO_2 > 8\,kPa$), low oxygen saturation (<90% on air), or the patient is tiring as indicated by rising respiratory rates, then admission to ITU is indicated. Patients with pre-existing lung disease present a significant challenge to intensive care staff, as weaning from ventilation is often prolonged and problematic.

RENAL DISEASE

Renal function deteriorates with age, but accelerated deterioration may occur in hypertension, diabetes, or after injudicious use of non-steroidals, for example in the elderly who have had a period of dehydration due to long periods of vomiting or diarrhoea. This manifests itself as either oliguria or anuria, and worsening urea and electrolytes.

Patients with established renal failure will be chronically anaemic owing to a reduction in erythropoietin production. A haemoglobin of <$90\,g/l$ is usual and the threshold for transfusion should be subsequently lowered. If the patient is on dialysis, postdialysis blood results are necessary prior to surgery and anaesthesia. In addition, surgery should be scheduled such that the heparin or epoprostenol (prostacyclin) that has been used to provide anticoagulation has been eliminated, i.e more than 4 hours postdialysis. The fistula for dialysis is usually in the forearm and should be protected from damage. Thus IV access and application of the BP cuff should be in the contralateral arm.

Because the kidney is responsible for the elimination of many drugs, renal dysfunction can result in prolonged drug half-life. Furthermore, kidney disease may cause hyperkalaemia, which can predispose to arrhythmias if excessive. A glucose/insulin infusion plus nebulized salbutamol can be used to drive the potassium down. In addition, the kidney is responsible for the elimination of water, and renal dysfunction can result in fluid retention and ultimately pulmonary oedema.

If at all possible, general anaesthesia should be avoided, but if this is impossible then agents with no renal elimination should be chosen. For example, atracurium is the drug of choice for muscle relaxation, as it is eliminated in the blood and liver by Hofman degradation. Mivacurium is a possible alternative. Uraemia is associated with slower gastric emptying, and these patients must be well fasted and on an H_2 antagonist, e.g ranitidine.

Suxamethonium causes a transient rise in plasma potassium and should be avoided if at all possible in patients with renal failure, as the patient may already have hyperkalaemia. Plasma potassium of $6\,mmol/l$ is associated with potentially fatal arrhythmias. Similarly, Ringer's or Hartmann's solutions are contraindicated because of their potassium content.

Great care must be taken with opiates as they are renally excreted. It may be possible to extend the regional technique in the postoperative period, e.g with an epidural, and avoid opiates altogether.

Whatever technique is chosen, there must be adequate intravascular fluid volume and minimal cardiovascular depression at all times, as kidney function in this group is often precarious and as much as possible should be preserved. Careful fluid balance should be maintained with scrupulous fluid balance charts. Urine output of $0.5\,ml/kg$ is the usual minimum volume desired in a healthy adult without renal disease, but less may be produced in the renal patient. A fluid load may produce the desired urine volume in a healthy patient but may cause overload and pulmonary oedema in the renal patient. Diuretics may be tried to promote urine production if fluid is accumulating. A CVP line is useful in major surgery where large blood loss and fluid shifts are anticipated.

LIVER DISEASE

The liver plays a key role in the metabolism of several drugs and the elimination of waste products. However, the liver has considerable reserves and extensive damage has to be done before dysfunction becomes apparent.

The liver produces many vital proteins, such as albumin. A low albumin is a bad prognostic sign and has implications for drug dosage, as several drugs bind to albumin, e.g. antiepileptics. A low albumin results in higher levels of free drug available in the plasma and greater therapeutic levels of some drugs, so dosages need to be reduced.

The liver is an important producer of coagulation factors and liver failure results in coagulopathy. This is obviously important if surgery is intended. A deranged coagulation screen may alert the surgeon to the possibility of uncontrollable haemorrhage during surgery and prophylactic coagulation products may be requested before surgery. Coagulopathy also has anaesthetic implications. Spinal and epidural anaesthesia are contraindicated as spinal haematomas can result in permanent paraplegia.

The liver is also a producer of glucose and liver failure may render the patient prone to hypoglycaemia. Regular blood glucose monitoring is therefore necessary.

Patients with liver disease should never be exposed to halothane, which in susceptible individuals will cause halothane hepatitis. However, this agent is rarely used in current practice.

Hepatorenal syndrome is a condition whereby jaundiced patients are at risk of developing renal failure. Several measures can be taken to prevent this. First, the patient is kept well hydrated, and second they are given agents that promote diuresis, e.g. mannitol.

Patients with chronic liver disease, e.g cirrhosis, may also have oesophageal varices, which can bleed. They may also have alcoholic cardiomyopathy, which renders them very unstable and prone to cardiac failure.

NEUROLOGICAL DISEASE

Traumatic head injuries, cerebral haemorrhages and tumours make up the majority of seriously ill patients presenting to the neurological unit. Many will require investigation, e.g. computed tomography (CT) or magnetic resonance imaging (MRI). Because these require the patient to remain still during the procedure, all but the most cooperative patients are anaesthetized.

The airway in brain-damaged patients is often lost and a Glasgow Coma Scale (Table 21.3)[1] of less than 8 is an indication for intubation and ventilation.

Table 21.3   Glasgow Coma Scale

Response	Score
Eye opening	
Spontaneous	4
To speech	3
To pain	2
Nil	1
Best motor response	
Obeys	6
Localizes	5
Withdraws (flexion)	4
Abnormal flexion	3
Extensor response	2
Nil	1
Verbal response	
Orientated	5
Confused conversation	4
Inappropriate words	3
Incomprehensible sounds	2
Nil	1

Many patients are admitted straight to ITU where, apart from the invasive monitoring discussed previously, neurological observations will be started, including conscious levels (Table 21.3) if not sedated, and intracranial pressures (ICP) if indicated. Patients who have had seizures, for example status epilepticus, may be paralysed but the brain may still be having epileptic discharges. Additional monitoring is required in the form of compressed spectral array and cerebral function monitors.

The aim of surgery for patients who are neurologically compromised is to provide as stable an anaesthetic as possible without great troughs or peaks of blood pressure. Thus a smooth induction, intubation and extubation is the goal, with a stable maintenance period in the middle. An opiate and muscle relaxant combination along with isoflurane is used in many units. An alternative technique is total intravenous anaesthesia (TIVA). Enflurane is contraindicated in patients with epilepsy because it reduces the threshold for seizures and can induce them in susceptible individuals.

The second aim of neurosurgical anaesthesia is to prevent raised ICP and to maintain cerebral perfusion pressure (CPP). CPP is the mean arterial pressure minus the ICP, and it will be reduced if the ICP rises. A reduced CPP will compromise cerebral blood flow and may cause a stroke. Normal ICP is

> **Box 21.1 Signs and symptoms of raised intracranial pressure**
>
> - Headache
> - Nausea and vomiting
> - Confusion
> - Altered consciousness
> - Bradycardia
> - Hypertension
> - Shift in midline seen on CT or MRI
> - Convulsions
> - Dilated and unreactive pupil ('blown pupil')
> - Contralateral hemiplegia
> - Apnoea

usually <15 mmHg, and if raised (Box 21.1) it can be reduced by a head-up position, hyperventilation to a $PaCO_2$ of approximately 3–4.0 kPa, inserting an intrathecal drain, or giving drugs such as mannitol, frusemide (furosemide), steroids or barbiturates. Cerebral blood flow may be monitored using transcranial Doppler techniques or jugular venous bulb oxygen saturation.

BLOOD DISORDERS

Anaemia and coagulation disorders are the blood disorders that cause the most concern to surgeons and anaesthetists.

A haemoglobin (Hb) of 100 g/l used to be taken as the gold standard for perioperative measurements. This is now acknowledged to be without an evidence base, and much lower limits are now acceptable.[2] A fit person can cope with an Hb of 80 g/l, but the threshold for transfusion changes if, for example, the patient has significant ischaemic heart disease, when he or she may need more oxygen-carrying capacity to compensate for the reduced coronary perfusion. Conversely, a person with renal failure rarely has an Hb above 90 g/l, and can cope with levels below this quite well. Signs that may indicate that transfusion is necessary are pallor, tachycardia and continuing blood loss. Symptoms that reveal a need for transfusion are postural dizziness, breathlessness and excessive tiredness.

Coagulopathy may be present in patients with end-stage liver disease, as discussed earlier, or as a result of disseminated intravascular coagulopathy (DIC). The latter is often due to huge blood loss and massive transfusion, which results in dilution of the coagulation factors. It requires the transfusion of coagulation products – fresh frozen plasma, platelets and cryoprecipitate. These may be given empirically in an emergency, or according to the coagulation results if there is time to wait for them.

THROMBOPROPHYLAXIS

Patients who are very ill, have had certain types of operations, for example orthopaedic or cancer surgery, are pregnant, obese, or have had long spells in hospital are prone to deep venous thrombosis and pulmonary embolism. They should be well hydrated and should have mechanical prophylaxis in the form of elasticated stockings or inflating boots. In addition, chemical prophylaxis should be considered in the absence of coagulopathy.[3] Currently, low molecular weight heparins such as enoxaparin and tinzaparin are used once daily by the subcutaneous route. If there is evidence that thrombosis has occurred, warfarin is started, but because it takes 2–3 days to become effective as measured by the international normalized ratio (INR), unfractionated heparin must also be started intravenously simultaneously, the levels of which are monitored with activated partial prothrombin time (APPT).

CASE EXAMPLES

Rheumatoid Arthritis

One of the best examples of multisystem disease is rheumatoid arthritis. This is an autoimmune disorder which can involve virtually all systems. Patients often present with joint pain or distortion requiring surgery.

Routine blood tests may reveal a chronic anaemia due both to the disease and the drugs the patient may be taking, e.g methotrexate. There is obviously a higher risk of perioperative transfusion if the proposed surgery is known to cause large blood loss. A chest X-ray may reveal lung disease. Pulmonary fibrosis, which will cause a restrictive airways disease (see Table 21.1), and rheumatoid nodules can reduce gas exchange. Pericardial effusions may also be diagnosed on the X-ray. If the neck and temporomandibular joints are involved, conventional intubation may be impossible owing to the lack of neck flexion or extension and limited mouth opening. Further, a cervical spine X-ray may show subluxation of the upper cervical vertebrae with cervical instability. Injudicious neck movement may cause these vertebrae to slip further on each other, with potential spinal cord transection. In these cases if a GA is necessary an awake fibreoptic intubation is indicated. Most anaesthetists will perform regional anaesthesia alone on rheumatoid patients if at all possible, as this removes potential intubation problems.

Many of these patients are on steroids, which must be given in normal doses preoperatively and supplemented with intravenous hydrocortisone if the prednisolone dosage is more than 10 mg daily.[4] Prednisolone may result in thin fragile veins, which makes venous access problematic. Some patients suffer from Sjögren's syndrome, which causes dry eyes, and care must be taken to protect the eyes during surgery. Finally, many patients may have already undergone joint replacement and should be moved gently and cautiously to prevent joint dislocation. Extra padding must be used in positioning them on the operating table, as their skin is very fragile and pressure areas must be protected.

Ms RB is a 58-year-old woman who has been admitted for an elbow replacement as her elbow has been deteriorating over the last 5 years and she can now hardly feed or wash herself. This is her fifth operation, as she has had her hips and shoulders operated on before. For the shoulder procedure, the anaesthetist had great difficulty intubating her and wrote this in her notes.

Apart from her rheumatoid disease, she is fit and well. Her medications include a non-steroidal anti-inflammatory agent, ibuprofen, plus prednisolone 5 mg daily, and her GP has also given her a proton-pump inhibitor, lansoprazole, to prevent gastric ulceration. Her Hb is 100 g/l and her urea and electrolytes are normal. An ECG was not thought necessary, but her chest and cervical spine were X-rayed.

On examination she weighs 60 kg and is 1.5 m tall. She admits to having 'terrible veins', and her neck is fairly fixed with little flexion or extension. She has a full set of teeth and the interincisor gap is only 2 cm. Her cervical spine X-ray reveals subluxation between the first and second cervical vertebrae. The anaesthetist explains that because of her neck problems and potential difficult airway, it would be best if she had an awake fibreoptic intubation.[5]

The perioperative practitioner has to set up a lot of equipment for a fibreoptic intubation. Apart from the fibreoptic laryngoscope, light source and monitor, he or she also needs to prepare a range of nasal tubes,

lubricating jelly and ancillary airways, e.g. Bermann or Ovasappian, in addition to the usual Guedel airways. An emergency cricothyroidotomy set should also be to hand. Some anaesthetists spray lidocaine (lignocaine) down the laryngoscope to provide anaesthesia. Others use nerve blocks in the neck. Drugs required include midazolam, a short-acting opiate like fentanyl, glycopyrrolate and lidocaine (lignocaine). A Magill forceps is handy to protract the tongue.

Some surgeons perform elbow replacements with the patient on the side. This involves many supports for the patient's hips and back, as well as the elbow support. Padding for the eyes, neck and contralateral elbow is needed. In addition, the IV cannula may not be accessible to the anaesthetist, so an extension set and a 3-way tap have to be inserted.

Pre-eclampsia

This condition affects 6–8% of all pregnant women and is of unknown origin. It is associated with hypertension and proteinuria, and affects many systems.[6] There is a generalized vasoconstriction which causes placental insufficiency and the fetus to be effectively starved in utero. This results in intrauterine growth retardation and occasionally placental infarction, which may lead to intrauterine death, particularly if the fetus is then subjected to the stress of labour. The vasoconstriction also affects the cerebral vasculature and, if severe, can cause neurological symptoms such as headache and visual disturbances. In a few women – 1 in 2000 pregnancies – convulsions may occur.

The renal vasoconstriction can cause glomerular dysfunction and loss of protein in the urine. Renal failure can ensue. The capillaries of these patients are extraordinarily leaky and they are often very oedematous. In addition, leaky pulmonary capillaries may make these women susceptible to pulmonary oedema, particularly if they are overloaded or in renal failure.

There is known to be a thromboxane/ prostaglandin imbalance. These two factors are involved in the coagulation pathway, and whether the patient is more prone to bleeding or thrombosis depends on which factor is more prevalent. In severe cases haemolysis, liver and platelet dysfunction may occur (HELLP syndrome – haemolysis, elevated liver enzymes and low platelets).

Most of these patients are started on oral antihypertensive agents, but if hypertension persists or there is evidence of cerebral, renal, placental or platelet dysfunction, the patient is delivered most commonly by caesarean section. Spinal anaesthesia is the preferred route. General anaesthesia is potentially hazardous in view of the hypertensive response to laryngoscopy and the oedematous larynx, which can cause difficulty in intubation. However, regional anaesthesia is contraindicated if the platelets fall below $80 \times 10^9/\text{dl}$, when the threat of spinal haematoma looms.

FR is a 30-year-old primigravida who was previously fit and well. A week before admission, when she was 33 weeks pregnant, she went to her GP complaining of headache and her BP was 140/85. There was a little proteinuria and the GP made an appointment to see her in a week. That morning she had a BP of 145/100, more proteinuria, and was markedly oedematous. She was immediately admitted to the maternity hospital, where she was monitored in the labour ward and given nifedipine and labetalol to reduce her BP, plus steroids (dexamethasone) to mature her baby's lungs. Her BP remained persistently high, with a diastolic of over 95. In addition, her urea and electrolytes began to deteriorate and her platelets fell from 180 the previous week to 100 on admission. The obstetricians decided to proceed to caesarean section as her pre-eclampsia was worsening.

She was premedicated with ranitidine, IV access was achieved, and she had a spinal anaesthetic inserted that contained heavy bupivacaine and diamorphine. The caesarean section was uneventful. She was taken to the high-dependency unit, where her fluid balance was strictly monitored. Her BP was controlled with oral labetalol and her analgesia achieved with intrathecal diamorphine. All her blood parameters improved the next day and she was discharged home 5 days later, although the baby stayed in the neonatal unit for 5 weeks.

SUMMARY

Caring for seriously ill patients or those with multi-system disease is very challenging as there may be conflicting requirements for each system. The team is often multidisciplinary and there should be realistic goals for both surgery and anaesthesia. High-dependency or intensive care is usually needed.

References

1. Sternbach GL. The Glasgow coma scale. J Emerg Med 2000; 19: 67–77.
2. Goldhill D, Boralessa H, Boralessa H. Anaemia and red cell transfusion in the critically ill. Anaesthesia 2002; 57: 527–529.
3. Scottish Intercollegiate Guidelines Network. Prophylaxis of venous thromboembolism. Edinburgh: SIGN; 2002.
4. Nicolson G, Burrin JM, Hall GM. Perioperative steroid supplementation. Anaesthesia 1998; 53: 1091–1104.
5. Popat M. Practical fibreoptic intubation. Oxford: Butterworth-Heinemann; 2001.
6. Mortl MG, Schneider MC. Key issues in assessing, managing and treating patients presenting with severe pre-eclampsia. Inter J Obstetric Anesth 2000; 9: 39–44.

Further reading

Aitkenhead AR, Rowbotham DJ, Smith G. Textbook of anaesthesia. Edinburgh: Churchill Livingstone; 2001.
Hampton JR. The ECG made easy. Edinburgh: Churchill Livingstone; 1999.
Singer M, Webb AR. Oxford handbook of critical care medicine. Oxford: OUP; 1996.

Websites

Neuromuscular blocking agents
http://www.users.dircon.co.uk/~rosebud/drugs/Neuromuscular-blockers.html

Chapter 22

Care of patients who have highly infectious disease

Gillian Stevenson

Key points

- Bloodborne viruses
- Hepatitis B and C
- Creutzfeldt-Jakob disease
- Tuberculosis
- Varicella zoster virus
- Human immunodeficiency virus

The objective of this chapter is to outline the risks to staff and patients from a variety of highly infectious diseases. It should be noted that guidance is continuously updated, and that a website search will ensure that practitioners' knowledge of local policies is dynamic.

BLOODBORNE VIRUSES (BBVs)

This section will discuss the most common BBVs. For the purposes of this chapter, BBVs will include human immunodeficiency virus (HIV), hepatitis B (HBV) and hepatitis C (HCV).

There are a number of issues that apply to all the BBVs, and these will be covered in this section. However, clinical features, diagnoses and post-exposure prophylaxis will be dealt with separately.

All hospitals should have their own policies for BBVs to ensure safe practice and the prevention of transmission to staff and patients.

As the status of patients with regard to any of these infections is generally unknown, it is essential that staff are aware of the risks from all blood and body fluids. Universal precautions must apply to all patients (see chapter on infection control principles).

The national guidance[1] on protection against BBVs advises that the following body fluids should be handled with the same precautions as blood:

- Cerebrospinal fluid
- Peritoneal fluid
- Pleural fluid
- Pericardial fluid
- Synovial fluid
- Amniotic fluid
- Semen
- Vaginal secretions
- Breast milk
- Any other body fluid containing visible blood, including saliva associated with dentistry
- Unfixed tissues and organs.

THE RISK OF TRANSMISSION OF BBVs

The risk of transmission of BBVs is greater from patient to healthcare worker, rather than the reverse. The risk to the healthcare worker is proportional to the prevalence of each virus in the general population. The infectious state of the patient and the type of injury can also affect the risk to the healthcare worker. The risks arise from patients who are carriers of any of these BBVs. It is essential that risk assessments be carried out for all procedures to be undertaken, rather than to focus on the patient's status.

The risk of acquiring occupationally acquired HBV in non-immune healthcare workers ranges from 2% to 40%, depending on the hepatitis e-antigen status of the patient. The risk from HCV is 3–10%, and for HIV the risk is 0.3%.[2] If a sharp is visibly contaminated with blood, and was used for venepuncture or the injury is deep, the risk is increased.

ACTION AFTER INJURY

All hospitals must have a postexposure policy which is in accordance with national guidance and which must be followed after any injury.[1]

The site of exposure should be washed immediately using hot water and soap, without scrubbing. Exposed mucous membranes, including conjunctivae, should be irrigated copiously with water (after first removing contact lenses, if worn). Puncture wounds should be allowed to bleed freely but must not be sucked. The injury should be reported promptly and advice on treatment sought immediately.

An accurate history should be obtained regarding the nature of the injury and the source patient. This information forms the risk assessment for further action. The information should include any possible indicators of BBV infection, including results of previous tests for HIV, hepatitis, and a medical history suggestive of any BBV infection.

The source patient should be asked to consent to testing for the BBV infection. This must include pretest discussion and obtaining the patient's consent to do so.

Postexposure prophylaxis will be covered separately for each of the BBVs.

It must be remembered that an injury can have a devastating effect on the injured person and their family: it is essential that they receive adequate support from management and the occupational health services.[3]

PREVENTION OF INJURIES

Many of the injuries that healthcare workers receive are preventable.

The reporting of injuries is very variable, so estimating the true incidence is difficult. Underreporting has been estimated at between 64% and 96%. Injuries are caused by recapping needles, dismantling equipment, accessing intravenous tubing and disposing of contaminated sharps.[2]

All sharp items must be disposed of into a sharps container, which must never be overfilled. When the sharps have reached the fill line the container must be sealed and disposed of promptly.

Needles should not be resheathed, as this is a recognized risk for acquiring a needlestick injury. Needles should only be removed from syringes when it is essential, e.g. when transferring blood into a container. Forceps should be used to remove the needle from the syringe.

REDUCING THE RISK DURING SURGICAL PROCEDURES[1]

Suture needles cause most of the injuries that occur during surgical procedures. The rate of injury varies between the different specialties and has been noted to be from 4% in orthopaedics to 10% for gynaecology. In gynaecology the rate of infection can vary from 10% for an abdominal hysterectomy to 21% for vaginal hysterectomy.

The main percutaneous injury that surgeons received was the puncturing of the non-dominant index finger: this is said to account for 50% of such injuries; 20% of injuries are caused by the operator to the assistant.

CHANGING PRACTICE[1]

To reduce the risk of exposure the following measures should be considered if they are not already the custom and practice:

- No more than one person should be working in an open cavity (unless of course it is essential)
- Use a hands-free technique where more than one person does not touch a sharp instrument simultaneously. Hand-to-hand passing of such instruments should be avoided
- Create a neutral zone for instruments to be transferred from person to person, e.g. a tray, kidney dish, or designated zone in the operative field
- Scalpels and needles should not be left exposed within the field
- Instruments rather than fingers should be used for retraction or while suturing
- Instruments should be used to remove blades and handle needles
- Sharp suture needles should be removed before the suture is tied
- Instruments rather than fingers should be used to tie sutures.

ALTERNATIVE EQUIPMENT

Blunt-tipped needles can reduce the incidence of glove puncture and injury, and although these are not suitable for suturing bowel and skin, they may be used for other aspects of abdominal closure. Staples should be considered as an alternative to suturing for bowel and skin closure.

REDUCING THE RISK OF BLOOD-SKIN CONTACT

See the section on use of gloves and protective clothing.

HEPATITIS B VIRUS (HBV)

Please note that precautions for prevention, isolation of the patient and care after a needlestick injury are covered in the generic BBV section. As with all surgical procedures a risk assessment should be carried out prior to the patient's arrival in theatre.

INTRODUCTION

Hepatitis B has a varying prevalence throughout the world. In Africa, parts of Asia, northern Canada and South America, approximately 8% of the population are surface antigen-positive. In countries such as the UK, most of western Europe and the USA the rate is less than 2%.[4]

In areas of high prevalence, hepatitis B virus causes significant morbidity and mortality, and has the ability to cause long-term carriage, resulting in cirrhosis and malignant changes in the liver.

CLINICAL FEATURES OF HEPATITIS (HBV AND HCV)

Features that may manifest include malaise, and anorexia with or without fever, which may be followed by jaundice. The liver will probably be enlarged and liver function tests will be abnormal. There may also be the presence of pale stools and dark urine.[4]

Hepatitis B has an insidious onset, during which there may be an urticarial-type rash and poly-arthralgia; the incubation period is 3–6 months.[6]

Complications that may follow HBV are acute fulminating hepatitis or persisting infection.

HBV and HCV cannot be distinguished clinically from one another[3] – this may only be done by specific testing.

VIROLOGY

Hepatitis B is a small envelope virus which contains partially double-stranded DNA.

Four major genes are contained within the DNA, each of which is coded for more than one protein. Hepatitis surface antigen is the major protein for the HBV. People who are HBV e-antigen positive are the most infectious.[4]

RISK GROUPS FOR HEPATITIS IN DEVELOPED COUNTRIES[5]

- Intravenous drugs abusers
- Homosexual men
- Sexual contacts of antigen-positive persons

- Residents in long-stay homes for the mentally handicapped (as a result of bites and scratches)
- Renal dialysis patients
- Recipients of multiple blood products
- Surgeons, dentists and morticians
- Infants of e-antigen positive mothers.

Other risk factors include tattooing and body piercing, which are related to inadequate disinfection of equipment.

RISKS TO STAFF

Occupationally acquired HBV is a significant risk in the USA. The Centers for Disease Control estimate that more than 100 healthcare workers with occupationally acquired HBV die each year in the USA.[7]

Although the figures in the UK do not mirror these, it is none the less essential that all staff carrying out exposure-prone procedures (EPP) be offered and accept HBV vaccination.

IMMUNIZATION

Effective vaccination programmes are vitally important to ensure that staff do not acquire what can be a life-threatening disease.[8,9] The vaccination consists of a course of three injections followed by an antibody test. Levels above 100 mIU/ml confer long-term protection. Approximately 10% of recipients do not produce an antibody response, perhaps related to age, weight and smoking. The response can also be affected if the vaccine is administered incorrectly, for example into the buttock.

NEEDLESTICK/SHARPS INJURY

The advice of the local occupational health department must be followed. The Department of Health guidance for after injury can be found in the BBV section (see earlier).

If a healthcare worker has been exposed to HBV-infected blood, postexposure prophylaxis should be considered. Guidance on this can be found in *Exposure to Hepatitis B Virus: Guidance on Post Exposure Prophylaxis*.[10] The risk of acquiring HBV from a sharp contaminated with blood from a patient who is HBV e-antigen positive is 1:3.

POSITIVE STAFF

Staff who are HBV surface antigen positive but e-antigen negative and who perform EPPs or clinical duties in a renal unit should be tested for viral load (hepatitis B virus DNA). Staff who have a viral load which is >103 genome equivalents per millilitre should be prevented from performing exposure-prone procedures. Both of the above groups are required to have their blood tested every 12 months.[11]

Hepatitis e-antigen-positive healthcare workers are not permitted to carry out EPPs. Any staff who are hepatitis B infected without being e-antigen positive and who refuse to have their viral load tested should not be permitted to carry out EPPs.

CONFIDENTIALITY OF HEALTHCARE WORKERS

Healthcare workers have the same right to confidentiality as any patient. However, where patients are or have been at risk it may be necessary in the public interest for the employer to gain access to confidential information.

NOSOCOMIAL TRANSMISSION OF HEPATITIS B

Transmission of HBV to patients from healthcare workers has been well documented. Incidents include the use of multidose vials,[12] transmission from a surgeon to a patient,[13] and a medical technician who infected five patients.[14]

TRANSMISSION VIA BLOOD TRANSFUSION

This has been a recognized risk for many years. In the UK, all donations issued for transfusion have been tested for HBV surface antigen since the early 1970s.[15] In an effort to reduce the chance of this happening, donor selection criteria aim to exclude people with recent risk factors for acquiring BBV infections.

HEPATITIS C

Hepatitis C (HCV) was discovered in 1989[16,17] as the cause of 90–95% of what was previously called post-transfusion non-A, non-B hepatitis. HCV is believed to be the most common cause of non-alcoholic liver disease in the USA.[18]

VIROLOGY

Hepatitis C virus is a single-stranded RNA virus. This differs from HBV, which is caused by a DNA virus. Antibody to the viral protein can be tested for in sera.[16] If it is diagnosed by the detection of antibodies to HCV then further tests should be done, as some assays have less than optimal specificity.[17] Confirmation is undertaken by detection of the HCV genome in serum by the polymerase chain reaction (PCR), and the presence of the virus implies a potential infection risk to others. There are at least six different types and 50 subtypes of rapidly mutating HCV.[19]

CLINICAL FEATURES

Infection is commonly followed by long-term carriage, with 60–70% of infected people developing chronic liver disease after 20–30 years. The incubation period is 2–4 months[19,20] and the infection is often subclinical and therefore goes undetected,[17] the individual being unaware that they have the infection.[21]

When infection is symptomatic it is identical to other forms of hepatitis[18] (see section on hepatitis B).

The majority of patients develop chronic active hepatitis with or without cirrhosis, which may appear in 20–50% of patients. Chronic hepatitis C has been linked to hepatocellular carcinoma. The remaining individuals may appear to be relatively healthy, although they may have some of the following symptoms: chronic fatigue, myalgias and arthralgias. In the USA, it has been reported that more than 8000 people die every year from complications related to HCV, and that the liver failure secondary to chronic hepatitis C is the major reason for liver transplantation.[21] The transplant eliminates the complications from cirrhosis, but reinfection of the graft with HCV is universal.

It is estimated that there are 100 million HCV carriers worldwide, with the prevalence in Europe being 0.5–2% of the general population.

RISK FACTORS FOR STAFF

The risk factor for infection parallels that of HBV. High rates are found among drug abusers, post transfusion (haemophiliacs), and to a lesser extent, haemodialysis patients. Drug use in infected women increases the risk of maternal transmission.[22] In 40–50% of diagnosed HCV cases the source is unknown. In contrast to HBV, the prevalence of HCV in healthcare workers appears to be no greater than in the general population. (For reduction in risks please see section on BBV.)

ACTION AFTER EXPOSURE

The risk to healthcare staff from a needlestick injury from a positive patient is 1:30.[23] It is essential that the injury is reported to enable the staff member to receive the correct follow-up (for initial treatment see section on BBV).

When an exposure from a known source is received the healthcare worker should be tested at 3 and 6 months for evidence of infection.[17] More than 97% of people who become infected with HCV will have detectable antibodies by 6 months after the exposure. In rare instances, however, in staff who are immunocompromised themselves (this could be illness or medication related) anti-HCV may not be detectable until 12 months after the incident. It is essential that such staff members are closely monitored for any possible illness.

Because the risk of acquiring HCV is small, the healthcare worker's activity should not be limited. If the patient's HCV status is unknown, local hospital policy should be followed, as there is no consensus as to whether their blood should be tested.

POSTEXPOSURE PROPHYLAXIS (PEP)

There is no postexposure prophylaxis for HCV, and immunoglobulin has not been shown to be effective in preventing HCV infection in exposed people.

In common with HIV, there is no vaccine for protection against this virus.

RISKS TO PATIENTS

There are risks to patients, who may acquire hepatitis C from healthcare staff who are carrying the virus. This has occurred during surgery,[24–27] and in Spain due to an anaesthetist with a drug habit[28] (see Bloodborne virus section).

HIV

Human immunodeficiency virus (HIV) is a member of the retrovirus family. It is responsible for HIV infection, which progresses to acquired immune deficiency syndrome (AIDS). It was first recognized in the early 1980s.[29]

CLINICAL FEATURES

After initial exposure to HIV most people develop antibody within 3 months.[30] There are three phases to HIV infection. The period between exposure and developing HIV antibody is called seroconversion and occurs 6–8 weeks after initial exposure. It is during this period that the individual may experience a 'flu-like' illness, lymphadenopathy, and possibly a rash. The rash is unusual and the lesions are ovoid and appear scuffed, but it is not itchy or painful. All the seroconversion illnesses resolve without specific treatment; however, in those whom illness occurs at this time, progression to AIDS is quicker.[29]

Following the seroconversion phase is the latent phase, and according to Bannister[29] this may last for 18 months to 15 years, with an average of 8 years. During this period the individual may be well most of the time. However, the total CD4 (T4) helper cell population slowly declines and the CD4 helper function becomes impaired. It is thought that this decline is exacerbated by each subsequent infection.

The last stage of HIV infection before AIDS onset is the symptomatic phase. When the sudden loss of CD4 cells increases, the latent phase is ending. A number of infections, both viral and bacterial, are common during this phase. Among these are herpes zoster, which can be severe, salmonella causing bacteraemia, and pneumococcal infection giving rise to pneumonia. Mucosal and skin infections are also seen, and among these are herpes simplex, and oral and genital candidiasis. With the falling CD4 count and the conditions that characterize immunodeficiency, AIDS can be diagnosed.

ROUTES OF TRANSMISSION

The routes of transmission in Africa and other developing countries are predominately heterosexual intercourse and vertical transmission (from infected mother to her child). However, in the more developed countries the main routes are shared contaminated drug injecting equipment and sexual intercourse between men.[29]

THE RISK OF TRANSMISSION TO HEALTHCARE STAFF

The risk to healthcare staff comes from exposure to blood and, in certain cases, other body fluids from infected patients (see section on BBVs). In addition to the list in the BBV section, HIV has been isolated from saliva, tears and urine. It is, however, only blood and blood products, semen, vaginal secretions, donor organs and tissues and breast milk that have been implicated in the transmission of infection.

The risks of transmission are greater from patients to staff. In healthcare, transmission may occur after percutaneous injury (e.g. needlestick or sharps injuries) that exposes the worker to the patient's blood. The risk for HIV is approximately 1:300 when the patient is HIV positive.

There is no vaccine for HIV. It is therefore imperative that staff are particularly careful when handling sharp items, or have such items around confused or disorientated patients.

The risk after a single mucocutaneous exposure (splashes into mucous membranes) to HIV is 1:2000.

ACTION FOLLOWING AN EXPOSURE

For initial first aid see the section on BBVs.

If the source patient is infected with HIV or is considered to be at risk but has not been tested, the UK Health Department's advice on postexposure prophylaxis for healthcare workers occupationally exposed to HIV should be followed.[31] These guidelines include advice on assessment of the risk, when postexposure prophylaxis would be recommended, and the choice of antiretroviral drugs.

Every hospital should have its own policy, which should include information on receiving advice, therapy, and how to obtain PEP rapidly. Advice should be available 24 hours a day. The decision regarding therapy should be made following a risk assessment of the incident and the exact clinical history of the source patient and their therapy to date. If the patient has experienced any drug therapy resistance, it is essential that the doctor prescribing the postexposure prophylaxis is aware of this.

Until there is evidence of the healthcare worker's having acquired HIV, their work practice need not be restricted as the risk is believed to be small, so that restrictions are not merited.[32]

HIV-INFECTED STAFF

Infected healthcare workers have an ethical and legal duty to protect the health and safety of their patients. They also have a right to expect their confidentiality to be respected.[33]

The Department of Health (DOH) guidance document on AIDS/HIV states that in the majority of healthcare procedures there is no risk of transmission of the virus from a worker to the patient.

However, the guidance also clearly states that the notable exception to this is where exposure-prone exposures are performed. When an injury to a healthcare worker occurs this could result in their blood contaminating the patient's open tissue, therefore HIV-infected healthcare workers must not perform any exposure-prone procedures.

The Expert Advisory Group on AIDS recommends that as far as is reasonable and practicable, patients who may have been at risk from such procedures should be notified and offered pretest discussions appropriate to their risk and an HIV antibody test.[33]

TRANSMISSIBLE SPONGIFORM ENCEPHALOPATHIES

Transmissible spongiform encephalopathies (TSE) include sporadic Creutzfeldt-Jakob disease (sCJD), variant CJD, Gerstmann-Straussler-Scheinker (GSS) disease, and fatal familial insomnia (FFI), all of which occur in humans and some other animal species. All of these diseases are caused by unconventional infectious agents which are different from other microbes.[34]

The important differences are:

- Unusual resistance to chemical and physical decontamination methods
- Serious disease which is usually fatal (there is no known treatment)
- The agents are not uniformly distributed in tissues of affected individuals but concentrated in neural tissues, including the brain, spinal cord and eye; lymphoreticular tissues, including tonsil and appendix, pose a lower risk and blood an even lower risk
- They are not highly contagious
- There have been no known cases of transmission of TSE to humans as a result of occupational exposure
- There is no screening or diagnostic test which can identify patients with these disorders.

All the transmissible spongiform encephalopathies cause degenerative brain disease. A common feature of all TSE is the appearance of microscopic vacuoles (holes) in the grey matter of the brain, giving it a spongelike appearance, hence the name spongiform encephalopathy. This section will discuss CJD and variant CJD.

All forms of CJD are associated with conformational change in a protein called the prion protein. The abnormal form of this protein accumulates in the brain and results in the death of nerve cells.[35]

CLINICAL FEATURES – SPORADIC CREUTZFELDT-JAKOB DISEASE (sCJD)

CJD is a progressive dementia characterized by spongiform encephalopathy. The agent is described as a filterable self-replicating agent.[36] The incubation period is said to range from 4 to 20 years; however, iatrogenic cases may have a shortened incubation period of 15 months to 2 years. The signs and symptoms include dementia, ataxia, mental confusion and myoclonic jerks. Diagnosis may be made on clinical grounds, but can only be confirmed after postmortem examination.

The commonest form of CJD is sporadic CJD, which affects about one per million of the population per annum and accounts for 85% of all cases of CJD. In the UK around 60 cases of sCJD are reported each year. Ten percent of cases occur as familial disease (familial CJD, GSS and FFI).

TRANSMISSION OF SPORADIC CJD

There is no evidence that any type of CJD can spread between people through normal social contact. Sporadic CJD has been transmitted between patients undergoing certain medical treatments. Transmission has occurred after neurological procedures, corneal graft operations, treatment with hormones prepared from human pituitary glands, and dura mater grafts.[40,41] These iatrogenic cases have probably occurred as a result of contamination of the instruments and the inability of decontamination processes to kill the prion protein.

VARIANT CREUTZFELDT-JAKOB DISEASE (vCJD)

This disease was first recognized in 1996. It is a new disease which is associated with the same transmissible agent that is responsible for bovine spongiform encephalopathy (BSE). vCJD is believed to be related to the consumption of contaminated bovine food products. Most of the population of the UK has probably been exposed to BSE, but there is no way of knowing how many people have been infected yet have no neurological symptoms or signs of disease. vCJD differs from other human TSE in that the transmissible agent also accumulates outside the central nervous system in lymphoid tissues throughout the body, e.g. tonsil, spleen and lymph nodes.[37–39]

Another notable difference between sCJD and vCJD is the age of onset. The median age of onset of disease for vCJD was 26 years and the median age at death 28 years, compared to 65 years for the median age at death in sporadic disease.[40] The youngest case was a 12-year-old and the oldest a 74-year-old. Before 1999 the oldest cases had been 53 years old. The mean duration of illness was 13 months.

TRANSMISSION OF vCJD

There has been no evidence yet that vCJD has been transmitted through surgical procedures, blood or tissue donation. However, as there are no screening tests to detect vCJD during its incubation, cases have not yet been identified.[34,35]

Precautionary measures have been introduced to reduce any potential risk of transmitting CJD through blood:

- People at risk of developing CJD are excluded from donating blood
- Since April 1999 all major blood products (e.g. factor VIII, immunoglobulins and anti-D for rhesus-negative pregnant women) have been manufactured from plasma donated outside the UK
- Since October 1999 blood donated in the UK has been processed to remove its white blood cells (leukodepletion).[42]

PRECAUTIONS AND PREVENTION OF TRANSMISSION

There is no epidemiological evidence to suggest that any particular precautions are required in most situations when caring for such patients; however, there are some specific guidelines related to invasive procedures and surgery.

When considering the precautions that may be required to prevent transmission a distinction should be made between those who are known or suspected of having CJD – i.e. those with clinical symptoms – and those who are potentially at risk of developing one of these diseases, i.e. asymptomatic but having a clinical or family history that places them in a risk group.

DEFINITIONS OF KNOWN, SUSPECTED AND AT-RISK PATIENTS[34]

Known patients are those who have been diagnosed as having CJD or a related disorder (sporadic CJD, vCJD, GSS, FFI). Suspected patients are those whose clinical symptoms are suggestive of CJD but where diagnosis has not been confirmed. At-risk patients are those who are potentially at risk of developing CJD or a related disorder:

- Recipients of hormone derived from human pituitary glands, e.g. growth hormone, gonadotrophin
- Recipients of human dura mater grafts
- People with a familial history of CJD, i.e. close blood relatives (parents, brothers, sisters, children, grandparents, grandchildren).

PRECAUTIONS REQUIRED DURING CLINICAL PROCEDURES ON KNOWN OR SUSPECTED CJD PATIENTS

- Whenever possible, procedures should be undertaken in an operating theatre
- Protective clothing should consist of a liquid-repellent gown over a plastic disposable apron, gloves, a mask and goggles or a face visor
- The procedure must be performed at the end of the list to allow for cleaning of the theatre
- Only a minimum number of staff should be present
- Single-use disposable instruments and equipment should be used. If this is not possible the instruments must not be reused
- Maintain a one-way flow of instruments.

All instruments and protective clothing used must be destroyed by incineration.

For certain items of expensive equipment, such as drills, etc., the infection team, neurosurgical staff and the manufacturer must be consulted before the scheduled surgery.

Instruments that have been used on a patient suspected of having CJD may be quarantined by secure storage in a rigid sealed container after use, until the diagnosis is confirmed. If the case is subsequently confirmed then the instruments must be destroyed by incineration. Only if a definitive alternative diagnosis is confirmed may the instruments be cleaned and decontaminated following the usual routine procedures.

PRECAUTIONS REQUIRED DURING CLINICAL PROCEDURES ON PATIENTS AT RISK OF DEVELOPING CJD

If the procedure involves the brain, spinal cord or eyes the precautions detailed above should be followed. If the procedure does not involve brain, spinal cord or eyes then the following precautions should be taken:

- Protective clothing as above, but may be reprocessed if not single use
- Single-use instruments and equipment where possible
- Reusable surgical instruments must not be reused until one of the recommended procedures has been carried out (see section on decontamination).

DECONTAMINATION AS RECOMMENDED IN THE NATIONAL GUIDANCE[34]

TSE are resistant to conventional decontamination methods. They are significantly affected by substances such as formalin and ethythlene oxide, and infectivity persists after autoclaving at conventional times and temperatures (e.g. 121°C for 15 minutes). TSE are also extremely resistant to high doses of ionizing and ultraviolet irradiation, and some residual activity has been shown to survive for long periods in the environment.

Decontamination should only be undertaken with the at-risk group, and as the agent is so resistant the emphasis must be on its removal by thorough cleaning. This should be followed by appropriate autoclaving or chemical treatment.

Methods recommended by the ACDP TSE are given below. For full details consult the guidelines.[34]

Chemical disinfectants

- 20 000 ppm available chlorine of sodium hypochlorite for 1 hour
- 2 M sodium hydroxide for 1 hour (known not to be completely effective)
- For histological samples only, 96% formic acid for 1 hour.

Gaseous disinfectants

There are none suitable.

Autoclaving

A porous load (high vacuum) steam sterilizer at 134–137°C for a single cycle of 18 minutes or six successive cycles of 3 minutes each must be used, although this is known not to be completely effective.

LABELLING AND TRANSPORTATION OF INSTRUMENTS

All instruments from any of the categories above must be clearly identified. Instruments used on known or suspected patients and those used on at-risk patients for brain, spinal cord or eye interventions must be labelled for disposal.

Items for reprocessing should be securely contained in a robust, leakproof container and transferred to the reprocessing unit or SSD by a designated person.

SAMPLE COLLECTION AND LABELLING

Protective clothing should be worn, trained personnel who are aware of the risks involved should collect the samples, and the specimen must be labelled with a biohazard sticker. The form should be completed in such a way as to maintain patient confidentiality.

Linen used on all these patients should be washed in accordance with current practice (DOH HSG (95) 18).[43]

SPILLAGES

Absorbent material should be used to soak up the spillage, and the operator should wear gloves and a disposable apron. All these items should be disposed of as clinical waste and should be incinerated.

CLINICAL WASTE

All waste must be dealt with in accordance with current guidance.

TUBERCULOSIS

The national guidelines for the control of tuberculosis in Scotland[43] define tuberculosis as 'disease in man by infection with *Mycobacterium* complex of organisms which may cause pulmonary and/or non-pulmonary disease'. These guidelines state that around 10% of those infected actually develop the disease, half within 1 year and the rest in the following 60 years.

The rate of tuberculosis fell in the UK as a result of chemotherapy in the 1940s and BCG immunization in the 1950s and 1960s. However, this decline ended in the 1980s and was followed by a small increase in reported cases. This, according to the Interdepartmental Working Group on Tuberculosis,[45] was due in part to demographic change, a consistently high rate among new immigrants, and the effects of poverty and homelessness. Only a small proportion is related to HIV in the UK.

The Interdepartmental Working Group on Tuberculosis[45] advise that all patients with suspected or confirmed pulmonary tuberculosis or tuberculosis of the larynx or respiratory tract, and all patients who are smear positive, should be considered potentially infectious until proved otherwise. Damani[46] extends this list to staff who have contact with patients attending respiratory medicine clinics and undergoing thoracic surgery. It is therefore important to obtain recent results before the patient is scheduled for surgery.

Patients who have suspected or proven tuberculosis and who are smear negative can be regarded as non-infectious for most practical purposes.

TRANSMISSION

Pulmonary (open) tuberculosis is spread via the respiratory route. In a person with infectious pulmonary tuberculosis airborne particles containing tubercle bacilli are shed while talking, sneezing and shouting.

ANAESTHETIC EQUIPMENT

Disposable anaesthetic circuits and filters must be used when a patient known to have open pulmonary tuberculosis is identified. This prevents contamination of the anaesthetic machine and potential cross-infection to other patients.

If contamination of the anaesthetic machine has taken place via the filters (this is a rare occurrence) it may be necessary to use formaldehyde gas for decontamination in sterile services. The equipment nearest the patient is most likely to be contaminated, e.g. face masks, tubing; if this is not single use, then decontamination will be required. This should be done by cleaning followed by thermal disinfection, preferably using a washer-disinfector (80°C).[46]

As disposable equipment should be used, it is not essential that the patient is last on the list as there is no risk to subsequent patients.

AEROSOL-GENERATING PROCEDURES

Bronchoscopy must not be carried out in an open ward area on a patient who may have tuberculosis.[45] This and similar procedures (induced sputum, medication by nebulizer) must be carried out in an appropriate area with adequate local exhaust ventilation.

Staff carrying out these procedures should wear a mask, and all unnecessary staff should be excluded.

If a room with air handling equipment is not available the procedure should be done at the end of the list or in the patient's own room. All these procedures relate to coughing, and so staff must also wear masks during extubation of the patient.

Large numbers of organisms may be exposed during excision and drainage of a closed tuberculous abscess, therefore masks should be worn for these operations.

DECONTAMINATION OF ENDOSCOPES

Transmission of *Mycobacterium tuberculosis* via endoscopes has been previously documented.[47] After cleaning, endoscopes must be disinfected in accordance with Department of Health guidelines, remembering to check the manufacturer's instructions for chemical compatibility. The solution varies from hospital to hospital, and so local infection control policy must be adhered to.

There are no special precautions for any other surgical instruments. They should be decontaminated and sterilized in the usual way.

DECONTAMINATION OF OPERATING ROOM SURFACES

No special precautions need to be taken.

DISPOSAL OF WASTE

Clinical waste from tuberculosis cases should be treated in accordance with national clinical waste guidelines.

STAFF SCREENING

As staff may be at risk of acquiring tuberculosis, they should be screened and offered protection with BCG vaccine prior to employment. Pre-employment screening should be carried out by the Occupational Health Department and should include a pre-employment questionnaire. Ayliffe et al[47] are of the opinion that the protection of staff is a legal responsibility for the employer. Philpott-Howard et al[49] suggest that any suspicious symptoms must be investigated with a medical examination, including a chest X-ray.

The symptoms that require investigation are a persistent cough with or without weight loss and anorexia or fever.[45] However, it should be recognized that BCG does not confer complete protection and therefore tuberculosis can still occur in vaccinated healthcare staff.[50]

POSITIVE STAFF

If a member of staff is identified with tuberculosis it is essential that there is cooperation between the infection control team, the attending physician and the Occupational Health Department, whether or not the disease has been occupationally acquired. Contact tracing of colleagues and patients should be undertaken.[50]

VARICELLA ZOSTER VIRUS

Chicken pox is an acute generalized viral disease caused by varicella zoster virus (VZV).[51]

CLINICAL FEATURES

The onset is sudden, with mild fever and a skin eruption that is initially maculopapular, and which then develops into a vesicular rash for 3–4 days and leaves a granular scab.

Herpes zoster (shingles) is a local reactivation of latent varicella infection in the dorsal root ganglia.[51,52]

COMPLICATIONS OF VZV

In children the infection is usually mild. In infants under 1 year and in adults there is a greater chance of pneumonia and encephalitis. This virus can cause complications in pregnant woman and the fetus or newborn. In the first trimester 10% of those infected may develop congential varicella syndrome. This consists of limb hypoplasia, microcephaly, cortical atrophy, chorioretinitis, cataracts and cutaneous scars.

Varicella in the neonate is a life-threatening disease, the mortality rate being perhaps as high as 40%. This occurs when the mother develops chickenpox within a week of delivery and no maternal antibody is developed in time to protect the neonate.[53]

About 28% of immunocompromised individuals who do not receive antiviral therapy may also develop varicella pneumonia, and death may result in 7% of these cases.

Disseminated VZV infection is more likely to occur in patients with lymphoma and leukaemia rather than other tumours. The rash appears after chemotherapy or irradiation.

RISKS TO OTHERS

Varicella zoster poses a threat to other patients, especially the immunocompromised, pregnant women, and infants in neonatal intensive care units.

Approximately 3–5% of healthcare staff are seronegative for antibodies to VZV and are at risk of acquiring the infection. In staff who are uncertain of their status or who have no history of varicella, serologic screening can be undertaken to ascertain who is susceptible.[54] It is therefore an advantage in areas where susceptible patients are cared for, that staff are aware of their own status. This should be part of the pre-employment screen.[55]

Staff who are seropositive are not at risk from VZV-seronegative individuals at work, or indeed at home. If a member of staff has antibodies and comes into contact with VZV they should continue at work.

Susceptible staff should not work with VZV patients; however, where they have been exposed to the virus they should not work with any high-risk patients (in many hospitals the policy states any patient) for 10 days after the first exposure until 21 days after the last possible exposure.[54,56] This would also apply if contact had been outside the hospital environment.

If a VZV patient requires surgery a history should be obtained from all the staff who will be involved with the patient.

CARING FOR THE VZV-POSITIVE PATIENT

Patients with VZV should, where possible, be discharged home. If this is not possible they must be isolated in a single room. They should not be in the operating department/reception/recovery with any other patients. To allow for ventilation clearance of the virus from the theatre environment such patients should be last on the list if at all possible.

IMMUNOCOMPROMISED STAFF

Staff who are HIV positive but do not have symptoms do not need to take particular precautions when nursing such patients. However, staff who have AIDS or other forms of immunosuppression who are antibody negative should discuss their work-related risks with the Occupational Health Department.[54]

TRANSMISSION

Controlling VZV in hospitals can prove very difficult for a number of reasons:

- Infected patients can excrete virus for several days before the onset of the rash, thereby unwittingly exposing others[51,52]

- Control measures may not be adhered to correctly
- Determining exposure can be very difficult, as some individuals may become infected via airborne transmission.

It is believed that there is less risk in the work situation than in the household environment.

References

1. Expert Advisory Group on AIDS and the Advisory Group on Hepatitis. Guidance for clinical health care workers: protection against infection with blood borne viruses. London: DOH; 1998.
2. APIC 1999 and APIC 1998 Guidelines Committees. Position paper: prevention of device-mediated bloodborne infections to health care workers. Am J Infect Control 1998; 26: 578.
3. Gershon RR, Flanagan PA, Karkashian C, et al. Healthcare workers' experience with post exposure management of blood borne pathogen exposures: a pilot study. Am J Infect Control 2000; 28: 421–428.
4. Bannister BA, Begg N, Gillespie SH. Infectious disease. Oxford: Blackwell Science; 1996: 183–206.
5. Shanson DC. Microbiology in clinical practice, 2nd edn. Bristol: Wright; 1989: 362–373.
6. Mims CA, Playfair JHL, Roitt IM, et al. Medical microbiology. London: Mosby; 1993: 25.1–25.30.
7. Louther J, Felden J, Rivera P, et al. Hepatitis B vaccination program at New York city hospital: seroprevalence, seroconversion and declination. Am J Infect Control 1998; 26: 423–427.
8. Rosen E, Rudensky B, Paz E, et al. Ten year follow-up of hepatitis B virus infection and vaccination status in hospital employees. J Hosp Infect 1999; 41: 245–250.
9. Evan B, Duggan W, Baker J, et al. Exposure of healthcare workers in England, Wales and Northern Ireland to blood borne viruses between July 1997 and June 2000: analysis and surveillance data. BMJ 2001; 322: 397–398.
10. PHLS. Exposure to hepatitis B virus: guidance on post exposure prophylaxis. Communicable Disease Report vol 9 review N9, p. R97. London: HMSO; August 1992.
11. National Health Service Executive. Hepatitis B infected healthcare workers: guidance on implementation of Health Service circular 2000/020. Leeds: HMSO; 2000. Online. Available: http://www.doh.gov.uk/nhsexec/hepatisb.htm
12. Kidd-Ljunggren K, Broman E, Ekuall H, et al. Nosocomil transmission of hepatitis B virus infection through multi-dose vials. J Hosp Infect 1999; 43: 57–62.
13. Harpaz R, Von Seidlein L, Averhoff F, et al. Transmission of hepatitis B virus to multiple patients from a surgeon without evidence of inadequate infection control. N Engl J Med 1996; 334: 549–554.
14. Ross R, Viazov S, Gross T, et al. Brief report: transmission of hepatitis C virus from a patient to an anaesthesiology assistant to five patients. N Engl J Med 2000; 343: 1851–1854.
15. Solden K, Ramsay M, Collins M. Acute hepatitis B infection associated with blood transfusion in England and Wales 1991–7: review of database. BMJ 1999; 318: 95.
16. Mims C, Playfair JHL, Roitt IM, et al. Medical microbiology. London: Mosby; 1993: 25.27–25.28.
17. Ayliffe GAJ, Fraise AP, Geddes AM, et al. Control of hospital infection. A practical handbook, 4th edn. London: Arnold; 2000; 211.
18. Schleupner CJ. Protecting recipients of blood and blood products. In: Wenzle R, ed. Prevention of nosocomial infections, 2nd edn. Baltimore: Williams and Wilkins; 1993; 341.
19. Center for Disease Control. Recommendations for prevention and control of hepatitis C virus. MMWR 1998; 47: 1040.
20. Philpott-Howard J, Casewell M. Hospital infection control policies and practical procedures. London: WB Saunders; 1995; 208.
21. McKeirnan SC. Hepatitis C. What do health care workers need to know? J Healthcare Safety Compliance Infect Control 2000; 14: 371–378.
22. Resti M, Azzari C, Galli I, et al. For the Italian Study Group on mother to infant hepatitis C virus transmission. Maternal drug use is a pre-eminent risk factor for mother to child hepatitis C virus transmission: results from a multicentre study of 1372 mother-infant pairs. J Infect Dis 2002; 185: 567–572.
23. Expert Advisory Group on AIDS and the Advisory Group on Hepatitis. Guidance for clinical healthcare workers: protection against infection with blood borne viruses. London: DOH; 1998.
24. Editorial. Hepatitis C virus transmission from health care worker to patient. Comm Dis Rep CDR Weekly 1995; 5: 121.
25. Esteban JI, Gomez J, Martell M, et al. Transmission of hepatitis B from a cardiac surgeon. N Engl J Med 1996; 334: 555–561.
26. Duckworth GJ, Heptonstall J, Aitkins C. Transmission of hepatitis C virus from a surgeon to a patient. Comm Dis Public Health 1999; 2: 188–192.

27. Brown P. Surgeon infects patient with hepatitis C. BMJ 1999; 319: 12–19.
28. Bosch X. Hepatitis C outbreak astounds Spain. Lancet 1998; 351: 1415.
29. Bannister B, Begg N, Gillespie S. Infectious disease. Oxford: Blackwell Science; 1996: 230–238.
30. Damani NN. Manual of infection control procedures. Oxford: OUP; 1997; 135.
31. UK Chief Medical Officer's Expert Advisory Group on AIDS/HIV. Post exposure prophylaxis. London: DOH; 2000.
32. Department of Health. AIDS/HIV infected healthcare workers guidance on the management of infected healthcare workers and patient notification. London: DOH; 1998.
33. Advisory Committee on Dangerous Pathogens Spongiform Encephalopathy Advisory Group. Transmissible spongiform encephalopathy agents: safe working and the prevention of infection. London: DOH; 1998.
34. DOH. Management of possible exposure to CJD through medical procedures. A consultation document. London: HMSO; 2001. Online. Available: http://www.doh.gov.uk/cjd/consultation
35. Beneson AS, ed. Control of communicable diseases in man, 16th edn. Washington, DC: American Public Health Association; 1995: 167–169.
36. Bruce ME, McConnell I, Will RG, et al. Detection of variant Creutzfeld–Jakob disease infectivity in extraneural tissues. Lancet 2001; 358: 208–209.
37. Ironside JW, Hilton D, Ghani A, et al. Retrospective study of prion-protein accumulation in tonsil and appendix tissues. Lancet 2000; 355: 1693–1694.
38. Hill AF, Butterworth RJ, Joiner S, et al. Investigation of variant Creutzfeld–Jakob disease and other human prion diseases with tonsil biopsy samples. Lancet 1999; 353: 183–189.
39. Creutzfeld–Jakob Disease Surveillance in the UK. Ninth annual report 2000. http://www.cjd.edac.uk/2000rep.html
40. Fishman M, Fort G, Mikolich D. Prevention of Creutzfeld–Jakob disease in healthcare workers. A case study. Am J Infect Control 1998; 26: 74–79.
41. Scottish Executive Health Department. Variant Creutzfeld–Jakob disease (vCJD): minimising the risk of transmission. NHS MEL 1999; 65, 31 August
42. DOH. Hospital laundry arrangements for used and infected linen. Health Service Circular (95)18. London: DOH; 1995.
43. Scottish Office. National guidelines for the control of tuberculosis in Scotland. Edinburgh: DOH; 1998.
44. Interdepartmental Working Group on Tuberculosis. The prevention and control of tuberculosis in the United Kingdom. London: DOH; 1998.
45. Damani NN. Manual of infection control procedures. Oxford: OUP; 1997; 149.
46. Ayliffe GAJ, Fraise AP, Geddes AM, et al. Control of hospital infection. A practical handbook, 4th edn. London: Arnold; 2000; 111.
47. Alvarado C, Reichelderfer M. APIC guidelines for the infection prevention and control in flexible endoscopy. Am J Infect Control 2000; 28: 138–155.
48. Philpott-Howard J, Casewell M. Hospital infection control policies and practical procedures. London: WB Saunders; 1995; 189.
49. Joint Tuberculosis Committee of the British Thoracic Society. Control and prevention of tuberculosis in the United Kingdom: code of practice 2000. Thorax 2000; 55: 887–901.
50. Damani NN. Manual of infection control procedures. Oxford: OUP; 1997; 104.
51. Fedson DS. Immunizations for health care workers and patients in hospitals. In: Wenzel R, ed. Prevention and control of nosocomial infections, 2nd edn. Baltimore: Williams and Wilkins; 1993: 251–252.
52. Bannister BA, Begg N, Gillespie SH. Infectious disease. Oxford: Blackwell Science; 1996; 245.
53. Ferson MJ, Bell SM, Robertson PW. Determination and importance of varicella immuno status of nursing staff in a children's hospital. J Hosp Infect 1990; 15: 347–351.
54. Philpott-Howard J, Casewell M. Hospital infection control policies and practical procedures. London: WB Saunders; 1995; 103.
55. Breuer J, Jefferies DJ. Control of viral infections in hospitals. J Hosp Infect 1990; 16: 191–221.

Chapter 23

Care of patients who are immunocompromised

Sarah Hart

CHAPTER CONTENTS

Key points

- Clinical implications of surgery to an immuno-compromised patient
- Risk assessment and clinical governance

INTRODUCTION

Immunocompromised patients are those whose immune systems are impaired, making them vulnerable to infection; this is also termed immunosuppressed. This chapter provides relevant information regarding the immune system, alterations to the immune system, microbiology, and the infections experienced by the immunocompromised patient. Risk assessment and management are included. These facts will allow the reader to identify patients' risk factors, and understand the potential problems associated with those risks. Care plans can be developed from these assessments which will assist in ensuring patients' safety during their perioperative care. Case studies are included to provide examples of risk assessment and care planning. All of this information needs to be read in conjunction with the other chapters in this book, as the principles contained in those chapters are all relevant for the immunocompromised patient.

Immunocompromised patients may be admitted to hospital for surgical interventions for three main reasons:

1. *Patients require surgical management for clinical problems, identical to immunocompetent patients.* For example, treatment may be required for planned

relatively minor surgery to improve quality of life, including operations such as hernia reduction, or the insertion of a percutaneous endoscopic gastrostomy (PEG) tube. Alternatively, there may be a need for emergency surgery, perhaps for bone fracture, appendectomy, or hip replacement for problems unrelated to the underlying immunosuppressive disease (see Case study 23.1).

2. *Patients require surgical intervention as part of a treatment programme.* Immunosuppression will occur during the treatment programme. For example, a patient suffers acute abdominal pain due to gastric lymphoma or acute obstruction as a result of bowel cancer. Diagnosis is made during exploratory laparotomy, leading to surgical excision of the diseased area. Such patients may be elderly, with poor nutritional status due to worsening signs and symptoms of disease, but will be generally immunocompetent.

A typical postoperative treatment plan for bowel cancer will be chemotherapy and radiotherapy, which may be followed by further surgery for resection of liver metastases. At the time of the second operation the patient will be significantly immunocompromised (see Case study 23.2).

3. *Patients are already immunocompromised, and require surgery as part of their treatment programme.* Surgery may be relatively minor, for example in a patient with cancer requiring endoscopic examination or lymph node biopsy, to assist in the diagnosis of symptoms such as rectal bleeding, chest disease or enlarged lymph nodes. Alternatively, surgery may be major, for example a patient with cystic fibrosis who has had long-term antibiotic and steroid therapy and who is receiving a heart-lung transplant. Similarly, a patient receiving a second renal transplant having previously been treated with ciclosporin and prednisolone (immunosuppressive therapy given to prevent graft rejection of the original kidney transplant).

Case study 23.1

A 50-year-old obese diabetic patient with breast cancer and bone metastases develops pain on movement. There is no history of trauma. Investigations show pathological fracture through the neck of femur.

Risk assessment
- Patient debilitated and in extreme pain. Bone is unlikely to heal naturally owing to the presence of bone metastases. Surgical fixation of fracture

required. Surgery to be undertaken as soon as possible. Research indicates the longer the preoperative stay in hospital the greater the possibility of acquiring a wound infection
- Restricted movement and mobility due to the fracture may cause the patient to develop deep vein thrombosis, chest infection and pressure sores
- Other risk factors include obesity, diabetes, and previous history of radiotherapy but not to the hip region
- Chemotherapy completed 4 months prior to fracture. Neutrophil and platelet counts have returned to normal but T-cell function generally takes longer to recover
- Patient immunocompromised owing to previous cancer therapy, which is compounded by history of diabetes and obesity.

Anaesthetic risk assessment
Patient: diabetic, obese, debilitated, anxious, in pain.

Care planning
- Informed consent
- Establish diabetes status, instigate glucose monitoring and insulin therapy (pre, during and post surgery)
- Pain control
- Psychological support
- Evaluate home circumstances to begin planning discharge
- Skin preparation
- Prevention of pressure sores (pressure-relieving mattress)
- Prevention of chest infection (physiotherapy, mobilize as soon as possible)
- Consider radiotherapy to area following recovery from surgery.

Reflective practice
Surgery improved this palliative care patient's quality of life, and meant that she could be discharged home.

Case study 23.2

A 50-year-old man has extensive sarcoma of the soft tissue of the left thigh. The treatment plan will include radiotherapy followed by five cycles of chemotherapy as an outpatient, followed by resection of the tumour.[1]

Risk assessment
- On registration, pain and anxiety were the main problems

- During the radiotherapy and chemotherapy the patient suffered varying degrees of nausea, vomiting, diarrhoea and mucositis, which were controlled by medication
- During the long preoperative period the patient's problems were dealt with as follows:
  1. Dietitian undertook regular assessment to assure adequate nutritional support.
  2. Psychological support was provided by the psychological support service.
  3. Social services, occupational therapy and physiotherapy provided discharge planning.
  4. Education to recognize and report side effects of therapy.

Care planning
- Patient booked to attend the preoperative outpatient clinic assessment clinic.
- Factors to be assessed included haemoglobin, white blood cells and platelets count:
  1. Suitability for anaesthetic
  2. Risk of endogenous infection, for example dental assessment.

During the preoperative assessment the patient was found to have a painful central venous line exit site, but was otherwise fit and anxious to proceed with the final stage of the treatment plan.

The central line was removed and the tip sent for microbiology testing with a swab from the exit site. Tip culture was negative, but the exit site swab was positive for methicillin-resistant *Staphylococcus aureus* (MRSA).

Patient was called back to the outpatients' department. A full MRSA screen was obtained and he was sent home with a 5-day treatment programme for MRSA eradication.

Surgery was booked once the decontamination treatment and one set of post-treatment swabs had been accomplished. Patient was booked into a single room and barrier nursing commenced. He was placed at the end of the theatre list. Prophylactic antibiotics were given immediately postoperatively and during the operation.

Perioperative care was completed satisfactorily, although drainage tubes remained in situ slightly longer than normal and wound healing was slow. The patient made a good recovery and was discharged home with district nurse support and continuing physiotherapy.

Reflective practice
In view of this patient's young, fit status at the time of diagnosis, an intensive integrated approach was his best chance of long-term survival.[1] During the treatment programme, invasive procedures, regular attendance in outpatients and treatment areas meant that he acquired MRSA. The preoperative assessment outpatient clinic allows problems such as MRSA colonization to be recognized and eradicated, thereby improving perioperative infection risks.

HOSPITAL-ACQUIRED INFECTION

In 1981 a national survey of hospital acquired infection (HAI) found that one in 10 patients acquired an infection while in hospital.[2] A later survey found little improvement.[3] Four major sites of infection were highlighted:

- Urinary tract infections 23.2% (catheterization increases risk)
- Surgical wound infections 10.7% (Table 23.1)
- Lower respiratory tract 22.9% (bronchopneumonia and pneumonia)
- Skin infections 9.6%. (invasive procedures increase risk).

Immunocompromised patients have an increased risk of HAI. Risk factors include the severity of any underlying disease, the use of invasive procedures, the presence of a medical device and the length of stay in hospital. Some immunocompromised patients have so many risk factors that an HAI cannot always be prevented.[5]

Sites of infection in immunocompromised patients differ from those of general hospitalized patients shown below. In neutropenia patients with haematological malignancies, for example, sites of infection were found to be:

- Bloodstream 45%
- Mouth, tonsils, pharynx 22%
- Respiratory tract 15%
- Skin and soft tissue 13%

Table 23.1 Traditional classification of surgical procedures and associated infection risks[4]

Surgical category	Infection risk (%)
Clean	1.5–4.2
Clean contaminated	<10
Contaminated	10–20
Dirty and infected	20–30

- Intravenous device related 5%
- Urinary tract 3%
- Others 2%.[6]

Recovery from HAI in immunocompromised patients is often found to be poor.[7]

PERIOPERATIVE HOSPITAL–ACQUIRED INFECTION

Whether or not an infection occurs after surgery depends on a completed interaction between

Table 23.2   Factors causing immunosuppression

Factors that cause immune defects	Examples	Resulting immune defect
Age	Elderly	Waning immune system. Ageing skin is more fragile and healing can be delayed[8,9] Physiological changes, e.g. decreased cough reflex, impaired circulation[10]
	Very young	Immature immune system
Disease	Acquired immune deficiency syndrome (AIDS)	Immune system damage by the human immunodeficiency virus (HIV), which can infect, damage and destroy T-cells
	Congenital immunodeficiencies	Born with an immune defect
	Bone marrow diseases, e.g. leukaemia, myeloma	Impaired immune system owing to disease damaging the bone marrow
	Diabetes mellitus	Defective phagocyte function Increased risk of vascular disease
	Autoimmune disease	Impaired immune system
Treatments	Cystic fibrosis, repeated courses of antibiotics and steroids	Damaged lungs Impaired immune response
	Cancer, i.e. radiotherapy and chemotherapy	Interferes with normal cell cycle function; neutrophils are the first blood cells affected
	Transplantation, e.g. cardiac, kidney, lung and pancreas	Impairs immune response by also reducing patient defence against infection
	Drugs such as ciclosporin, steroids and azathioprine given to prevent graft rejection Bone marrow or stem cell transplantation Conditioning drugs to remove functioning bone marrow prior to transplantation, plus antirejection drugs following transplant	Impairs immune response. Reduces the body's defence against infection
	Steroids	Reduce inflammatory response, increasing risk of infection
	Splenectomy	Reduced ability to mount an immune response[11]
Malnutrition	Oesophageal or stomach cancer, which inhibits eating	Essential for wound healing and maintenance of immunological function
	Eating disorders	As above
	Prolonged fasting, i.e. pre and post surgery	As above
Invasive procedures	Central venous catheters Urinary catheters Surgical wounds	Invasive devices that bypass the body's natural immune system
Damaged skin	Pressure sores, burns, leg ulcers	Breach of the skin, which is a natural barrier to infection[12]
Damaged mucous membrane	Mucositis, colitis, lung damage	Damage to a natural barrier to infection

any of the following:

- Patient-related factors – immunity, nutritional status, and complications such as diabetes and chest disease
- Wound – size, trauma and platelet count
- Surgical intervention – length and type of surgery
- Microbiological – presence, concentration and virulence of microorganisms
- Foreign devices – drains, catheters
- Antibiotic prophylaxis – choice, presence of resistant organisms
- Drains, tracheostomy, PEG, colostomy, urostomy, skin flaps, prostheses.

IMMUNITY

Immunity is a mechanism whereby the body recognizes something as foreign and is able to eliminate or control the potential damage that the foreign object may cause.

Three main functions of the immune system include:

- Immune surveillance to recognize damaged or foreign cells
- Defence against microorganisms
- Removal of used or damaged cells.

Impairment of the immune system may be caused by a number of factors (Table 23.2). Examples and reasons for the defects are included in the table.

COMPONENTS OF THE IMMUNE SYSTEM

The immune system is made up of many different cells (cellular immunity) and proteins (humeral immunity). The most important components are listed in Table 23.3. The various causes of immuno-compromisation mean that patients will have different defects, and these defects will differ in their severity. For example, a patient who is HIV positive will have a less severe T-cell defect than one with AIDS, and a patient with newly diagnosed lymphoma, leukaemia or myeloma, or a patient undergoing intensive chemotherapy, will have several defects which will be more severe than those in a similar patient who has completed their treatment and whose disease is in remission.

The components described in Table 23.3 are also involved in wound healing.[14] Tissue damage stimulates the release of inflammatory mediators such as prostaglandins and histamine. These cause nearby blood vessels to become more permeable and to vasodilate (chemotaxis), which allows proteins and a variety of enzymes, growth factors and nutrients from the blood vessels to bathe the wound. The combination of the inflammatory response and the local presence of these substances causes cells of the immune system to be attracted to the injury site. These cells (neutrophils and macrophages) cleanse the wound by removing by phagocytosis any damaged or unwanted cells, such as microorganisms. Pus formation at the site of a wound is caused by dead cells, bacteria and immune cells.

Table 23.3   Components of the immune system

Components	Immune function
Cellular immunity	
T lymphocytes (T-cells) concerned with the production of cytokines, in particular interleukins	Activation of leucocytes to phagocytose microorganisms
B lymphocytes (B-cells) concerned with the production of antibody	Activation of B lymphocytes to produce antibody
	Assist in phagocytosis by leucocytes
Leucocytes (macrophages, neutrophils)	Phagocytosis of bacteria
	Activity enhanced by complement and specific antibody
	Improves wound healing[13]
Humeral immunity	
Antibody (immunoglobulins)	Proteins that facilitate phagocytosis
Complement	Proteins that facilitate phagocytosis
Interleukin (in particular interleukin 2)	Proteins that activate the immune response

The inflammatory response is the beginning of wound healing. This response produces localized signs and symptoms of heat, swelling, erythema and pain. These symptoms are similar to the signs and symptoms of infection. Patients who are immunocompromised are often unable to produce a normal inflammatory response and may therefore not experience the normal signs of infection. Such patients may also encounter delayed healing following surgical interventions. Increased scarring may also be a problem.[15]

Immunocompromised patients may develop infections other than wound infections, in particular chest and urinary infections. Systemic infections such as these can alter the inflammatory and healing process in other sites, which can increase the incidence of wound infection in septic patients.[16]

NON-SPECIFIC IMMUNITY

There are non-specific immune factors that also have to be considered in perioperative practice, which help to reduce the risk of infection. Table 23.4 lists those non-specific immune factors that are most likely to be affected by surgery.

MICROBIOLOGY

Immunocompromised patients will develop infections from microorganisms that affect immunocompetent patients. Table 23.5 shows the most common microorganisms that cause hospital-acquired infections. Immunocompromised patients will also be at risk of developing infections from opportunistic microorganisms that do not normally cause infection (Table 23.6).

Table 23.4 Non-specific immunity

Non-specific immunity	Infection risk	Prevention of infection
Respiratory tract Hair and mucus (traps inhaled particles) Cough reflex prevents aspiration of inhaled particles Ciliated epithelium moves inhaled particles from lungs	Chest infection, which will be increased by mechanical ventilation	Physiotherapy Careful analgesia to facilitate physiotherapy
Digestive tract Acidity of gastric fluids destroys ingested bacteria Normal flora of bowel discourages growth of pathogens by competing for nutrients	Translocation of bacteria from digestive system	Reduce length of fasting as far as reasonably possible. Appropriate use of food supplements and enteral feeding until the patient can return to a normal diet
Skin Physical barrier	Breaks in skin allow bacteria to enter, causing infection	Hygiene, Physiotherapy Attention to pressure areas Limit invasive procedures
Bladder Constant flushing of urine eliminates bacteria from bladder Acidity of urine discourages growth of bacteria	Urinary infection risk increased by catheterization[17]	Good fluid intake Closed urinary drainage system Handwashing
Mouth and eyes Saliva and tears prevent adherence of bacteria	Stomatitis Local infection leading to systemic or secondary infection Eye infection Irreversible eye damage	Adequate fluid intake Oral hygiene Mouth washes[18] Eye care

Although any pathogenic or opportunistic organisms can cause infection, Table 23.6 shows the major opportunistic microorganisms that cause infection in immunocompromised patients. Risk factors include central vascular catheters, hyperalimentation, colonization by a causative organism, and the use of broad-spectrum antibiotics.

Antibiotic-resistant microorganisms are of particular concern[21] and can include a wide variety of bacteria[22] and fungi.[23] Resistant organisms which are particularly associated with perioperative care include:

- Methicillin-resistant *Staphylococcus aureus* (MRSA). Analysis of a year's surveillance of surgical site infections found that half of the infections were caused by *Staphylococcus aureus*, and 67% of these were MRSA.[19] Analysis of bacteraemia found

Table 23.5 Microorganisms that are a common cause of hospital-acquired infection

Microorganism	Common disease	Reservoir	Prevention
Staphylococcus aureus	Wound infections (cause of up to 80% of wound infection[19]) Bacteraemia	Hands of staff, skin of patients, the environment	Handwashing, optimum personal hygiene, clean environment
Staphylococcus epidermidis	Intravenous line infections	Hands of staff, skin of patients, and the environment	Handwashing, optimum personal hygiene, clean environment
Streptococcus pyogenes	Wound infection	Throats and hands of staff and patients	Handwashing, clean environment
Escherichia coli	Urinary and wound infection	Bowel, and the environment	Handwashing, clean environment
Klebsiella	Wound, septicaemia and respiratory infections	Moist, inanimate environment	Handwashing, clean dry environment
Pseudomonas aeruginosa	Urinary, septicaemia and wound infections	Moist, inanimate environment	Handwashing, clean dry environment

Table 23.6 Common microorganisms that can cause infections in the immunocompromised patient

Microorganism	Disease	Reservoir	Prevention
Aspergillus	Pneumonia	Dust and soil	Clean environment, dust control during building or renovation work
Candida (*Candida albicans* is the commonest species causing disease)	Septicaemia	Colonization of mouth, intestinal tract and vagina increased following antibiotics	Aseptic technique, good hygiene, correct use of antibiotics
Pneumocystis carinii	Pneumonia	Environment	Prophylaxis
Legionella (one of many potential waterborne organisms[20])	Pneumonia	Water supply by inhalation, ingestion and surface absorption	Correct cleaning and maintenance of water supply Correct maintenance of water temperature
Cytomegalovirus (CMV)	Pneumonia	Person to person, reactivation of latent infection	Antiviral prophylaxis
Cryptococcus	Profuse intractable diarrhoea	Water supply Farm and domestic animal bowels	Clean water supply, handwashing after handling animals
Mycobacterium tuberculosis	Lung, bone, lymph node disease	Infected persons. Reactivation of latent infection	Vaccination
Salmonella, Listeria	Food poisoning, septicaemia, meningitis	Food, unclean kitchen and kitchen equipment	Cleanliness, adequate cooking of food
Herpes simplex/zoster	Central nervous infection	Latent infection	Antiviral prophylaxis

that in some regions 50% of all *Staphylococcus aureus* bacteraemias were caused by MRSA.[24]

- Vancomycin-resistant *Enterococcus faecum* (VRE). Major cause of endocarditis, urinary tract infection, intra-abdominal and pelvic infection and soft tissue infection.[25]

SOURCES OF MICROORGANISMS ASSOCIATED WITH WOUND INFECTIONS

Preoperative

- Exogenous infection acquired from other patients, hospital environment, visitors and staff. Risk increases with the length of the preoperative hospital stay
- Endogenous infection from the patient's own normal flora.

At the time of surgery

- Airborne from the environment,[25] for example inadequate functioning air conditioning or poor control of movement within theatre, or from staff[26]
- Endogenous spread from the patient's own skin
- Exogenous spread from the theatre staff's hands, etc. Inanimate objects such as theatre trolley, table, lights, etc.

Postoperative

Drains, catheters, dressings and lotions due to poor aseptic technique.

- Haematogenous seeding from bowel, lung, mucous membranes
- Pre-existing infection at site other than surgical wound, for example urinary infection, colitis and mucositis.

Although the presence of bacteria in wounds delays healing, most chronic wounds progress towards healing.[27]

MICROBIOLOGICAL DIAGNOSIS

Infections occurring in immunocompromised patients are often associated with morbidity and mortality and prompt accurate diagnosis is essential.[28]

The laboratory diagnosis of infection in immunocompromised patients is challenging.[29] Results have to be interpreted to establish the clinical significance of the microorganisms detected.[30] All signs and symptoms of infection or deteriorating health must be fully investigated. Microbiological investigations should include swabs, blood cultures, urine, pus, aspirate and biopsies. Serum testing for antigen and antibody is helpful in suspected infections such as cytomegalovirus (CMV), herpes and hepatitis. Diagnosis can be assisted by radiographic investigations, and in some cases invasive procedures are required, for example fibreoptic bronchoscopy with bronchoalveolar lavage (BAL) to investigate infections with agents such as *Aspergillus* and *Mycobacterium*.

Gram-negative bacteria remain a leading cause of perioperative hospital-acquired infection, in particular ventilation-associated pneumonia and catheter-associated urinary infection, whereas Gram-positive bacteria are responsible for the majority of wound, bacteraemia and line-associated infections.[31]

ANTIBIOTIC THERAPY

When neutropenic patients have signs and symptoms of infection, antibiotics should be commenced as soon as possible. Generally it is preferable to treat suspected infections where the cause is unknown using a combination of antibiotics. Antibiotics should be given for long enough to ensure complete eradication of the infection. Selection of the most appropriate drug involves consideration of safety, proven efficiency, toxic effects, cost, and the underlying condition of the patient.

Most patients are prescribed antibiotics on an empirical basis for all suspected or known infections, as microbiological identification of the causative organism(s) can take 48 hours. The choice of whether the drug will have a narrow or a broad spectrum and be given singly or in combination will be decided after clinical assessment and a review of microbiological results of what is the most likely causative organism. Speed is essential, as outcome is directly related to early and appropriate therapy. Immunocompromised patients are generally given high-dose drugs via the intravenous route. Toxic drugs should be monitored by blood level testing[32] and the dose adjusted accordingly.[33]

Broad-spectrum antibiotics predispose to fungal infections. Antibiotics suppress the growth of normal commensal bacteria and thereby promote the overgrowth with fungal organisms.[34]

The emergence of microorganisms resistant to antimicrobial drugs may be due to their excessive use for human and veterinary purposes, treatment at subtherapeutic levels, poor patient compliance, transfer of genetic material coding for antimicrobial resistance between organisms, or more commonly cross-infection from one patient to another.

Antimicrobial-resistant microorganisms may colonize sites such as skin, wounds, sputum, tracheostomies, or cause infection. Immunocompromised patients, or those with wounds or invasive devices who are already colonized with antimicrobial resistant organisms, are more likely to develop infections.

Infection with antimicrobial-resistant microorganisms can be more difficult to treat effectively or may prove fatal. The Department of Health[35,36] has set out actions for the National Health Service. These include:

- Minimize morbidity and mortality due to antimicrobial resistant infection
- Control antimicrobial-resistant organisms
- Facilitate more efficient and effective use of NHS resources.

These goals can be achieved by:

- Strengthening the prevention and control of infection
- Optimizing antimicrobial prescribing
- Improving surveillance of infection and monitoring antimicrobial usage to provide the information base for action.[37]

PERIOPERATIVE RISKS OTHER THAN INFECTION

Although the risk of infection is probably the major risk experienced by the immunocompromised patient, factors other than those already mentioned in Table 23.2 that need to be considered include the following:

1. *Platelet count*. For many patients who have a reduced white cell count there is a corresponding reduction in the platelet count. Similarly, in patients with myeloma, for example, platelet counts may be normal but abnormal paraproteins may cause platelets and coagulation factors to malfunction, predisposing the patient to bleed.

Thrombocytopenia is defined as a platelet count of less than $50 \times 10^9/L$ of blood. The normal

platelet count is $250–500 \times 10^9/L$ blood. This is particularly marked in patients with haemato-oncology-associated diseases and treatments, e.g. leukaemia. Any trauma to the skin that penetrates the dermis, e.g. surgical wound or cannulation, will result in bleeding. The immediate response will be for the blood vessels to constrict to stop the flow of blood; this action will be assisted by the coagulation cascade instigated by platelets that are in contact with the damaged blood vessels, to form a plug which stops the bleeding and holds the wound edges together.[38] Reduced platelet count will lead to delayed healing, increased wound drainage, and may predispose the patient to a wound infection.

The patient's platelet count must be monitored during the perioperative period and platelet transfusion can be given. Platelets are normally given when:

- There is active bleeding whatever the count
- Platelet count $10 \times 10^3/L$
- Platelet count $<20 \times 10^9/L$ without bleeding, but with a temperature of $38°C$
- Platelet count $>10 \times 10^9/L$ and $<50 \times 10^9/L$ and suspected platelet dysfunction
- Platelet count $>50 \times 10^9/L$ prior to minor invasive procedure
- Platelet count $>75 \times 10^9/L$ prior to or following major invasive procedure
- Septicaemic patients may need platelets even if their platelet count is $>20 \times 10^9/L$.

Careful assessment and management of patients with thrombocytopenia is essential. Thrombocytopenia is a factor which identifies patients at greater risk of complications.[39] It is essential that surgery does not increase the ill health of thrombocytopenic patients.

2. *Radiotherapy*. Radiotherapy causes damage to the intracellular components of living cells, which can result in the disruption of cell division and lead to cell death. This is the desired effect on abnormal cancer cells, but at the same time normal cells can also be affected. Skin damage that occurs at the time of radiotherapy treatment would not be expected to heal until the radiotherapy treatment is completed. The nearer surgery is scheduled to the completed radiotherapy treatment the greater the risk of delayed healing of the surgical wound.

3. *Fungating wounds*. Tumour infiltration of the skin may be due to direct invasion of local tumours or through metastatic spread. This causes capillary damage, which can result in rupture, or occlusion,

leading to necrosis of the skin, which may lead to fungating wounds. Generally fungating wounds do not heal. Chronic wounds will inevitably be contaminated with bacteria, which does not generally delay wound healing.[40] Surgical intervention is generally not an option: care relies on holistic assessment, psychosocial support, and the use of appropriate dressings and wound care products.

RISK ASSESSMENT

Risk management is an indispensable part of good practice and should be an integrated part of all patient care. Risk assessment identifies and thereby highlights potential hazards of an activity, the likelihood that harm will result from that activity, and the procedures to be followed. This process ensures that appropriate safety measures are in place to reduce the likelihood of complications arising in the first place, or if it does occur the risk will be reduced to an acceptable level.

It is only by carrying out risk assessments that working systems and processes can be monitored and adapted at patient level to ensure that a safe and effective care plan is negotiated.

Integrated care pathways are a valuable tool to improve clinical effectiveness and quality of care. Integrated care pathways help to ensure a consistent, coordinated pattern of care, which can also

Table 23.7   Risk assessment

Assessment factor	Risk	Potential problem
Past medical history	Anaesthetic risk	Lungs, i.e. asthma Heart, i.e. cardiac failure
	Colonized with antibiotic-resistant organism, e.g. VRE, MRSA	Endogenous infection
	Clotting problems	Deep vein thrombosis Haemorrhage
Current medical treatment (as above plus)	Antibiotic	Suppress normal flora, predisposing to the acquisition of HAI with increased pathogenicity
	Steroids (arthritis)	Immune suppression
	Current wound, i.e. fungating	Haematogenous seeding of bacteria
	Diabetic	Reduce normal inflammatory response
Nutritional status	Obesity	Anaesthetic risk May delay healing owing to reduced availability of oxygen to the surgical wound
	Malnutrition	Infection risks Delayed healing
Communication skills	Language	Inhibits informed consent
	Hearing	A fully informed patient is more likely to cooperate with treatment
	Intelligence level	
Patient strengths and coping abilities	Mobility (arthritis)	Chest infection, deep vein thrombosis, pressure sore
Social support/resources	Friends and family help the patient cope with treatment and care	Lack of support/resources increases stress and anxiety
Spiritual and cultural needs	Provision increases patients' wellbeing	Lack increases stress and anxiety
Psychological issues	Stress	Stress increases immune defect[42]
	Sexuality	Psychological problems increase
	Body image (mastectomy, colostomy)	stress and anxiety

produce information for clinical audit, guideline development, and for managing change.[41]

PERIOPERATIVE RISK ASSESSMENT

Immunosuppression is a complex state, determined by a number of factors. Risk assessment involves consideration of these factors to establish the degree of risk.

Assessment would include:

- The extent and duration of immunosuppression
- The underlying cause
- Planned treatment
- The presence of invasive devices (urinary and intravenous devices, endotracheal tubes, etc.)
- Damage to natural barriers to infection (skin, mucous membranes)
- Metabolic abnormalities, malnutrition.

Other general assessment factors that have to be considered for all patients, but which are especially important for the immunocompromised patient, can be found in Table 23.7, which outlines the assessment factors, the risks and potential problems for the patient.

PREVENTION OF PERIOPERATIVE COMPLICATIONS

Any invasive procedure carries a risk of infection, which may be serious in persons with healthy immune systems but can be life threatening in the immunocompromised. Prevention of infection is related to a combination of:

- Preoperative preparation
- Surgical technique
- Perioperative prophylaxis
- Postoperative care
- Surveillance
- Audit
- Education, training and supervision.

PREOPERATIVE CARE

For planned surgery, preoperative outpatient clinics allow for a full risk assessment to be undertaken and remedial therapy given.[43]

All the healthcare workers involved in the patient's care, and the patient themselves, must be made aware of the risk and time allowed to discuss those risks.[44] The patient must be re-evaluated at the time of admission by nursing, clinicians and anaesthetic staff.

For essential surgery the decision to proceed is usually relatively straightforward. However, with elective surgery the patient needs to evaluate their quality of life without surgery against the high risk of treatment. If the patient is given a full explanation of the planned treatment their cooperation will be ensured.

Anxiety can produce alterations in immune function that will affect recovery from surgery and wound healing. Psychological support is important for all patients during the perioperative period, but is essential for immunocompromised patients.[45]

NURSING CARE

Immunocompromised patients require skilled nursing care. The attributes of nurses and the components that provide quality care as described by such patients include:

- Professional knowledge
- Continuity
- Attentiveness
- Coordination
- Partnership
- Individualization
- Rapport
- Caring.[46]

Handwashing

Handwashing is considered the single most important intervention to prevent hospital-acquired infection (HAI). Hands must be decontaminated immediately before and after each direct patient care contact. The choice of handwashing method depends on the task being undertaken.

Handwashing procedure:

1. Remove jewellery and wristwatch; roll up sleeves
2. Clean hands; use an alcohol hand rub, which must come into contact with all surfaces of the hand
3. Dirty hands: wet hands with hand hot water, apply non-medicated liquid soap, rub on all surfaces of hand for at least 10–15 seconds; rinse, and dry with a good-quality paper towel
4. Prior to an aseptic technique (surgical scrub): as above using an antimicrobial soap preparation instead of the liquid non-medicated soap. Washing must include the hands and forearms.

For clean hands, alcoholic hand rubs and antimicrobial preparations appear superior to liquid soap in reducing bacterial counts. Alcoholic hand rubs and antimicrobial soap preparations have similar actions.[47] Alcoholic hand rubs have the advantage of being quick and convenient, as well as less damaging to skin.[48] Studies to evaluate handwashing have found poor practice, especially among medical staff.[49]

Segregation

Immunocompromised patients must be segregated from patients known to be infected.

Environment

Environment, equipment and food must be of a clean standard.

Endogenous infections

Endogenous infections are more difficult to prevent. Good hygiene, including mouth care, is helpful.

OPERATING THEATRE

Basic building requirements for operating theatres apply to all patients regardless of their immune status. Similarly, theatre practices should be of the same high standard for all patients. Requirements include restrictions on movement within the theatre, separation of clean and dirty areas and equipment; and strict attention to asepsis. Further information can be obtained from NHS Estates CD ROM *Building Better Healthcare*.[50,51]

Other important issues include the following:

• Ventilation reduces postoperative infection, with ultraclean ventilation being used for orthopaedic surgery. There is controversy regarding the need for specialized ventilation for minimally invasive surgery. Recommendations exist for the insertion of central venous lines.[52] However, for laparoscopic interventions it is less clear. As a laparoscopic operation may need to be converted to an open procedure the ventilation must also be appropriate for unplanned subsequent procedures.[53]

• Surgical instruments must be prepared in a sterile services department that complies with UK Medical Devices Regulations 1994 and 3017. EEC Council Directive 93/42/EEC Legislation L169.

• Instruments must have a total traceability system.[54]

• Benchtop sterilizers must only be used for dropped solid instruments where a replacement is not available.[55]

• Equipment that cannot be autoclaved must be disinfected using an automatic washer-disinfector; the disinfectant must have antiviral, antibacterial, antituberculosis and antispore properties.

• Single-use instruments must not be reused.[56]

POSTOPERATIVE CARE

Some immunocompromised patients, such as bone marrow and stem cell transplant patients, are normally cared for in a clean environment (reverse barrier nursing, protective isolation).[57] Following surgery, immunocompromised patients may be admitted into recovery. Although some recovery units have single rooms, these are generally kept for infected patients. Few recovery departments have sufficient rooms to segregate immunocompromised patients. Generally immunocompromised patients are placed at the end of the ward next to patients who are known not to have a contagious infection. Understaffing, overcrowding and a mix of patients will increase the risk of cross-infection in recovery.[58]

Prevention of infection can be assisted in the following ways:

• Direct transfer of infection can be prevented by the use of colour-coded aprons which are changed between patients, careful handwashing before and after patient contact, and thorough cleaning of shared equipment.

• Airborne transfer is more difficult to control and is particularly difficult during bedmaking,[59] or when, for example, other patients have productive coughs.

• Strict aseptic technique should be used when handling wounds, drains and catheters. Immunocompromised patients being cared for in intensive care are of special concern, as 25% of all hospital infections are attributed to intensive care units,[21] many of which are due to endogenous infection.[60]

• Compliance with intravenous devices policies, as central venous devices are the major cause of bacteraemia.[42]

• Compliance with urinary catheterization policy, as catheterization is the main cause of urinary infection.[17]

- Attention to patient hygiene, in particular mouth care.[61]
- Prevention of skin damage, especially pressure sores.[62]
  - Optimum pain control.
  - Physiotherapy and early mobilization.

SURGICAL ANTIMICROBIAL PROPHYLAXIS

Surgical antimicrobial prophylaxis aims to prevent or decrease the incidence of postoperative wound infections by reducing the bacterial load of potentially pathogenic bacteria to a level that cannot overwhelm the patient's natural immune defence system. Although prophylaxis has been seen to decrease the incidence of infection rates[63] there is concern regarding:

- The considerable costs of the drugs
- Inappropriate use, which adds pressure on microbial ecology within the hospital
- Inappropriate use, including choice, timing, administration and duration of prophylaxis
- Increased risk of the development of antimicrobial resistance, which is associated with poor clinical outcome and increased treatment costs.[64]

Prophylaxis can reduce postoperative rates for many surgical procedures, especially if the antimicrobial drugs are administered at the appropriate time and for the correct duration. Prophylactic drugs must be safe, cost effective, and offer optimal bactericidal activity against all pathogens, both aerobic and anaerobic, Gram-positive and Gram-negative bacteria that are likely to contaminate the surgical wound.

When choosing the appropriate drugs, individual hospitals should take into consideration current national guidelines, local infection control problems, and the type of surgery and the individual's circumstances.

FACTORS THAT INCREASE IMMUNOCOMPROMISED PATIENTS' RISK OF INFECTION

Ventilation

Ventilation-associated pneumonia (VAP) arises following endotracheal intubation and mechanical ventilation and is a frequent nosocomial infection in intensive care units. Patients with reduced defences against infection are particularly susceptible to chest infections, as bacterial colonization of the respiratory tract is normally removed by the phagocytic white cells found in the mucous membranes of the respiratory system. Damage to the mucous membrane during intubation increases the risk of VAP.[65]

Whereas VAP is often due to the endogenous spread of the patient's own normal flora, other causes include airborne spread of organisms such as *Staphylococcus*, and cross-infection due, for example, to healthcare workers not washing their hands before and after each patient contact.

Prevention includes compliance with careful handwashing policy. It is suggested that compliance is especially low in coronary care units, generally because of staff shortages.

Tracheostomy care

A tracheostomy is a surgical opening in the anterior wall of the trachea; this is a common procedure that may be undertaken as a temporary measure at the time of major surgery, or as a permanent procedure following total laryngectomy, and is relatively common in patients with head and neck cancers. Surgical intervention may be in association with radiotherapy and chemotherapy.

Tracheostomy care includes the use of humidified oxygen, suctioning, mouth care, regular changing of the tracheostomy tube in patients with copious secretions, and wound management.

Prevention of infection includes the use of sterile suction catheters and gloves, sterile nebulizers using sterile water, and strict aseptic techniques when handling new tracheostomies.

Pain control

Optimal perioperative pain control reduces the incidence of complications after major surgery. Complications such as deep vein thrombosis, chest infection or pressure sores may occur if pain control is not managed correctly. Too much analgesia will sedate the patient, which will hinder physiotherapy; too little will make the patient reluctant to cooperate with physiotherapy. Similarly, severe pain has an effect on the sympathetic nervous system and the neuroendocrine stress response, which can have a detrimental affect on components of the blood and body.

It is essential that during the preoperative informed consent discussions the patient is given a realistic understanding of the pain that they should expect. Greater fear and distress prior to surgery is associated with a slower and more complicated recovery.[66] If they are well informed, the patient's anxiety may be reduced. This may mean they will be able to cooperate more fully with decisions related to postoperative pain control, as it is important to prevent pain rather than allowing it to become established. Fully informed patients will report the first signs of pain, as they will understand that it is unlikely to recede without analgesia.

Assessment of pain is essential to identify all the factors involved in the patient's experience of pain. Assessment must begin before surgery and continue through to discharge.[67] Monitoring allows for evaluation of the effectiveness of pain control interventions. As many surgical procedures involve more than one incision site, pain is assessed more accurately using an assessment chart.

Alternatives to medication can assist the patient to cope with pain. This may be achieved by teaching patients coping and relaxation techniques.

The use of epidural analgesia has increased, as it has been found to provide good postoperative pain relief.[68] Complications, although rare, include haematoma, dural tap and infection.[69] Infection is a potential problem and may present as a superficial infection at the entry site, with inflammation, erythema, discharge or pain.

Deep infection includes the presence of pus in the epidural space or infection of the central nervous system, i.e. meningitis or abscess.

Prevention includes:

- Strict aseptic techniques during insertion and subsequent manipulation
- Close monitoring, surveillance and audit of epidural catheters, to allow for analysis of the number of infections and risk factors.

EDUCATION AND TRAINING OF STAFF

Blood transfusion

Transfusion of blood and blood products to correct clinical abnormalities is an essential part of care. Contamination of blood and blood products is uncommon, but can occur during donation, collection, processing, storage or administration of the product. For immunocompromised patients the resulting septicaemia can be fatal. The most common cause is skin contamination from the donor at the time of venesection, or from the hands of staff handling the donation. Signs and symptoms of infection are rapid, with rigors, chills, fever, nausea, vomiting, pain and hypotension. Treatment must be immediate by stopping the transfusion, treating symptoms, taking microbiological samples and considering prescribing antibiotics. The remainder of the transfusion must be tested to establish the cause of the contamination's complications.

Other problems associated with blood and blood product transfusions are the same for all patients, and include acute haemolytic reaction due to incompatibilities in the ABO blood grouping, acute respiratory distress syndrome following large amounts of blood, air embolism, and circulatory overload. Prevention of problems includes strict aseptic technique, careful checking of the product, and regular observation of the patient.

Minimizing operative blood loss by meticulous haemostasis to reduce the number of blood transfusions is essential,[70] as it has been suggested that blood transfusions can lead to transfusion-induced immunosuppression.[71]

Nutritional support

An adequate diet is essential for critical care patients[72] as it provides the nutrients for immune products such as cytokines, which are essential for wound healing and the prevention of infection. Postoperative oral supplements improve nutritional status, reduce the use of antibiotics and improve quality of life in malnourished patients.[73]

Nutritional support supplements a patient who is unable to maintain their nutritional status by their usual diet. In the perioperative period this includes both enteral and parenteral feeding. Animal studies suggest that parenteral nutrition promotes bacterial translocation from the gut.[74] Human studies suggest this theoretical concern is unfounded.[75]

Total parenteral nutrition (TPN) is the direct intravenous infusion of sterile fluids containing all nutrients to meet the patient's daily needs. Feeding is via a central venous catheter for patients with a non-functioning or inaccessible GI tract who are likely to be nil by mouth for 5 days or longer, for example following major abdominal surgery.

Parenteral feeding has the disadvantage of increasing the risk of infection, as the TPN solution encourages the growth of microorganisms. Strict aseptic technique is essential, with the TPN solution being infused via a dedicated IV catheter lumen which is not used for any other procedures, such as drug administration, monitoring or blood taking.

Enteral feeds are commercially prepared feeds that can be given as a bolus, as an intermittent or continuous infusion via a gravity drip set, or pump assisted. Feeding can be administered via the following routes:

- Nasogastric – using a fine-bore enteral tube via the nose into the stomach, which is suitable for short-term postoperative use
- Gastrostomy – via a PEG tube held in position by a flange or balloon for patients requiring long-term feeding
- Jejunostomy – a fine-bore feeding tube into the jejunum, for patients with upper gastrointestinal surgery.

Close monitoring of the patient is essential and includes careful fluid balance, haematology and biochemical blood testing.

Evidence that inadequate nutrition does exist,[76] prompt identification of nutritional problems and rapid interventions are essential to increase the chances of optimum wound healing.[77]

Environmental cleanliness

Good hygiene is essential for preventing HAI.[78] Since 2000 hospital Trusts have been inspected by the Patient Environment Action Teams (PEATs) to assess their level of patient facilities. Infection control factors included in these inspections included cleanliness, tidiness, general decoration, support services, furniture and food. Following each inspection each Trust is scored between 1 and 4, and given a colour code – green for high quality, yellow for acceptable, red for poor. Action plans are agreed and further inspections check on progress.[79]

Cleaning of the operating theatre is particularly important to reduce contamination as far as is practically possible.[25]

EDUCATION AND TRAINING

All staff involved with patient contact must receive education, training and supervision related to the prevention of HAI.[78] A comprehensive appraisal system is essential for assessing and monitoring clinical performance. Appraisal provides an objective opinion of practice and identifies both strengths and areas for development.[80]

POLICIES

Evidence-based policies provide the basis of good practice by establishing evidence-based guidelines[81] which are relevant to the hospital where they are being used. National guidelines can be adapted at local level.[78] It is essential that all staff are aware of the relevant policies for their work, and have received education, training and supervision to ensure those policies are implemented and followed.[82]

Policies provide a basis for audit and feedback of the findings to staff.[83]

Barriers to evidence-based practice include time constraints, limited access to the literature, lack of training in information seeking and critical appraisal skills, practical versus intellectual knowledge, and inappropriate work environments that discourage information seeking. It is important that perioperative practitioners are encouraged to learn the skills to practise evidence-based care to ensure the patient is provided with the best care available.[84]

CLINICAL GOVERNANCE

Clinical governance is a system by which an organization is directed and controlled, at its most senior levels, in order to achieve its objectives and its standards of accountability, probity and openness. To achieve the objectives of clinical governance, independent and organizational review has to be undertaken.

Clinical governance provides the framework through which healthcare facilities are accountable for making a continuous effort to improve the quality of service and creating an environment in which high-quality clinical care can be instigated and maintained.[35] Clinical governance includes infection control.

SURVEILLANCE

Surveillance, which involves data collection, analysis and feedback to clinicians, is central to detecting, treating and ultimately reducing infection rates. Surveillance identifies areas of concerns, which enables Trusts to target prevention activities effectively.[85] It also allows comparisons with other studies.[86] Surveillance has been shown to decrease infection rates, decrease morbidity and save money.[87]

Nationally, the Nosocomial Infection National Surveillance Scheme (NINSS) has enhanced surveillance, producing strong comparative data that can be used as a benchmark of performance.

Two important NINSS surveys which have produced very worthwhile information include:

- A 2-year analysis of bacteraemia which indicated that there was a significant variation in rates, with 9.0 per 1000 patient days in general intensive care, compared with 4.9 in haematology, 0.8 in general surgery and 0.5 in general medicine.[19]
- Surgical site infection rates, with an average of 10.6 infections per 100 operations for large bowel surgery, compared to 2.5 for total hip replacement and 1.9 for abdominal hysterectomy.[19]

Surveillance must include postdischarge surveillance,[88] as it has been seen that between 50 and 70% of surgical wound infections occur after discharge.[89]

AUDIT

Audit is an essential and important aspect of infection control. Any part of patient care can be audited. Audit allows for monitoring and critical evaluation of working practices, identifying problem areas, and provides evidence of improvements in practice. The Department of Health[78] suggests that national guidelines provide a focus for audit and feedback to staff.

CONCLUSION

Surgical management is an essential part of care of the immunocompromised patient, and if undertaken with caution and expertise can assist in their recovery and long-term survival. Every effort must be made to ensure that the death rate following surgery continues to decrease.[90]

Surgical management of immunocompromised patients requires special consideration, which includes:

- Careful and thorough preoperative evaluation and assessment of risk
- Preoperative preparation
- Optimum intraoperative techniques
- Prudent postoperative care
- Superlative rehabilitation
- Continuous assessment and treatment of complications.

References

1. Sondak VK, Robertson JM, Sussman JJ, et al. Preoperative idoxuridine and radiation for large soft tissue sarcomas: clinical results with five year follow up. Ann Surg Oncol 1998; 5: 106–112.

2. Meers PD, Ayliffe GAJ, Emerson AM. Report of the national survey of infection in hospitals 1980. J Hosp Infect 1981; 2(Suppl): 23–28.

3. Emmerson AM, Enstone JE, Griffin A, et al. The second national prevalence survey of infection in hospital – overview of the results. J Hosp Infect 1996; 32: 175–190.

4. Mangram AJ, Horan TC, Pearson ML, et al. The Hospital Infection Control Practices Advisory Committee. Guidelines for prevention of surgical site infection. Control Hosp Epidemol 1999; 20: 247–278.

5. Taylor K, Plowman R, Roberts JA. The challenge of hospital acquired infection. London: National Audit Office; 2001.

6. Glauser MP, Calandra T. Infections in patients with hematologic malignancies. In: Glauser MP, Pizzo PA, eds. Management of infections in immunocompromised patients. London: WB Saunders: 2000; 148–188.

7. Garrouste-Orgeas M, Chevret S, Mainardi JL, et al. A one year prospective study of nosocomial bacteraemia in ICU and non ICU patients and its impact on patient outcome. J Hosp Infect 2000; 44: 203–213.

8. Denham JW, Ackland SP, Burmeister B, et al. Causes for increased myelosuppression with increasing age in patients with oesophageal cancer treated by chemo/radiotherapy. Eur J Cancer 1999; 35: 921–927.

9. Swift ME, Burns AL, Gray KL, et al. Age-related alterations in the inflammatory response to dermal injury. J Invest Dermatol 2001; 117: 1027–1035.

10. Crossley KB, Peterson PK. Infections in the elderly. In: Mandell GL, Bennett JE, Dolan R, eds. Principles and practice of infectious diseases, 4th edn. New York: Churchill Livingstone; 1995: 2737–2741.

11. Waghorn DJ. Overwhelming infection in asplenic patients: current best practice preventative measures are not being followed. J Clin Pathol 2001; 54: 214–218.

12. Parker L. Applying the principles of infection control to wound care. Br J Nurs 2000; 9: 394–396.

13. Canturk NZ, Esen N, Vural B, et al. The relationship between neutrophils and incisional wound healing. Skin Pharmacol Appl Skin Physiol 2001; 14: 108–116.

14. Gillitzer R, Goebeler M. Chemokines in cutaneous wound healing. J Leukocyte Biol 2001; 69: 513–521.

15. Baxter CR. Immunologic reaction in chronic wounds. Am J Surg 1994; 167: 12S–14S.

16. Rico RM, Ripamonti R, Burns AL, et al. The effect of sepsis on wound healing. J Surg Res 2002; 102: 193–197.

17. Department of Health. Guidelines for preventing infections associated with the insertion and maintenance of short-term indwelling urethral catheters in acute care. J Hosp Infect 2001; 47: S39–S46.

18. Bill K. The importance of mouth care. Nurs Standard 2000; 14: 57–61.

19. Public Health Laboratory Service. Surveillance of surgical site infection in English hospitals 1997–1999. London: Central Public Health Laboratory Service, 2000.

20. Emmerson AM. Emerging waterborne infections in healthcare settings. Emerg Infect Dis 2001; 7: 272–276.

21. Trilla A. Epidemiology of nosocomial infection in adult intensive care units. Intens Care Med 1994; 20: S1–S4.

22. Jugo J, Kennedy R, Crowe MJ, et al. Trends in bacteraemia on the haematology and oncology units in UK tertiary referral hospitals. J Hosp Infect 2002; 50: 48–55.

23. Kremery V, Barnes AJ. Non-*Albicans candida* spp. Causing fungaemia: pathogenicity and antifungal resistance. J Hosp Infect 2002; 50: 243–260.

24. Lewis CM, Zervos MJ. Clinical manifestations of enterococcal infection. J Clin Microb Infect Dis 1990; 9: 111–117.

25. Faure O, Fricker-Hidalgo H, Lebeau B, et al. Eight-year surveillance of environmental fungal contamination of hospital operating rooms and haematological units. J Hosp Infect 2002; 50: 155–160.

26. Lankester BJ, Bartlett GE, Garneti N, et al. Direct measurement of bacterial penetration through surgical gowns: a new method. J Hosp Infect 2002; 50: 281–285.

27. Thomson PD. Immunology, microbiology and the recalcitrant wound. Ostomy Wound Manage 200; 46: 77S–82S.

28. Gillespie T, Masterton RG. Investigation of infection in the netropenic patient. J Hosp Infect 1998; 38: 77–99.

29. Bille J. Laboratory diagnosis of infections in febrile neutropenic or immunocompromised patients. Inter J Antimicrob Agents 2000; 16: 87–89.

30. Correa L, Pittet D. Problems and solutions in hospital-acquired bacteraemia. J Hosp Infect 2000; 46: 89–95.

31. Eggimann P, Pittet D. Nonantibiotic measures for the prevention of Gram-positive infections. Clin Microb Infect 2001; 7: 91–99.

32. Eltaway AT, Bahnassy AA. Aminoglycoside prescription, therapeutic monitoring and nephrotoxicity at a university hospital in Saudi Arabia. J Chemo 1996; 8: 278–282.

33. Ismail R, Hag AH, Azman M, et al. Therapeutic drug monitoring of gentamicin: a 6-year follow-up audit. J Clin Pharmacol Therapy 1997; 22: 21–25.

34. Pizzo PA, Robichaud KJ, Gill FA. Empiric antibiotics and antifungal therapy for cancer patients with prolonged fever and granulocytopenia. Am J Med 1982; 72: 101–111.

35. Department of Health. Standing Medical Advisory Committee. The path of least resistance. London: HMSO; 1998.

36. Department of Health. UK antimicrobial resistance strategy and action plan. London: HMSO; 2000.

37. NHS Executive. Resistance to antibiotics and other antimicrobial agents. Leeds: NHS Executive; 1999.

38. Ofoso FA. The blood platelet as a model for regulating blood coagulation on cell surfaces and its consequences. Biochemistry 2002; 67: 47–55.

39. Dominietto A, Raiola AM, van Lint MT, et al. Factors influencing haematological recovery after allogenic haemopoietic stem cell transplant: graft-versus-host disease, donor type, cytomegalovirus infection and cell dose. Br J Haematol 2001; 112: 219–227.

40. Dow G, Brown A, Sibbald RG. Infection in chronic wounds: controversy in diagnosis and treatment. Ostomy Wound Manag 1999; 45: 23–27.

41. Selwood K. Integrated care pathways: an adult toll in paediatric oncology. Br J Nurs 2000; 9: 34–38.

42. Romeo C, Cruccetti A, Turuaco A, et al. Monocyte and neutrophil activity after minor surgical stress. J Paed Surg 2002; 37: 741–744.

43. Singh S, Manji M. A survey of pre-operative optimisation of high-risk surgical patients undergoing major elective surgery. Anaesthesia 2001; 50: 988–990.

44. Sullivan RJ, Menapace LW, White RM. Truth telling and patient diagnosis. J Med Ethics 2001; 27: 192–197.

45. Fehder WP. Alterations in immune response associated with anxiety in surgical patients. Clinical Forum for Nurse Anaesthetists 1999; 10: 124–129.

46. Radwin L. Oncology patients' perceptions of quality nursing care. Res Nurs Health 2000; 23: 179–190.

47. Lucet JC, Rigaud MP, Mentre F, et al. Hand contamination before and after different hand hygiene techniques: a randomized clinical trial. J Hosp Infect 2002; 5: 276–280.

48. Pereira LJ, Lee GM, Wade KJ. An evaluation of five protocols for surgical handwashing in relation to skin condition and microbial counts. J Hosp Infect 1997; 36: 49–65.

49. Karabey S, Ay P, Derbentli S, et al. Handwashing frequencies in an intensive care unit. J Hosp Infect 2002; 50: 36–41.

50. NHS Estates. Building better health care 2. Policy guidance. CD-ROM. Norwich: The Stationery Office; 2001.

51. Ayliffe GAJ, Fraise AP, Gedded AM, et al. Control of hospital infection. A practical handbook, 4th edn. London: Arnold; 2000.

52. Department of Health. Guidelines for preventing infections associated with the insertion and maintenance of central venous catheters. J Hosp Infect 2001; 47: A47–S67.

53. Humphreys H, Taylor EW. Operating theatre ventilation standards and the risk of postoperative infection. J Hosp Infect 2002; 50: 85–90.

54. NHS Executive. Decontamination of medical devices. London: DOH; 2000.

55. Medical Devices Agency. Single-use medical devices: implications and consequences of reuse. London: DOH; 2000: DB2000(04).

56. Medical Devices Agency. Guidance on the purchase, operation and maintenance of vacuum benchtop steam sterilizers. London: DOH; 2000: DB2000(05).

57. Mallett J, Dougherty L. Barrier nursing: nursing the infectious or immunosuppressed patient. In: Mallett J, Dougherty L. The Royal Marsden Hospital manual of clinical nursing procedures, 5th edn. Oxford: Blackwell Science; 2000: 44–122.

58. Anderson BM, Lindemann R, Bergh K, et al. Spread of methicillin-resistant *Staphylococcus aureus* in a neonatal intensive unit associated with understaffing, overcrowding and mixing patients. J Hosp Infect 2002; 50: 18–24.

59. Shiomori T, Miyamoto H, Makishima M. Evaluation of bedmaking-related airborne and surface methicillin resistant *Staphylococcus aureus* contamination. J Hosp Infect 2002; 50: 30–35.

60. Weinstein RA. Epidemiology and control of nosocomial infection in adult intensive care units. Am J Med 1991; 91: 179S–184S.

61. Miller M, Kearney N. Oral care for patients with cancer: a review of the literature. Cancer Nurs 2001; 24: 241–254.

62. Rycroft-Malone J, Duff L. Developing clinical guidelines: issues and challenges. J Tissue Viability 2002; 10: 144–149.

63. Wenzel RP. Perioperative antibiotic prophylaxis. N Engl J Med 1992; 326: 327–339.

64. Talon D, Mourey F, Touratier S, et al. Evaluation of current practices in surgical antimicrobial prophylaxis before and after implementation of local guidelines. J Hosp Infect 2001; 49: 193–198.

65. Koeman M, van der Ven AJAM, Ramsay G, et al. Ventilation-associated pneumonia: recent issues on pathogenesis, prevention and diagnosis. J Hosp Infect 2001; 49: 155–162.

66. Kiecolt-Glaser JK, Page GG, Marucha PT, et al. Psychological influences on surgical recovery. Perspectives from psychoneuroimmunology. Am Psychol 1998; 53: 1209–1218.

67. Kremer MJ. Surgery, pain and immune function. Clinical Forum for Nurse Anaesthetists 1999; 10: 94–100.

68. Buggy DJ, Smith G. Epidural anaesthesia and analgesia: better outcome after major surgery. BMJ 1999; 319: 530–531.

69. Dawson SJ, Small H, Logan MN, et al. Case control study of epidural catheter infections in a district general hospital. Comm Dis Public Health 2000; 3: 300–302.

70. Dresner SM, Lamb PJ, Shenfine J, et al. Prognostic significance of peri-operative blood transfusion following radical resection of oesophageal carcinoma. Eur J Sug Oncol 2000; 25: 492–497.

71. Craig SR. Effect of blood transfusion on survival after esophagogastrectomy for carcinoma. Ann Thoracic Surg 1998; 66: 356–361.

72. Stotts NA, Washington DF. Nutrition: a critical component of wound healing. Clin Iss Crit Care Nurs 1990; 1: 585–594.

73. Beattie AH, Prach AT, Baxter JP. Postoperative oral nutritional supplementation improved nutritional status and quality of life in malnourished patients. Gut 2000; 46: 813–818.

74. Alverdy JC, Aoys E, Moss GS. Total parenteral nutrition promotes bacterial translocation from the gut. Surgery 1988; 104: 185–190.

75. Sedman PC, MacFie J, Palmer MD, et al. Preoperative total parenteral nutrition is not associated with mucosal atrophy or bacterial translocation in humans. Br J Surg 1995; 82: 1663–1667.

76. Rollins H. Nutrition and wound healing. Nurs Standard 1997; 11: 49–52.

77. Johnson LJ. Nutrition and wound healing. Sem Perioper Nurs 1993; 2: 238–242.

78. Department of Health. Standard principles for preventing hospital-acquired infections. J Hosp Infect 2001; 47: S21–S37.

79. Tyson A. The clean hospital programme and infection control. Br J Infect Control 2002; 3: 17.

80. Metcalf C. The importance of performance appraisal and staff development: a graduate nurses perspective. Inter J Nurs Pract 2001; 7: 54–56.

81. Cullin TL, McColle E. Review: nursing care driven by guidelines improves some process measures and patient outcomes. Evidence-Based Nurs 1999; 2: 87–90.

82. Thomson L, Cullum N, McColl E, et al. Effects of clinical guidelines in nursing, midwifery and the therapies: a systematic review of evaluation. Qual Health Care 1998; 7: 183–191.

83. National Audit Office. The management and control of hospital acquired infection in acute NHS Trusts in England. London: The Stationery Office; 2000.

84. DiCenso A, Cullum N, Ciliska D. Implementing evidence-based nursing: some misconceptions. Evidence-Based Nurs 1998; 1: 38–39.

85. Smyth ET, Emmerson AM. Surgical site infection surveillance. J Hosp Infect 2000; 45: 173–184.

86. Finkelstein R, Rabino G, Kassis I, et al. Device-associated, device-day infection rates in an Israeli adult general intensive care unit. J Hosp Infect 2000; 44: 200–205.

87. Emmerson AM. The impact of surveys on hospital infection. J Hosp Infect 1995; 30: 421–440.

88. Stockley JM, Allen RM, Thomlinson DF, et al. A district general hospital's method for post-operative infection surveillance, including post-discharge follow-up, developed over a five-year period. J Hosp Infect 2001; 49: 48–54.

89. Holtz TH, Wenzel RP. Post-discharge surveillance for nosocomial wound infections: a brief review and commentary. J Epidemiol 1992; 121: 182–205.

90. Goldacre MJ, Griffith M, Gill L, et al. In-hospital death as fraction of all deaths within 30 days of hospital admissions for surgery: analysis of routine statistics. BMJ 2002; 324 (7345): 1069–1070.

Further reading

Ayliffe GAJ, Fraise AP, Gedded AM, et al. Control of hospital infection. A practical handbook, 4th edn. London: Arnold; 2000.

Glauser MP, Pizzo PA, eds. Management of infections in immunocompromised patients. London: WB Saunders, 2000; 148–188.

Mims CA, Playfair JHL, Roitt IM, et al. Medical microbiology. Baltimore: Williams and Wilkins; 1993.

Grundy M, ed. Nursing in haematological oncology. Edinburgh: Baillière Tindall; 2000.

Mallett J, Dougherty L. Barrier nursing: nursing the infectious or immunosuppressed patient. In: Mallett J, Dougherty L. The Royal Marsden Hospital manual of clinical nursing procedures, 5th edn. Oxford: Blackwell Science; 2000.

Naylor W, Laverty D, Mallet J, eds. The Royal Marsden Hospital manual of wound management in cancer care. Oxford: Blackwell Science; 2001.

Chapter 24

The mental health needs of perioperative patients

Mark Sewart

'Men are disturbed not by things, but by the views which they take of them.'

Epictetus, 1st Century AD.

Key points

- The role of public attitudes and the media in mental health and illness
- Principal psychiatric disorders and interventions
- Mental health law
- The perioperative patient with mental illness

INTRODUCTION

'At any one time one adult in six suffers from one or other form of mental illness. In other words, mental illnesses are as common as asthma. They range from more common conditions such as deep depression to schizophrenia, which affects fewer than one person in a hundred. Mental illness is not well understood, it frightens people and all too often it carries a stigma'.[1]

This statement comes from the foreword to the *National Service Framework for Mental Health*, a document that by its very existence should highlight the need for reform of mental health services. If the statistics it uses accurately reflect the prevalence of mental health problems, then on average one in six patients being cared for in the perioperative environment may be actively experiencing some form of mental disorder. Furthermore, other statistics suggest that for every three patients with a known mental health problem there will be a fourth who either suffers from an undiagnosed mental disorder or who is unwilling to declare their problems.[2]

A possible view is that patients in the operating theatres are experiencing a challenge to their mental health – stress-induced anxiety – and this may become a problem for those who struggle to cope with stress. The basic, instinctive notion that mental health is indivisible from physical health has been expressed in many forms for millennia. Minimizing the psychological distress caused by physical therapies is quite properly the concern of anyone committed to a holistic approach to care planning and delivery.[3]

No-one should indulge in partisanship over the professional group highlighted in this story. In a study commissioned by the United Kingdom Central Council for Nursing, Midwifery and Health Visiting, a member of a service user focus group reported that 'Non-mental health trained nurses never take your physical complaints seriously, they always think it is part of your mental state'.[4]

Box 24.1   Case study: Misdiagnosis of a patient with mental health problems

The following story is, regrettably, a true one.

A gentleman with a severe and enduring mental health problem experienced a sudden onset of acute abdominal pain. He managed to get to the A&E department, where he was seen by a surgical registrar. The patient's notes had been obtained and reviewed by the registrar prior to his examination of the patient, and he noted that the patient was known to have a psychotic disorder. After the initial enquiry as to the problem, the registrar's response to the patient was: 'Go away and come back when you're prepared to tell us what the problem really is'.

Within 24 hours of the patient returning home, in a distressed, bewildered and profoundly uncomfortable state, he was admitted as an emergency with a perforated appendix. The story might have ended there, but unfortunately, as a result of his treatment, the patient became mentally unwell. Despite having been relatively stable prior to the incident, the experience of his visit to A&E and the emergency surgery triggered his psychosis. In his subsequent paranoid delusional state he believed that the hospital staff were trying to kill him.

RECOGNIZING THE PROBLEM

In 1997 a Joint Working Party of the Royal College of Psychiatrists and the Royal College of Surgeons published a report on the psychological care of surgical patients.[5] The notion is not a new one – although the report's references were impeccably current, other references to relieving the anxiety and distress caused by surgery go back more than half a century, yet the biggest problem in addressing the psychological distress caused by surgery is still the belief that psychological problems are intangible, individual, and 'all in the mind' – and therefore not worthy of serious consideration. Undoubtedly it is 'normal' to experience fear and anxiety when facing surgery. Equally, it would be normal to experience pain from a broken leg but no objections would be raised to giving analgesia. Therefore, it would not seem unreasonable to offer some relief of a patient's psychological distress in the same circumstances.

ATTITUDES

Tackling prejudice, both overt and subconscious, is the cornerstone of an effective and relevant approach to the mental health of perioperative patients. Prejudices are often a product of the society we live in and become subliminally absorbed into our belief systems. Thus they become so embedded in our psyche that they can be difficult or impossible to deal with, even when challenged directly. So it is with mental health issues – for example, a practitioner might conjure up a variety of images if he or she knew that a particular patient on an operating list were a 'known schizophrenic'. The image often owes more to fictional – usually violent – characters who feature all too prominently in cinema and television. The better-informed practitioner might see a frightened and vulnerable individual who will need to be managed with warmth, sensitivity and understanding so that he or she can emerge from their surgical experience intact, in terms of both their physical and their mental health.

Equally, in a society that relies on labels ('diabetic', 'epileptic', 'schizophrenic'), it is quite possible to understand how a whole patient group can be stigmatized. The traditional concept of 'madness' is consistent with the stereotypes and caricatures that society loves to perpetuate. Indeed, in a 1996 survey it was found that almost half of national press coverage of mental health issues linked mental disorders with violence and criminal behaviour.[6] However, people who exhibit the kinds of behaviours that might reinforce these stereotypes probably represent less than 1% of the total number of people in the UK with mental health problems.

In conceptualizing mental health it is possible to view it as a continuum, ranging from serious mental illness at one end to complete holistic wellness at the other.[7] Subscription to this sort of model requires that all of us accept that everybody is somewhere on that continuum. It therefore follows that there can never be any justification in the view – however subconscious – that mental illness is something that happens to somebody else. Nevertheless, it is hard for society, and even sometimes healthcare professionals, to get away from the stereotypical caricature of 'madness'.

THE MEDIA

It is always easy to blame the media when particular groups in society are misrepresented, and yet the media are there to report the news. The media's attitude to mental disorder can best be summed up by one of their own clichés, which itself hints at madness. It is said that if a dog bites a man that is not news, but if a man bites a dog – now that is news. So it is with mental disorder, and most particularly schizophrenia. If a 'schizophrenic' has a good day, week month or year that is not news. If a 'schizophrenic' attacks people then that is news. The fact that a person is more likely to sustain a physical attack from someone with no discernible mental health problems at all, than from someone with a psychotic mental disorder, gains no column inches whatsoever. Of course, the statistics that support this may not be an accurate reflection of the incidence of mental illness in the population as a whole, but are certainly an issue for mental health service users themselves, who feel disadvantaged and stigmatized. In a MIND survey, 60% of patients with a diagnosed mental illness felt media coverage was to blame for the discrimination they experienced.[8]

It is interesting also to note that other adverse events – train crashes for example – usually prompt the media into redressing the balance with expert opinion as to the safety of rail travel. The media rarely seems inclined, however, to draft a credible mental health expert to put the isolated actions of a few disturbed and psychotic people into perspective. If the aspiration implicit in the National Service Framework for Mental Health is to destigmatize those with mental disorders, then unfortunately, although the media could be a powerful ally, they are unlikely to divine much in the way of newsworthy material in such a campaign.

PRINCIPAL DISORDERS

Before embarking on an exploration of typical disorders of mental health it is worth noting that mental disorders rarely conform to textbook definitions. Because at present the origins of most mental disorders are more a matter of speculation than specification, it would be foolish to try and be overly prescriptive and definitive herein. Broadly speaking, mental disorders may be subdivided into two groups, referred to as 'psychotic disorders' and 'anxiety and depressive disorders', which in the past were termed 'psychoses' and 'neuroses'.[9] The former are best described by conditions such as schizophrenia and manic (bipolar) depression. The latter are usually characterized by anxiety, depression, stress disorders (e.g. post-traumatic stress disorder) and any manifestation of phobia.

Consistency in the classification of mental health disorders is sometimes complicated by the fact that there are two slightly different reference works in common use – the World Health Organization's International Classification of Disease part 10 (ICD 10) and the Diagnostic and Statistical Manual edition IV (DSM-IV). In this text the majority of diagnostic material and symptomatology is based on DSM-IV, except where otherwise indicated.

DIAGNOSIS

As with many physical disorders, mental disorders rarely fit neatly into any kind of diagnostic pattern. To make a diagnosis, certain key criteria must be met. Not all of the listed symptoms need be present, provided a certain number – which varies according to the disorder – are present.

PSYCHOTIC DISORDERS

Schizophrenia

'Schizophrenia' is a word that is slowly beginning to fall into disuse, as it is generally regarded as an umbrella term for a wide range of psychotic conditions rather than a definitive diagnosis. It is also probably the most misunderstood and misrepresented word in the health lexicon. Despite deriving from the Greek for 'split mind', the classic stereotype of schizophrenia as the individual with two separate, 'Jekyll and Hyde' personalities is, sadly, instantly recognizable to the general population and largely incomprehensible to mental health professionals. In an attempt to separate the various presentations, DSM-IV gives four subtypes of schizophrenia: paranoid, catatonic, disorganized and undifferentiated.[10] For the purposes of this chapter a broad, generic example is described.

Schizophrenia is thought to be organic in origin, although research is ongoing to identify the definitive pathology of the condition. It is believed to occur as a result of imbalances in chemical neurotransmitters in the brain, leading to a disorder which is characterized by symptoms that fall into two groups, referred to as positive and negative signs (Table 24.1).[11]

Hallucinations are commonly auditory, but may be visual or experienced through smell, taste or touch, or indeed any combination of the senses, sometimes giving the individual a complete sensory experience that is more real to them than reality itself. Thus auditory hallucinations are typically described as being louder and 'more real' than simply hearing one's own thoughts. However, most people's 'voices' are idiosyncratic and unique, often being described as having someone following immediately behind you and talking into your ear, or like carrying around a backpack with stereo speakers attached. The voices are not always hostile, but most typically are derogatory, threatening, and derisive of the hearer, chipping away at their confidence and self-esteem at one end of the spectrum and rendering them helpless with fear at the other.

Table 24.1   Positive and negative signs for schizophrenia

Positive	Negative
Hallucinations	'Flat' emotional response
Delusions	Poverty of speech
Behavioural disorganization	Social withdrawal and isolation
Hostility	Lack of spontaneity or interests
Disorganized or chaotic thoughts	Impaired concentration

Delusions are not unique to psychotic disorders, but feature in those who hear voices, most frequently as some form of explanation, or 'irrational rationalization' of the voices. For example, where bereavement has triggered the psychosis the voice or voices may seem to belong to the deceased relative or loved one. However, to take another example from many, individuals claiming to hear voices from the radio or TV may equally be struggling to find an explanation for the source of the voices. If the intensity of the voices overwhelms the part of the brain responsible for interpreting speech, the brain may be unable to differentiate between what someone on the TV is saying and what the individual is hearing, causing the hearer to believe – or at least be unable to fully refute the belief – that the person on TV is talking to them, or about them. This latter point is important. Many of those who hear voices know full well that they are a part of their disorder, and that no matter how real they seem they are not; and yet, as the voices are often with them most or all of the time, it is impossible to deny them completely. This phenomenon of incorporating fragments of reality into the unreality of individual perception potentially renders the sufferer extremely vulnerable while undergoing general anaesthesia. The altered perceptions may be many times more disturbing to someone who is already predisposed to a unique interpretation of reality.

As a consequence of hallucinations and delusions individuals may find their ability to deal with the routine minutiae of everyday life severely impaired. This is usually noted in the other positive signs of disorganized and chaotic behaviour. Where the delusions involve paranoid elements the person may become untrusting of or even hostile to others, if those others are believed to be acting against the person.

Negative symptomatology follows on from these precursors, causing the individual to withdraw from social and family groupings and attempt to grapple with their inner turmoil alone. The sheer effort required to learn to live with these symptoms leaves the individual exhausted, which further contributes to their inability to function effectively.

Typically, during periods of stability the individual may have insight into their condition. Unfortunately, the psychopathology of schizophrenia usually means that if they become unwell again that insight is lost.

Bipolar affective disorder

Depression as a concept should need no introduction. Clinical depression, however, is often a complex and intangible concept and features across the spectrum of mental disorders. Depression, which includes as its principal characteristic psychotic symptoms, interwoven with extremes of elation and misery – polarized moods – is referred to as bipolar affective disorder. Previously this disorder was known as 'manic depression' or 'manic depressive psychosis'. The key features of this disorder are the polarized extremities of mood. Other symptomatologies may often be confused with schizophrenia, leading to overlapping diagnoses. The classic features of bipolar affective disorder during the manic phase are as follows:

- Hallucinations – usually auditory
- Delusions – grandiose as below or persecutory
- Grandiose delusions and behaviours
- Euphoria and elation
- Evidence of thought disorder – pressure of speech, incongruence, rhyming and puns
- Sleep disturbances
- Irritability and demanding behaviour
- Violence (rarely) and aggression
- Lack of insight
- Vulnerability to suggestion and exploitation.

There is usually some evidence of thought disorder, often characterized by pressure of speech, a problem often evident in children where, simply put, the brain is working faster than the mouth can move. There are further clues contained in speech, such as inadvertent puns and 'clang association', which is typically understood to mean the juxtaposition of inappropriate words, phrases or concepts. Other evidence to support the diagnosis may be gained from observed irritability, insomnia, demanding behaviour, aggression or violence.

The transition between euphoria and elation and a state of hopelessness and misery is as individual as the person experiencing it, although it is in terms of days or weeks rather than hours. At the other end of the spectrum, symptomatology during the depressive phase is as follows:

- Insomnia/hypersomnia, interrupted sleep and, classically, early morning wakening
- Listlessness and fatigue
- Constipation
- Weight loss
- Loss of appetite/overeating

- Extreme low mood – becoming lower as the day progresses
- Anhedonia (inability to find enjoyment or pleasure in anything)
- Hopelessness, guilt, self-blame
- Thoughts of suicide
- Agitation and impeded motor functioning.

During periods of depression the individual may experience a level of hopelessness and despair that goes beyond suicidal – indeed, the danger time is when an individual is on the transition from depression and becoming relatively well. The same is true when they are coming down from a period of euphoria, often with the aid of medication. During the euphoric phase they believe they can take on the world. It is only when they come down – or are brought down – from that high that they realize their situation. Representatives of 'user groups' have described the phenomenon as 'suddenly realizing what an awful life you have', although the language is usually more colourful. It should be unsurprising, therefore, that such people are at a greater risk of suicide.

Other psychoses

There are believed to be a number of distinct psychotic conditions which have in the past been grouped together as 'schizophrenia'. Indeed, there is growing evidence of psychotic symptoms overlapping into the classic neuroses, further complicating diagnosis and definitive treatment. Whereas it is usual for there to be some identifiable cause of physical problems that may be treated, in mental health the cause is most frequently unknown and therefore the clinical management is reduced to treating the symptoms. This is often where the mental health nurse can step in, using generic and specialist nursing skills to 'help the client help themselves' and offer the sort of emotional and psychological support that is necessary.

Disorders that appear to mimic schizophrenia but which lack some of the definitive diagnostic criteria are termed schizotypal or schizoaffective disorders. These diagnoses may ultimately be refined into schizophrenia, but as a key diagnostic criterion for schizophrenia is for symptoms to persist longer than 6 months, psychotic episodes of lesser duration followed by a return to premorbid levels of functioning may well attract an initial diagnosis of schizotypal or schizoaffective disorder. Equally, episodes of this nature sometimes occur once or twice only, leaving the individual fully recovered. This illustrates one of the key drivers behind the move to make a firm diagnosis of schizophrenia with great caution. The erroneous perception is that once someone is diagnosed as schizophrenic they have no hope of recovery or a normal life. Therefore, clinicians need to be in no doubt whatsoever before they hang such an evocative and stigmatizing label on anyone.

Drug-induced psychosis normally results from drug use but sometimes occurs as a result of alcohol problems. A full recovery is possible provided the dependence is successfully treated. As with schizo-affective disorders there is a need to be aware that, once fully rehabilitated, individuals who have experienced drug induced psychosis need never exhibit psychotic symptoms again, although they may carry an increased risk.

ANXIETY AND DEPRESSIVE DISORDERS (NEUROSES)

These conditions are not without their stigma – who has not heard or indeed used the term 'neurotic' in a disparaging and derogatory way? There are those who make light of this group, referring to them as the 'worried well'. This is grossly unreasonable. Disorders such as anxiety and depression can be severely disabling, and an unsympathetic and perfunctory approach from healthcare professionals can exacerbate the distress and misery experienced by this group.

Anxiety

Anxiety is a concept with which every perioperative practitioner should be familiar. Most anxiety disorders can be seen to be extensions of common, everyday anxieties made worse by an order of magnitude. For example, walking through a busy area may cause the average person to become more vigilant and alert. In such circumstances a sufferer of one of the anxiety disorders may become highly distressed, even paralysed with fear, and yet the physiological responses involved are initially identical. It is the inability of the individual with the anxiety disorder to cope with those responses that fuels the fear, the panic and the subsequent behaviours, leaving them overwhelmed with feelings ranging from profound dread to abject terror. It is thought that everyday anxieties may develop into abnormal and disabling conditions as a result of

many factors: environmental, social, occupational, bereavement and so forth.

Anxiety may present in such a way that anyone would be able to identify it, or it may quite inexplicably disable someone who has never appeared overtly anxious. It is quite possible for apparently physical symptoms to have arisen from an anxiety state owing to autonomic arousal. An individual may not consciously feel 'anxious' but may be displaying physical symptoms which are indeed due to an anxiety imperceptible to that individual. This phenomenon can often be problematic. Imagine attending your GP complaining of headaches, nausea, dizziness and palpitations. You may attribute these to any number of physical ailments, but anxiety is likely to be at the very bottom of the list, if it features at all. Yet this very characteristic should serve to demonstrate that mental and physical well-being really is indivisible. Furthermore, theatre staff and their colleagues on the surgical wards need to be aware that there are physiological effects of anxiety that may cause real physical problems. 'Prolonged anxiety leads to increased protein breakdown, decreased wound healing, decreased immune response, increased risk of infection, and fluid and electrolyte balance disturbance'.[12]

Anxiety may be subdivided into categories which derive from their principal presenting symptomatologies:

- Generalized anxiety disorder
- Panic disorders
- Obsessive-compulsive disorder
- Phobias.

However, there may be features from more than one recognized disorder. Physical symptoms of anxiety may include some or all of the following:

- Headache
- Dizziness
- Flushing
- Palpitations
- Sweating
- Dry mouth
- Diarrhoea
- Frequency of micturition.

Hypochondria or hypochondriasis is an anxiety disorder, features of which can often be seen in other diagnoses. From the list of physical symptoms above it should be easy to see that it would be quite possible to rationalize physical symptoms as something life threatening and terminal, or simply enough of a cause of distress to warrant repeated presentations for help. The phenomenon of somatization – i.e. giving physical expression to feelings of anxiety, guilt, self-hatred, etc. – is not restricted to hypochondriasis and may be seen as a feature of many disorders, principally with an anxiety base but also across the spectrum of mental health problems. Nevertheless, for those enduring such an experience it can be distressing, frightening, and of course painful. How much more distressing, frightening and painful would it be for them to be told they were imagining it all? It is not unusual for the patient to accept that they may be exaggerating the symptoms, and whereas this is useful to exclude a delusional component it may do little to relieve the patient's distress.

Phobias Phobias are well known, but little understood, phenomena. Arachnophobia, claustrophobia, agoraphobia and many others are words that have passed into common, if often inappropriate, usage. In a piece bluntly entitled 'A Survey of Pre-operative Fear', Ramsay[13] found that there was a high response rate to enquiries regarding fear and anxiety before surgery. As a registrar in anaesthetics, Ramsay may have been sobered by the fact that, by a large margin, most patients actually feared the anaesthetic more than the surgery.[13]

It is quite possible, however, to become phobic about anything, and hospital and needle phobias are common. Phobias are sometimes linked with panic attacks, in that both conditions are examples of autonomic anxiety responses to stimuli. Panic attacks may differ, however, in that the trigger may not be apparent to the individual, whereas the phobic patient knows what it is they fear. They commonly also know that that fear is irrational, but as with many mental disorders there is not necessarily a functioning link between knowing something and really believing it.

Depression

Depression is surprisingly common. In fact, studies suggest that clinical depression will affect one in four men and one in two women at some point in their lives. What sets clinical depression apart from 'everyday' depression is severity and duration. A diagnosis of depression may be made if three key symptoms are present: persistent low mood, anhedonia (an absence of the ability to experience pleasure) and fatigue, combined with four other

symptoms associated with depression, which may include some of the following:

- Irritability
- Preoccupation and withdrawal
- Reduced libido
- Appetite changes
- Sleep changes
- Poor concentration
- Loss of interest/inattentiveness
- Guilt.

Furthermore, the period of depression should have lasted for at least 2 weeks before definitive diagnosis is made.

The World Health Organization believes that by 2020 depression will be second only to heart disease in terms of its burden on health care worldwide. Furthermore, UK government figures suggest that 30% of the workforce will experience a mental health problem each year, with the majority being anxiety and depression disorders.[14]

Depression as a concept rather than a specific condition is problematic in mental health because it has the ability to straddle the whole area. Mild to moderate depression is classically the sort of condition that can be handled in a primary care setting and offers a reasonable prognosis, whereas depression can become a functional part of psychosis. Indeed, depression is often a secondary diagnosis in psychotic disorders.

Eating disorders

A great deal of attention is paid to eating disorders in the media, which is somewhat ironic as the media arguably have some responsibility for the stereotypical images that fuel these disorders. The two principal disorders of note are anorexia nervosa and bulimia. The former is characterized by early onset, predominantly but not exclusively in girls aged 12–18, and normally begins with obsessive behaviour regarding eating, reducing consumption to near starvation levels. The behaviour is as a result of a perception by the individual that they do not meet the standards that society appears to them to have set. The latter is typically later in onset, if derived from a similar motivation, and may have developed from earlier anorexia. There are similarities between the eating disorders and body dysmorphic disorder. However, this condition more often relates to specific features of the body rather than its overall size and shape. It may have an element of hypochondriasis and, in common with that condition, can often lead to repeated presentation to medical services.

It cannot be stressed enough that, for people experiencing any kind of mental disorder, their perception of reality is their reality, and although it might be proper to challenge it in a controlled, careful manner, a blunt, direct dismissal of their feelings or beliefs is likely to erect barriers rather than serve any useful therapeutic function.

SUICIDE AND SELF-HARM

The risk of suicide in the general population is relatively low. However, the risk among those experiencing mental health problems is significantly increased. Standard 7 of the National Service Framework for Mental Health addresses the issue of suicide directly. The government's own target, based on *Saving Lives: Our Healthier Nation,* is to reduce suicides by one-fifth by 2010–15. The National Service Framework itself observes that in an average primary care group based on a population of 100 000 one could expect 10 suicides per year. However, it goes on to point out that of those 10, only 2 or 3 are likely to be currently known to mental health services.[15] It might be argued that those 2 or 3 represent the 'one-fifth' in the government's target.

Suicide is a hugely complex issue. Very often even the act itself leaves behind a great deal of uncertainty, and coroners are reluctant to record a verdict of suicide unless it is absolutely incontrovertible. In fact, there are at least three subtypes within what the general population perceive as suicide, namely completed suicide, parasuicide and attempted suicide.

Completed suicide is usually preceded by certain observable behaviours. There is likely to be evidence of extreme low mood, although the 'public face' of someone contemplating suicide may not indicate the severity of the lowered mood. There may be 'boat burning' behaviour – giving away treasured possessions, terminating relationships, etc. The individual may even actively tell people of their plans, although this is often also a feature of parasuicide. The fact that 7 or 8 out of every 10 people who commit suicide are not currently known to mental health services is significant. It points to an urgent need for a greater understanding of mental health issues across the range of healthcare disciplines and in the general population as a whole.

Parasuicide is usually characterized by what appears to be a suicide attempt, the circumstances of which have features indicative of a wish by the person involved to be discovered or otherwise rescued. This sort of behaviour has been described as 'a cry for help', which should not be dismissed or ignored. Sadly, there is always the risk of an unintended lethal outcome.

Attempted suicide is generally regarded to mean a genuine attempt that proves unsuccessful. Considering the likely state of mind of someone who genuinely tries to kill themselves – they most likely consider themselves a failure – the fact that they failed even to commit suicide successfully will do nothing to enhance their self-esteem and places them at high risk of further attempts.

Self-harm often appears alongside suicide but should really be considered as a separate entity. The individual who presents with multiple superficial lacerations to the wrists and forearms is unlikely to have sustained those injuries as a result of attempted or parasuicide. Self-harming behaviour is a complex issue in its own right and is used to relieve stress or distress. The example above is the more obvious face of self-harm and is often referred to as 'self-mutilation'. However, other types of self-harm exist, such as self-neglect, self-poisoning, or even addiction, in the context of the addiction being considered self-destructive. The causes are as complex as the presentations, but most frequently involve some form of abuse and deprivation in childhood, which leads to extremely low self-worth and the use of self-destructive behaviours to externalize the feelings of worthlessness.

PERSONALITY DISORDER

Personality disorders are said to be present when there is no other evidence of any functional mental illness and yet there is still evidence of dysfunctional or maladaptive behaviour. It has thus reopened the 'nature or nurture' debate, the ongoing discussion about whether or not an individual is born with a predisposition to certain behaviours or whether they have been learned in early life. These behaviours are often problematic, and although they may appear similar to recognized mental disorders it is often possible to exclude them in reaching a diagnosis of personality disorder. The terms psychopath and sociopath are no longer used, but were previously attributed to those diagnosed with some form of personality disorder.

In the field of mental health there are those who practise on the basis that personality disorder is not a mental illness, and therefore nothing can be done for someone so diagnosed. Conversely, some believe that improvements may be achievable, principally through non-medical interventions. In an echo of the attention that focused on schizophrenia, the public perception of personality disorder is inescapably a preoccupation with dangerous and severe or antisocial personality disorders. However, there are many other manifestations, and as with all disorders, both physical and mental, there are an infinite number of levels of severity, combinations, dual and multiple diagnoses that may affect the individual. Elements of personality disorder, for example, may be present in someone with an organic mental health disorder. DSM-IV lists 11 personality disorders, including 'personality disorder not otherwise specified'. Of the 10 others it is interesting to note that some echo the organic disorder they mimic, for example 'schizotypal personality disorder'. It should therefore be easy to see that definitive diagnosis in mental health is always challenging – where does mental illness end and personality disorder begin?

INTERVENTIONS

The medical model is only one of many that may be utilized in considering the treatment and management of people with mental health problems, but it serves well to understand the pharmacology of mental health. Patients often expect the doctor to give them a pill that will make them better. Although there are pharmaceutical aids to treatment, the expectations of the client can be a barrier to effective clinical management where other non-medicinal treatments and strategies are indicated. Other methods cover a range of interventions involving medicine, nursing, psychology and occupational therapy, as well as other professions allied to medicine.

PHARMACOLOGY

To maintain perspective on the scale of mental health issues it is noteworthy that in 1996, for example, 25% of drugs prescribed on the NHS were for mental health problems.[16] Treatment of mental disorders by medication depends on there being some organic pathology for the medication to act on. Schizophrenia, for example, is believed by many to occur as a result of higher than usual levels of dopamine in the brain. This permits the transmission of more information than the receiving part of the brain can process, resulting in hallucinatory phenomena, cognitive dysfunction and chaotic behaviour. Administration of an appropriate antipsychotic preparation can successfully modify dopamine reception or absorption in the brain, resulting in reduced symptomatology. However, most antipsychotic medications induce dramatic side effects, which can have a greater impact on the individual than the symptoms the medication was intended to alleviate. Small wonder, then, that there is a reluctance among clients to take this kind of medication. In the past this was usually interpreted as non-compliance stemming from the client's disorder, but there is now an increased understanding of the importance of weighing management of symptoms against quality of life, resulting in greater sensitivity and flexibility in prescribing. One client known to the author summed up the difficulties he encountered by saying that he could stop the voices by taking the prescribed amount of his medication, but in so doing the side effects would effectively stop him. Therefore, contrary to his medical advice, he modified his dosages by trial and error until he found a level that allowed him to cope with reduced symptoms and still maintain a 'normal' level of functioning.

Antipsychotic medication is divided into two types, typical and atypical. Typical antipsychotics are the older drugs, such as chlorpromazine and haloperidol. Then there are the newer atypical drugs, such as olanzapine and risperidone. People with serious and enduring mental health problems are likely to have tried examples of both types. The most troublesome side effects of the typical antipsychotics were what are termed extrapyramidal side effects – essentially drug-induced parkinsonism. Unfortunately, once someone has developed these side effects they often persist, even if the medication is changed to an atypical drug. However, even the newer drugs have their problems. Olanzapine, for example, can cause a significant increase in appetite, resulting in weight gain. Nutritional advice has always been offered to clients with psychosis, but such advice has taken on a new importance since the introduction of this particular drug.

Perioperative patients who may be taking antipsychotic and adjunctive medications may be at higher risk during anaesthesia owing to certain interactions. Furthermore, patients with psychosis may often also be being treated for secondary disorders, such as depression and anxiety.

As with antipsychotics, antidepressants are similarly subdivided, but into three, and it is the action of the drug that is used for differentiation. The older antidepressants are the tricyclics and the MAOIs or monoamine oxidase inhibitors. Tricyclics act by blocking enzymes in the brain which are believed to be impairing neurotransmission. Examples are amitriptyline, clomipramine and dosulepin (dothiepin).

MAOIs are seldom used in current practice because of their inefficiency and side effects. As the name suggests, they act by inhibiting the enzyme monoamine oxidase A, which is one of those thought to be primarily responsible for impairing neurotransmission.

Newer preparations are referred to as selective serotonin reuptake inhibitors (SSRI). This group act more specifically than the other preparations, focusing on the levels of the neurotransmitter enzyme serotonin in the brain. Blockading the synaptic receptors for serotonin increases the available serotonin in the synaptic space. Examples of SSRIs are fluoxetine (better known as Prozac), paroxetine and sertraline.

In order to ensure the safety and appropriate care of patients under active pharmacological treatment for mental health problems it is important to have an understanding of the actions of psychiatric drugs, particularly in relation to any potential interactions that might occur with anaesthetics, analgesics and other drugs commonly used in the operating department. If it is known that a patient is on such treatment an understanding that there are potential dangers should at least prompt practitioners to check whether there are any significant contraindications or interactions of note. To help

Table 24.2 The principal known drug interactions in surgery and anaesthesia

Drug	Interaction	Drug
Antipsychotics	Increased hypotensive effects	Anaesthetics and antihypertensives
	Increased sedative effects	Opioid analgesics, anxiolytics and hypnotics
	Increased ventricular arrhythmias	Antiarrhythmics
	Possible risk of arrhythmias and/or convulsions	Certain antibiotics
	Convulsive threshold lowered	Antiepileptics
	Risk of ventricular arrhythmias	Antihistamines and β-blockers
	Increased extrapyramidal side effects	Antiemetics
	Increased side effects	Antimuscarinics
Antidepressants	Risk of neurotoxicity with use of more than one	Antidepressants
	Hypertension and arrhythmias	Adrenaline (epinephrine) (local anaesthetics containing adrenaline appear safe)
	Increased plasma concentrations < >	Antipsychotics, some anxiolytics and hypnotics and β-blockers
	Possible increase in coagulation effects	Anticoagulants
	Lowered convulsion threshold	Antiepileptics
	Risk of arrhythmias	Antihistamines and β-blockers
	Sedative effects	
	Hypertension and overstimulation of the central nervous system	Dopaminergics
	Increased effects on central nervous system	Lithium
	Risk of convulsions (with tramadol)	Opioid analgesics
	Reduced effect of sublingual preparations	Nitrates
Anxiolytics and hypnotics	Enhanced sedative effect	Anaesthetics, opioid analgesics, antidepressants, antipsychotics, antihistamines, β-blockers and muscle relaxants
	May increase plasma levels of the anxiolytic/hypnotic	Antibiotics
	Increased hypotension	Antihypertensives

facilitate this, Table 24.2 summarizes the principal known interactions.

COMMUNICATION

There may be little the practitioner feels able to do for people with actual or potential mental problems encountered in the operating department. Certainly the bulk of academic work on the reduction of anxiety and induced stress quite rightly focuses on the preoperative and postoperative phases, and it is here that the most valuable work can be done. However, there is a continual move towards day-case and particularly local anaesthetic surgery, which is starting to erode the mystery of what lies behind the operating room door. There is more opportunity for a patient-focused approach to care with patients undergoing procedures using local anaesthesia. Furthermore, perioperative practitioners often develop a high level of interpersonal skills because of the pressures of working within a team in such a challenging area, and because of the relatively short time that they have to gain the patient's trust and confidence.

It is often of limited value to recommend particular approaches to interpersonal behaviour. It may be more useful to ensure that practitioners are adequately informed about mental health issues and for them then to use that information to modify their approach to interpersonal relationships. In other words, it is not possible to teach practitioners how to talk to people with mental health problems. However, if practitioners approach all patients from a position of unconditional positive regard and respect for them as human beings, then a working knowledge of mental health issues may enable them to use their existing communication skills more effectively.

Because of either the symptoms of the disorder or the debilitating nature of the side effects, people who are receiving treatment may present with additional communication problems. The importance of unconditional positive regard for the patient cannot be understated. As one patient put it, 'just because we take antipsychotics, it doesn't mean we take "stupid pills" as well'. 'Unconditional positive regard'[17] is a phrase most often attributed to psychologist Carl Rogers and, as stated earlier, the spirit of it is to approach all patients from a position of respect and an acknowledgement of their fundamental worth as human beings. Two related facets of interpersonal relationships that are brought into sharp focus by the perioperative experience are 'locus of control' and the 'power differential'. Locus of control refers to the abdication of responsibility to another and is representative of the classic notion of 'your life in their hands'. This will inevitably cause some anxiety even in the best-prepared patient, and is supported by the fact that most studies of perioperative anxiety suggest that the anaesthetic provokes more anxiety than the surgery itself.[18] Power differential can be seen in many settings. For example, it exists between senior and junior members of any group of people, theatre staff included, and is central to any hierarchical structure. For many years the power differential between doctors and patients was seen as something of a gulf, whereas in a more contemporary light that gap is narrowing. Yet in the context of locus of control how much more power could one human being exercise over another than to render them unconscious, unable even to breathe for themselves, and to keep them in that state for a lengthy period? Therefore, anything that minimizes the psychological impact of that key, immediate preoperative period will be a positive contribution to the total care of that patient.

MENTAL HEALTH LAW

The current Mental Health Act of 1983 (MHA 83) is based largely on the Act of 1959, which itself drew heavily on earlier legislation.[19] At the time of writing, MHA 83 is under review pending the drafting of new legislation. Much has happened in clinical mental health practice and the society such practice seeks to serve in the last 19 years, and a great deal of the legislation attracts considerable debate and criticism in the contemporary setting.

Certain sections of MHA 83 permit treatment to be carried out against the wishes of the client who is the subject of the section. However, the only treatment that may be given is that prescribed by the patient's consultant psychiatrist, or another doctor who is approved under section 12 of the Act, and must relate specifically to the client's mental illness. In short, the fact that a mental health client is detained in accordance with a section of MHA 83 does not mean that they forfeit all of their rights in terms of consent to treatment – only very specific, targeted treatments may be given for specific expected outcomes in relation to a client's mental health, and only for specified periods. This may also include the use of electroconvulsive therapy (ECT).

ECT

ECT is still indicated in the management of major depressive disorders, and despite the controversy that has always surrounded the treatment there is enough empirical evidence to support its continued use. In some operating departments there may be a requirement for theatre staff to participate in ECT. Some hospitals have dedicated ECT facilities or even dedicated staff, but the infrequency with which this treatment is utilized means that it is uneconomical for smaller hospitals to sustain such a service.

ECT is believed to act on the brain in the same way as antidepressants, but more efficiently and without the side effects of the available drugs. ECT itself has side effects, the most common of which is short-term memory loss, but it is still regarded as a valid treatment. Informal patients, i.e. those who are not detained in hospital, must give their consent for treatment. This consent is usually well informed owing to the collaborative, patient-centred care planning that occurs in mental health. Patients who are subject to detention and treatment under the Mental Health Act do not surrender all of their rights to refuse treatment. Where ECT has been prescribed and is to be carried out against the patient's will it can only proceed when the appropriate paperwork is complete and available. Patients may be given treatment against their wishes while they are detained under sections 2 or 3 of MHA 83. As ECT is usually carried out over a period of 8 to 12 treatments it is unlikely someone would be having ECT on a section 2, as this is only for 28 days. Such planned care would in all likelihood prompt a review and application for a section 3 where appropriate. Section 58 of MHA 83 allows for specified treatments, including ECT, to be given with either the patient's consent or a second opinion by a doctor appointed by the Mental Health Act Commission, the body that oversees the application of MHA 83 in practice. It is therefore important that theatre staff asked to assist in carrying out ECT

treatment familiarize themselves with the paperwork in exactly the same way as they would with a consent form. Patients undergoing ECT should be accompanied by a qualified mental health nurse, who should be able to produce the relevant form. It is advisable to ensure that mental health units are supplied with preoperative checklists (many have devised their own in partnership with theatre staff), which should indicate that the relevant forms – Form 38 for patients who consent and Form 39 if a second opinion has had to be sought – have been correctly completed and are available.

Caring for distressed and frightened people undergoing this procedure will always be a challenge. Provided the theatre staff take a gentle and sympathetic approach and are mindful of the legal aspects and cognisant of the nature of the patient's illness, then the psychological impact of the experience can be minimized as far as possible.

CONCLUSION

If the practitioner believes that care should be continuous and unbroken throughout a patient's hospital stay, then he or she should understand the mental health needs of their patients if they wish to deliver truly holistic care. On the other hand, if the practitioner has succumbed to the quantitative, output-driven, automated, depersonalized, conveyorbelt approach to care that may be the result of long waiting lists and short deadlines, then such concerns will be of marginal relevance.

The Joint Working Party of the Royal College of Surgeons and the Royal College of Psychiatrists recommends that links be forged between perioperative and mental health professionals.[4] A wider understanding of the issues discussed in this chapter will go some way to forging such links. The contents of this chapter can be used to inform and enhance practitioners' approaches to the care of their patients in the furtherance of quality care delivery in the operating department.

References

1. Department of Health. A national service framework for mental health. London: HMSO; 1999.
2. Jenkins R, Bebbington P, Brugha TS, et al. British psychiatric morbidity survey. Br J Psychiatry 1998; 173: 4–7.
3. Harrison A. The mental health needs of patients in physical care settings. Nurs Standard 2001; 15: 47–56.
4. United Kingdom Central Council for Nursing, Midwifery and Health Visiting. The nursing, midwifery and health visiting contribution to the continuing care of people with mental health problems: a review and UKCC action plan. London: UKCC; 2000.

5. Joint Working Party of the Royal College of Surgeons of England and Royal College of Psychiatrists. The psychological care of surgical patients CR55. London: Royal College of Surgeons of England and Royal College of Psychiatrists; 1997.

6. Ward G. Making headlines. London: Health Education Authority; 1997.

7. Lancaster J. Adult psychiatric nursing. New York: Medical Examination Publishing; 1988.

8. Read J, Baker S. Not just sticks and stones: a survey of the stigma, taboos and discrimination experienced by people with mental health problems. London: MIND; 1996.

9. Gibb RC, Macpherson GJD. A common language of classification and understanding. In: Thompson T, Mathias P, eds. Lyttle's mental health and disorder, 3rd edn. Edinburgh: Baillière Tindall; 2000

10. American Psychiatric Association. Diagnostic and statistical manual of mental disorders, 4th edn. Washington, DC: American Psychiatric Association; 1994.

11. Rethink. What is schizophrenia? Rethink. Online. Available: http://www.rethinkcarers.org/standard.asp?id=50 Surrey.

12. Martin D. Pre-operative visits to reduce patient anxiety: a study. Nurs Standard 1996; 10: 33–38.

13. Ramsay M. A survey of pre-operative fear. Anaesthesia 1972; 27: 396–402.

14. Office for National Statistics. Surveys of psychiatric morbidity in Great Britain. Report Three – Economic activity and social functioning of adults with psychiatric disorders. Norwich: The Stationery Office; 1995.

15. Department of Health. Saving lives: our healthier nation. London: HMSO; 1998.

16. Department of Health. Statistics of prescriptions dispensed in FHSAs: England 1985–1995. London: HMSO; 1996.

17. Rogers CR. On becoming a person: a therapist's view of psychotherapy. New York: Houghton Mifflin; 1961.

18. Mitchell M. Psychological preparation for patients undergoing day surgery. Ambul Surg 2000; 8: 19–29.

19. Jones R. Mental Health Act manual, 6th edn. London: Sweet and Maxwell; 1999.

Further reading

Birchwood M, Tarrier N. Psychological management of schizophrenia. Chichester: Wiley; 1994.

Rogers CR. On becoming a person: a therapist's view of psychotherapy. New York: Houghton Mifflin; 1961.

Thompson T, Mathias P, eds. Lyttle's mental health and disorder, 3rd edn. Edinburgh Baillière Tindall; 2000.

Acknowledgements

The following are sincerely thanked for their support and guidance: Mr P Goward, Mr S Hemingway and Mr S Chady, Department of Mental Health and Learning Disabilities, Nursing School of Nursing and Midwifery, University of Sheffield; Mr G Cockshutt, Mental Health Training and Consultancy.

Chapter 25

Transplantation

Peter Mercer

Key points

- Donor registers
- Brainstem death
- Donation
- Post-transplant complications
- Immunosuppression and rejection

HISTORY

In 1996 organ transplantation passed its golden jubilee. It was in 1946 that the first renal isograft transplant operation was undertaken in Boston, Massachusetts. Since that time further milestones have been achieved, with the first liver transplant being performed in the USA by Dr Thomas Starzl and the first heart transplant by Dr Christiaan Barnard in South Africa, in 1967.

In the UK the first transplants were performed of a liver at Addenbrooke's Hospital in Cambridge in 1968, the first heart at Papworth Hospital in Cambridge in 1979, and the first kidney at King's College Hospital in 1965.

In the intervening years transplantation has become a tried and tested mode of treatment for patients with a wide variety of conditions. This chapter will seek to address the infrastructure that supports transplantation in the UK. It will explain the role and responsibilities of the regulatory body Unrelated Live Transplant Regulatory Authority (ULTRA), and that of UK Transplant. It will address the pathways for organ donation and for organ recipients across the transplant types. Consideration will be given to the surgical management of patients and the medical follow-up, including post-transplant complications. Immunosuppressive therapy will also be addressed.

TERMINOLOGY

Transplantation can be performed between varying combinations of donors and recipients in an attempt to maximize the usage of donated organs and their availability to suitable recipients. To clarify the groupings the following terminology is commonly used:

- *Allograft*: a transplant performed most commonly between individuals of the same species but not genetically identical
- *Autograft*: transplant performed from one tissue site to another in the same individual, e.g. skin grafting
- *Isograft*: transplant performed most commonly between individuals who are of the same species and are genetically identical, as in identical twins
- *Xenograft*: transplant performed most commonly between individuals who are not of the same species and not genetically identical, for example pig to human transplantation
- *Cadaveric*: this term is applied to donors who are confirmed as brain dead according to strict criteria
- *Living donor*: this term is applied to donors who are alive and who may or may not be related to the potential recipient. This is mostly commonly seen in renal transplantation
- *Orthotopic*: the diseased organ is removed and replaced by the transplanted organ lying in the normal anatomical position
- *Heterotopic*: the transplanted organ is placed in a different anatomical position from normal.

ROLE OF UK TRANSPLANT

The UK Transplant Support Service Authority (UKTSSA) was set up as a Special Health Authority (SHA) in 1991 to support transplant activities on a national basis. The Authority is funded by the Department of Health. Following a review of the role and function of the UKTSSA in 2000, it was decided that changes were necessary to meet the changing nature of transplant activities. These changes included:

- Improving and increasing organ procurement
- Supporting transplant coordinators
- Maintenance of the National Transplant Database
- Clinical audit activity
- User Advisory Groups reorganization
- Improving IT systems and support.

To manage this process UKTSSA was renamed UK Transplant. The infrastructure to implement the corporate and business plans was reorganized to assist in delivering changes over a 5-year period.

The day-to-day function of UK Transplant is managed from its headquarters in Bristol, from where the national waiting list for all transplant recipients is maintained. This enables matching of donor organs to suitable recipients.

NATIONAL TRANSPLANT DATABASE

All of the renal, liver and cardiothoracic transplant centres are obliged to provide information and data on patients being referred for transplantation or organ donation. The data are collected at local Trust level and subsequently transferred in paper or electronic format to UKT for entry into the National Database. This contains in excess of 30 years' worth of data on all patients in the UK, and is managed by the Data Executive at UK Transplant.

The database is used to inform NHS, Royal College and transplant community users on many elements of patient assessment, operation and follow-up. Statistical analyses of the data are available to assist clinical staff in transplant units in making informed decisions regarding patient care.

Access to the database is being extended to include local users, who can interrogate it via the Internet. This information can subsequently be used to inform research, audit and clinical governance activity. Evidence of the benefits of such extensive data collection can be seen in organ-specific audits, the Transplant Activity Audit and the UKT Annual Report. These are available via the UK Transplant website, http://www.uktransplant.org.uk

ORGAN DONOR REGISTER

The NHS Organ Donor Register, opened in 1993, is managed by staff at UK Transplant in Bristol. The intention of the Register is to capture as many

members of the public as possible who are prepared to state their desire to donate organs at the
time of death. Entry is gained by registration at GP
surgeries or by completion of a form when applying for a driving licence via DVLA.

The Register is used to assist transplant coordinators when they are discussing organ donation
possibilities with clinicians and relatives. Similar to
the 'donor card', it confirms the stated intentions of
the potential organ donor while leaving the ultimate decision of whether to proceed to donation
with close relatives or spouses. At present more
than 8 million people are registered with the Organ
Donor Register.

ROLE OF ULTRA

The Unrelated Live Transplant Regulatory Authority
(ULTRA) was set up following the publication of
the Human Organ Transplant Act 1989 and, under
guidance from the Department of Health, is responsible for approving transplant operations. This
gives legal sanction to all transplants involving a
living donor who is not a close blood relative of the
recipient.

The membership of ULTRA comprises doctors,
nurses, scientists and others who take informed
ethical decisions on the suitability of a donor to
donate an organ to another. After a full medical
assessment of the potential donor's suitability, an
independent assessor becomes involved. The assessor works separately from members of the transplant team to clarify the degree of knowledge and
insight each donor has into the risks, benefits and
reasons for donating. Following an interview the
assessor completes a summary report which seeks
to ensure donation is made free from coercion or
exploitation.

Specifically, what ULTRA needs to know is:

- That the donor has not been paid to donate and
  that no other pressure has been brought to bear
- That the doctor who asks for approval from
  ULTRA is acting on behalf of the donor
- That both donor and recipient have been seen by
  an independent assessor and have been fully
  informed by the doctors responsible for both that:
  - the donor understands the nature and risks
    involved in donating an organ
  - consent is freely and fully given
  - the donor understands that consent can be
    withdrawn at any time before the operation.

WHAT IS BRAINSTEM DEATH?

Conditions under which diagnosis of brain stem
death should be made are as follows:

The prospective donor should fulfil the following preconditions and necessary exclusions.

Preconditions

1. There should be no doubt that the patient's
condition is due to irredeemable brainstem death of
known aetiology. If a patient has suffered primarily
from a cardiac arrest, hypoxia or severe circulatory
insufficiency with an indefinite period of cerebral
hypoxia, or is suspected of having cerebral air or fat
embolism, it may take longer to establish the diagnosis and be confident of the prognosis. In some
patients the primary pathology may only be discovered by continuing clinical observation and
investigation.

2. The patient is on a ventilator because spontaneous respiration has been inadequate or ceased
altogether. Possible causes of apnoea should be
excluded, for example neuropathic, neuromuscular
and myopathic syndromes that may occur in the
context of intensive therapy and may cause
problems weaning from a ventilator. Additionally,
neuromuscular blocking agents and the persistent
effects of hypnotic or narcotic drugs must have been
excluded as a cause of respiratory inadequacy or failure. The persistent effects of such drugs should be
excluded by elicitation of deep tendon reflexes or by
the demonstration of adequate neuromuscular conduction with a conventional nerve stimulator.

Necessary exclusions The patient is deeply unconscious. There should be no evidence that this state is
due to depressant drugs.

Narcotics, hypnotics and tranquillizers may have
prolonged action, particularly when hypothermia
coexists or in the context of renal or hepatic failure.
In some patients hypoxia may have followed ingestion of a drug, but in this situation the criteria for
brainstem death will not be applicable until such
time as the drug effects have been excluded as a
continuing cause of unresponsiveness.

Primary hypothermia as a cause of unconsciousness must have been excluded.

Potentially reversible circulatory, metabolic and
endocrine disturbances must have been excluded
as the cause of continuing unconsciousness.

Although it is recognized that these disturbances
are a likely accompaniment of brainstem death (e.g.

hypernatraemia, diabetes insipidus) they must be excluded as a cause rather than an effect of that condition. As an effect they do not preclude the diagnosis of brainstem death.

ORGAN DONATION

UK Transplant oversees the process of organ donation at a national level in the UK. Organ donors are identified in A&E departments, general intensive care units and neurosurgical critical care units. Donors can be identified by nursing, medical or transplant coordinators. To assist in this process, UK Transplant has specific criteria to clarify the status of the donor.

General criteria

- Age 0–75 years
- Absolute contraindications:
  - Human immunodeficiency virus (HIV)
  - Creutzfeldt-Jakob disease (CJD)
- Seek special advice in cases of:
  - Untreated sepsis
  - IV drug abuse
  - Malignancy
  - High-risk groups
- Irreversible brainstem damage identified
- Maintained on external respiratory ventilation as a result of:
  - Intracerebral haemorrhage
  - Trauma
  - Cerebral anoxia
  - Biopsy-proven brain tumour.

Specific criteria

Heart–lung donation
- Age up to 65 years maximum
- No history of specific respiratory disease
- Accurate smoking history
- Good O_2/CO_2 gas exchange
- Good living compliance with ventilation.

Kidney donation
- Age 2–75 years maximum
- No history of specific renal disease
- Adequate renal function
- No long-standing history of insulin-dependent diabetes mellitus
- HLA matching required.

Liver donation
- Age up to 75 years maximum
- No history of evidence of liver disease or injury
- No chronic alcohol abuse
- Adequate liver function.

Additional criteria

- Lack of objection established from the legal next of kin or designated person, and a Coroner's consent where applicable.

CLINICAL TESTS FOR BRAINSTEM DEATH

1. The pupils are fixed and dilated and do not react to light.
2. Absent corneal reflex (care is taken not to damage the cornea).
3. The vestibular ocular reflexes are absent (no eye movements occur) during the slow injection of 50 ml of ice-cold water over 1 minute in each external auditory meatus in turn. Clear access to the tympanic membrane must be established by direct inspection and the neck must be flexed at 30°. The performance of this manoeuvre may be prevented on one side but this does not invalidate the diagnosis of brainstem death.
4. No motor responses (that arise from the cranial nerve distribution) can be elicited on stimulation of any body area. There is no limb response to supraorbital ridge pressure.
5. There is no cough or gag reflex to bronchial stimulation by a suction catheter placed down the trachea.
6. No respiratory movements during apnoea test (refer to apnoea test specifics).

Specifics of the apnoea test

- The patient should be preoxygenated with 100% oxygen for 10 minutes prior to testing.
- During the test it is necessary for the arterial carbon dioxide to exceed the threshold for respiratory stimulation, that is, $PaCO_2$ should reach 6.65 kPa (50 mmHg).
- Disconnect the patient from ventilator but continue oxygenation by administering 6 L/min via a fine-bore catheter down the endotracheal tube.
- Observe the patient for 10 minutes for any respiratory effort, and a repeat blood gas analysis should be taken to ensure $PaCO_2$ has risen above 6.65 kPa (50 mmHg).
- Reconnect patient to the ventilator.

Patients with pre-existing chronic respiratory disease who may be responsive to supranormal levels of carbon dioxide and depend upon hypoxic drive are special cases and should be managed in conjunction with an expert in respiratory disease.

WHO CAN PERFORM BRAINSTEM TESTS?

The diagnosis of brainstem death should be made by at least two medical practitioners who have been registered for more than 5 years, are competent in this field and who are not members of the transplant team. They may carry out the two sets of tests separately or together.

REPETITION OF TESTING

The tests are repeated to remove the risk of observer error. The timing of the interval between the two sets is a matter for clinical judgement but should be adequate for all those directly concerned. The interval between the tests will depend on the primary pathology, the clinical course of the disease and the progress of the patient.

COMMON CLINICAL PROBLEMS OF THE BRAINSTEM DEAD PATIENT

- Hypothermia
- Hypotension/hypertension
- Endocrine disturbances
- Electrolyte imbalance
- Arrhythmias
- Hypoxia
- Coagulopathy
- Neurogenic pulmonary oedema.

CARDIOVASCULAR CHANGES

Hypertension

Causes Massive increases in circulating catecholamines are associated with brainstem death, resulting in increases in heart rate, blood pressure, cardiac output and systemic vascular resistance (SVR). This period of intense autonomic activity can be followed by hypotension.

Management If hypertension is sustained sodium nitroprusside (SNP) titrated to a maximum of 4 mg/kg/min until normotension is achieved. The goal is to maintain normotension.

Hypotension

Causes Loss of vasomotor tone, myocardial depression and hypovolaemia due to loss of thyroid function and the actions or loss of actions of ACTH. Blood loss, diuretics and diabetes insipidus (see below) also affect it, resulting in poor organ perfusion with potential ischaemia and ischaemia-related injuries. Also ECG abnormalities, changes including ST segment and T-wave changes, atrial and ventricular arrthymias and conduction abnormalities.

Management Replace preoperative fluid loss, such as urine output. Crystalloid replacement may be dextrose 4% or saline 0.25% with the addition of K+ 20 mmol. Fluids should be infused with a warming coil wherever possible. Colloids should only be used to adjust filling pressures. Blood of the same type may be given to keep Hb >10.

Inotropes Dopamine 3–5 mg/kg/min if all else fails in the face of a normal SVR. The goal is to provide cardiac stability, normotension, and hence adequate organ perfusion.

Pulmonary changes

Causes Intense vasoconstriction as a result of hormone/catecholamine storm may lead to acute left ventricular failure. This is also thought to be the underlying basis for pulmonary oedema, by disrupting pulmonary capillary membranes. Other causes may be trauma, aspiration or sputum retention, resulting in high pulmonary artery (PA) pressures, pulmonary oedema, and poor tissue and organ perfusion.

Management
- Physiotherapy (including bagging and suction)
- Frequent turning and bronchial toilet
- High tidal volume 12–15 ml/kg
- Add PEEP <5
- Sputum for Gram stain
- Correct CO_2 and FiO_2
- Frequent arterial blood gases
- Avoid excessive crystalloid infusion
- Bronchoscopy.

Goal
- PaO_2 >11.0 kPa
- SaO_2 >98%
- $PaCO_2$ 4.5–5.5 kPa
- FiO_2 <40%
- Clear chest X-ray
- Audible good clear air entry.

Endocrine disturbances – diabetes insipidus

Causes   Lack of antidiuretic hormone due to cerebral ischaemia/trauma, resulting in polyuria causing gross hypovolaemia and electrolyte imbalance. Common electrolyte disturbances experienced are hypokalaemia, hypocalcaemia and hypernatraemia. Serum osmolarity will be elevated and urine osmolarity will be low.

Potential consequences are:

- Cardiac arrhythmias
- Poor cardiac contractility
- Asystole.

Management
- Do not fluid deplete.
- Instigate fluid replacement therapy (in some centres dextrose 5%/nasogastric water is used)

Goal   Normalize urine output and concentration.

Hyperglycaemia

Cause   Reduced insulin secretion, sympathetic storm and the addition of inotropes/dextrose-containing fluids to treat vascular changes and hyponatraemia, resulting in high blood sugars.

Management   Utilize a sliding scale IV insulin regimen, the goal of which is to maintain a blood sugar level between 4 and 6 mmol/l.

Haematological changes – coagulopathy

Cause   The ischaemic brain and the resultant catecholamine storm releases fibrinolytic agents into the circulation, resulting in the presentation of a disseminated intravascular coagulation (DIC)-type picture.

THE ORGAN DONATION PROCESS

To ensure the organ donation process is managed effectively, the involvement of donor procurement coordinators is usually required. The role and responsibilities of such coordinators vary widely across the UK. Generally, the transplant coordinator will be contacted to assist in supporting the family of the potential donor to make an informed decision about whether or not to proceed to donate. They are in a position to advise on the potential medical management of the donor. Additionally, the coordinator can assist in the process of obtaining consent to donate.

Consent

There are two specific forms of consent acknowledged by the worldwide transplant community.

Presumed consent is the practice of presuming that unless the potential donor has specified that they do not want their organs taken after death, they become available for transplantation. Countries such as Belgium and Austria operate according to the 'presumed consent' rule. This is also called the 'opt out': by signing a register at their Town Hall, which is maintained on a national database accessible to all transplant coordinators, patients confirm that they have consciously chosen not to offer their organs for transplantation.

Informed consent is the practice of obtaining specific 'informed' permission from the relatives or spouse of the potential donor to proceed to donation. This practice is commonly seen in the UK and the rest of Europe. This is also called the 'opt-in' rule. An example of 'opting in' is seen in the joining of the organ donor register or signing of an organ donor card in the UK. In this instance the general public choose to offer their organs and identify their wishes explicitly.

However, refusal to consent to organ donation continues to present a major problem for the transplant community. Refusal occurs in up to 50% of those asked in North America, Europe and Australia. Reasons include:

- Inability to accept the patient's death
- Poor approach from those requesting donation
- Belief that the operation will mutilate the donor's body
- Cultural beliefs
- Religious beliefs.

In these circumstances a well trained, experienced and knowledgeable practitioner may manage to obtain consent. Most often the donor coordinator can fulfil this role. The ability to act effectively with thorough informed communication, empathy for the relatives and the potential donor, and a clear plan for the donation process can make the obtaining of consent a more productive and well managed process. It is essential that support and guidance are available to the clinical staff throughout this process.

SEQUENCE OF EVENTS FOR MULTIORGAN DONATION

1. The suggestion of organ donation should be raised following the completion of the second set of

brainstem death tests (some families may offer donation prior to testing).

2. Contact the on-call transplant coordinator for advice on the clinical suitability of the potential donor.

3. If the potential donor is to be referred to the Coroner their permission must be sought before donation can take place. The consultant or the transplant coordinator may do this.

4. On completion of the second set of brainstem death tests the family must be informed of the declaration of death. It would then be appropriate to offer the option of organ and tissue donation and the family's wishes documented in the medical notes or on a form stating lack of objection.

5. At this point the transplant coordinator is available to meet and to counsel the next of kin, answering any questions they may have. The coordinator is also available to act as a resource/ supporter for the staff.

6. Prior to or after meeting the next of kin the coordinator will complete a comprehensive physical examination and assessment of the potential donor and ascertain their current cardiovascular, pulmonary and metabolic status. This information will be used to assess the viability of the various organs.

7. The following blood samples will be required:
- 10 ml of blood in a plain blood tube for virology screening
- 3 ×10 ml of blood in citrated blood containers for tissue typing.

8. Further information that will be required:
- Blood group
- Urea and electrolytes
- Liver function tests
- Arterial blood gases
- Clotting studies
- Height and weight
- Chest X-ray
- ECG
- Culture and sensitivity screens – wounds, sputum, urine.

9. On completion of the overall assessment the transplant coordinator will register the donor with UKT. Identification of recipients will then commence for organ placement. This may take a considerable period (many hours), as recipients may be located throughout the UK or Europe.

10. Once a recipient(s) has been identified, a theatre time will be negotiated with the local theatre staff.

11. The transplant teams will come directly to the theatre department on their arrival.

12. In theatre the donor will continue to be fully monitored, ventilated, and receive all ongoing infusions.

13. Support from the anaesthetist will be required for approximately 2 hours of surgery, in order to maintain the donor's ventilatory and cardiovascular status. Muscle paralysing agents and prophylactic antibiotics will be administered. A general anaesthetic may sometimes be given to maintain CVS stability, but is not always required as the patient has been certified brainstem dead.

14. During the operation the transplant coordinator is available to inform and support all staff, and may act as a circulator for the transplant team. The coordinator also liaises with recipient transplant centres and completes required documentation.

15. Postoperatively, the transplant coordinator will perform last offices with assistance from theatre staff (in accordance with local hospital policy, and any family wishes wherever possible).

16. The donor family will be able to contact the coordinator at any time, and if it is their wish they will receive a letter thanking them for their decision to donate their loved one's organs, and also information about the outcome of the donation. Any information is treated with the strictest of confidence, and any correspondence kept anonymous and handled by the transplant coordinator.

17. The transplant coordinator will also write to the staff members involved in the care of the patient, thank them for supporting the family, and inform them of the outcome of the organ donation.

ORGAN DONORS

There are two potential sources of organs for donation and subsequently transplantation. The primary source is the cadaveric donor. In this case the donor will have been declared brainstem dead according to strict criteria. In these cases the cause of death is likely to have been related to head injury, intracerebral haemorrhage or, in rare cases, a primary brain tumour. The donor is maintained on a life support system so that the circulation is maintained. These are termed 'heart-beating donors'. The donor is taken to theatre in a controlled manner and the circulation interrupted to allow the removal of either one or several organs.

The second type of cadaveric donor is termed the asystolic or non-heart beating donor. In this case the donor has suffered cardiopulmonary problems resulting in death. A typical scenario is the patient who does not recover from a cardiopulmonary resuscitation attempt. In these cases organs can be donated for transplantation following a short delay, which confirms that circulatory function has definitely stopped. Once confirmed, perfusion of the organs (usually the kidney) can begin, although this type of donation is not without its problems. Cessation of circulation starts a process whereby oxygenated blood no longer reaches the kidney. As a result, ischaemic damage to the tissue occurs. Thus the transplant surgeon must act quickly to remove the kidneys and cold-perfuse them, reducing the tissues' requirement for oxygen and nutrients.

However, even in the most competent hands the resultant damage caused by the 'warm ischaemia' time leads to an inferior degree of postoperative function in the transplanted kidney. It is possible, however, to support the recipient with courses of dialysis until the kidney recovers.

The second type of organ donor is the 'living donor'. This option has arisen as a viable alternative for patients who primarily require kidney transplantation and, more rarely, liver and lung transplantation. As the supply of cadaveric organ donors has declined, so the transplant community has developed living donation as safe, effective option for certain individuals.

Living donation is almost unique in the field of medicine in that the procedure performed on a donating patient is not for their benefit and has physical disadvantages. In light of this risk the work-up of both donor and recipient must be performed to exacting standards. The ethical issues to be dealt with are not inconsiderable and include:

- Individual autonomy
- Altruism
- Evidence of lack of coercion.

ASSESSMENT EXAMPLE – RENAL TRANSPLANT

Kidney transplantation was first performed to treat patients with end-stage renal disease (ESRD). ESRD is a chronic, progressive process that results in the loss of irreplaceable nephrons within the kidney. Although the kidney can increase the functional capacity of surviving nephrons, this compensatory response can act to hide underlying advanced nephron damage. Thus, once symptoms and clinical signs become apparent there can be minimal surviving levels of functioning renal tissue; commonly renal function, measured by glomerular filtration rate (GFR), will have fallen to 15% of normal.

At this stage renal transplantation becomes the optimal treatment option for most patients. To facilitate this process, patients must undergo a series of tests and interviews to assess their suitability for transplantation.

This basic assessment programme can be modified to include additional investigations to ensure accurate assessment of any coexisting disease likely to hinder transplant surgery or postoperative recovery. In practice, this will include the exclusion of cardiac, respiratory, gastrointestinal and infective problems.

Once a full assessment has been performed, the patient will be seen by a nephrologist and a renal transplant surgeon to determine their suitability for entry to the transplant waiting list. This whole process is managed by the renal recipient transplant coordinator, who acts as a liaison between the transplant centre and the patient and family.

The transplant coordinator is responsible for ensuring all tests are performed, that results are available, that the patient is fully informed regarding the process, and that support is offered to guide the candidate to an informed decision.

1. History
   - Full medical history – renal disease, other diseases/operations
   - Medications
   - Blood transfusions
   - Allergies
   - Family and social history
   - Smoking
   - Alcohol/drug intake or abuse.
2. Physical examination
   - Full clinical examination
     - Central nervous system
     - Peripheral vascular system
     - Abdomen
     - Weight measurement.
3. Routine investigations
   - Full blood count
   - Blood group
   - Red cell antibodies screen
   - Urea and electrolytes
   - Liver function tests
   - Calcium/phosphate
   - Fasting lipids
   - Viral screen: HIV, hepatitis B, C, CMV, herpes, EBV

4. Chest X-ray
5. ECG
6. Urine screen for culture.

Causes of end-stage renal disease

- Diabetes mellitus
- Hypertension
- Glomerulonephritis
- Pyelonephritis
- Polycystic kidney disease
- Vascular disease of the kidney
- Obstruction of the kidney.

Clinical signs of renal disease

- Oliguria (reduced urinary volume)
- Lethargy/malaise
- Fluid retention
- Loss of appetite/weight
- Nausea, vomiting
- Nocturia.

CARDIAC TRANSPLANTATION

Cardiac transplantation offers patient survival of greater than 85% at 1 year post transplant. In keeping with all types of transplantation, careful assessment of each patient must be performed.

Specific criteria to be considered include:

- End-stage heart disease – life expectancy 6–12 months
- Age <65 years (investigated on physiological, not always chronological age)
- Coexistent disease
- Absence of infection
- Psychosocial stability
- Diabetes with significant end-organ damage
- Obesity
- Alcohol/drug/tobacco misuse
- Severe peripheral vascular disease.

Indications

- Reduced left ventricular ejection fraction – without evidence of reversible ischaemia not likely to respond to valvular surgery
- Significant exercise limitation, VO_2max (peak exercise oxygen uptake) <14 ml/kg/min.

The aim of heart transplantation is to increase the life expectancy of the severely ill patient beyond that of patients treated medically or with conventional surgery, and to increase exercise performance and quality of life.

Contraindications

The generally accepted contraindications are not absolute but relative. The aim is to utilize a limited resource in the best way possible.

Relative contraindications:

- Age >60 years
- Renal impairment (creatinine clearance <50 ml/min)
- Hepatic dysfunction not attributed to congestion (including deranged coagulation)
- Any evidence of diabetic microvascular complications
- Pharmacologically irreversible pulmonary hypertension (PVR >4 Wood units)
- History of malignancy
- Chronic infection (e.g. hepatitis positivity)
- Psychosocial problems likely to be exaggerated by high-dose steroids.

HEART-LUNG TRANSPLANTATION

Indications

As with liver transplantation, cardiac and pulmonary transplantation offers a life-saving opportunity to patients with end-stage disease.

Cardiac indications
- Cardiomyopathy
- Coronary artery disease
- Valvular heart disease
- Congenital heart defects
- Retransplantation.

Pulmonary indications
- Emphysema/obstructive pulmonary disease
- Pulmonary fibrosis
- Alpha-Antitrypsin deficiency
- Pulmonary hypertension*
- Cystic fibrosis*
- Congenital defects.*

*Cardiopulmonary indications are given above.

LUNG TRANSPLANTATION

Lung transplantation poses unique challenges to clinical teams because, unlike other types of organ transplant, the transplanted organ is required to function immediately it is transplanted, and secondly, it is readily open to external bacteria and pathogens via the airway. As a result, selection and management of potential candidates must be especially rigorous.

Specific criteria to be considered include:

- Coronary disease
- Hypertension
- Renal dysfunction
- Age <65 years
- Diabetes
- Obesity
- Alcohol/drug/tobacco misuse.

Absolute contraindications:

- Steroid intolerance as seen in gastrointestinal or musculoskeletal complications
- Septic lung disease
- AIDS.

LIVER TRANSPLANTATION

Indications

Liver transplantation is the sole treatment currently available for end-stage liver dysfunction. This can be in the acute phase following paracetamol hepatoxicity or non-paracetamol drug-induced liver failure, or the chronic phase as detailed below.

Chronic phase indications
- Primary biliary cirrhosis
- Primary sclerosing cholangitis
- Autoimmune hepatitis
- Alcoholic liver disease
- Chronic hepatitis (hepatitis B, C)
- Liver malignancy
- Cholangiocarcinoma
- Epithelioid haemangioendothelioma.

There is a range of other indications for possible liver transplantation.

Liver transplantation now offers patient survival rates that vary between 80 and 85% at 1 year post operation. The major limiting factor for all organ types remains the availability of suitable donor organs. As a result, the selection process needs to be rigorous. There are a number of important considerations for any patient being presented as a candidate for transplantation. These include:

- Timing of referral
- Prognosis
- Complications
- Quality of life.

Contraindications
- AIDS
- Cardiopulmonary disease
- Age >70 years
- Coexistent infection outside extrahepatic biliary
- Liver tumour (needs specific consideration of tumour type)
- Active alcohol/drug abuse
- Portal venous system thrombosis: needs specific medical consideration
- Pulmonary hypertension: needs specific medical consideration.

PANCREATIC TRANSPLANTATION

Pancreatic transplantation is relatively rare in both Europe and the USA. Approximately 5–10% of all transplants performed involve the pancreas. Pancreatic transplantation is undertaken when insulin secretion by the pancreas is affected. The resulting deficiency of insulin leads to type 1 (insulin-dependent) diabetes. In this case, patients require regular insulin injections to control their blood glucose levels.

Indications

- Recurrent hypoglycaemic episodes
- Previous kidney transplant
- End-stage kidney failure requiring simultaneous kidney/pancreas transplant for ongoing diabetes.

SURGICAL PROCEDURE

The transplant coordinator is a central figure throughout this period. He or she is responsible for the precise timing of both donor and recipient operations, and is required to communicate effectively with the surgical teams, who are often operating in different hospitals many miles apart. The coordinator must ensure that each operation runs smoothly and effectively. Any complications or delays must be anticipated where possible to allow readjustment of the scheduling of procedures. Additionally, transport arrangements to move the donor organ to the receiving hospital must also be meticulously planned to minimize the potential ischaemic damage to the organ.

Throughout the surgical procedure it is the responsibility of the transplant coordinator to manage the care of the relatives and staff. This is usually shared with surgical medical colleagues who can give accurate and up-to-date information and feedback to relatives and staff on the outcome of surgery. The opportunity for questions and answers where possible is an essential element of both donor and recipient surgical procedures, and must be carried out in an empathetic and sensitive manner. It requires time and experience to be completed successfully, but can make a very significant difference to the overall outcome for those who are closely involved, both professionally and emotionally.

Following the start of the donor operation the surgical team must work quickly and efficiently to remove the donated organs. Most commonly the heart and/or lungs are removed first. This is because these organs are the most susceptible to ischaemic damage, caused by stopping the oxygen and blood supply. It follows that the liver, then the pancreas and then the kidneys are removed. It is important that the organs are adequately cooled in ice, and a preservation fluid is used to safeguard the organ from ischaemic damage during transportation to the receiving hospital.

Each organ reacts differently to the insult of removal. However, it is essential that the transplant surgeons aim to minimize the so-called 'cold ischaemic time', i.e. the period between the cessation of blood supply in the donor to the re-establishment of blood supply in the recipient. Commonly the acceptable cold ischaemic time for each organ is:

- Kidney: <24 hours
- Liver: 12 hours
- Pancreas: 6–12 hours
- Heart and lungs: 4–6 hours.

There is a variety of surgical team preferences when using a fluid to preserve the organ. Most commonly used in the UK are UW (University of Wisconsin) solution and Euro Collins solution. Both contain a mix of glucose and additives to support the deoxygenated tissues.

Once the surgical procedure on the recipient commences the focus of the operation is toward ensuring minimal bleeding and that the anastomosis of veins and arteries is accurately and neatly performed. Attention to detail at this stage is essential to maximize the postoperative recovery of the transplanted organ. To assist this process the surgeon can utilize cardiopulmonary bypass (CPB). CPB is always used in heart and heart-lung operations. It is also an option during single lung and liver operations. CPB ensures the patient can be maintained in a stable state during the operation. The surgical field can be maintained to allow the surgeon free and ready access to the anastomotic site without fear of the view being reduced by bleeding.

POST-TRANSPLANT COMPLICATIONS

Principles

In all cases of organ transplantation the postoperative management of the patient requires a focused, knowledgeable and responsive approach to the identification and treatment of complications. There are a number of complications, which have the potential to affect any patient regardless of organ type. They are summarized here.

Surgery Complications following surgery are relatively rare. The main concern for the surgical team is bleeding. As vessels are resected and repaired so damage to small and large vessels occurs. Bleeding that is not adequately managed can lead to several life-threatening situations, including:

- Hypotension
- Tachycardia
- Reduced haemoglobin
- Coagulopathy.

Early detection and treatment of bleeding in the operating theatre can minimize the effects on the patient and the transplanted organ. However, should bleeding persist the risk of coagulation-related problems increases. These include thrombosis of vessels, embolus formation and anastomotic breakdown. Again, early detection of these complications can minimize their effect.

Intensive care Following the recipient operation the patient returns to the intensive care unit for close monitoring and manipulation of their therapy. The complications that can potentially affect the patient at this stage are common to all types of transplant operation, and include:

- Respiratory dysfunction
- Cardiac dysfunction – arrthymias, hypotension
- Fluid imbalance
- Renal dysfunction
- Electrolyte imbalance.

The surgical, medical and nursing teams work closely together to manage the patient through the first few days post operation. Commonly the patient will remain in the intensive care unit until a stable physical and psychological state is reached. They must be breathing spontaneously on room or low levels of oxygen. They must have a stable heart rate and blood pressure. Renal function must be acceptable in terms of fluid and electrolyte balance. Fluid and food intake must have commenced either orally or via nasogastric feeding. Typically a patient will be kept in the ICU for approximately 2–4 days.

TISSUE TYPING/IMMUNOLOGY

For transplantation to be successful a number of major issues must be considered with regard to the matching of donor and recipient to ensure the optimal outcome.

Major histocompatibility complex (MHC)

The major histocompatibility complex is an area of genetic material found on chromosome 6 in humans. It is responsible for the immune system's response to foreign tissue. A series of specific molecules are involved in this process, known as human leukocyte antigens (HLA). They are categorized as class 1, identified as HLA-A, -B and -C, and class II, identified as HLA-DP, -DQ and -DR. It is the interaction between these class I and class II molecules and T lymphocytes (T cells) that causes a rejection response between the recipient and the transplanted organ to be initiated.

Tissue typing

To limit the extent of the rejection response, research into identifying the interaction between these cells has been performed. This has demonstrated that where HLA can be compared between donated organ and recipient prior to transplantation, it is possible to predict better survival outcomes for patients. This process of tissue typing has been utilized in the field of kidney transplantation to minimize the immune response to the transplanted organ. Kidney transplantation is the most appropriate field for tissue typing owing to the extended cold ischaemia times in this area. This allows donor and recipient sera to be compared accordingly.

To maximize the overall potential for matching donor and recipient HLA as closely as possible, a central system operated in the UK, and managed by UK Transplant in Bristol, are responsible for matching donors and recipients across the country.

ABO blood group matching

Research has demonstrated that minimizing graft rejection is essential to patient survival. Central to this is ensuring that organs and recipients are matched according to the ABO criteria applied during the process of blood transfusion. Thus group A donor blood or organs can be given to group A recipients, but not group O or B blood. Only group O (the universal donor) blood can be given to A or B group patients.

Lymphocytotoxic cross–match

To minimize the recipient response to the donor organ, an additional process called lymphocytotoxic cross-matching is performed. This process involves comparing the recipient's blood samples with donor blood or lymph tissue. This is performed in the presence of complement. As a result, a reaction between antigen/antibody and complement occurs.

This reaction is measured and used to determine which donor and recipient can be safely matched. Complicating factors for this process include previous transplants, blood transfusion or pregnancy. In this instance, increased numbers of antibodies are generated, making cross-matching more difficult. In patients who have received any of the above, the chances of receiving a transplant are reduced according to the degree of mismatch.

Transplant rejection

Transplantation of any organ is a complicated process that poses a series of challenges to clinical teams, perhaps the biggest single challenge being the management of the rejection process.

Rejection is the result of a series of actions and reactions within the body's immune system, which is responsible for monitoring 'foreign' bodies within the body. This includes viruses, bacteria and transplanted organs. In response to a foreign entity the immune system kickstarts a series of events to get rid of the interloper. This process is called rejection and is categorized in three ways:

1. Hyperacute rejection   This is a rare process in transplantation today. However, hyperacute rejection occurs where antibodies in the recipient's bloodstream very rapidly attack antigens detected as a result of sensitization to the donor organ, that is, sensitization through ABO incompatibility or MHC incompatibility.

2. Acute rejection   This process can occur in any transplant type, most often during the early weeks and months post transplantation. The early phase is most problematic, as it is during this period that there is a need to strike the right balance between immunosuppression, thereby avoiding rejection, and avoiding side effects from the immunosuppression therapy. Acute rejection can be managed by increasing the dose of the main immunosuppressant, by administering doses of intravenous corticosteroid, or by antibody therapy.

3. Chronic rejection The process of chronic rejection occurs over a more protracted time frame, typically months and usually years post transplant. There are a variety of contributory processes to this, which vary according to transplant type. These are:

– Infection – viral, bacterial and fungal
– Repeated episodes of acute rejection, poorly controlled
– Long-term immunosuppression side effects
– High blood pressure
– Diet/obesity.

Detection of acute and chronic rejection also varies according to transplant type. However, certain general principles apply that include:

– Routine measurement of clinical signs – observing for hypertension, pyrexia, tachycardia
– Routine imaging of organ – CT scanning, chest X-ray
– Ultrasound, echocardiography
– Routine blood monitoring for major organ function:
    – Urea and electrolytes
    – Fasting lipids
    – Liver function tests
    – Blood glucose
    – Full blood count
    – Eosinophil counts
– Histological examination of organ tissue samples
– Close psychological observation of patient wellbeing and response to treatment.

Immunosuppression

The key to a successful outcome in transplantation is management of the rejection process via an effective immunosuppressive regimen tailored to the individual patient. The challenge for the clinical team is to strike a balance between suppression of the immune response, drug-specific side effects such as nephrotoxicity, and non-specific immunosuppression with the consequences of infection and malignancy. In response to this challenge a series of complex and novel treatment strategies have been used.

However, the basis of most treatment protocols lies in the so-called 'triple therapy' regimen. Triple therapy comprises three pharmaceutical elements, ciclosporin, azathioprine and corticosteroids.

Ciclosporin First used for clinical practice in 1978, it is the mainstay of standard immunosuppression. It works by inhibiting lymphocyte proliferation, and does have significant side effects and drug interactions. Therefore, usage must be carefully managed to ensure optimal therapy, avoiding nephrotoxicity, hypertension and hyperlipidaemia.

Azathioprine The second drug of choice is azathioprine, first used in clinical practice in 1962. It works by inhibiting RNA and DNA synthesis and blocking interleukin-2 (IL-2) production. It also requires careful administration as it can have a suppressant effect on white blood cells and bone marrow.

Corticosteroids Corticosteroids were first introduced to clinical practice in the 1960s. They have potent immunosuppressant and anti-inflammatory properties but cannot be used as the sole immunosuppressive drug. Corticosteroids function by interfering with T-cell and macrophage-derived cytokines. This drug must also be managed carefully to minimize unwanted side effects, such as weight gain, peptic ulceration and diabetes.

Additionally, there are different drugs that can supplement 'triple therapy' in specific patients. These include polyclonal antilymphocyte preparations such as antithymocyte globulin (ATG), which acts to eliminate circulating T lymphocytes, monoclonal antilymphocyte preparations such as OKT3 and Campath I, which also act to eliminate T lymphocytes, and macrolide antibodies such as rapamycin, which also block the cell proliferation process.

The principles behind any combinations of these therapies is to eliminate acute rejection, minimize side effects in the short and long term, and finally moderate the chronic rejection process. As a result they must be carefully administered and monitored to ensure maximal effectiveness.

ADDITIONAL COMPLICATIONS

Any type of organ transplant is at risk of several types of additional complications. Generally these are related to the medical management of the patient.

Infection

After the initial dose of immunosuppression infection remains a lifetime risk for the patient, who must have their immunosuppression in order to survive and not reject the transplanted organ. However, the immune system is also responsible for protecting the body from the multitude of viral, fungal and bacterial organisms circulating in the atmosphere. It is therefore essential that a careful balance be maintained between adequate immunosuppression, whereby the body can detect and fight these organisms appropriately without support from drugs, and oversuppression, where the body is open to infection and may need intervention in the form of drugs to prevent significant complications. Both medical team and patient must be vigilant for evidence of infection through regular screening to ensure any complicating factors are avoided. This is particularly important during the first postoperative year, when the patient has a requirement for significant levels of immunosuppression.

Malignancy

Immunosuppressive regimens have progressed significantly over the years in terms of efficacy and reduced side effects, but they continue to present a major risk to all patients because of their potential association with the development of cancers in the long term. As with infections, it is essential that the patient be closely monitored for any early evidence of developing cancers. Early intervention confers the best chance of success in treating any malignancy, particularly in immunosuppressed patients.

Cardiovascular disease

Another risk factor associated with immunosuppression relates to the development of cardiovascular changes in either the coronary or the peripheral circulation. Immunosuppressive drugs are known to cause changes in the body that increase blood pressure (hypertension), circulating blood lipids (hyperlipidaemia) and circulating blood glucose (hyperglycaemia). As a result the patient requires close monitoring in the long term. Follow-up focuses on issues such as diet, weight loss, appropriate medication and good self-care, avoiding smoking and reducing alcohol intake.

Cardiovascular disease is of particular concern in cardiac patients, as changes in the vasculature of the coronary arteries can occur at any time and can lead to a significant reduction in cardiac performance. Therefore, monitoring needs to be particularly rigorous to detect changes as early as possible to allow for treatment modification.

General

The transplant operation and its long-term management lays the patient open to complications such as osteoporosis, anaemia, obesity, skin problems and a variety of other minor complaints. Additional medication and medical management may be required to minimize these unwanted effects.

Bibliography

Allen RD, Chapman JR. A manual of renal transplantation. London: Arnold; 1994.

Alter MJ. Epidemiology of hepatitis C. Hepatology 1997; 26: 625–655.

Bay WH, Herbert LA. The living donor in kidney transplantation. Ann Inter Med 1987; 106: 719–727.

British Transplant Society. United Kingdom guidelines for living donor kidney transplantation. London: British Transplant Society; 2000.

Cohen B, Wright C. A European perspective on organ procurement. Breaking down the barriers to organ donation. Transplant 1999; 68: 985–990.

Costanzo MR. Selection and treatment of candidates for heart transplantation. Sem Thoracic Cardiovasc Surg 1996; 3: 113–125.

Danovitch GM. Handbook of kidney transplantation, 3rd edn. Philadelphia: Lippincott Williams and Wilkins; 2001.

Dark JH, Patterson MD, Al-Jilaihawi AN, et al. Experimental en bloc double lung transplantation. Ann Thoracic Surg 1986; 42: 394–398.

Department of Health. A code of practice for the diagnosis of brainstem death, including guidelines for the identification and management of potential organ and tissue donors. London: DOH; 1998.

Department of Health. An investigation into conditional organ donation. London: DOH; 2000.

Department of Health. Unrelated Live Transplant Authority. Report 1995–1998. London: DOH; 1999.

Devlin J, O'Grady J. Indications for referral and assessment in adult live transplantations: a clinical guideline. British Society of Gastroenterology. Guidelines in Gastroenterology; 2000.

Edwards BS, Rodenheffer RJ. Prognostic features in patients with congestive cardiac failure and selection criteria for cardiac transplantation. Congestive heart failure and cardiac transplantation. Mayo Clin Proceed 1992; 69: 485–492.

Fabbri A, Bryan AJ, Sharples LD, et al. Influence of recipient and gender on outcome after heart transplantation. J Heart Lung Transplant 1992; 11: 701–707.

Gore SM, Cable DJ, Holland AJ. Organ donation from intensive care units in England and Wales: two year confidential audit of deaths in intensive care. BMJ 1992; 304: 349–355.

Hood RM, Arnold HS, Calhoon JH. Techniques in general thoracic surgery: single lung transplantation. Philadelphia: Lea and Febiger; 1993: 161–168.

Intensive Care Society. Donation of organs for transplantation. The management of potential organ donors. A manual for the establishment of local guidelines. Oxford: Intensive Care Society; 1999.

Losse B. Indications and selection criteria for cardiac transplantation. Thoracic Cardiovasc Surg 1990; 38: 276–279.

Michelson P. Presumed consent to organ donation: ten years' experience in Belgium. J R Soc Med 1996; 89: 663–666.

British Medical Association. Organ donation in the 21st century: time for a consolidated approach. London: BMA; 2000.

Roels L, Deschoolmeester G, Vaurenterghein Y. A profile of people objecting to organ donation in a country with presumed consent law: data from the Belgian National Registry. Transplant Proceed 1997; 29: 1473–1475.

Shapiro AM, Lakey JR, Ryan EA, et al. Islet cell transplantation in seven patients with type 1 diabetes mellitus using a glucocortoid – free immunosuppressive regimen. N Engl J Med 2000; 343: 230–238.

UK Transplant. Donor audit report 1990–1999. Bristol: UK Transplant; 2001.

UK Transplant. Annual report 2000–2001. Bristol: UK Transplant; 2001.

UK Transplant Co-ordinators' Association. Religious and cultural issues. Information for healthcare professionals. London: UKTCA; 1998.

Waters PF. Lung transplantation: recipient selection. Sem Thoracic Cardiovasc Surg 1992; 4: 73–78.

Further reading

Abbas AK, Lichtman AH, Potter JS. Cellular and molecular immunology, 4th edn. Philadelphia: WB Saunders; 2000.

Abecassis M, Blei AT, Flamm S. Liver transplantation. In: Stuart FP, Abecassis M, Kaufman DB, eds. Organ transplantation. Texas: Landes Bioscience; 2000: 169–207.

Caplan AL. Ethical policy issues in the procurement of cadaver organs for transplantation. N Engl J Med 1984; 311: 981–983.

Kings Fund. A question of give and take: improving supply of donor organs for transplantation. London: Kings Fund Institute; 1994: 37–42.

Kumar V, Cotran R, Robbins SL, eds. Basic pathology, 6th edn. Philadelphia: Lippincott; 1999.

Morris PJ. Kidney transplantation: principles and practice, 4th edn. Philadelphia: WB Saunders; 1994.

First MR. Transplantation in the nineties. Transplant 1992; 53: 1–11.

Schofield PM, Corris PA. Management of heart and lung transplant patients. London: BMJ Books; 1998.

Tortora GJ, Grabowski SR. Principles of anatomy and physiology. New York: Wiley; 1996.

Recommended websites

UK Transplant
www.uktransplant.org.uk

European Transplant Coordinators Organization
www.etco.org

United Network for Organ Sharing (UNOS)
www.unos.org

Collaborative Transplant Study
www.cts.med.uni-heidelberg.de

European Liver Transplant Registry
www.eltr.org

British Medical Association
www.bma.org.uk

UK Transplant Coordinators Association
www.uktca.org.uk

British Liver Trust
www.britishlivertrust.org.uk

National Kidney Federation
www.kidney.org.uk

British Transplant Society
www.bts.org.uk

For Patient's Perspective
www.heart-transplant.co.uk

Index

Please note that page references to major mentions of topics are in **bold** print, whereas any references to non-textual matter, e.g. boxes, figures or tables, are in *italics*

Journals of related interest

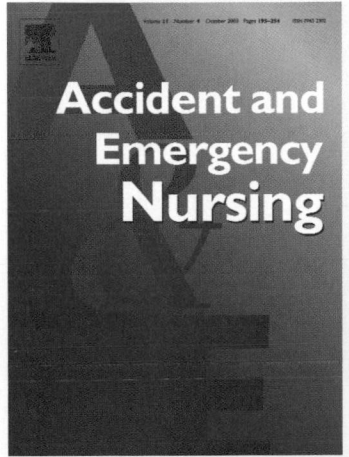

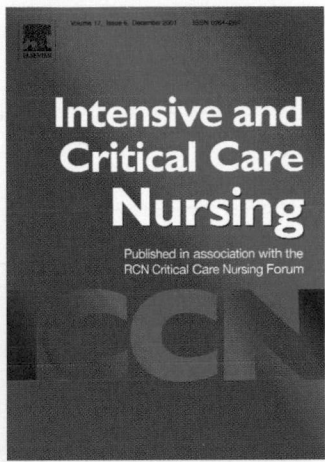

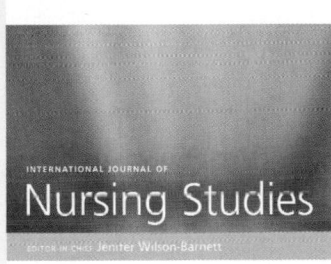